4TH EDITION

ILLUSTRATED DENTAL EMBRYOLOGY, HISTOLOGY, AND ANATOMY

MARGARET J. FEHRENBACH, RDH, MS

Oral Biologist and Dental Hygienist
Adjunct Instructor, Bachelor of Applied Science Degree, Dental Hygiene Program,
Seattle Central College, Seattle, Washington
Educational Consultant and Dental Science Technical Writer, Seattle, Washington

TRACY POPOWICS, PhD

Associate Professor, Department of Oral Health Sciences
School of Dentistry, University of Washington, Seattle, Washington

ELSEVIER
SAUNDERS

ELSEVIER
SAUNDERS

3251 Riverport Lane
Maryland Heights, Missouri 63043

ILLUSTRATED DENTAL EMBRYOLOGY, HISTOLOGY, AND ANATOMY,
FOURTH EDITION   ISBN: 978-1-4557-7685-6
Copyright © 2016, 2011, 2006, 1997 by Saunders, an imprint of Elsevier, Inc.

Notices

Knowledge and best practice in this field are constantly changing. As new research and experience broaden our understanding, changes in research methods, professional practices, or medical treatment may become necessary.

Practitioners and researchers must always rely on their own experience and knowledge in evaluating and using any information, methods, compounds, or experiments described herein. In using such information or methods they should be mindful of their own safety and the safety of others, including parties for whom they have a professional responsibility.

With respect to any drug or pharmaceutical products identified, readers are advised to check the most current information provided (i) on procedures featured or (ii) by the manufacturer of each product to be administered, to verify the recommended dose or formula, the method and duration of administration, and contraindications. It is the responsibility of practitioners, relying on their own experience and knowledge of their patients, to make diagnoses, to determine dosages and the best treatment for each individual patient, and to take all appropriate safety precautions.

To the fullest extent of the law, neither the Publisher nor the authors, contributors, or editors, assume any liability for any injury and/or damage to persons or property as a matter of products liability, negligence or otherwise, or from any use or operation of any methods, products, instructions, or ideas contained in the material herein.

International Standard Book Number: 978-1-4557-7685-6

Content Strategist: Kristin Wilhelm
Content Development Manager: Ellen Wurm-Cutter
Content Development Specialist: Joslyn Dumas
Publishing Services Manager: Julie Eddy
Project Manager: Jan Waters
Design Direction: Ashley Miner

Printed in the U.S.A.

Last digit is the print number: 9   8   7   6   5   4   3   2

REVIEWERS

JANITA COPE, RDH, MS

Associate Professor
Dental Hygiene
Oregon Tech
Klamath Falls, Oregon

JEFFREY R. SMITH, DMD

Instructional Program Manager
Dental Programs
Florida State College at Jacksonville
Jacksonville, Florida

PREFACE

OVERVIEW

This textbook provides an extensive background for student dental professionals in the area of oral biology as well as dental professional program graduates who need to take competency examinations or update their background knowledge in this area. The textbook strives to integrate the clinical aspects of dentistry with the basic science information that is key to its successful performance by the dental professional.

The textbook is divided into four units: **Orofacial Structures, Dental Embryology, Dental Histology,** and **Dental Anatomy.** The textbook was organized into units to accommodate differing curriculum; thus, the units do not have to be presented in any specific order. However, the first unit on orofacial structures serves as an outstanding review for the students before further study in oral biology, which is also presented in this textbook.

FEATURES

Each of the four units of this textbook consists of several chapters, with each chapter building on the preceding ones in that unit. Each chapter begins with an objectives listing. This serves as a checkpoint for students to test their understanding of the chapter's content. In addition, each chapter contains key terms. The terms listed are highlighted in blue when presented for the first time in the textbook. Terms used in other chapters are also bolded for increased emphasis of important concepts. Pronunciations of these terms are provided in the glossary.

The chapters contain figures that incorporate both microscopic and clinical photographs, and also useful tables and boxes. Most of the photographs are original to this textbook and come from the personal collection of Margaret J. Fehrenbach and the Dr. Bernhard Gottlieb Collection (see Acknowledgments). The fine illustrations of the dentitions are original to this textbook, as are most of the other ones in the other areas of oral biology.

Within each chapter are discussions of clinical considerations of the topic covering various treatment situations; these allow for an increased integration of the basic science information into everyday practice for the dental professional. Each chapter contains cross-references to figures and other chapters so that the reader can review or investigate interrelated subjects. The content of this edition incorporates additional input from students and educators as well as the latest information from scientific studies and experts.

The textbook concludes with a bibliography, a complete glossary f key terms using short easy-to-remember phrases with pronunciation guide, and appendices that contain a review of anatomic nomenclature, units of measurement, permanent tooth measurements, and developmental information for the dentitions.

EVOLVE

A companion **Evolve website** is available for both students and instructors. It can be accessed directly at http://evolve.elsevier.com/Fehrenbach/illustrated.

INSTRUCTOR RESOURCES

- *Image Collection:* All of the images from the textbook are available electronically and they can be downloaded and used in PowerPoint or other classroom lecture formats.
- *Test Bank:* Approximately 600 objective-style questions—multiple-choice, true/false, matching, short answer—are available with accompanying objective mapping, rationales, and page/section references for textbook remediation.
- *TEACH Instructor's Resource Manual:* This resource includes detailed lesson plans, PowerPoint lecture outlines, classroom activities, and the answers to the workbook activities.

STUDENT RESOURCES

- *Practice Quizzes:* Approximately 200 multiple-choice questions are available in an instant-feedback format and they are mapped to objectives with rationales for correct and incorrect answers. Page-number references are also included for remediation.
- *Histology Matching Game:* This learning game has drag-and-drop exercises for histological identification of images.
- *Review & Assessment Questions:* Approximately 450 review/assessment short-answer questions for discussion, review, and/or assessment.
- *Supplemental Considerations—Additional Material:* Information available on topics of interest to specific chapters that build on the core chapter discussion and enrich learning.
- *Tooth Identification Exercises:* Matching exercises that correlate a photo of an actual permanent tooth with its tooth number and description are available for the students, including instant feedback for self-assessment.
- *WebLinks:* Robust listings of additional web resources are included in supplement chapter discussions.

ADDITIONAL RESOURCES

The companion **Workbook for Illustrated Dental Embryology, Histology, and Anatomy** is also available for student use. The workbook features activities such as structure identification exercises, glossary exercises, tooth drawing exercises, infection control guidelines for extracted teeth, and review questions. Patient examination procedures for extraoral and intraoral structures, the dentition, and occlusal evaluation have been added to integrate the clinical aspects of dentistry with the basic science information within the included clinical exercises. Case studies are also present for each unit as well as removable flashcards using the original illustrations of the permanent dentition from the textbook.

This textbook is coordinated with the *Illustrated Anatomy of the Head and Neck* by Margaret J. Fehrenbach and Susan W. Herring and it can be considered a companion textbook to complete the curriculum in oral biology. Many of the figures are also presented in the *Dental Anatomy Coloring Book*, edited by Margaret J. Fehrenbach.

Margaret J. Fehrenbach
Tracy Popowics

ACKNOWLEDGMENTS

We would like to thank Content Strategist, Kristin Wilhelm, Content Development Specialist, Joslyn Dumas, and the rest of the staff at Elsevier for making this textbook possible. In addition, we would like to thank Heidi Schlei, RDH, BS, Instructor, Waukesha County Technical College, Milwaukee, Wisconsin, for her clinical insights as well as Susan Herring, PhD, Professor of Orthodontics, School of Dentistry, University of Washington, Seattle, Washington, for her overall support. Also used in the compilation of this text was material on orthodontic therapy from Dona M. Seely, DDS, MSD, Orthodontic Associates of Bellevue, Washington.

Most of the elegant microscopic sections that are original to this textbook are from the Dr. Bernhard Gottlieb Collection, courtesy of James E. McIntosh, PhD, Professor Emeritus, Department of Biomedical Sciences, Baylor College of Dentistry, Dallas, Texas. Bernhard Gottlieb was a Viennese physician and dentist (1886-1950) who taught at Baylor College and authored hundreds of scientific articles and four textbooks. Most importantly, he is responsible for the beginnings of oral histology. He is also acknowledged to be the first dental professional to integrate basic science information with clinical dental treatment. We are proud to continue his legacy in this manner.

Finally, we would like to thank our families, colleagues, and students.

Margaret J. Fehrenbach
Tracy Popowics

CONTENTS

UNIT I OROFACIAL STRUCTURES, 1

1 **Face and Neck Regions, 1**
Face and neck, 1
Face regions, 1
Frontal, orbital, and nasal regions, 1
Infraorbital and zygomatic regions, 2
Buccal region, 2
Oral region, 2
Mental region, 2
Neck regions, 6

2 **Oral Cavity and Pharynx, 9**
Oral cavity properties, 9
Oral cavity divisions, 9
Oral vestibules, 9
Jaws, alveolar processes, and teeth, 10
Oral cavity proper, 14
Pharnygeal divisions, 17

UNIT II DENTAL EMBRYOLOGY, 18

3 **Prenatal Development, 18**
Prenatal development, 18
Preimplantation period, 20
Embryonic period, 22
Second week, 23
Third week, 24
Fourth week, 27
Fetal period, 31

4 **Face and Neck Development, 32**
Facial development, 32
Stomodeum and oral cavity formation, 33
Mandibular arch and lower face formation, 34
Frontonasal process and upper face formation, 35
Maxillary process and midface formation, 36
Upper and lower lip formation, 36
Cervical development, 38
Primitive pharynx formation, 38
Branchial apparatus formation, 38

5 **Orofacial Development, 43**
Orofacial development, 43
Palatal development, 43
Primary palate formation, 43
Secondary palate formation, 44
Palate completion, 44

Nasal cavity and septum development, 45
Tongue development, 45
Body of tongue formation, 45
Base of tongue formation, 47
Completion of tongue formation, 49

6 **Tooth Development and Eruption, 51**
Tooth development, 51
Initiation stage, 53
Bud stage, 54
Cap stage, 54
Bell stage, 60
Apposition and maturation stages, 62
Root development, 66
Root dentin formation, 66
Cementum and pulp formation, 66
Multirooted tooth development, 67
Periodontal ligament and alveolar process development, 68
Primary tooth eruption and shedding, 68
Permanent tooth eruption, 70

UNIT III DENTAL HISTOLOGY, 77

7 **Cells, 77**
Cell properties, 77
Cell anatomy, 77
Organcllcs, 79
Inclusions, 81
Cell division, 81
Extracellular materials, 81
Intercellular junctions, 83

8 **Basic Tissue, 85**
Basic tissue properties, 85
Epithelium properties, 86
Epithelium histology, 86
Epithelium classification, 86
Epithelium regeneration, turnover, and repair, 87
Basement membrane properties, 89
Basement membrane histology, 89
Connective tissue properties, 89
Connective tissue histology, 90
Connective tissue classification, 91
Connective tissue proper, 92
Specialized connective tissue properties, 93

Cartilage properties, 93
Bone properties, 94
Blood properties, 98
Muscle properties, 100
Muscle classification, 100
Skeletal muscle histology, 101
Nerve tissue properties, 101
Nerve tissue histology, 101
Nervous system, 103

9   Oral Mucosa, 104
Oral mucosa properties, 104
Lining mucosa, 104
Masticatory mucosa, 105
Specialized mucosa, 105
Epithelium of oral mucosa, 106
Lamina propria of oral mucosa, 108
Oral mucosa regional differences, 109
Labial mucosa and buccal mucosa, 110
Alveolar mucosa, 111
Ventral surface of the tongue and floor of the
mouth, 111
Soft palate, 112
Hard palate, 112
Attached gingiva, 112
Tongue and lingual papillae properties, 113
Filiform lingual papillae, 117
Fungiform lingual papillae, 117
Foliate lingual papillae, 117
Circumvallate lingual papillae, 117
Oral mucosa pigmentation, 118
Oral mucosa turnover, repair,
and aging, 119

10   Gingival and Dentogingival Junctional
Tissue, 123
Gingival tissue properties, 123
Gingival tissue anatomy, 123
Gingival tissue histology, 124
Dentogingival junctional tissue properties, 125
Dentogingival junctional tissue histology, 126
Dentogingival junctional tissue development, 130
Dentogingival junctional tissue turnover, 130

11   Head and Neck Structures, 133
Head and neck structures, 133
Gland properties, 133
Salivary gland properties, 133
Thyroid gland properties, 140
Lymphatics properties, 141
Lymph nodes, 142
Intraoral tonsillar tissue properties and histology, 143
Nasal cavity properties, 143
Nasal cavity histology, 144
Paranasal sinuses properties, 145
Paranasal sinuses histology, 145
Paranasal sinuses development, 146

12   Enamel, 147
Enamel properties, 147
Enamel matrix formation, 149
Enamel matrix maturation, 150
Enamel histology, 152

13   Dentin and Pulp, 158
Dentin-pulp complex, 158
Dentin properties, 158
Dentin matrix formation, 159
Dentin matrix maturation, 160
Mature dentin components, 160
Dentin types, 161
Dentin histology, 166
Aging dentin, 167
Pulp properties, 167
Pulp anatomy, 167
Pulp histology, 168
Pulp zones, 169
Aging pulp, 170

14   Periodontium: Cementum, Alveolar
Process, and Periodontal Ligament, 172
Periodontium properties, 172
Cementum properties, 172
Cementum development, 174
Cementum histology, 174
Cementum types, 175
Cementum repair, 175
Alveolar process properties, 179
Jaw development, 179
Jaw anatomy and histology, 180
Periodontal ligament properties, 187
Periodontal ligament cells, 187
Periodontal ligament fiber groups, 188

UNIT IV DENTAL ANATOMY, 193

15   Overview of Dentitions, 193
Dentitions, 193
Tooth types, 193
Tooth designation, 193
Dentition periods, 194
Primary dentition period, 194
Mixed dentition period, 195
Permanent dentition period, 195
Dental anatomy terminology, 197
General dental terms, 197
Tooth anatomy terms, 198
Orientational tooth terms, 200
Tooth form, 203
Considerations for dental anatomy study, 205

16   Permanent Anterior Teeth, 207
Permanent anterior teeth properties, 207
Permanent incisors, 209

General features of permanent incisors, 209
Permanent maxillary incisors, 212
Permanent mandibular incisors, 217
Permanent canines, 220
General features of permanent canines, 220
Permanent maxillary canines, 223
Permanent mandibular canines, 225

17 Permanent Posterior Teeth, 228
Permanent posterior teeth properties, 228
Permanent premolars, 230
General features of permanent premolars, 230
Permanent maxillary premolars, 233
Permanent mandibular premolars, 238
Permanent molars, 244
General features of permanent molars, 244
Permanent maxillary molars, 246
Permanent mandibular molars, 254

18 Primary Dentition, 262
Primary teeth properties, 262
Primary incisors, 265
Primary canines, 267
Primary molars, 268

19 Temporomandibular Joint, 272
Temporomandibular joint properties, 272
Joint bones, 272
Temporal bone, 272
Mandible, 272

Joint capsule, 274
Joint disc, 274
Joint movement, 275

20 Occlusion, 281
Occlusion properties, 281
Centric occlusion, 281
Arch form, 283
Dental curvatures and angulations, 284
Centric stops, 286
Centric relation, 286
Lateral and protrusive occlusion, 287
Mandibular rest position, 288
Primary occlusion, 289
Malocclusion, 290
Malocclusion classification, 291

BIBLIOGRAPHY, 299
GLOSSARY, 301
APPENDIX A: ANATOMIC POSITION, 314
APPENDIX B: UNITS OF MEASURE, 315
APPENDIX C: TOOTH MEASUREMENTS, 316
APPENDIX D: TOOTH DEVELOPMENT, 319
INDEX, 321

CHAPTER 1

Face and Neck Regions

Additional resources and practice exercises are provided on the companion Evolve website for this book:
http://evolve.elsevier.com/Fehrenbach/illustrated.

●●● LEARNING OBJECTIVES

1. Define and pronounce the key terms in this chapter.
2. Locate and identify the regions and associated surface landmarks of the face on a diagram and a patient.
3. Integrate the clinical considerations for the surface anatomy of the face into patient examination and care.

4. Locate and identify the regions and associated surface landmarks of the neck on a diagram and a patient.
5. Integrate the study of surface anatomy of the neck into patient examination and care.

FACE AND NECK

Dental professionals must be comfortably familiar with the surface anatomy of the face and neck as discussed in this introduction to **Unit I** to provide comprehensive dental care. The superficial features of the face and neck provide essential landmarks for many of the deeper anatomic structures.

Examination of these accessible features on a patient, both by visualization and palpation, can give information about the health of deeper tissue. Some degree of variation in surface features can be considered within a normal range. However, a change in a surface feature in a patient may signal a condition of clinical significance and must be noted in the patient record, as well as correctly followed up by the examining dental professional. Thus, the variations among individuals are not what should be noted but the changes in a particular individual.

Some of these surface changes in the features of the face and neck may be due to underlying developmental disturbances. Knowledge of the surface features of the face and neck additionally helps dental professionals to understand the associated developmental pattern. **Unit II** describes the development of the face and neck and associated developmental disturbances. However, other visible surface changes may be due to underlying associated histologic tissue changes. In **Unit III**, the histology of the face and neck is correlated with its visible surface features. Thus, dental professionals need to study face and neck surface structures before continuing further in the study of dental embryology and histology, as well as dental anatomy, as presented in **Unit IV**.

In this textbook, the illustrations of the face and neck, as well as any structures associated with them, are oriented to show the head in anatomic position (see **Appendix A**), unless otherwise noted. This is the same position as if the patient in a clinical setting is viewed straight on while sitting upright in the dental chair.

FACE REGIONS

The face and neck surface is divided into regions, as is the head itself. Within each region are certain surface landmarks. It is important to practice finding these landmarks in each region using a personal mirror while referring to this textbook, as well as the **Workbook for Illustrated Dental Embryology, Histology, and Anatomy**, in order to improve your skills of examination. Later, locating them on peers and then on patients in a clinical setting will add a real-world level of competence.

The **regions of the face** include: the frontal, orbital, nasal, infraorbital, zygomatic, buccal, oral, and mental regions (Figure 1-1). **Lymph (limf) nodes** are located in certain areas of the face and head and, when palpable, should be noted in the patient record (Figure 1-2, also see Figure 11-16).

FRONTAL, ORBITAL, AND NASAL REGIONS

The **frontal (frun-tal) region** of the face includes the forehead and the area above the eyes (Figure 1-3). In the **orbital (or-bit-al) region** of the face, the eyeball and all its supporting structures are contained in the **orbit (or-bit)** of the skull which is the bony eye socket.

The main feature of the **nasal (nay-zil) region** of the face is the **external nose** (Figure 1-4). The **root of the nose** is located between the eyes, and the tip is the **apex of the nose**. Inferior to the apex on

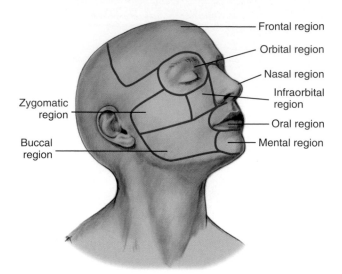

FIGURE 1-1 Regions of the face: Frontal, orbital, infraorbital, nasal, zygomatic, buccal, oral, and mental. (Adapted from Fehrenbach MJ, Herring SW: *Illustrated anatomy of the head and neck*, ed 4, St Louis, 2012, Saunders/Elsevier.)

each side of the nose is a nostril, or **naris** (**nay**-ris) (plural, **nares** [**nay**-rees]). The nares are separated by the midline **nasal septum** (**sep**-tum). The nares are also bounded laterally by winglike cartilaginous structures, each **ala** (**ah**-lah) (plural, **alae** [ah-**lay**]) of the nose.

INFRAORBITAL AND ZYGOMATIC REGIONS

The **infraorbital** (in-frah-**or**-bit-al) **region** of the face is located inferior to the orbital region and lateral to the nasal region (see Figure 1-3). Farther laterally is the **zygomatic** (zy-go-**mat**-ik) **region**, which overlies the bony support for the cheek, the **zygomatic arch**. The zygomatic arch extends from just below the lateral margin of the eye toward the middle part of the external ear.

Inferior to the zygomatic arch and just anterior to the external ear is the **temporomandibular** (tem-poh-ro-man-**dib**-you-lar) **joint (TMJ)**. This is the location where the upper skull forms a joint with the lower jaw (see Figure 19-1). The movements of the joint occur when the mouth is opened and closed using the lower jaw or the lower jaw is moved to the right or left. To palpate the lower jaw moving at the TMJ on a patient, a finger is placed into the external ear canal during movement.

BUCCAL REGION

The **buccal** (**buk**-al) **region** of the face is composed of the soft tissue of the cheek (see Figure 1-3). The cheek forms the side of the face and is a broad area of the face between the nose, mouth, and ear. Most of the upper cheek is fleshy, mainly formed by a mass of fat and muscles. One of these muscles forming the cheek is the strong **masseter** (**mass**-et-er) **muscle**, which is palpated when a patient clenches the teeth together (see Figure 19-8, *A*). The sharp angle of the lower jaw inferior to the earlobe is termed the **angle of the mandible** (**man**-di-bl).

The **parotid salivary** (pah-**rot**-id sal-i-ver-ee) **gland** has a small part that can be palpated on a patient in the buccal region as well as in the zygomatic region (Figure 1-5, see Figure 11-7). Thus, the parotid is located irregularly from the zygomatic arch down to the posterior border of the lower jaw.

ORAL REGION

The **oral region** of the face has many structures within it, such as the lips and oral cavity (Figure 1-6, see Figures 2-2 and 2-11). The upper and lower lips are fleshy folds that mark the gateway of the oral cavity proper. The **vermilion** (ver-**mil**-yon) **zone** of each lip has a darker appearance than the surrounding skin, with the lips outlined from the surrounding skin by a transition zone, the **mucocutaneous** (moo-ko-ku-tay-nee-us) **junction** at the vermilion border. Between the vermilion zone and the inner oral cavity is the intermediate zone.

On the midline of the upper lip extending downward from the nasal septum is a vertical groove, the **philtrum** (**fil**-trum). The philtrum terminates in a thicker area of the midline of the upper lip, the **tubercle** (**too**-ber-kl) **of the upper lip**. Underlying the upper lip is the upper jaw, or **maxilla** (mak-**sil**-ah) (Figure 1-7, *A*). The bone underlying the lower lip is the lower jaw, or **mandible** (Figure 1-7, *B*). For more information on the jaws, see a detailed discussion in **Chapter 2**. The upper and lower lips meet at each corner of the mouth at the **labial commissure** (**lay**-be-al **kom**-i-shoor).

Disruption of the vermilion zone may make it hard to determine the exact location of its mucocutaneous junction at the vermilion border between the lips and the surrounding skin (Figure 1-8). These changes may be due to scar tissue from past traumatic incidents, developmental disturbances, or cellular changes in the tissue, such as those that occur with solar damage. These changes may also represent a more serious condition, such as cancer; however, this can be verified only with tissue biopsy and microscopic examination. If disruption is initially only from solar damage, protection of the lips (especially the lower lip) with sunscreen is important because sun exposure increases the risk of cancerous changes. The risk of cancerous changes with the lips can be increased with chronic alcohol and tobacco use.

If disruption of the vermilion zone and its mucocutaneous junction at the vermilion border has been caused by a traumatic incident, noting it in the patient record is important given that the rest of the oral cavity may be affected. If this change is part of a past history of a cleft lip, this also needs to be noted (see Figure 4-8).

MENTAL REGION

The chin is the major feature of the **mental** (**men**-tal) **region** of the face. The bone underlying the mental region is the mandible, or lower jaw. The midline of the mandible is marked by the **mandibular symphysis** (man-**dib**-you-lar **sim**-fi-sis) (see Figure 4-5).

On the lateral aspect of the mandible, the stout, flat plate of the **ramus** (**ray**-mus) (plural, **rami** [**rame**-eye]) extends upward and backward from the body of the mandible on each side (see Figure 1-7, *B*, and Figure 1-9). At the anterior border of the ramus is a thin, sharp margin that terminates in the **coronoid** (**kor**-ah-noid) **process**. The main part of the anterior border of the ramus forms a concave forward curve, the **coronoid notch**.

The posterior border of the ramus is thickened and extends from the angle of the mandible to a projection, the **mandibular condyle** (**kon**-dyl) with its neck. The articulating surface of the condyle is the head of mandibular condyle within the TMJ. Between the coronoid process and the condyle is a depression, the **mandibular notch**.

The face can be divided vertically into thirds, and this perspective is considered the **vertical dimension of the face** (see Figure 1-3).

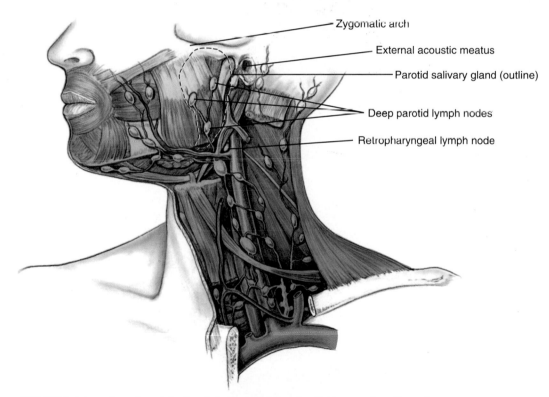

A

B

FIGURE 1-2 Lymph nodes of the head. **A,** Superficial nodes. **B,** Deep nodes. (From Fehrenbach MJ, Herring SW: *Illustrated anatomy of the head and neck,* ed 4, St Louis, 2012, Saunders/Elsevier.)

FIGURE 1-3 Landmarks of the frontal, orbital, infraorbital, zygomatic, buccal, and mental regions, as well as the three divisions of the vertical dimension of the face (see also Figure 1-10). (From Fehrenbach MJ, Herring SW: *Illustrated anatomy of the head and neck,* ed 4, St Louis, 2012, Saunders/Elsevier.)

FIGURE 1-4 Landmarks of the nasal region with the nasal septum highlighted *(dashed lines).* (From Fehrenbach MJ, Herring SW: *Illustrated anatomy of the head and neck,* ed 4, St Louis, 2012, Saunders/Elsevier.)

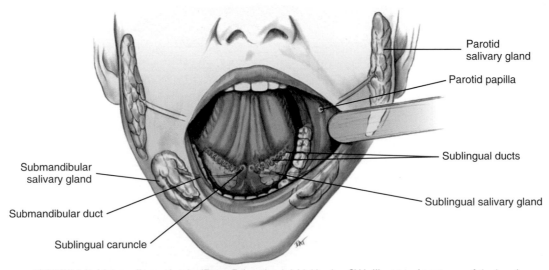

FIGURE 1-5 Major salivary glands. (From Fehrenbach MJ, Herring SW: *Illustrated anatomy of the head and neck,* ed 4, St Louis, 2012, Saunders/Elsevier.)

FIGURE 1-6 Upper and lower lips with the vermilion zones and mucocutaneous junctions at the vermilion borders. (From Fehrenbach MJ, Herring SW: *Illustrated anatomy of the head and neck,* ed 4, St Louis, 2012, Saunders/Elsevier.)

FIGURE 1-8 Disruption of vermilion zone and its mucocutaneous junction at the vermilion border on the lower lip due to solar damage. (Courtesy of Margaret J. Fehrenbach, RDH, MS.)

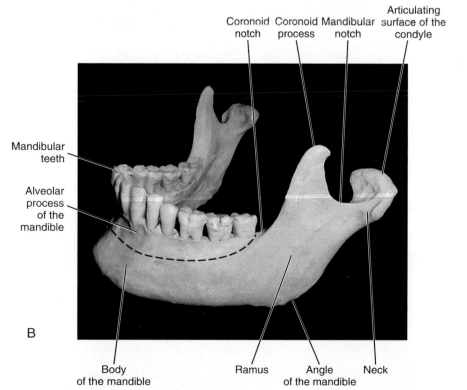

FIGURE 1-7 Landmarks of the maxilla **(A)** and mandible **(B)**. (From Fehrenbach MJ, Herring SW: *Illustrated anatomy of the head and neck,* ed 4, St Louis, 2012, Saunders/Elsevier.)

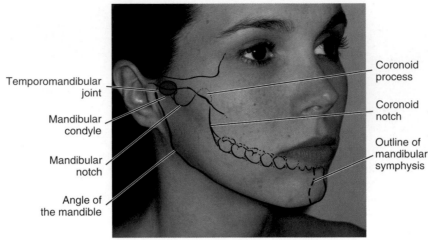

FIGURE 1-9 Landmarks of the mandible integrated with overlying facial features. (From Fehrenbach MJ, Herring SW: *Illustrated anatomy of the head and neck,* ed 4, St Louis, 2012, Saunders/Elsevier.)

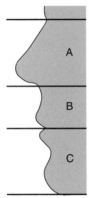

FIGURE 1-10 Golden Proportions of the face with its three divisions illustrating the considerations of vertical facial dimension: *Nasal height (A)* is related to *maxillary height (B)* as 1.000:0.618; sum of nasal height and maxillary height (A + B) are related to *mandibular height (C)* as 1.618:1.000; mandibular height *(C)* is related to maxillary height *(B)* as 1.000:0.618; orofacial height (B + C) is related to nasal height *(A)* as 1.618:1.000. Note that each ratio is 1.618, which is integral to these guidelines. These guidelines can also be used when considering the esthetics of the related smile. See also Figure 1-3.

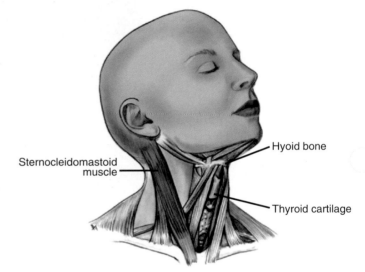

FIGURE 1-11 Landmarks of the neck region. (From Fehrenbach MJ, Herring SW: *Illustrated anatomy of the head and neck,* ed 4, St Louis, 2012, Saunders/Elsevier.)

A discussion of vertical dimension allows a comparison of the three divisions of the face for functional and esthetic purposes using the **Golden Proportions,** which is a set of guidelines (Figure 1-10 and see Figure 1-3). Loss of height in the lower third, which contains the teeth and jaws, can occur in certain circumstances, causing pronounced changes in the functions as well as esthetics of the orofacial structures (see Figure 14-22).

NECK REGIONS

The **regions of the neck** extend from the skull and lower jaw down to the clavicles and sternum (Figure 1-11). Lymph nodes are located in certain areas of the neck and, when palpable on a patient, should be noted in the patient record (Figure 1-12). The regions of the neck can be divided further into different cervical triangles using the large bones and muscles located in the area.

The large strap muscle, the **sternocleidomastoid** (stir-no-klii-do-mass-toid) **muscle (SCM),** is easily palpated on each side of the neck

of a patient (see Figure 1-11), with its borders dividing the neck into further regions. At the anterior midline is the **hyoid** (hi-oid) **bone,** which is suspended in the neck. Many muscles attach to the hyoid bone, which controls the position of the base of the tongue. Also found in the anterior midline and inferior to the hyoid bone is the **thyroid cartilage** (thy-roid kar-ti-lij), which is the prominence of the "voice box," or **larynx** (lare-inks). The vocal cords, or ligaments of the larynx, are attached to the posterior surface of the thyroid cartilage.

The **thyroid gland,** an endocrine gland, can also be palpated on a patient within the midline cervical area (Figure 1-13 and see **Chapter 11**). Thus, the thyroid gland is located inferior to the thyroid cartilage, at the junction of the larynx and the trachea. The **parathyroid** (par-ah-thy-roid) **glands** are also endocrine glands that located close to or within the posterior aspect of each side of the thyroid gland but cannot be palpated in a patient. The **submandibular** (sub-man-dib-you-lar) **salivary gland** and the **sublingual** (sub-ling-gwal) **salivary gland** can also be palpated in a patient in the neck region (see Figure 1-5 and Figure 11-7).

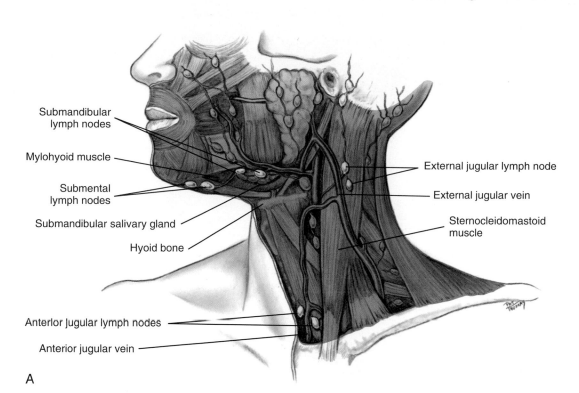

Submandibular
lymph nodes

Mylohyoid muscle

Submental
lymph nodes

Submandibular salivary gland

Hyoid bone

External jugular lymph node

External jugular vein

Sternocleidomastoid
muscle

Anterior jugular lymph nodes

Anterior jugular vein

A

Digastric muscle

Jugulodigastric
lymph node

Hyoid bone

Superior deep cervical lymph nodes

Internal jugular vein

Jugulo-omohyoid lymph node

Interior deep cervical
lymph nodes

Sternocleidomastoid muscle (cut)

Accessory lymph nodes

Accessory nerve

Omohyoid muscle

Supraclavicular lymph node

Clavicle (cut)

Thoracic duct

B

FIGURE 1-12 Lymph nodes of the neck. **A,** Superficial cervical nodes. **B,** Deep cervical nodes. (From Fehrenbach MJ, Herring SW: *Illustrated anatomy of the head and neck,* ed 4, St Louis, 2012, Saunders/ Elsevier.)

FIGURE 1-13 Thyroid gland. (From Fehrenbach MJ, Herring SW: *Illustrated anatomy of the head and neck,* ed 4, St Louis, 2012, Saunders/Elsevier.)

Oral Cavity and Pharynx

Additional resources and practice exercises are provided on the companion Evolve website for this book: ⓔ
http://evolve.elsevier.com/Fehrenbach/illustrated

●●● LEARNING OBJECTIVES

1. Define and pronounce the key terms in this chapter.
2. Locate and identify the divisions and associated surface landmarks of the oral cavity on a diagram and a patient.
3. Integrate the clinical considerations for the surface anatomy of the oral cavity into patient examination and care.

4. Outline the divisions of the pharynx and identify them on a diagram.
5. Integrate the study of surface anatomy of the visible divisions of the pharynx into patient examination and care.

ORAL CAVITY PROPERTIES

A dental professional must be totally committed to improving the overall health of every patient. In order to accomplish this, dental professionals must be particularly knowledgeable about their main area of focus, the oral cavity, and the adjacent throat or pharynx and its health. To visualize this area of focus successfully, it is important to know the boundaries, terminology, and divisions of the oral cavity and the pharynx as discussed in this second chapter of **Unit I**. Later, **Unit II** describes the development of oral tissue and associated developmental disturbances. Following that, **Unit III** describes the underlying histology of orofacial tissue that gives them many characteristic surface features. Later, **Unit IV** discusses dental anatomy.

Some degree of variation can be possible in the oral cavity and visible divisions of the pharynx. However, a change in any tissue or associated structure in a patient may signal a condition of clinical significance and must be noted in the patient record, as well as correctly followed up by the examining dental professional. Thus, it is not the variations among individuals that should be noted but the changes in a particular individual.

In this textbook, the illustrations of the oral cavity and pharynx, as well as any structures associated with them, are oriented to show the head in anatomic position (see **Appendix A**), unless otherwise noted. This is the same as if the patient in a clinical setting is viewed straight on while sitting upright in the dental chair.

ORAL CAVITY DIVISIONS

The oral cavity is divided into the vestibules, jaws and alveolar processes, teeth, and oral cavity proper. Within each part of the oral cavity are certain surface landmarks. It is important to practice finding these surface landmarks in the oral cavity using a personal mirror while referring to this textbook, as well as the **Workbook for Illustrated Dental Embryology, Histology, and Anatomy**, in order to improve skills of examination. Later, locating them on peers and then on patients in a clinical setting adds a real world level of competence.

An understanding of the divisions of the oral cavity is aided by knowing its boundaries; many structures of the face and oral cavity mark the boundaries of the oral cavity (Figure 2-1). The lips of the face mark the anterior boundary of the oral cavity, and the pharynx or throat is the posterior boundary. The cheeks of the face mark the lateral boundaries, and the palate marks the superior boundary. The floor of the mouth is the inferior border of the oral cavity.

Many oral structures are identified with orientational terms based on their relationship to other orofacial structures, such as the facial surface, lips, cheek, tongue, and palate (see Figure 2-1). Those structures closest to the facial surface are termed facial (fay-shal). Those facial structures closest to the lips are termed labial (lay-be-al). Those facial structures close to the inner cheek are termed buccal (buk-al). Those structures closest to the tongue are termed lingual (ling-gwal). Those lingual structures closest to the palate are termed palatal (pal-ah-tal).

ORAL VESTIBULES

The upper and lower horseshoe-shaped spaces in the oral cavity between the lips and cheeks anteriorly and laterally and the teeth and their soft tissue medially and posteriorly are considered the vestibules (ves-ti-bules), both maxillary and mandibular (Figure 2-2). These oral vestibules are lined by a mucous membrane, or oral mucosa (mu-ko-sah). The inner parts of the lips are lined by a pink labial mucosa.

The labial mucosa is continuous with the equally pink buccal mucosa that lines the inner cheek. However, both the labial and buccal mucosa may vary in coloration, as do other regions of the oral mucosa, in individuals with pigmented skin (see Figure 9-23).

The buccal mucosa covers a dense pad of underlying fat tissue at the posterior part of each vestibule, the buccal fat pad. The buccal fat pad acts as a protective cushion during mastication (mass-ti-kay-shin), or chewing. On the inner part of the buccal mucosa, just opposite the maxillary second molar, is a small elevation of tissue called the parotid papilla (pah-rot-id pah-pil-ah). The parotid papilla protects the opening of the parotid duct (or Stensen duct) of the parotid salivary gland (see Figures 1-5 and 11-7).

Deep within each vestibule is the vestibular fornix (ves-tib-u-lar fore-niks), where the pink labial mucosa or buccal mucosa meets the redder alveolar mucosa (al-vee-o-lar mu-ko-sah) at the mucobuccal (mu-ko-buk-al) fold. The labial frenum (free-num) (plural, frena [free-nah]) is a fold of tissue located at the midline between the labial mucosa and the alveolar mucosa on the upper and lower dental arches.

On the surface of the labial and buccal mucosa is a common variation, Fordyce (for-dice) spots (or granules) (Figure 2-3, A). These are visible as small, yellowish elevations on the oral mucosa. They represent deeper deposits of sebum from trapped or misplaced sebaceous gland tissue, usually associated with hair follicles. Most of the population has these harmless small bumps; however, they become more prominent with age due to thinning of the overlying tissue.

Another variation noted on the buccal mucosa is the linea alba (al-bah) (see Figure 2-3, B). This is a white ridge of hyperkeratinization (or calloused tissue) that extends horizontally at the level where the maxillary and mandibular teeth come together and occlude; similar ridges of white tissue can sometimes be present on the tongue perimeter. An excess amount of this whitened ridge on either the buccal mucosa or tongue can be associated with certain oral parafunctional habits (see Figure 9-7).

JAWS, ALVEOLAR PROCESSES, AND TEETH

The jaws, the maxilla and mandible, are deep to the lips and within the oral cavity (Figure 2-4 and see Figure 1-7). The maxilla consists of two maxillary bones that are sutured together during development. The maxilla has a nonmovable articulation with many facial and skull bones, and each maxillary bone includes a body and four processes. Each body of the maxilla (mak-sil-ah) is superior to the teeth and contains the maxillary sinus (mak-si-lare-ee sy-nus). In contrast, the mandible is a single bone with a movable articulation with the temporal bones at each temporomandibular joint (TMJ). The heavy horizontal part of the lower jaw inferior to the teeth is the body of the mandible.

The alveolar process, or alveolar bone, is the bony extension for both the maxilla and mandible that contain each tooth socket of the teeth or alveolus (al-vee-oh-lus) (plural, alveoli [al-vee-oh-lie]) (see Figure 14-14). The facial surface of the alveolus of each canine, the vertically placed canine eminence (kay-nine em-i-nins), is especially prominent on each side of the maxilla. All the teeth are attached to the bony surface of the alveoli by the fibrous periodontal (pare-ee-o-don-tl) ligament (PDL), which allows some slight tooth movement within the alveolus while still supporting the tooth.

Each of the mature and fully erupted teeth consists of both the crown and the root(s) (Figures 2-5 and 2-6). The crown of the tooth is composed of the extremely hard outer enamel (ih-nam-l) layer and

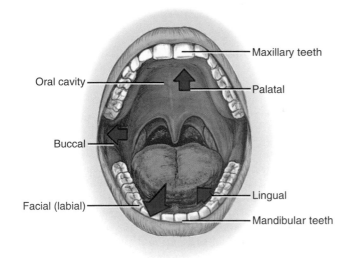

FIGURE 2-1 Oral cavity and the jaws with the designation of the orientational terms *(arrows)* facial, labial, buccal, palatal, and lingual. (From Fehrenbach MJ, Herring SW: *Illustrated anatomy of the head and neck,* ed 4, St Louis, 2012, Saunders/Elsevier.)

Labels: Maxillary teeth, Oral cavity, Palatal, Buccal, Facial (labial), Lingual, Mandibular teeth

FIGURE 2-2 Vestibules of the oral cavity with its landmarks. (From Fehrenbach MJ, Herring SW: *Illustrated anatomy of the head and neck,* ed 4, St Louis, 2012, Saunders/Elsevier.)

Labels: Parotid papilla, Buccal mucosa, Labial mucosa, Maxillary vestibule, Alveolar mucosa, Mucobuccal fold, Mandibular vestibule

Maxillary teeth

Buccal mucosa with Fordyce spots

Dorsal surface of tongue

A

Maxillary teeth

Linea alba

Lateral surface of tongue

Buccal mucosa

B

FIGURE 2-3 Buccal mucosa and labial mucosa with possible variations. **A,** With Fordyce spots visible as small, yellowish elevations. **B,** With the linea alba visible as a white ridge of hyperkeratinization that extends horizontally at the level where the teeth occlude, with a similar white ridge on the lateral surface of the tongue. (Courtesy of Margaret J. Fehrenbach, RDH, MS.)

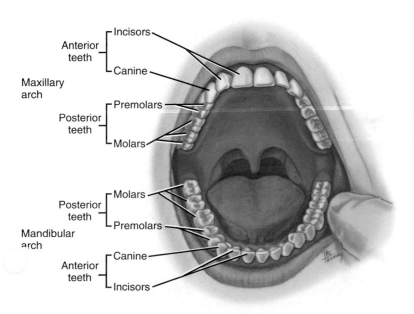

Incisors

Anterior teeth

Canine

Maxillary arch

Premolars

Posterior teeth

Molars

Molars

Posterior teeth

Premolars

Mandibular arch

Canine

Anterior teeth

Incisors

FIGURE 2-4 Diagram of the dental arches with its permanent teeth and its landmarks.

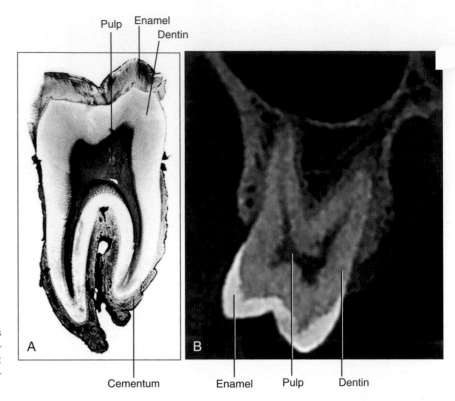

FIGURE 2-5 Distribution of the various tissue types of the tooth. **A,** Gross specimen of tooth cross-sectioned. **B,** Radiograph of tooth. (From Nanci A: *Ten Cate's oral histology,* ed 8, St Louis, 2013, Mosby/Elsevier.)

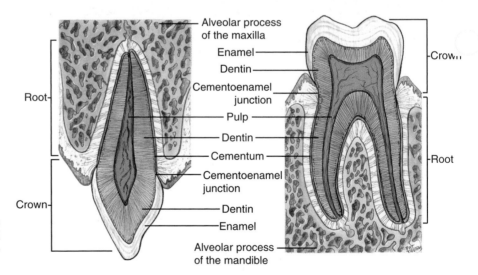

FIGURE 2-6 Diagram of an alveolar process of both a single-rooted tooth and a multirooted tooth showing the crown and root as well as associated tissue types.

the moderately hard inner **dentin** (den-tin) layer overlying the **pulp** of the tooth. The pulp is the soft innermost layer in the tooth. The moderately hard dentin continues to cover the soft tissue of the pulp of the tooth in the root(s), but the outermost layer of the root(s) is composed of **cementum** (see-**men**-tum). The bonelike cementum is the part of the tooth that attaches to the periodontal ligament, which then attaches to the alveolus of bone, holding the tooth in its socket.

DENTAL ARCHES

The alveolar processes with the teeth in the alveoli are also called **dental arches**, the **maxillary arch** and **mandibular arch** (see Figure 2-4). The teeth in the maxillary arch are the **maxillary teeth**, and the teeth in the mandibular arch are the **mandibular teeth**.

Just distal to the last tooth of the maxillary arch is a tissue-covered elevation of the bone, the **maxillary tuberosity** (too-beh-**ros**-i-tee). Similarly, on the lower jaw is a dense pad of tissue located just distal to the last tooth of the mandibular arch, the **retromolar** (re-tro-**mo**-ler) **pad**. The tooth types in both arches of the teeth of children, or **primary teeth**, include **incisors** (in-**sigh**-zers), **canines** (**kay**-nines), and **molars** (**mo**-lerz).

Adult teeth, or **permanent teeth**, also include all the same tooth types as the primary teeth, as well as **premolars** (pre-**mo**-lerz). The teeth in the front of the mouth, the incisors and canines, are considered **anterior teeth**. The teeth located toward the back of the mouth, the molars and premolars, if present, are considered **posterior teeth**. The permanent maxillary anterior teeth are supplied by the anterior superior alveolar artery, with the permanent maxillary posterior teeth by the posterior superior

FIGURE 2-7 Variation of exostoses *(arrows)* on the facial surface of the maxillary arch. (Courtesy of Margaret J. Fehrenbach, RDH, MS.)

FIGURE 2-8 Variation of bilateral mandibular tori *(arrows)* on the lingual surface of the mandibular arch. (Courtesy of Margaret J. Fehrenbach, RDH, MS.)

alveolar artery; all of the permanent mandibular teeth are supplied by branches of the inferior alveolar artery. Additionally, the maxillary teeth are drained by the posterior superior alveolar vein, with mandibular teeth drained by the inferior alveolar vein. Later **Unit IV** discusses the dental anatomy of each tooth of both dentitions, primary and permanent.

Clinical Considerations with Alveolar Process

A variation present usually on the facial surface of the alveolar process of the maxillary arch is **exostoses** (eks-ox-**toe**-seez). They are localized developmental growths of bone with a possible hereditary etiology, and which may be associated with occlusal trauma (Figure 2-7, see **Chapter 20**). They may be single, multiple, unilateral, or bilateral raised hard areas, located in the premolar to molar region covered by oral mucosa, appearing on radiographs as radiopaque (light) areas. They may interfere with radiographic analysis, as well as restorative and periodontal therapy, and thus must be noted in the patient record.

Another similar variation present on the lingual aspect of the mandibular arch is the **mandibular torus** (**tore**-us) (plural, **tori** [**tore**-eye]) (Figure 2-8). Each torus is a developmental growth of bone with a possible hereditary etiology similar to exostoses and may also be associated with bruxism (grinding). They are usually present bilaterally in the area of the premolars and can present surface clefting, appear lobulated or nodular, or even contact each other over the midline.

Mandibular tori are covered in oral mucosa and vary in size. They are slow growing and asymptomatic lesions, which may be seen on radiographs as radiopaque (light) masses. They may interfere with speech, oral hygiene procedures, radiographic film placement and analysis, as well as prosthesis therapy of the mandibular alveolar process. The patient may require reassurance of their background, and they must be noted in the patient record.

GINGIVAL TISSUE

Surrounding the maxillary and mandibular teeth in the alveoli and covering the alveolar processes are the soft tissue gums, or **gingiva** (jin-ji-vah) (or more accurately, but not commonly by the dental community, *gingivae*), composed of a firm pink mucosa (Figure 2-9). The gingival tissue that tightly adheres to the alveolar process surrounding the roots of the teeth is the **attached gingiva**. The line of demarcation between the firmer and pinker attached gingiva and the movable and redder alveolar mucosa is the scallop-shaped **mucogingival** (mu-ko-jin-ji-val) **junction**.

Alveolar mucosa

Mucogingival junction

Attached gingiva

Maxillary teeth

Mandibular teeth

FIGURE 2-9 Gingival tissue and its landmarks on the maxillary arch, with the mucogingival junction highlighted *(dashed line)*. (From Fehrenbach MJ, Herring SW: *Illustrated anatomy of the head and neck,* ed 4, St Louis, 2012, Saunders/Elsevier.)

At the gingival margin of each tooth is the marginal gingiva (or free gingiva), which forms a cuff above the neck of the tooth (Figure 2-10). The free gingival (jin-ji-val) groove separates the marginal gingiva from the attached gingiva. This outer groove varies in depth according to the area of the oral cavity; the groove is especially prominent on mandibular anterior teeth and premolars. At the most coronal part of the marginal gingiva is the free gingival crest.

The interdental (in-ter-den-tal) gingiva is the gingival tissue between adjacent teeth adjoining attached gingiva, with each individual extension being an interdental papilla (pah-pil-ah). The attached gingiva may have areas of melanin (mel-a-nin) pigmentation, especially at the base of the interdental papillae (see Figure 9-23). The

inner surface of the gingival tissue with each tooth faces a space, the gingival sulcus (sul-kus).

ORAL CAVITY PROPER

The inside of the mouth is known as the oral cavity proper (Figure 2-11). The space of the oral cavity is enclosed anteriorly by both the maxillary arch and mandibular arch. Posteriorly, the opening from the oral cavity proper into the pharynx or throat is the fauces (faw-seez).

The fauces are formed laterally on each side by the anterior faucial (faw-shawl) pillar and the posterior faucial pillar. The palatine

FIGURE 2-10 Close-up of the gingival tissue and its landmarks with the location of the gingival sulcus noted *(arrow)*. (From Fehrenbach MJ, Herring SW: *Illustrated anatomy of the head and neck*, ed 4, St Louis, 2012, Saunders/Elsevier.)

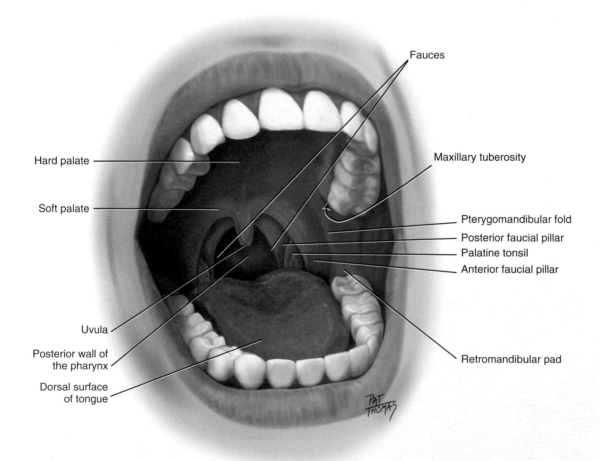

FIGURE 2-11 Oral cavity proper and the landmarks that form its boundaries. (From Fehrenbach MJ, Herring SW: *Illustrated anatomy of the head and neck*, ed 4, St Louis, 2012, Saunders/Elsevier.)

tonsils (pal-ah-tine ton-sils) are located between these folds of tissue created by underlying muscles and are what patients call their "tonsils," which can become enlarged when involved with inflammation (see Figure 11-18). Included within the oral cavity proper are the palate, tongue, and floor of the mouth.

PALATE

Within the oral cavity proper is the roof of the mouth or palate (pal-it). The palate separates the oral cavity from the nasal cavity. The palate has two parts: anterior and posterior (Figure 2-12, see Figure 5-5). The firmer anterior part is considered the hard palate.

A midline ridge of tissue on the hard palate is the median palatine raphe (ra-fee), which overlies the bony fusion of the palate. A small bulge of tissue at the most anterior part of the hard palate, lingual to the anterior teeth, is the incisive (in-sy-ziv) papilla. Directly posterior to this papilla are palatine rugae (ru-gee), which are firm, irregular ridges of tissue radiating from the incisive papilla and raphe.

The looser posterior part of the palate is considered the soft palate (see Figure 2-11). A midline muscular structure, the uvula (u-vu-lah) of the palate, hangs down from the posterior margin of the soft palate. The pterygomandibular (teh-ri-go-man-dib-you-lar) fold extends from the junction of hard and soft palates down to the mandible, just behind the most distal mandibular tooth, and stretches when the mouth is opened wider. This fold covers a deeper fibrous structure and separates the cheek from the throat.

Clinical Considerations with Palate

A variation noted on the midline of the hard palate is the palatal torus, which is similar to the mandibular torus in presentation and etiology (Figure 2-13). The torus can interfere if prosthesis therapy of the maxillary alveolar process is considered. It needs to be noted in the patient record, and patients may need to be reassured as to its background. More serious pathology of the palate, such as a history of cleft palate, also needs to be recorded because of its impact on dental care (see Figure 5-6).

TONGUE

The tongue is a prominent feature of the oral cavity proper (Figure 2-14). The posterior one-third is the pharyngeal part of the tongue, or base of the tongue. The base of the tongue attaches to the floor of the mouth. The base of the tongue does not lie within the oral cavity proper but within the oral part of the throat (discussed later in the chapter). The anterior two-thirds of the tongue is the body of the tongue, which lies within the oral cavity proper. The tip of the tongue is the apex of the tongue.

The top, or dorsal surface of the tongue, has a midline depression, the median lingual sulcus, corresponding to the position of a midline fibrous structure deeper in the tongue and fusion tissue area. Certain surfaces of the tongue have small, elevated structures of specialized mucosa, the lingual papillae, some of which are associated with taste buds (see Figures 9-16 to 9-20). Taste buds are the specialized organs of taste.

The slender, threadlike, whitish lingual papillae are the filiform (fil-i-form) lingual papillae, which give the dorsal surface its velvety texture. The reddish, smaller mushroom-shaped dots on the dorsal surface are the fungiform (fun-ji-form) lingual papillae. Farther posteriorly on the dorsal surface of the tongue, and more difficult to see clinically, is an inverted V-shaped groove, the sulcus terminalis (ter-mi-nal-is). The sulcus terminalis separates the base from the body of the tongue, demarcating a line of fusion of tissue during the tongue's development.

The 10 to 14 larger mushroom-shaped lingual papillae, the circumvallate (serk-um-val-ate) lingual papillae line up along the anterior side of the sulcus terminalis on the body. Where the sulcus terminalis points backward toward the throat is a small, pitlike depression, the foramen cecum (for-ay-men se-kum). Even farther posteriorly on the dorsal surface of the base of the tongue is an irregular mass of tissue, the lingual tonsil (see **Chapter 11**).

The side or lateral surface of the tongue has vertical ridges, the foliate (fo-le-ate) lingual papillae (Figure 2-15).

The underside, or ventral surface of the tongue, has large visible blood vessels, the deep lingual veins, which pass close to the surface (Figure 2-16). Lateral to each deep lingual vein is the plica fimbriata (pli-kah fim-bree-ay-tah) (plural, plicae fimbriatae [pli-kay fim-bree-ay-tay]) with fringelike projections.

FLOOR OF THE MOUTH

The floor of the mouth is located in the oral cavity proper, inferior to the ventral surface of the tongue (Figure 2-17). The lingual frenum is a midline fold of tissue between the ventral surface of the tongue and the floor of the mouth.

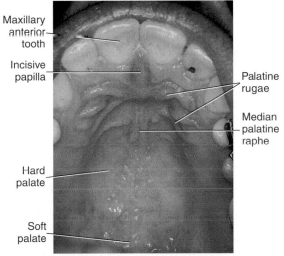

FIGURE 2-12 Palate and its landmarks. (From Fehrenbach MJ, Herring SW: *Illustrated anatomy of the head and neck,* ed 4, St Louis, 2012, Saunders/Elsevier.)

Labels: Maxillary anterior tooth; Incisive papilla; Hard palate; Soft palate; Palatine rugae; Median palatine raphe

FIGURE 2-13 Variation of the palatal torus *(arrow)* on the midline of the hard palate. (Courtesy of Margaret J. Fehrenbach, RDH, MS.)

Epiglottis

Palatine tonsil

Lingual tonsil

BASE

Foramen cecum

Circumvallate lingual papillae

Sulcus terminalis

BODY

Median lingual sulcus

Filiform lingual papillae

Fungiform lingual papillae

A Apex of the tongue

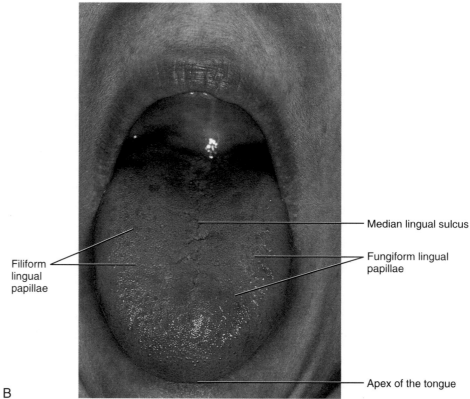

Median lingual sulcus

Filiform lingual papillae

Fungiform lingual papillae

Apex of the tongue

B

FIGURE 2-14 Dorsal surface of the tongue with its landmarks. **A,** Diagram. **B,** Clinical view. (From Fehrenbach MJ, Herring SW: *Illustrated anatomy of the head and neck,* ed 4, St Louis, 2012, Saunders/Elsevier.)

Upper lip

Dorsal surface

Lateral surface

Ventral surface

Apex of the tongue

Foliate lingual papillae   Body   Base

FIGURE 2-15 Lateral surface of the tongue with its landmarks. (From Fehrenbach MJ, Herring SW: *Illustrated anatomy of the head and neck,* ed 4, St Louis, 2012, Saunders/Elsevier.)

A ridge of tissue on each side of the floor of the mouth, the sublingual (sub-ling-gwal) fold, joins in a V-shaped configuration extending from the lingual frenum to the base of the tongue. The sublingual folds contain openings of the sublingual duct from the sublingual salivary gland (see Figures 1-5 and 11-7). The small papilla, or sublingual caruncle (kar-unk-kl), at the anterior end of each sublingual fold contains openings of the submandibular (sub-man-dib-you-lar) duct and sublingual duct (or Wharton duct and Bartholin duct, respectively) from both the sublingual as well as the submandibular salivary gland.

PHARNYGEAL DIVISIONS

The oral cavity proper provides the entrance into the deeper structure of the throat, or pharynx (fare-inks). The pharynx is a muscular tube that has both respiratory and digestive system functions. It has three divisions: nasopharynx, oropharynx, and laryngopharynx (Figure 2-18).

The division of the pharynx that is superior to the level of the soft palate is the nasopharynx (nay-zo-fare-inks), which is continuous with the nasal cavity. The division that is between the soft palate and the opening of the larynx is the oropharynx (or-o-fare-inks). The oropharynx is considered the oral part of the pharynx and is visible for the most part to the dental professional. The fauces, discussed earlier, marks the boundary between the oropharynx and the oral cavity proper. Only part of the nasopharynx is visible during an intraoral examination by a dental professional (see Figure 2-11). Finally, the laryngopharynx (lah-ring-gah-fare-inks) is the more inferior division of the pharynx, close to the laryngeal opening. To examine the more extensive parts of the nasopharynx, as well as the laryngopharynx or even the oropharynx in some patients, special diagnostic tools are needed.

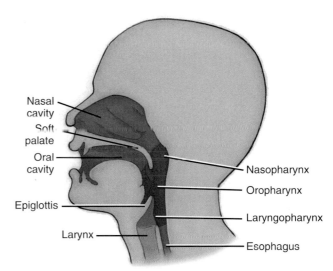

FIGURE 2-18 Midsagittal section of the head with the divisions of the pharynx and associated regions. (From Fehrenbach MJ, Herring SW: *Illustrated anatomy of the head and neck,* ed 4, St Louis, 2012, Saunders/Elsevier.)

FIGURE 2-16 Ventral surface of the tongue with its landmarks. (From Fehrenbach MJ, Herring SW: *Illustrated anatomy of the head and neck,* ed 4, St Louis, 2012, Saunders/Elsevier.)

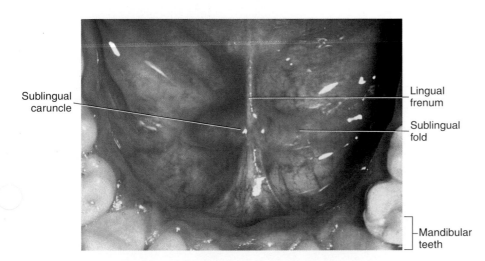

FIGURE 2-17 Floor of the mouth with its landmarks. (From Fehrenbach MJ, Herring SW: *Illustrated anatomy of the head and neck,* ed 4, St Louis, 2012, Saunders/Elsevier.)

CHAPTER **3**

Prenatal Development

e Additional resources and practice exercises are provided on the companion Evolve website for this book: http://evolve.elsevier.com/Fehrenbach/illustrated.

●●● LEARNING OBJECTIVES

1. Define and pronounce the key terms in this chapter.
2. Outline the preimplantation period, including the major events that occur during this first week of prenatal development.
3. Integrate a study of the preimplantation period of prenatal development into the development of the orofacial structures and the clinical considerations due to developmental disturbances associated with these structures.
4. Outline the second week of prenatal development during the embryonic period, including the major events that occur.
5. Outline the third week of prenatal development during the embryonic period, including the major events that occur.
6. Outline the fourth week of prenatal development during the embryonic period, including the major events that occur.
7. Integrate the study of the embryonic period of prenatal development into orofacial development and the clinical considerations due to developmental disturbances associated with these structures.
8. Outline the fetal period of prenatal development, including the major events that occur after the fourth week until birth within this period.
9. Integrate the study of the fetal period of prenatal development into orofacial development and the clinical considerations due to developmental disturbances associated with these structures.
10. Identify the structures present during prenatal development on a diagram.

PRENATAL DEVELOPMENT

Dental professionals need to have an understanding of the major events of prenatal development in order to understand the development of the structures of the face, neck, and oral cavity and the underlying relationships among these structures. Embryology (em-bre-ol-ah-jee) is the study of prenatal development and is introduced in this first chapter of **Unit II**.

Prenatal (pre-nay-tal) development begins with the start of pregnancy and continues until the birth of the child; the 9 months of gestation is usually divided into 3-month time spans, or trimesters. Prenatal development consists of three distinct successive periods: preimplantation period, embryonic period, and fetal period (Table 3-1). The preimplantation period and the embryonic period make up the first trimester of the pregnancy, and the fetal period constitutes the last two trimesters.

Each of the structures of the face, neck, and oral cavity has a primordium (pry-more-de-um), the earliest indication of a tissue type or an organ during prenatal development. This information about the embryologic background of a structure also helps in the appreciation

of any clinical considerations that may occur in these structures due to developmental disturbances.

Clinical Considerations for Prenatal Development

Developmental disturbances that involve the orofacial structures as well as other parts of the body can include congenital malformations (kon-jen-i-til mal-for-may-shins) (or birth defects), which are evident at birth. Most of these occur during both the preimplantation period and the embryonic period and thus involve the first trimester of the pregnancy (discussed later in this chapter). Such malformations occur in 3 out of 100 cases and are one of the leading causes of infant death. This does not include anatomic variants, which are common, such as variation in the lesser details of a bone's shape. Amniocentesis (am-nee-o-sen-tee-sis) (or amniotic fluid test [AFT]) is a prenatal diagnostic procedure to detect chromosomal abnormalities where the amniotic fluid is removed and its fetal cells are grown for microscopic study of the chromosomes as well as sampled for determination of other fetal complications.

TABLE 3-1	Prenatal Development Periods*		
PREIMPLANTATION PERIOD	**EMBRYONIC PERIOD**		**FETAL PERIOD**
First Week	Second to Eighth Week		Third to Ninth Month

Zygote

Disc

Embryo

Blastocyst

Embryo

Folded Embryo

Fetus

| Fertilization and implantation | Induction, proliferation, differentiation, morphogenesis, and maturation (see Table 3-3) | Maturation |

*The structure size is not accurate or comparative.

Malformation can be due to genetic factors, such as chromosome abnormalities or environmental agents and factors. These environmental agents and factors involved in causing malformations can include infections, drugs, and radiation and are considered to be **teratogens** (ter-ah-to-jens) (Table 3-2). Women of reproductive age should wisely avoid teratogens to protect the developing infant from possible congenital malformations (discussed later in this chapter).

Malformations in the face, neck, and oral cavity range from a serious cleft in the face or palatal region to small deficiencies of the soft palate or developing cysts underneath an otherwise intact oral mucosa. Dental professionals should remember that any orofacial congenital malformations discovered when examining a patient are usually understandable and traceable to a specific time in the embryologic development of the individual. Thus, the dental professional must initially understand the development of an individual's orofacial region, including its sequential process to later understand any associated pathology present.

TABLE 3-2	Known Teratogens Involved in Congenital Malformations
TERATOGEN	**DESCRIPTION**
Drugs	Ethanol, tetracycline, phenytoin sodium, lithium, methotrexate, aminopterin, diethylstilbestrol, warfarin, thalidomide, isotretinoin (retinoic acid), androgens, progesterone
Chemicals	Methylmercury, polychlorinated biphenyls
Infections	Rubella virus, syphilis spirochete, herpes simplex virus, human immunodeficiency virus
Radiation	High levels of ionizing type*

*Diagnostic levels of radiation, such as in the dental setting, should be avoided with pregnant women unless for a dental emergency but there has not been any direct link to congenital malformations.

Sperm (enlarged)

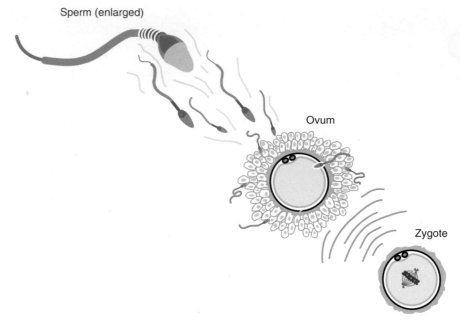

Ovum

Zygote

FIGURE 3-1 Sperm fertilizes the ovum and unites with it to form the zygote after the process of meiosis and during the first week of prenatal development. Both the chromosomes of the ovum and sperm are involved in the process.

PREIMPLANTATION PERIOD

The first period of prenatal development, the **preimplantation** (pre-im-plan-**tay**-shin) **period**, takes place during the first week after conception (see Table 3-1). At the beginning of the first week, conception takes place where a woman's **ovum** (**oh**-vum) is penetrated by and united with a man's **sperm** during **fertilization** (fur-til-uh-**zay**-shun) (Figure 3-1). This union of the ovum and sperm subsequently forms a fertilized egg, or **zygote** (**zy**-gote).

During fertilization, the final stages of **meiosis** (my-**oh**-sis) occur in the ovum. The result of this process is the joining of the ovum's chromosomes with those of the sperm (see **Chapter 7**). This joining of chromosomes from both biologic parents forms a new individual with "shuffled" chromosomes. To allow this formation of a new individual, the sperm and ovum are joined, resulting in the proper number of chromosomes (diploid number of 46). If both these cells, sperm and ovum, instead carried the full complement of chromosomes, fertilization would result in a zygote with *two times* the proper number, resulting in severe congenital malformations and prenatal death (see later discussion).

This situation of excess chromosomes is avoided with meiosis, because, during their development in the gonads, this process enables the ovum and sperm to reduce by one-half the usual number of chromosomes (to haploid number of 23). Thus, the zygote has received half its chromosomes from the woman and half from the man, with the resultant genetic material a reflection of both biologic parents. The photographic analysis of a person's chromosomes is done by orderly arrangement of the pairs in a **karyotype** (**kare**-e-oh-tipe), with the sex known by the presence of either having *XX* chromosomes for a woman or *XY* for a man (Figure 3-2).

After fertilization, the zygote then undergoes mitosis, or individual cell division, that splits it into more and more cells due to **cleavage** (**kleve**-ij) (see Table 7-2). After initial cleavage, the solid ball of cells becomes a *morula*. Because of the ongoing process of mitosis and secretion of fluid by the cells within the morula, the zygote now becomes a **blastocyst** (**blas**-tah-sist) (or blastula) (Figure 3-3). The rest of the first week is characterized by further mitotic cleavage, in which the blastocyst splits into smaller and more numerous cells as it undergoes successive cell divisions by mitosis.

Thus, mitosis is a process that takes place during tissue growth or regeneration, which is different from meiosis that takes place during

Metaphase chromosomes

Karyotype

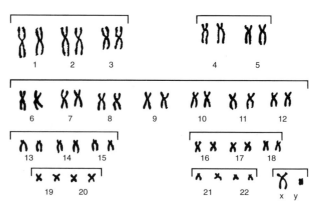

FIGURE 3-2 Example of a karyotype demonstrating a photographic analysis of the chromosomes, with its orderly arrangement of the pairs. This karyotype is of a man since it has both *X* and *Y* chromosomes because the presence of the *Y* determines maleness.

FIGURE 3-3 Zygote undergoing mitotic cleavage to form a blastocyst that travels to become implanted in the endometrium of the uterus.

FIGURE 3-4 Blastocyst. **A,** Consists of both an embryoblast layer and trophoblast layer. **B,** Cross section. **C,** Photomicrograph of sections of blastocysts recovered from the endometrium of the uterus at 4 days. (From Moore KL, Persaud TVN, Torchia MG: *The developing human: clinically oriented embryology,* ed 10, St Louis, 2015, Saunders/Elsevier.)

fertilization as discussed (see Table 7-2). Mitosis that occurs during cell division is the self-duplication of the chromosomes of the parent cell and their equal distribution to daughter cells. The result is that the daughter cells have the same chromosome number and hereditary potential as the parent cells. As it grows by cleavage, the blastocyst travels from the site where fertilization took place to the uterus.

By the end of the first week, the blastocyst stops traveling and undergoes **implantation** (im-plan-**tay**-shin) and thus becomes embedded in the prepared endometrium, the innermost lining of the uterus on its back wall. After a week of cleavage, the blastocyst consists of a layer of peripheral cells, the **trophoblast** (**trof**-oh-blast) **layer**, and a small inner mass of embryonic cells, or **embryoblast** (**em**-bre-oh-blast) **layer** (Figure 3-4). The trophoblast layer later gives rise to important prenatal support tissue. The embryoblast layer later gives rise to the embryo during the prenatal period that follows the embryonic period.

Clinical Considerations for Preimplantation Period

If any disturbances occur in the basic process of meiosis during fertilization, major congenital malformations result from the chromosomal abnormality, which occur in 1 out of 10 cases. An example of this is **Down syndrome** (or trisomy 21) where an extra chromosome number 21 is present after meiotic division (Figure 3-5). This syndrome presents with certain orofacial features that include a flat, broad face with

FIGURE 3-5 Down syndrome from an extra chromosome number 21 presents with noted orofacial features as well as various levels of mental disability. (From Zitelli BJ, Davis HW: *Atlas of pediatric physical diagnosis,* ed 6, St Louis, 2012, Mosby/Elsevier.)

widely spaced eyes, flat-bridged nose, epicanthic folds, oblique eyelid fissures, furrowed lower lip, tongue fissures, lingual papillae hypertrophy, and various levels of mental disability. An arched palate and weak tongue muscles lead to an open mouth position with protrusion of the tongue of the usual size, and articulated speech is often difficult. It may also involve increased levels of periodontal disease, delayed tooth eruption, and fewer teeth present with microdontia.

Implantation of the zygote may also occur outside the uterus with an ectopic (ek-**top**-ik) pregnancy, most occurring within the fallopian tube. This disturbance has several causes but is usually associated with factors that delay or prevent transport of the dividing zygote to the uterus, such as scarred uterine tubes due to pelvic inflammatory disease. In the past, ectopic pregnancies ruptured causing loss of the embryo and threatening the life of the pregnant woman but now they are successfully treated with medications.

EMBRYONIC PERIOD

The second period of prenatal development, the embryonic (em-bre-on-ik) period, extends from the beginning of the second week to the end of the eighth week (see Table 3-1). Certain physiologic processes or spatial and temporal events called *patterning* occur during this period, which are considered key to the further development (Table 3-3). These physiologic processes include induction, proliferation, differentiation, morphogenesis, and maturation (discussed next). These processes cause the structure of the implanted blastocyst to become, with further development, an embryo (em-bre-oh). These physiologic processes also allow the teeth and associated orofacial structures, as well as other organ structures, to develop in the embryo (see Table 6-1).

The first physiologic process involved during prenatal development is the process of induction (in-**duk**-shin), the action of one group of cells on another, which leads to the establishment of the developmental pathway in the responding tissue. Over time, the populations of embryonic cells vary in the competence of their response to induction. Just what triggers cells to develop into structures from cellular interactions is only beginning to be understood, but many developmental disturbances can result from a failure of induction, leading to a further failure of initiation of certain embryologic structures. Induction can also occur in the later stages of development when the structure just increases in size, but these time periods do not seem to be as sensitive.

Another type of physiologic process that follows induction as well as the other processes is the dramatic process of proliferation (pro-lif-er-**ay**-shin), which is controlled levels of cellular growth present during most of prenatal development. Later, migration of these proliferated cells also occurs. Finally, growth also occurs as a result of an accumulation of cellular byproducts.

Growth may be by appositional (ap-oh-**zish**-in-al) growth, in which tissue enlarges by the addition of layers on the outside of a structure. In contrast, growth may be by interstitial (in-ter-**stish**-il) growth, which occurs from deep within a tissue type or organ. Hard tissue growth (such as mature bone or hard dental tissue) is usually appositional, whereas soft tissue (such as skin or gingival tissue) increases by interstitial growth. Some tissue types (such as cartilage and immature bone tissue) use both types of growth to attain their final mature size.

It is important to note that growth is not just an increase in overall size, like a balloon being blown up, but it involves differential rates for the different internal tissue types and organs. An example of this varied rate of growth is tooth eruption in a child, which occurs over many years, allowing for the associated growth of the jaws that surround and support the teeth.

In the process of differentiation (dif-er-en-she-**ay**-shun), a change occurs in the embryonic cells, which are identical genetically but later become quite distinct structurally and functionally. Thus, cells that perform specialized functions are formed by differentiation during the embryonic period. Although these functions are minimal at this time, the beginnings of all major tissue types, organs, and organ systems are formed during this period from these specialized cells.

Differentiation occurs at various rates in the embryo. Many parts of the embryo are affected: cells, tissue types, organs, and systems. Various terms describe each one of these types of differentiation, and it is important to note the specific delineation between each of them. Cytodifferentiation (site-oh-dif-er-en-she-**ay**-shun) is the development of different cell types. Histodifferentiation (his-toe-dif-er-en-she-**ay**-shun) is the development of different histologic tissue types within a structure. Morphodifferentiation (mor-foe-dif-er-en-she-**ay**-shun) is the development of the differing morphology (mor-**fol**-ah-je), which makes up its structure or shape, for each organ or system.

During the embryonic period, the complexity of the structure and function of these cells increases. This is accomplished by morphogenesis (mor-fo-**jen**-is-is), which is the process of development of specific tissue structure or shape. Morphogenesis occurs due to the migration or proliferation of embryonic cells, which is followed by the inductive interactions of those cells. As previously mentioned, induction continues to occur throughout the embryonic period as a result of the new varieties of cells interacting with each other, producing an increasingly complex organism.

Finally, the physiologic process of maturation (ma-cher-**ray**-shin) of the tissue types and organs begins during the embryologic period and continues later during the fetal period. It is important to note that the physiologic process of maturation of the individual tissue types and organs also involves the processes of proliferation, differentiation, and morphogenesis. Thus, maturation is not the attainment of just the correct adult size but also the correct adult structure and function of tissue types and organs.

An embryo is recognizable by the eighth week of prenatal development, which is the end of the embryonic period. This chapter discusses only the major events of the second, third, and fourth weeks of the embryonic period. The remaining weeks of prenatal development, which are pertinent to dental professionals, are addressed in

TABLE 3-3	Developmental Processes
PROCESS	**DESCRIPTION**
Induction	Action of one group of cells on another that leads to the establishment of the developmental pathway in the responding tissue
Proliferation	Controlled cellular growth and accumulation of byproducts
Differentiation	Change in identical embryonic cells to become distinct structurally and functionally
Morphogenesis	Development of specific tissue structure or differing form due to embryonic cell migration or proliferation and inductive interactions
Maturation	Attainment of adult function and size due to proliferation, differentiation, and morphogenesis

Chapters 4 and 5, which describe the more detailed development of the orofacial structures.

SECOND WEEK

During the second week of prenatal development within the embryonic period, the implanted blastocyst grows by increased proliferation of the embryonic cells, with differentiation also occurring resulting in changes in cellular morphogenesis; every ridge, bump, and recess now indicates these increased levels of cellular differentiation. This increased number of embryonic cells creates the embryonic cell layers (or germ layers) within the blastocyst. A bilaminar (by-lam-i-nar) embryonic disc is eventually developed from the blastocyst and appears as a three-dimensional but flattened, essentially circular plate of bilayered cells (Figure 3-6).

FIGURE 3-6 Blastocyst forming the bilaminar embryonic disc. **A,** Consisting of the epiblast layer and hypoblast layer surrounded by the amniotic cavity and yolk sac. **B,** Photomicrograph of longitudinal section of an embedded 14-day embryo. (From Moore KL, Persaud TVN, Torchia MG: *The developing human: clinically oriented embryology,* ed 10, St Louis, 2015, Saunders/Elsevier.)

FIGURE 3-7 Bilaminar embryonic disc with primitive streak resulting in bilateral symmetry.

The bilaminar embryonic disc (or disk) has both a superior and inferior layer. The superior epiblast (ep-i-blast) layer is composed of high columnar cells, and the inferior hypoblast (hi-po-blast) layer is composed of small cuboidal cells. After its creation, the disc is suspended in the uterus's endometrium between two fluid-filled cavities, the amniotic (am-nee-ot-ik) cavity, which faces the epiblast layer, and the yolk sac, which faces the hypoblast layer and serves as initial nourishment for the disc. The bilaminar embryonic disc later develops into the embryo as prenatal development continues.

Even later, the placenta (pla-sen-tuh), a prenatal organ that joins the pregnant woman and developing embryo, develops from the interactions of the trophoblast layer and endometrial tissue. The formation of the placenta and the developing umbilical circulation permit selective exchange of soluble bloodborne substances between them. This includes oxygen and carbon dioxide as well as nutritional and hormonal substances.

THIRD WEEK

During the beginning of the third week of prenatal development within the embryonic period, the primitive streak forms within the bilaminar disc (Figure 3-7). This furrowed, rod-shaped thickening in the middle of the disc results from an increased proliferation of cells in the midline area. The primitive streak causes the disc to have bilateral symmetry (sim-me-try), with a right half and left half; most of the further development of each half of the embryo mirrors the other half. If looked at from a top view, the embryo would resemble the sole of a shoe with the head end wider than the tail end and with a slightly narrowed middle.

In addition, during the beginning of the third week, some cells from the epiblast layer move or migrate toward the hypoblast layer only in the area of the primitive streak (Figure 3-8). These migratory cells locate in the middle between the epiblast and hypoblast layers and become mesoderm (mes-oh-derm), an embryonic connective tissue, as well as embryonic endoderm (en-doe-derm). Mesodermal cells have the potential to proliferate and differentiate into diverse types of connective tissue, forming cells such as fibroblasts, chondroblasts, and osteoblasts (see **Chapter 8**).

With three layers present, the bilaminar embryonic disc has thickened into trilaminar (try-lam-i-nar) embryonic disc (Figure 3-9). Thus, the trilaminar embryonic disc has three embryonic cell layers. With the creation of the new embryonic cell layers of mesoderm and embryonic endoderm, the epiblast layer is now considered ectoderm (ek-toe-derm). At the same time, the hypoblast layer has been displaced by the cells migrating into the primitive streak and now becomes extra-embryonic endoderm.

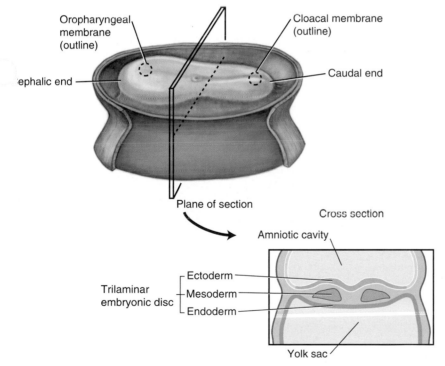

FIGURE 3-8 Bilaminar embryonic disc with migration of the epiblast layer cells toward the hypoblast layer to form the new mesoderm layer.

FIGURE 3-9 After the formation of the middle layer of mesoderm, the resulting trilaminar embryonic disc consists of the ectoderm, mesoderm, and endoderm. The cephalic and caudal ends of the disc are associated with the oropharyngeal and cloacal membranes *(dashed circles)*.

Within the trilaminar embryonic disc, each embryonic cell layer is distinct from the others and thus gives rise to specific tissue (Table 3-4, see Table 8-1). The ectoderm gives rise to the skin epidermis, the central nervous system (CNS), and other structures. The mesoderm gives rise to connective tissue, such as skin dermis, cartilage, bone, blood, muscle, and other associated tissue. The endoderm gives rise to the respiratory epithelium and cells of glands.

Mesoderm and associated tissue are found in all areas of the future embryo except at certain embryonic membranes at both ends of the embryo and the pharyngeal pouches (discussed later in this chapter).

In these areas without mesoderm present, both the ectoderm and endoderm fuse together, thereby preventing the migration of mesoderm between them.

Because the trilaminar embryonic disc has undergone so much growth during the past 3 weeks, certain anatomic structures of the disc become apparent. The disc now has a **cephalic** (se-fal-ik) **end**, or head end. At the cephalic end, the oropharyngeal membrane forms, which consists of only ectoderm externally and endoderm internally, without any intermediate mesoderm. This membrane is the location of the future primitive mouth or stomodeum of the embryo and thus

TABLE 3-4	Development of Embryonic Cell Layers			
	ECTODERM	**MESODERM**	**ENDODERM**	**NEURAL CREST CELLS***
Origin	Epiblast layer	Migrating cells from epiblast layer	Migrating cells from epiblast layer	Migrating neuroectoderm
Histologic features	Columnar	Varies	Cuboidal	Varies
Future structures	Epidermis; sensory epithelium of the eyes, ears, nose, nervous system, and neural crest cells; mammary and cutaneous glands	Dermis, muscle, bone, lymphatics, blood cells and bone marrow, cartilage, reproductive, and excretory organs	Respiratory and digestive system linings, liver, and pancreatic cells	Components of nervous system pigment cells, connective tissue proper, cartilage, bone, and certain dental tissue

*Neural crest cells from the neuroectoderm are included, but they are not present in the embryonic disc until the later part of the third week; neural crest cells are considered to be a *fourth embryonic cell layer* by embryologists.

the beginning of the digestive tract (see Figure 4-1). The disc also has a **caudal** (kaw-dal) **end**, or tail end (see Figure 3-9). At the caudal end, the cloacal membrane forms, which is the location of the future anus, or terminal end of the digestive tract.

During the latter part of the third week, the CNS begins to develop in the embryo (Figure 3-10). Many steps occur during this week to form the beginnings of the spinal cord and brain (see Table 8-7). First, a specialized group of cells differentiates from the ectoderm and is now considered **neuroectoderm** (noor-oh-ek-toe-derm). These cells are localized to the **neural** (noor-al) **plate** of the embryo, which is a central band of cells that extends the length of the embryo, from the cephalic end to the caudal end. This plate undergoes further growth and thickening, which cause it to deepen and invaginate inward, forming the **neural groove**.

Near the end of the third week, the neural groove deepens further and is surrounded by the **neural folds**. As further growth of the neuroectoderm occurs, the **neural tube** is formed during the fourth week by the neural folds undergoing **fusion** (fu-zhin) at the most superior part. The neural tube forms the future spinal cord as well as other neural tissue of the CNS (see Table 3-4).

Other areas of the embryo also undergo fusion during the third week and in subsequent weeks, as the embryo develops, but the process occurs differently depending on the structures involved. In the case of the neural tube (and also the palate as discussed in **Chapter 5**), the process of fusion, as the name implies, can be the joining of two separate surfaces on the embryo (Figure 3-11). However, in the case of facial fusion, the process of fusion can also include the elimination of a groove between two adjacent processes appearing as swellings on the same surface of the embryo. In these cases, merging of underlying tissue and cell migration into the groove produces the joining of the facial processes (see Figures 4-3 and 4-4).

In addition, during the third week, another specialized group of cells, the **neural crest cells (NCCs)**, develop from neuroectoderm (Figure 3-12). These cells migrate from the crests of the neural folds and then join the mesoderm to form **mesenchyme** (mes-eng-kime). The mesenchyme is involved in the development of many face and neck structures, such as the branchial arches, because they differentiate to form most of the connective tissue of the head.

On reaching their predetermined destinations, the NCCs undergo differentiation into diverse cell types that are, in part, specified by local environmental influences. Embryologists consider the NCCs to be a *fourth embryonic cell layer* (see Table 3-4). In future development, these cells become involved in the formation of components of the nervous system, melanocyte pigment cells, connective tissue proper, cartilage, bone, and certain dental tissue by becoming a specialized type of mesenchyme,

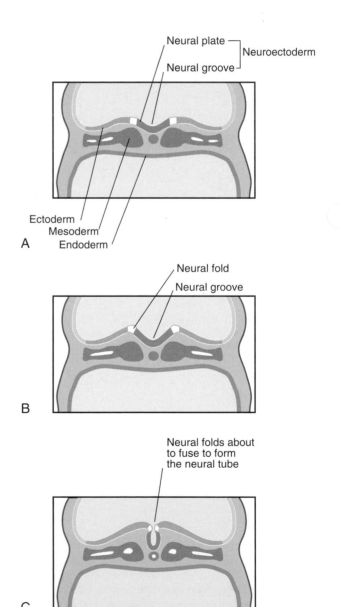

FIGURE 3-10 Central nervous system of the embryo beginning t form. **A,** Formation of the neuroectoderm from the ectoderm with the neural plate that thickens to form the neural groove. **B,** Neural groove deepens to become surrounded by the neural folds. **C,** Neural folds meet and fuse, forming the neural tube.

FIGURE 3-11 Process of fusion that can have the joining of swellings or tissue from *different* surfaces of the embryo, which occurs with the neural tube, upper lip, and palate. This is unlike the fusion with the joining of swellings or tissue on the *same* surface of the embryo that occurs on the face (see Figure 4-4).

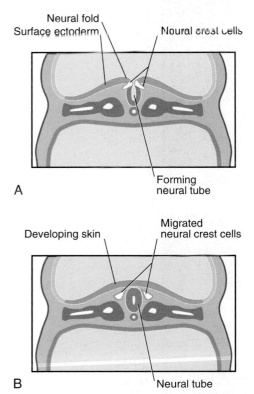

FIGURE 3-12 Neural crest cells from the neural folds **(A)** will migrate and join with the mesoderm to form the mesenchyme **(B)** to affect tissue development.

ectomesenchyme, such as the formation of the pulp, dentin, cementum, alveolar process, and periodontal ligament (see Figure 6-1). Thus, NCCs are essential in formation of most oral and dental tissue, xcept for the enamel and certain types of cementum, as well as the levelopment of the face and neck (see **Chapters 4, 5, and 6**).

By the end of the third week, the mesoderm additionally differentiates and begins to divide on each side of the tube into 38-paired cuboidal segments of mesoderm, forming the **somites** (**so**-mites)

(Figure 3-13). The somites later appear as distinct elevations on the surface of the sides of the embryo and continue to develop in the following weeks of prenatal development, giving rise to most of the skeletal structures of the head, neck, and trunk, as well as the associated muscles and dermis of the skin.

FOURTH WEEK

During the fourth week of prenatal development within the embryonic period, the trilaminar embryonic disc undergoes anterior (cephalic) and lateral **embryonic folding**, which places forming tissue types into their proper positions for further embryonic development, as well as producing a somewhat tubular embryo (Figure 3-14). This folding results from extensive proliferation of the ectoderm and differentiation of basic tissue and occurs mainly at the cephalic end, where the brain will form. This cephalic tissue grows beyond the oropharyngeal membrane to overhang the developing heart.

Folding due to increased growth occurs not only at the cephalic end but also at the caudal end and at the sides of the embryo simultaneously. As a result of this folding, the positions of the embryonic cell layers take on a more recognizable placement for the further development of the embryo.

Thus, after folding of the disc, the endoderm lies inside the ectoderm, with mesoderm filling in the areas between these two layers. This movement of the embryonic cell layers forms one long, hollow tube lined by endoderm from the cephalic end to the caudal end of the embryo—specifically, from the **oropharyngeal** (or-oh-fah-**rin**-je-al) **membrane** to the **cloacal** (klo-**ay**-kal) **membrane**. This tube is the future digestive tract and is separated into three major regions: foregut, midgut, and hindgut.

The anterior part of this tube is the **foregut** (**fore**-gut), which forms the primitive pharynx, or primitive throat, and includes a part of the primitive yolk sac as it becomes enclosed with folding (see Figure 4-10). The two more posterior parts, the **midgut** (**mid**-gut) and **hindgut** (**hinde**-gut), respectively, form the rest of the mature pharynx, as well as the remainder of the digestive tract (see Figure 2-18). During development of the digestive tract, four pairs of pharyngeal pouches will form from evaginations on the lateral walls lining the pharynx (see Figure 4-11).

Finally, during the fourth week, the face and neck begin to develop, with the primitive eyes, ears, nose, oral cavity, and jaw areas. The development of the face and neck is discussed in **Chapter 4**, and the development of the associated oral cavity is described in **Chapters 5 and 6**.

Clinical Considerations for Embryonic Period

Because the beginnings of all essential external and internal structures are formed during the embryonic period, this is considered the most critical period of prenatal development. Thus, developmental disturbances occurring during this period may give rise to major congenital malformations of the embryo (as discussed earlier).

One syndrome that can occur within this period is **ectodermal dysplasia** (ek-toe-derm-al dis-**play**-ze-ah), which involves the abnormal development of one or more structures from ectoderm (Figure 3-15). This syndrome has a hereditary etiology and presents with abnormalities of the teeth, skin, hair, nails, eyes, facial structure, and glands, because these are derived from ectoderm or associated tissue. There may be partial or complete anodontia, the absence of some or all teeth in each dentition, and the teeth that are present for either dentition frequently have developmental disturbances (see **Chapter 6**). Partial or full dentures are used for both functional and esthetic purposes,

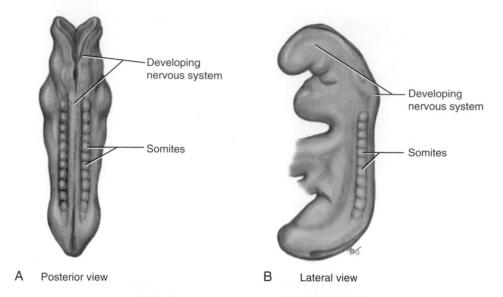

A   Posterior view

B   Lateral view

FIGURE 3-13 Differentiated mesoderm gives rise to the somites. **A** and **B,** Somites are located on both the sides of the developing nervous system. **C,** View of 13-somite embryo at around 24 days. (From Moore KL, Persaud TVN, Torchia MG: *The developing human: clinically oriented embryology,* ed 10, St Louis, 2015, Saunders/Elsevier.)

FIGURE 3-14 Trilaminar embryonic disc has folded into the embryo. **A** and **B,** Disc now has undergone embryonic folding as a result of extensive growth of the ectoderm, and there is development of the brain with spinal cord, heart, and digestive tract. **C,** With this folding, the endoderm is now inside the ectoderm, with the mesoderm filling in the areas between the two tissue types, except at the two embryonic membranes as shown on cross section. (From Moore KL, Persaud TVN, Torchia MG: *The developing human: clinically oriented embryology,* ed 10, St Louis, 2015, Saunders/Elsevier.)

but need to be reconstructed periodically as the jaws continue to grow; implants may be considered after growth halts if bone levels of each remaining alveolar process are adequate.

If there is failure of migration of the NCCs to the facial region, **Treacher Collins (tree-**chur **kol-**inz) **syndrome (TCS)** (or mandibu-ofacial dysostosis) develops in the embryo (Figure 3-16). This results in failure of specific areas of orofacial development, presenting with downward slanting eyes, underdeveloped zygomatic bone, drooping lateral lower eyelids, and conductive hearing loss, with malformed or

absent ears as well as dental developmental disturbances, such as ano-dontia, enamel dysplasia, and micrognathia (small lower jaw).

In addition, if teratogens are present during the active differentia-tion of a tissue type or organ, after crossing from pregnant woman by way of the placenta, this can raise the incidence of congenital malfor-mations. An example of an infective teratogen for the embryo is the virus causing **rubella** (roo-**bell**-ah), which can result in cataracts, car-diac defects, and deafness. Another infective teratogen is the bacterial spirochete causing **syphilis** (**sif**-i-lis), *Treponema pallidum,* because

FIGURE 3-15 Ectodermal dysplasia is marked by the abnormal development of ectodermal structures resulting in certain facial features and an absence of teeth, or anodontia (partial in this case). (Courtesy of Margaret J. Fehrenbach, RDH, MS.)

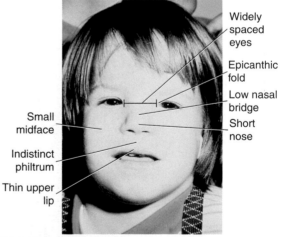

FIGURE 3-17 Dental anomalies from syphilis, an infective teratogen. **A,** Hutchinson incisors. **B,** Mulberry molar. (From Ibsen OAC, Phelan JA: *Oral pathology for dental hygienists*, ed 6, St Louis, 2014, Saunders/Elsevier.)

FIGURE 3-16 Treacher Collins syndrome from the failure of migration of the neural crest cells to the facial region in the embryo presents with areas without complete orofacial development, having marked features, including micrognathia (small lower jaw). (From Kaban LB, Toulis MJ: *Pediatric oral and maxillofacial surgery*, ed 1, Philadelphia, 2004, Saunders/Elsevier.)

it produces defects in the incisors (Hutchinson incisor) and molars (mulberry molar), as well as blindness, deafness, and possible paralysis if not treated (Figure 3-17, see **Chapters 16 and 17**).

An example of the result of a teratogenic drug effect during the embryonic period is fetal (fete-il) alcohol syndrome (FAS) (Figure 3-18). High levels of ethanol ingested by a pregnant woman cross the placenta and can result in prenatal and postnatal growth deficiency, mental disabilities, and other facial disturbances, such as small head circumference, low nasal bridge, short nose, small midface, widely spaced eyes with epicanthic folds and eyelid fissures, indistinct philtrum, and thin upper lip. Oral changes, such as crowding of the dentition, mouth breathing, anterior open bite, and associated gingivitis, may occur, possibly because of an increased finger sucking habit. However, the effects of alcohol on prenatal development can include much more than those defining criteria, and prenatal exposure to alcohol can potentially impact development at almost any point in the pregnancy, from embryonic through fetal development.

Direct exposure to high levels of radiation can act as an environmental teratogen during the embryonic period. Radiation may injure embryonic cells, resulting in cell death, chromosome injury, and delay of mental and physical growth. The severity of embryonic damage

Widely spaced eyes
Epicanthic fold
Low nasal bridge
Short nose
Small midface
Indistinct philtrum
Thin upper lip

FIGURE 3-18 Fetal alcohol syndrome presents with noted orofacial features and various levels of mental disability. This syndrome is caused by the pregnant women's excessive use of ethanol during the embryonic period. (From Streissguth AP, Landesman-Dwyer S, Martin JC, et al: Teratogenic effects of alcohol in humans and laboratory animals, *Science* 209:353-361, 1980. Copyright 1980; American Association for the Advancement of Science.)

is associated with the absorbed dose, the dose rate, and the state of embryonic or fetal development at the time of exposure.

However, congenital abnormalities have not been directly linked to a diagnostic level of radiation, such as that used in the dental setting. Scattered radiation from a radiographic examination of the oral cavity administers a dose of only a few millirads to a pregnant woman, which is not known to be teratogenic to an embryo. Nevertheless, even this small dose should be avoided during pregnancy unless an emergency situation requires it; proper protective precautions should be used with all patients at all times as well as with the administering dental professionals.

Failure of fusion of the neural tube results in neural tube defects of the tissue overlying the spinal cord, such as the meninges, vertebral arches, muscles, and skin. One type of neural tube defect is spina bifida (spi-nah bif-ah-dah), characterized by defects in the vertebral arches and various degrees of disability. Nutritional and environmental factors can also have an important role as teratogens in causing neural tube defects; folic acid supplements are now being recommended during pregnancy to help prevent this defect as well as cleft lip and cleft palate (see Figures 4-8 and 5-6).

FETAL PERIOD

The final period of prenatal development, the fetal period, follows the embryonic period (see Table 3-1). It encompasses the beginning of the ninth week or third month continuing to the ninth month, with the maturation of existing structures occurring as the embryo enlarges to become a fetus (fete-is). This process involves not only the physiologic process of maturation of the individual tissue types and organs but also further proliferation, differentiation, and morphogenesis, as discussed before with the development of the embryo.

Although developmental changes with the fetus are not as dramatic as those that occur during the embryonic period, they are important because they allow the newly formed tissue types and organs to function. Even though the embryo has been breathing since the third week of prenatal development, by the end of the fourth month, the fetal heartbeat and fetal movements are also present.

Clinical Considerations for Fetal Period

Systemic tetracycline antibiotic therapy of the pregnant woman can act as a teratogenic drug during the fetal period. This therapy can result in tetracycline (tet-rah-si-kleen) stain within the child's primary teeth that are developing at that time. This intrinsic yellow to

FIGURE 3-19 Lingual view of the permanent maxillary anterior teeth with tetracycline stain caused by the ingestion of the drug by a child during the time of development of the permanent dentition. Veneer restorative crowns have been placed on the facial surface of the affected teeth for esthetic reasons. Many times vital whitening (or bleaching) may also be effective to some extent, evening out the tooth color. (Courtesy of Margaret J. Fehrenbach, RDH, MS.)

yellow-brown discoloration of the teeth can occur in slight, moderate, or severe degrees, as the antibiotic becomes chemically bound to the dentin for the life of the tooth, and because of the transparency of overlying enamel, this stain is easily visible.

The adult's permanent teeth may also be affected, similarly to the primary teeth, if the drug is given to a child during their development (Figure 3-19). If the permanent teeth are involved, treatment may require full-coverage crowns or veneers to improve the appearance of the teeth, although, in some cases, vital tooth whitening may even out the discoloration. Thus, this type of antibiotic therapy should be avoided if possible in pregnant women and children. Studies also show that overuse of amoxicillin in children with ear and respiratory infections may be involved in pitting and intrinsic stain in the permanent tooth enamel, resulting in enamel dysplasia (see Box 6-1, O, P).

CHAPTER 4

Face and Neck Development

ⓔ Additional resources and practice exercises are provided on the companion Evolve website for this book: http://evolve.elsevier.com/Fehrenbach/illustrated.

●●●● LEARNING OBJECTIVES

1. Define and pronounce the key terms in this chapter.
2. Outline the events that occur during facial development, describing each step in its formation.
3. Identify the structures present during facial development on a diagram.
4. Integrate the study of the facial development into understanding the observed orofacial structures and the clinical considerations due to developmental disturbances of these structures.

5. Outline the events that occur during neck development, describing each step in its formation.
6. Identify the structures present during neck development on a diagram.
7. Integrate the study of neck development into understanding the observed orofacial structures and the clinical considerations due to developmental disturbances of these structures.

FACIAL DEVELOPMENT

Dental professionals must have a clear understanding about the development of the face to further relate the underlying structural relationships to any developmental disturbances that may be present.

The face and its associated tissue begin to form during the fourth week of prenatal development within the embryonic period (Figure 4-1 and Box 4-1). During this time, the rapidly growing brain of the embryo bulges over the oropharyngeal membrane and developing heart (Figure 4-2). The area of the future face is now squeezed between the developing brain and heart with the formation of the three embryonic layers and resultant embryonic folding (see Figure 3-14).

All three embryonic layers are involved in facial development: ectoderm, mesoderm, and endoderm (Table 4-1). Early development of the face is also dominated by the proliferation and migration of ectomesenchyme, derived from neural crest cells (NCCs) (see **Chapter 3** for more discussion).

Facial development includes the formation of the primitive mouth, mandibular arch, maxillary process, frontonasal process, and nose. Facial development depends on the five major facial processes (or prominences) that form during the fourth week and surround the primitive mouth of the embryo: single frontonasal process and paired maxillary and mandibular processes (Figure 4-3). Thus, these facial processes become the centers of growth for the face. If the adult face is divided into thirds—upper face, midface, and lower face—these parts roughly correspond to the three centers of facial growth. The upper face

is derived from the frontonasal process, the midface from the maxillary processes, and the lower face from the mandibular processes.

The facial development that starts in the fourth week will be completed later in the twelfth week within the fetal period. The face changes shape considerably as it grows from being an embryo to forming into a fetus. Thus, overall facial proportions develop during the later fetal period. It is important to note that the development of the associated oral structures is occurring at the same time as discussed in **Chapters 5 and 6**.

Most of the facial structures develop by fusion of swellings or tissue on the *same* surface of the embryo (Figure 4-4). A cleft, or furrow, is initially located between these adjacent swellings due to proliferation, differentiation, and morphogenesis (see Table 3-3). However, with most facial fusion, these furrows are usually eliminated as the underlying mesenchyme migrates into the furrow, making the embryonic facial surface smooth. This migration takes place because adjacent mesenchyme grows and merges beneath the external ectoderm during the maturation of the structure. In some cases, a slight groove or line maybe left on the facial surface, showing where the fusion of the swellings took place. Differing from this type of fusion that takes place on the facial surface is the type of fusion that occurs during development of the upper lip and palate (see Figure 3-11). In contrast to most facial fusion, upper lip and palatal fusion involves the fusion of swellings or tissue from *different* surfaces of the embryo, such as that which occu with the fusion of the neural tube (see Figure 3-10, *C*).

The overall growth of the face is in both an inferior and anterior direction in relationship to the cranial base. The growth of the

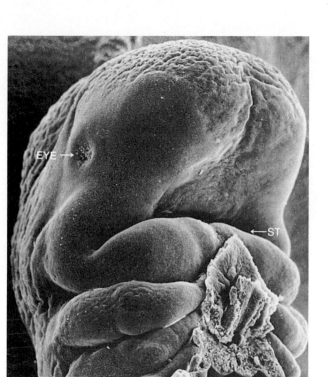

FIGURE 4-1 Scanning electron micrograph of the embryo at the fourth week, showing the developing face with its stomodeum (*ST*) and lens placode for the eye as well as the developing brain. (Nearby anterior placed developing heart has been cut away to display the branchial arches.) (From Hinrichsen K: The early development of morphology and patterns of the face in the human embryo, *Adv Anat Embryol Cell Biol* 98:1-79, 1985.)

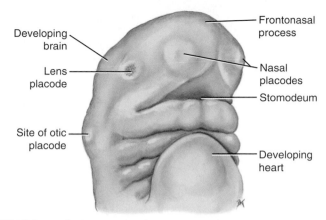

FIGURE 4-2 Embryo at the fourth week of prenatal development showing the developing brain, the forming face from the growth of the frontonasal process with its stomodeum and placodes, and the developing heart.

BOX 4-1	**Facial Development within Fourth Week of Prenatal Development**

Developmental Events Overview (Not in Precise Order of Occurrence)

- Disintegration of the oropharyngeal membrane of stomodeum enlarges the primitive mouth, allowing access to the primitive pharynx
- Mandibular processes fuse to form mandibular arch, which then uses to form the mandible and lower lip
- Frontonasal process forms and gives rise to the nasal placodes, nasal pits, medial and lateral nasal processes, and intermaxillary segment to form the nose and primary palate
- Maxillary process forms from mandibular arch on each side of the stomodeum
- Maxillary processes fuse with each medial nasal process to form upper lip and with each mandibular arch to form the labial commissures

TABLE 4-1	**Embryonic Orofacial Development**	
EMBRYONIC STRUCTURES	**ORIGIN**	**FUTURE STRUCTURES**
Stomodeum	Ectodermal depression enlarged by disintegration of oropharyngeal membrane	Oral cavity proper
First branchial arch (aka *mandibular arch*)	Fused mandibular processes and neural crest cells	Lower lip, lower face, mandible with associated tissue (other arch derivatives shown in Table 4-2)
Maxillary process(es)	Superior and anterior swelling(s) from mandibular arch and neural crest cells	Midface, upper lip sides, cheeks, secondary palate, posterior part of maxilla with associated tissue, zygomatic bones, part of temporal bones
Frontonasal process	Ectodermal tissue and neural crest cells	Medial and lateral nasal processes
Nasal pits	Nasal placodes	Nasal cavities
Medial nasal process(es)	Frontonasal process medial to nasal pits	Middle of nose, philtrum region, intermaxillary segment
Intermaxillary segment	Fused medial nasal processes	Anterior part of maxilla with associated tissue, primary palate, nasal septum
Lateral nasal process(es)	Frontonasal process lateral to nasal pits	Nasal alae

upper face is initially the most rapid, in keeping with its association with the rapidly developing brain. Subsequently, the forehead ceases to grow significantly after age 12. In contrast, the midface and lower face grow more slowly over a prolonged period of time and finally cease to grow late in puberty. Much later, the eruption of the permanent third molars at approximately 17 to 21 years of age marks the end of the major growth of the lower two-thirds of the face. The underlying facial bones, also developing at this time, depend on centers of bone formation by intramembranous ossification (see Figure 8-12).

STOMODEUM AND ORAL CAVITY FORMATION

At the beginning of the fourth week, the primitive mouth has become the **stomodeum** (sto-mo-de-um) (or stomatodeum), which initially appeared as a shallow depression in the embryonic surface ectoderm at its cephalic end (see Figures 4-1 and 4-2).

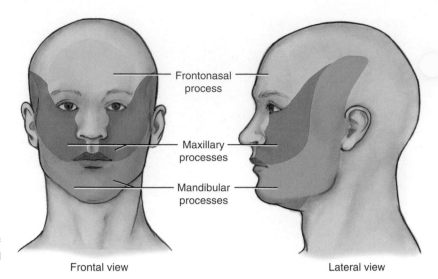

FIGURE 4-3 Adult face with its embryonic derivatives of the five facial processes: single frontonasal process and paired maxillary and mandibular processes.

Frontonasal process

Maxillary processes

Mandibular processes

Frontal view

Lateral view

FIGURE 4-4 Facial fusion can involve the elimination of a furrow between two adjacent swellings of tissue on the *same* surface of the embryo. This fusion process differs from that of the neural tube, upper lip, and palatal fusion, which is the fusion of two separate structures from two *different* surfaces (see Figure 3-11).

At this time, the stomodeum is limited in depth by the oropharyngeal membrane (see Figure 3-14). This temporary membrane, consisting of external ectoderm overlying endoderm, was formed during the third week of prenatal development. The membrane also separates the stomodeum from the primitive pharynx. The primitive pharynx is the cranial part of the foregut, which is the beginning of the future digestive tract.

The first event in the development of the face during the latter part of the fourth week of prenatal development is disintegration of the oropharyngeal membrane (Figure 4-5). With this disintegration of the membrane, the primitive mouth is increased in depth and enlarges across the surface of the midface. Access now occurs through the stomodeum between the internal primitive pharynx and the outside fluids of the amniotic cavity that surrounds the

embryo. In future development, the stomodeum will give rise to the oral cavity, which will be lined by oral epithelium, derived from ectoderm as a result of embryonic folding. Additionally, the oral epithelium derived from ectoderm and associated underlying mesodermal tissue will give rise to the teeth and associated tissue types as discussed in **Chapter 6** (see Figure 6-1).

MANDIBULAR ARCH AND LOWER FACE FORMATION

After formation of the stomodeum but still within the fourth week, two bulges of tissue appear inferior to the primitive mouth: the two **mandibular** (man-**dib**-you-lar) **processes** (see Figure 4-5). These processes consist of a core of mesenchyme formed in part by NCCs that migrated to the facial region to join with the mesoderm; they are covered externally by ectoderm and internally by endoderm.

These paired mandibular processes then fuse at the midline to form the **mandibular arch**, the developmental form of the future lower dental arch, the mandible. After fusion, the mandibular arch then extends as a band of tissue found inferior to the stomodeum and between the developing brain and heart. In the midline, on the surface of the mature bony mandible, is the mandibular symphysis, indicating where the mandible is formed by fusion of right and left mandibular processes (see Figure 1-9). The mandibular arch and its associated tissue are the first parts of the face to form after the stomodeum, separating it from the developing cardiac bulge.

The mandibular arch is also considered the *first branchial arch* (discussed later in this chapter). Thus, this tissue depends on NCCs for its formation, as do all the other more inferior five branchial arches. During the growth of the mandibular arch, **Meckel cartilage** (mek-el kar-ti-lij) forms within each side of the arch (see Figure 5-3, *A-B*). Most of this cartilage disappears as the bony mandible forms by intramembranous ossification lateral to and in close association with the cartilage; yet, a small part makes a contribution to it (see **Chapters 5 and 8**). Also, the cartilage participates in the formation of the middle ear bones.

In future development, the developing mandibular arch directly gives rise to the lower face, including the lower lip. Thus the mandibular arch will also give rise not only to the mandible, but additionally its mandibular teeth and associated tissue. The mandible of the embryo initially

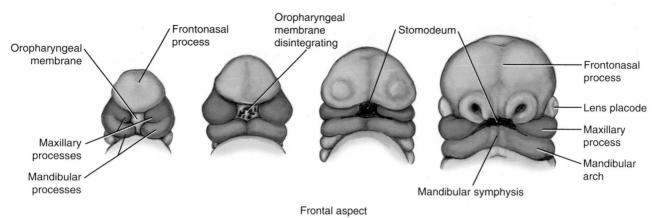

Oropharyngeal
membrane

Frontonasal
process

Oropharyngeal
membrane
disintegrating

Stomodeum

Frontonasal
process

Lens placode

Maxillary
process

Maxillary
processes

Mandibular
arch

Mandibular
processes

Mandibular symphysis

Frontal aspect

FIGURE 4-5 During the third to fourth week, disintegration of the oropharyngeal membrane enlarges the stomodeum of the embryo and allows access between the primitive mouth and the primitive pharynx. The frontonasal process also enlarges, helping to form the nasal region. Mandibular processes give rise to the maxillary processes and then fuse together at the mandibular symphysis, forming the mandibular arch inferior to the enlarged stomodeum.

appears underdeveloped, but it achieves its more characteristic mature prominent form as it develops further during the fetal period (see Figures 4-5 and 4-3, respectively).

The mesoderm of the mandibular arch forms the muscles of mastication (masseter, temporalis, and pterygoids), as well as some palatal muscles and suprahyoid muscles (see Figure 19-8). Because these muscles are derived from the mandibular arch, they are innervated by the first arch nerve, the trigeminal nerve or fifth cranial nerve (see Table 13-3). The mandibular arch is also involved in the formation of the tongue (see Figure 5-9).

During the fifth to sixth week, primitive muscle cells from the mesoderm in the mandibular arch begin to differentiate. These primitive muscle cells become oriented to the site of origin and insertion of the masticatory muscles that they will form. By the seventh week, the mandibular muscle mass has enlarged, and the cells have begun to migrate into the areas where they will begin to differentiate into the four muscles of mastication as discussed. Muscle cell migration occurs before bone formation in the facial area.

By the tenth week, the mandibular muscle masses have become well organized bilaterally into the four muscles of mastication. Nerve branches from the trigeminal nerve are incorporated early in these muscle masses. The muscle cells of the masseter and medial pterygoid muscles have formed a vertical sling that inserts into the site that will form the angle of the mandible. The temporalis muscle cells have differentiated in the temporal fossa and are inserting into the developing coronoid process. The lateral pterygoid muscle cells, which arise from the infratemporal fossa, extend horizontally into the mandibular condyle and disc of the temporomandibular joint.

FRONTONASAL PROCESS AND UPPER FACE FORMATION

During the fourth week, the frontonasal (frun-to-nay-zil) process also forms as a bulge of tissue at the most cephalic end of the embryo and is the cranial boundary of the stomodeum (see Figure 4-2). In future development, the frontonasal process gives rise to the upper face, which includes the forehead, bridge of the nose, primary palate, nasal septum, and all structures associated with the medial nasal processes.

PLACODE DEVELOPMENT

On the outer surface of the embryo are placodes, which are rounded areas of specialized, thickened ectoderm found at the location of developing special sense organs. The facial area of the embryo has two lens placodes (plak-odz), which are initially located fishlike on each side of the frontonasal process (see Figures 4-1 and 4-2). Later in development, these lens placodes migrate medially from their lateral positions and form the future eyes and associated tissue.

The two otic (o-tik) placodes are even more laterally and posteriorly placed and form pits that create the future internal ear and the associated tissue as they appear to rise to their mature position as a result of their relative growth. Parts of the nearby branchial apparatus of the embryonic neck later form the external and middle ear (discussed later in this chapter).

In addition to the lens and otic placodes, the two nasal (nay-zil) placodes form in the anterior part of the frontonasal process, just superior to the stomodeum, during the fourth week (see Figure 4-2). These button-like structures form as bilateral ectodermal thickenings that later develop into olfactory epithelium for the sensation of smell, located in the mature nose.

NOSE AND PARANASAL SINUS FORMATION

During the fourth week, the tissue around the nasal placodes on the frontonasal process undergoes growth, thus starting the development of the nasal region and the nose. The placodes then become submerged, forming a depression in the center of each placode, the nasal pits (or olfactory pits) (Figure 4-6). These nasal pits later develop into the nasal cavity (Figure 4-7, A, and see Figure 11-19).

Deepening of the nasal pits produces a nasal sac that grows internally toward the developing brain. At first, the nasal sacs are separated from the stomodeum by the oronasal (or-oh-nay-zil) membrane. This temporary membrane disintegrates, bringing the nasal and oral cavities into communication in the area of the primitive choanae, posterior to the developing primary palate. At the same time, the superior, middle, and inferior nasal conchae are developing on the lateral walls of the developing nasal cavities.

Frontal aspect

Lateral aspect

Medial nasal process

Nasal pit

Lateral nasal process

Medial nasal process

Lateral nasal process

Maxillary process

Medial nasal processes fusing with each other

Medial nasal process fusing with maxillary process on each side

Lateral nasal process

Philtrum

Upper lip

Philtrum

FIGURE 4-6 Development of the nose from the fusion of the medial and lateral nasal processes; also showing the formation of the upper lip from the medial process fusing with the maxillary process on each side of the stomodeum.

Some of the paranasal sinuses develop later during the fetal period, and others develop after birth. All form as outgrowths of the walls of the nasal cavities and become air-filled extensions of the nasal cavities in the adjacent bones, such as in the maxilla and the frontal bone (see Figure 11-21).

The middle part of the tissue growing around the nasal placodes appears as two crescent-shaped swellings located between the nasal pits. These are the medial nasal processes (see Figure 4-6). In future development, the medial nasal processes will fuse together externally to form the middle part of the nose from the root of the nose to the apex of the nose, as well as the tubercle of the upper lip and philtrum (see Figures 1-4 and 1-6).

The paired medial nasal processes also fuse internally and grow inferiorly on the inside of the stomodeum, forming the intermaxillary (in-ter-mak-si-lare-ee) segment (or premaxillary segment) by the end of the seventh week of prenatal development (see Figure 4-7, *B and C*, and see Figure 5-1). The intermaxillary segment is involved in the formation of certain maxillary teeth (incisors) and associated structures, such as the primary palate and nasal septum.

On the outer part of the nasal pits are two other crescent-shaped swellings, the lateral nasal processes (see Figure 4-6). In future development, the lateral nasal processes form the alae of the nose, and the fusion of the lateral nasal, maxillary, and medial nasal processes forms the nares (see Figure 1-4). The embryonic nose remains visually flat, however,

until the fetal period, when facial development is completed and it has its more mature elevated appearance.

MAXILLARY PROCESS AND MIDFACE FORMATION

During the fourth week of prenatal development, within the embryonic period, an adjacent swelling forms from increased growth of the mandibular arch on each side of the stomodeum, the maxillary (mak-si-lare-ee) process. Subsequently, each maxillary process will grow superiorly and anteriorly around the stomodeum (see Figure 4-5). Because it is formed from the mandibular arch, the maxillary process is also formed from mesenchyme provided by NCCs that joined with the mesoderm.

In future development, the maxillary processes will form the midface. This includes the sides of the upper lip, cheeks, secondary palate, and posterior part of the maxilla with its canines, certain posterior teeth, and associated tissue. This tissue also forms the zygomatic bones and parts of the temporal bones.

UPPER AND LOWER LIP FORMATION

During the start of the sixth week of prenatal development, the upper lip begins formation when each maxillary process fuses with each

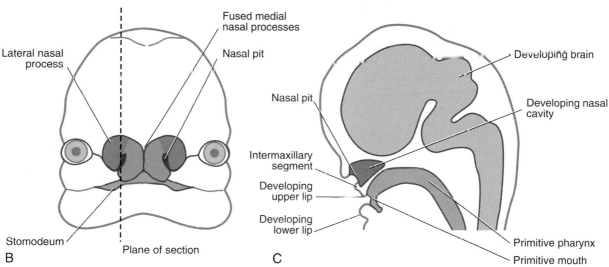

Lateral nasal process

Medial nasal process

Groove separating the maxillary process from the lateral nasal process

Maxillary process

Groove separating the maxillary process from the medial nasal process

Fused medial nasal processes

Nasal pit

Lateral nasal process

Nasal pit

Developing brain

Developing nasal cavity

Intermaxillary segment

Developing upper lip

Developing lower lip

Stomodeum

Plane of section

Primitive pharynx

Primitive mouth

B

C

FIGURE 4-7 Embryo at 6 weeks. **A,** Photograph of forming upper and lower lip. **B** and **C,** Sagittal sections of the head showing the development of the intermaxillary segment from the fusion of medial nasal processes on the inside of the stomodeum. (**A,** Courtesy of K.K. Sulik from Nanci A: *Ten Cate's oral histology,* ed 8, St Louis, 2013, Mosby.)

medial nasal process on both sides of the stomodeum, which are brought into proximity by proliferation of the NCCs-derived mesenchyme (see Figures 4-6 and 4-7, A). Thus, the maxillary processes contribute to the sides of the upper lip, and the two medial nasal processes contribute to the philtrum (see Figure 1-6).

This fusion of these processes to form the upper lip is similar to the fusion of the neural tube and palate because it takes place between two processes on *different* surfaces on each side of the face (see Figure 3-11). The maxillary and medial nasal processes grow toward one another, and fusion initially occurs at the ectodermal surfaces where the processes contact one another. The fused ectodermal tissue is temporarily trapped between the joining processes and later disappears so that the mesenchyme is continuous across the fused medial nasal and maxillary processes. Fusion of these processes to form the upper lip is completed during the end of the seventh week of prenatal development when the grooves between the processes are obliterated. The maxillary processes on each side of the developing face partially fuse with the mandibular arch on each side to create each labial commissure, with the mandibular arch already forming the lower lip.

Clinical Considerations for Upper Lip Development

Failure of fusion of the maxillary process with the medial nasal process can result in cleft (kleft) lip, with varying degrees of disfigurement and disability present in the upper lip (Figures 4-8 and 4-9). The ectodermal tissue trapped within the fusing processes may also fail to disappear. Thus the mesenchyme is prevented from growing together across the two processes. This disturbance may be hereditary or associated with environmental factors. It also may be isolated or associated with other developmental abnormalities, such as cleft palate (see Figure 5-6, *C-E*). Cleft lip occurs in about 1 in 1000 cases. The cleft results from a failure of the mesenchyme to grow beneath the ectoderm to obliterate any grooves between

Unilateral cleft lip   Bilateral cleft lip

FIGURE 4-8 Two main types of cleft lip deformities, unilateral and bilateral clefts.

FIGURE 4-9 Unilateral cleft lip that is located at the side of the midline of the oral cavity where the facial processes failed to fuse. (Courtesy of Margaret J. Fehrenbach, RDH, MS.)

these processes, or even a deficiency or absence of mesenchyme in the area.

These clefts of the lip can be located at one side or both sides of the upper lip; it may be unilateral or bilateral and may vary from a notch in the vermilion zone of the upper lip (incomplete cleft) to more severe cases (complete cleft) that extend into the floor of the naris and through the alveolar process of the maxilla.

Cleft lip is more common and more severe in men, and it is more commonly unilateral and on the left side. It can complicate nursing and feeding of the child as well as present challenges with speech development and facial appearance, and it may increase oronasal infection levels. It is treated by oral and plastic surgery, with dental intervention; however, speech and hearing therapy may also be needed.

CERVICAL DEVELOPMENT

The development of the neck parallels the development of the face over time, beginning during the fourth week of prenatal development within the embryonic period and completed during the fetal period (Figure 4-10, A). The neck and its associated tissue develop from the primitive pharynx and the branchial apparatus, which will be discussed in the next sections. Dental professionals must understand the development of the neck to relate its underlying structural relationships to any developmental disturbances that may be present.

PRIMITIVE PHARYNX FORMATION

The beginnings of the hollow tube of the embryo are derived from the anterior part of the foregut and will form the primitive pharynx (fare-inks), which is the future oral part of the pharynx, or oropharynx (see Figure 4-10, B, and see Figure 2-18). The foregut is originally derived from the endoderm embryonic cell layer (see Figure 3-14). The primitive pharynx widens cranially where it joins the primitive mouth or later, the stomodeum, and narrows caudally as it joins the esophagus. The endoderm of the pharynx lines the internal parts of the branchial arches and passes into balloon-like areas of the pharyngeal pouches (discussed later in this chapter). However, this same endoderm does not come to line the oral cavity proper or nasal cavity. Instead, the oral cavity proper and nasal cavity are both lined by ectoderm as a result of embryonic folding.

The caudal part of the primitive pharynx forms the esophagus, which leads to the stomach. A ventral outgrowth forms the laryngopharynx, larynx, and trachea and ends in the superior part of the developing lungs. The developing thyroid gland is also an anterior outpocket from the ventral wall of the pharynx (see Figure 11-14).

BRANCHIAL APPARATUS FORMATION

Discussed earlier, the branchial apparatus (brang-ke-al ap-pah-ra-tis) (or pharyngeal apparatus) consists of the branchial arches, branchial grooves and membranes, and pharyngeal pouches.

During the fourth week of prenatal development, stacked bilateral swellings of tissue appear inferior to the stomodeum and include the mandibular arch. These are the branchial arches (or pharyngeal arches), with the mandibular arch being the first branchial arch and the other more inferior arches numbered in craniocaudal sequence (Figure 4-11, and see Figure 4-10, A). These branchial arches consist of six pairs of U-shaped bars of which the central core consists of mesenchyme derived from mesoderm invaded by NCCs, now referred to as ectomesenchyme. This neural-derived mesenchyme condenses to form a bar of cartilage in each arch. Each branchial arch is also covered externally by ectoderm, except for the first arch because it forms anterior to the oropharyngeal membrane. In addition, each branchial arch is lined internally by endoderm and supports the lateral walls of the primitive pharynx.

The branchial arches are located bilaterally, oriented in an anterior-posterior direction on the embryo, bending to surround and support the lateral walls of the developing pharynx. It is important to note that the fifth branchial arch is often so rudimentary that often it is absent or it is included within the fourth branchial arch. The branchial arches will give rise to important structures of the face and neck (see Table 4-2).

Each paired branchial arch has its own developing cartilage, nerve, vascular, and muscular components within each mesenchymal core. The first two pairs of arches develop to the greatest extent of all the arches and are also the only ones specifically named. In general, these first two pairs of arches form the midface and lower face, respectively, and the lower four pairs of arches are involved in the formation of the structures of the neck.

The first branchial arch, which is also known as the mandibular arch, and its associated tissue were described earlier and include Meckel cartilage. Forming within the second branchial arch, which is also known as the hyoid (hi-oid) arch, is cartilage similar to that of the mandibular arch, Reichert (rike-ert) cartilage. Most of it disappears during development; however, parts of it are responsible for a middle ear bone, a process of the temporal bone, and parts of the hyoid bone.

Second branchial groove

Third branchial arch

Second branchial arch

Developing heart

Somites

Maxillary process

Mandibular process

Lens placode

Nasal placode

Stomodeum

A

Developing brain

Primitive pharynx

Foregut

Stomodeum

Developing heart

B

FIGURE 4-10 Embryo during the fourth week of prenatal development. **A,** Photograph. **B,** Diagram. Internally, the foregut gives rise to the primitive pharynx, which will form the oropharynx. (From Moore KL, et al: *The developing human: clinically oriented embryology,* ed 10, St Louis, 2015, Saunders.)

Additionally, the perichondrium surrounding Reichert cartilage gives rise to the ligament of the hyoid bone. The mesoderm of the hyoid arches helps form the muscles of facial expression, the middle ear muscles, and a suprahyoid muscle. Because these muscles are derived from the hyoid arches, these structures are all innervated by the nerve of the second arches, which is the facial nerve or

seventh cranial nerve. The hyoid arches, along with the third and fourth branchial arches, are also involved in formation of the tongue (see Figure 5-9).

During the seventh week, the muscle cells from the mesoderm of the hyoid arches have begun to differentiate. These muscle cells then begin to migrate over the mandibular muscle masses. By the tenth

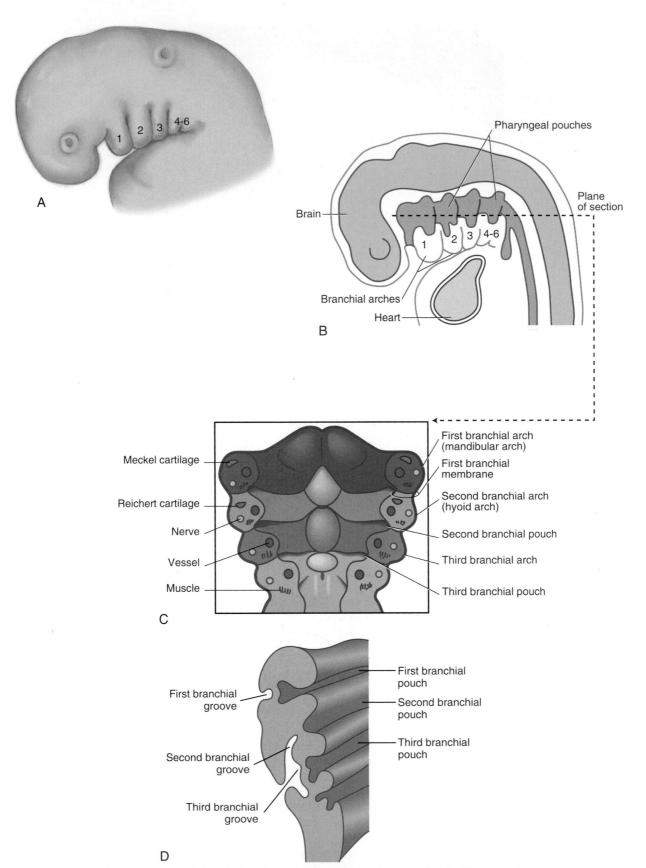

FIGURE 4-11 Embryo during the fourth week of prenatal development. **A** to **D,** Diagrams of two sections with the six branchial arches highlighted along with corresponding pouches and grooves.

TABLE 4-2	Branchial Arches and Derivative Structures	
ARCHES	FUTURE NERVES AND MUSCLES	FUTURE SKELETAL STRUCTURES AND LIGAMENTS
First arches (aka *mandibular arches*)	Trigeminal nerve, muscles of mastication, mylohyoid and anterior belly of digastric, tensor tympani, tensor veli palatini muscles	Malleus and incus of middle ear, including anterior ligament of the malleus, spheno-mandibular ligament, and parts of sphenoid bone (see also Table 4-1)
Second arches (aka *hyoid arches*)	Facial nerve, stape-dius muscle, muscles of facial expression, posterior belly of the digastric muscle, stylo-hyoid muscle	Stapes and parts of malleus and incus of middle ear, stylohyoid ligament, styloid process of the tempo-ral bone, lesser cornu of hyoid bone, upper part of body of hyoid bone
Third arches	Glossopharyngeal nerve, stylopharyngeal muscle	Greater cornu of hyoid bone, lower part of body of hyoid bone
Fourth through sixth arches	Superior laryngeal branch and recurrent laryngeal branch of vagus nerve, levator veli palatini muscles, pharyngeal constrictors, intrinsic muscles of the larynx	Laryngeal cartilages

TABLE 4-3	Pharyngeal Pouches and Derivative Structures
POUCHES	FUTURE STRUCTURES
First pouches	Tympanic membrane (with first branchial groove), tympanic cavity, mastoid antrum, auditory tube
Second pouches	Crypts and lymphatic nodules of the palatine tonsils
Third and fourth pouches	Parathyroid and thymus glands

pharyngeal pouches, gives rise to a definitive mature structure of the head and neck (discussed later in this chapter).

To accomplish this the first branchial groove becomes deeper to the extent that the ectoderm of the branchial groove contacts the endoderm of the pharyngeal pouches. At this time, only a thin, double-layered membrane, the first branchial membrane (or pharyngeal membrane), separates the groove from the pouches, although mesenchyme later separates these two layers. This membrane, with its three layers, develops into the tympanic membrane (eardrum). Thus, the first groove forms the external auditory meatus. Other branchial membranes appear in the bottom of each of the four branchial grooves, although, in contrast, they are only temporary structures.

By the end of the seventh week, the last four branchial grooves are obliterated as a result of a sudden spurt of growth experienced by the pair of hyoid arches, which grow in an inferior direction and eventually form the neck. This obliteration of grooves gives the mature neck a smooth surface contour.

At the same time, four well-defined pairs of **pharyngeal** (fah-rin-je-il) **pouches** develop as endodermal evaginations from the lateral walls lining the pharynx (see Figure 4-11). The pouches develop as balloon-like structures in a craniocaudal sequence between the branchial arches. The fifth pharyngeal pouches are absent or rudimentary. Many structures of the face and neck are developed from the pharyngeal pouches (Table 4-3).

The first pharyngeal pouches form between the first and second branchial arches and become the auditory tubes. The palatine tonsils are derived from the lining of the second pharyngeal pouches and also from the pharyngeal walls. The parathyroid glands and thymus gland are derived from the lining of the third and fourth pharyngeal pouches. Additionally, a part of the thymus gland is of ectodermal origin.

The growth and development of the thymus is not complete at birth. The thymus is a relatively large lymphatic organ during the perinatal period and then later starts to diminish in relative size during puberty. By adulthood, the thymus located at the superior part of the breastbone is often scarcely recognizable; however, it still is functioning by secreting thymic hormones and by maturing T-cell lymphocytes (see Figure 8-16).

Clinical Considerations for Branchial Apparatus Development

Most congenital malformations in the neck originate during transformation of the branchial apparatus into its mature derivatives. Some of these are a result of the persistence of parts of the branchial apparatus that usually disappear during development of the neck and its associated tissue.

week, the muscle cells have migrated superiorly all over the face, forming a thin sheet of muscle masses. Both superficial and deep groups of muscle fibers eventually develop from these muscle masses and become attached to the newly differentiating bones of the facial skeleton as the muscles of facial expression. The nerve from the facial nerve is incorporated early in these muscle masses.

The **third branchial arch** has an unnamed cartilage associated with it. This cartilage will be responsible for the formation of parts of the hyoid bone. The only muscle to be derived from the mesoderm of each third arch is a pharyngeal muscle. Each pair of arches is innervated by the glossopharyngeal nerve or ninth cranial nerve.

Both the **fourth branchial arch** and the **sixth branchial arch** also have unnamed cartilage associated with them. These arches fuse and participate in the formation of most of the laryngeal cartilages. The mesoderm of these arches is associated with the muscles of the larynx and pharynx. These structures are innervated by the ninth and tenth cranial nerves, although the nerves of these arches are branches of the vagus nerve or tenth cranial nerve.

Between neighboring branchial arches, external grooves are noted on each side of the embryo. These are the **branchial grooves** (or pharyngeal grooves or branchial clefts) (see Figure 4-11). Only the first branchial groove, which is located between the first and second branchial arches at approximately the same level as the first

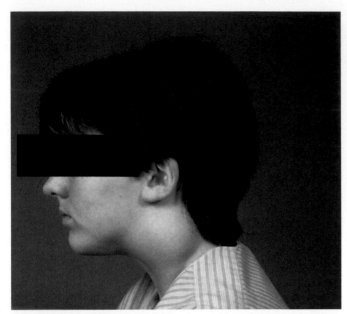

FIGURE 4-12 A branchial cleft cyst from the second arch, which is associated with a slowly enlarging, painless swelling on the lateral surface of the neck. These large cysts often lie free in the neck just inferior to the angle of the mandible, but they may develop anywhere along the anterior border of the sternocleidomastoid muscle as in this case. (From Moore KL, et al: *The developing human: clinically oriented embryology,* ed 10, St Louis, 2015, Saunders.)

The second branchial grooves occasionally do not become obliterated, and thus parts remain to form a branchial cleft cyst (Figure 4-12). These cysts may drain through sinuses along the neck but may also remain free in the lateral neck tissue just inferior to the angle of the mandible and anywhere along the anterior border of the sternocleidomastoid muscle. These cysts do not become apparent until they produce a slowly enlarging painless swelling that may be associated with small pits and skin tags that may involve fluid drainage from a sinus tract. The cyst is treated by surgical excision or, more recently, sclerotherapy.

CHAPTER 5

Orofacial Development

Additional resources and practice exercises are provided on the companion Evolve website for this book:
http://evolve.elsevier.com/Fehrenbach/illustrated.

●●● LEARNING OBJECTIVES

1. Define and pronounce the key terms in this chapter.
2. Outline the events that occur during palatal development, describing each step of its formation.
3. Integrate the study of palatal development into understanding the present structure and the clinical considerations due to developmental disturbances involved in palatal development.
4. Identify the structures present during palatal development on a diagram.
5. Outline the events that occur during nasal cavity and nasal septum development.
6. Integrate the study of nasal cavity and nasal septum development into understanding the present structure.
7. Identify the structures present during nasal cavity and nasal septum development on a diagram.
8. Outline the events that occur during the tongue development, describing each step of its formation.
9. Integrate the study of tongue development into understanding the present structure and the clinical considerations due to developmental disturbances involved in tongue development.
10. Identify the structures present during tongue development on a diagram.

OROFACIAL DEVELOPMENT

This chapter continues with embryonic orofacial development, starting from where the sequence left off with the development of the stomodeum, face, and neck in **Chapter 4** (see Figures 4-1 and 4-2 and also Box 4-1). Thus, this chapter discusses the development of the associated orofacial structures, including the palate, nasal septum, nasal cavity, and tongue, with tooth development being discussed in **Chapter 6**. The orofacial structures discussed in this chapter develop during the fourth week to the twelfth week of prenatal development, spanning the later part of the embryonic period and early part of the fetal period. However, the development of other orofacial structures (such as the jaws, temporomandibular joint, and salivary glands) is discussed with their associated histology in later chapters.

Dental professionals must have a clear understanding about the development of the oral structures to relate to their present structure as well as to any developmental disturbances that may be present.

PALATAL DEVELOPMENT

The formation of the palate, initially in the embryo and later in the fetus, takes place over several weeks of prenatal development (Table 5-1). The formation of the palate starts during the fifth week of prenatal development within the embryonic period from two separate embryonic structures: primary palate and secondary palate. The palate is then completed later during the twelfth week within the fetal period. The palate is developed in three consecutive stages: formation of the primary palate, formation of the secondary palate, and completion of the final palate.

The completion of the final palate involves the fusion of swellings or tissue from *different* surfaces of the embryo to meet and join, similar to that of the fusion of the neural tube and the components of the upper lip (see Figure 3-11). In contrast, most of the other structures of the orofacial region develop by the joining of swellings or tissue on the *same* surface of the embryo, which leads to the elimination of furrows between the facial processes (see Figure 4-4).

PRIMARY PALATE FORMATION

During the fifth week of prenatal development and still within the embryonic period, the intermaxillary segment forms (Figure 5-1, *A*). The intermaxillary segment arises as a result of fusion of the two medial nasal processes internally within the embryo (see Figure 4-7). The intermaxillary segment is an internal wedge-shaped mass that extends inferiorly and deep to the nasal pits on the inside of the stomodeum. It initially serves as a partial floor of the nasal cavity and the nasal septum.

The intermaxillary segment also gives rise to the **primary palate** (pal-it) (or primitive palate). At this time, the primary palate serves still as only a partial separation between the developing oral cavity proper and the nasal cavity (see Figure 5-1, *B*). In future development, the primary palate will form the premaxillary part of the maxilla, which is the anterior one-third of the hard palate. This smaller part of the hard palate is located anterior to the incisive foramen and will contain certain maxillary anterior teeth (incisors) (see Figure 2-12). The formation of the primary palate completes the first stage of palate development.

SECONDARY PALATE FORMATION

During the sixth week of prenatal development, within the embryonic period, the bilateral maxillary processes give rise to two **palatal** (pal-ah-tal) **shelves** (or lateral palatine processes) (Figures 5-2, 5-3, *A-B*, and 5-4). These shelves grow inferiorly and deep on the inside of the stomodeum in a vertical direction, along both sides of the developing tongue. The tongue is forming on the floor of the primitive pharynx at this time, and as it grows, it initially fills the common nasal and oral cavity (tongue development is discussed later in this chapter).

TABLE 5-1	Palatal Development
TIME PERIOD	**PALATAL STRUCTURES INVOLVED**
Fifth to sixth week	Primary palate: Intermaxillary segment from fused medial nasal processes
Sixth to twelfth week	Secondary palate: Fused palatal shelves from maxillary processes
Twelfth week	Final palate: Fusion of all three processes

As the developing tongue muscles begin to function, the tongue contracts and moves out of the way of these developing palatal shelves; thus, the tongue avoids being an obstacle to the future fusion of the palatal shelves by moving both anteriorly and inferiorly. This process is aided by the growth of the lower jaw primordium. The movement of the tongue makes it now confined solely to the oral cavity proper and out of the developing nasal cavity, which is completed around the eighth week of prenatal development.

Because of unknown shelf-elevating forces, the palatal shelves, after growing in a vertical direction, "flip" up in a superior direction within a few hours of the movement of the tongue. Thus, the shelves move into a horizontal position, which is now superior to the developing tongue. Next, the two palatal shelves elongate and move medially toward each other, meeting to join, and then fusing to form the **secondary palate**.

The secondary palate will give rise to the posterior two-thirds of the hard palate, which contains certain maxillary anterior teeth (canines) and posterior teeth, all located posterior to the incisive foramen (Figure 5-5). It The secondary palate also gives rise to the soft palate and its uvula. The median palatine raphe within the mucosa lining and the deeper median palatine suture on the adult maxillary bone indicate the line of fusion of the palatal shelves.

PALATE COMPLETION

The formation of the secondary palate is completed during the second stage of palate development. To complete the palate, the posterior part of the primary palate meets the secondary palate due to increased growth, and these structures gradually fuse in an anterior to posterior direction (see Figures 5-2, 5-3, *A-B*, and 5-4). When these three processes completely fuse, they form the final palate, including the hard and soft palate,

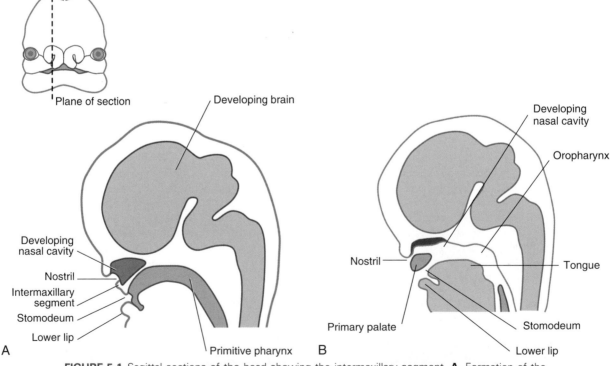

FIGURE 5-1 Sagittal sections of the head showing the intermaxillary segment. **A,** Formation of the intermaxillary segment from the fusion of the two medial nasal processes on the inside of the stomodeum of the embryo. **B,** Intermaxillary segment forms into the primary palate, which serves as a partial separation between the developing oral and nasal cavities.

during the twelfth week of prenatal development. Now, the mature oral cavity becomes completely separated from the nasal cavity, which has begun to undergo development of its nasal septum (discussed next).

Bone formation (or ossification) has already begun in the anterior hard palate by the time palatal fusion is completed (see **Chapter 8**). In contrast, in the more posterior soft palate, mesenchyme from the first and second branchial arches migrates into the area to form the palatal muscles that will be involved in swallowing and speech (discussed later in this chapter).

The small paired nasopalatine canals persist after development near the median plane of the mature palate at the site of the junction of the primary palate and the secondary palate (see Figure 5-5, *A-B*). These canals are represented in the mature hard palate by the incisive foramen beneath the incisive papilla, which is the common opening for the bilateral nasopalatine canals. An irregular suture extends from the incisive foramen to the alveolar process of the maxilla between the maxillary lateral incisor and canine teeth on each side. It demarcates where the primary and secondary palates fused. This bony fusion is completed within the first year of birth, with the overlying epithelium already fused by that time.

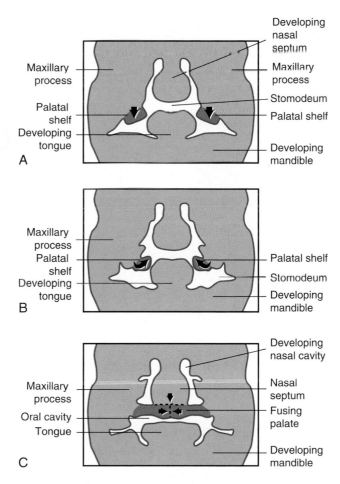

FIGURE 5-2 Developing palate is highlighted in a coronal section through the developing head. **A,** Palatal shelves formation from the maxillary process deep on the inside of the stomodeum. The growing shelves are vertical *(arrows)* and the position of the developing tongue is between the shelves. **B,** Palatal shelves grow in a horizontal direction toward each other, after "flipping" in a superior direction *(arrows),* to form the secondary palate. **C,** Fusion of the three processes *(arrows)* to complete the final palate in the fetus: Primary palate with two palatal shelves to form the secondary palate.

Failure of fusion of the palatal shelves with the primary palate and/or with each other results in **cleft (kleft) palate** with varying degrees of disability (Figure 5-6). This disturbance may be hereditary or associated with environmental factors. Cleft palate occurs 1 in 2500 cases. It may also be isolated or associated with other abnormalities, such as cleft lip (Figure 5-7); however, it may involve only the soft palate or may extend through to the hard palate. Isolated forms of cleft palate are less common than cleft lip and are more common in women, unlike cleft lip, which is more common in men. **Cleft uvula (u-vu-lah)** is the least complicated form of cleft palate (Figure 5-8).

Complications can include difficulty with nursing or feeding the child, increased oronasal infections, and challenges with speech development and appearance. Treatment includes oral and plastic surgery with dental intervention; however, speech and hearing therapy may also be necessary.

NASAL CAVITY AND SEPTUM DEVELOPMENT

The nasal cavity forms in the same time frame as the palate, from the fifth to twelfth week of prenatal development. It will later serve as part of the respiratory system (see Figure 11-19). The future nasal septum of the nasal cavity is also developing when the palate is forming. The structure of the nasal septum, similar to the primary palate, is a growth from the fused medial nasal processes (see Figures 5-2, 5-3, *A-B,* and 5-4). The tissue types that form the nasal septum will grow inferiorly and deep to the medial nasal processes and superior to the stomodeum.

The vertical nasal septum then fuses with the horizontally oriented final palate after it forms. This fusion begins in the ninth week and is completed by the twelfth week. With the formation of the nasal septum and final palate, the paired nasal cavity and the single oral cavity in the fetus become completely separate. The nasal cavity and the oral cavity also undergo development of different types of mucosa, such as respiratory mucosa and oral mucosa, respectively (see **Chapters 9 and 11**).

The developing nasal septum has considerable influence on determining the final orofacial form. It transmits septal growth "pull and thrust" to facial bones, such as the maxilla, as it expands its vertical length—a dramatic sevenfold amount between the tenth week of prenatal development and subsequent birth.

TONGUE DEVELOPMENT

The tongue develops during the fourth to eighth weeks of prenatal development (Table 5-2). It develops from independent swellings located internally on the floor of the primitive pharynx, formed by the first four branchial arches (see Table 4-2).

Specifically, the body of the tongue develops from the first branchial arch, and the base of the tongue originates later from the second, third, and fourth branchial arches. The furrows between these swellings are eliminated by fusion similar to that on the facial surface with proliferation, migration, and merging of the mesenchyme inferior to the ectoderm into the furrows (see Figure 4-4).

BODY OF TONGUE FORMATION

During the fourth week of prenatal development, within the embryonic period, the tongue begins its development. The tongue development begins as a triangular median swelling, the **tuberculum impar**

FIGURE 5-3 Photomicrographs of the coronal section through the developing head showing the palatal shelves during the formation of the secondary palate at the seventh week (**A**) and then the ninth week (**B** and **C**). Note that the position of the tongue, forming palate, and nasal septum (with its nasal cavity), which changes over time. The palatal shelves have moved into a horizontal position superior to the tongue, and now a final palate will be fully completed with fusion and the nasal and oral cavities will be separate. The teeth in the future dental arches *(arrows)*, mandibular bone, and Meckel cartilage are also developing during this same time period. (**A** and **B**, From Nanci A: *Ten Cate's oral histology*, ed 8, St Louis, 2013, Mosby; **C**, From personal collection of Major M. Ash, Jr.)

(too-**ber**-ku-lum **im**-par) (or median tongue bud) (Figure 5-9, *A-B*). The single tuberculum impar is located in the midline and is formed on the mandibular arch, which is considered the first branchial arch, at the floor of the primitive pharynx within the embryo's conjoined nasal and oral cavities (see Figure 4-11).

Later, two oval **lateral lingual** (ling-gwal) **swellings** (or distal tongue buds) develop on each side of the tuberculum impar (see Figure 5-9, *A-B*). It is important to note that these anterior swellings are from the further growth of mesenchyme of the mandibular arch.

The paired lateral lingual swellings grow in size and merge with each other.

Then the two fused swellings overgrow and encompass the disappearing tuberculum impar to form the anterior two-thirds of the mature tongue, the body of the tongue, which lies within the oral cavity proper. The median lingual sulcus is a superficial demarcation of the line of fusion of the two lateral lingual swellings, as well as of a deeper fibrous structure (see Figure 2-14). Thus, the tuberculum impar itself does not form any recognizable part of the mature tongue.

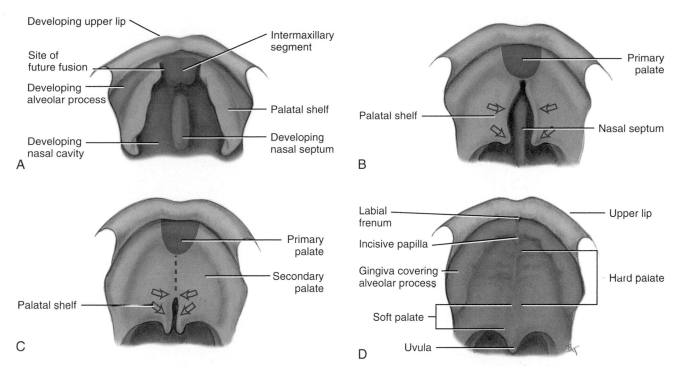

FIGURE 5-4 Development of the palate and nasal septum from an inferior view. Early stages of development of both the palate with its palatal shelves and the intermaxillary segment **(A)**, formation of primary palate **(B)**, nasal septum fusion with the final palate **(C)** in order to separate the nasal and oral cavities completely **(D)**. Note that growth of the palatal shelves is indicated by *arrows* in **B** and **C** with their fusion from anterior to posterior.

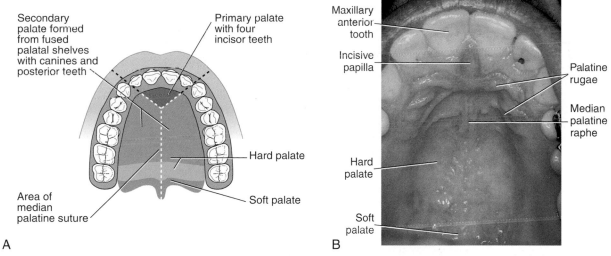

FIGURE 5-5 Adult palate with its derivative developmental structures, such as the permanent teeth. **A,** Diagram with suture areas highlighted *(dashed lines)*. **B,** Mature palate with associated embryologic landmarks. (Part B courtesy of Margaret J. Fehrenbach, RDH, MS.)

Around the lingual swellings, the cells degenerate forming a sulcus, which frees the body of the tongue from the floor of the mouth, except for the attachment of the midline lingual frenum (see Figure 2-17).

BASE OF TONGUE FORMATION

Immediately posterior to these fused anterior swellings, the **copula** (kop-u-lah) becomes evident (see Figure 5-9, *B*). The single midline copula is formed from the fusion of mesenchyme of mainly the third and parts of the fourth branchial arch. The copula gradually overgrows the hyoid arch, which is considered the second branchial arch. This overgrowth will form the posterior one-third of the mature tongue, the base of the tongue.

Even farther posterior to the copula is the projection of a third median swelling, the **epiglottic** (ep-ee-glot-ik) **swelling**, which develops from the mesenchyme of the posterior parts of the fourth branchial arches (see Figure 5-9, *B*). This swelling marks the development of the most posterior region of the tongue and site of the future epiglottis.

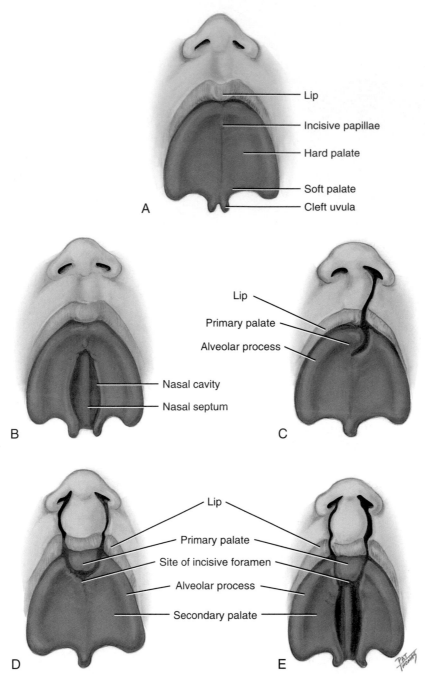

Lip

Incisive papillae

Hard palate

Soft palate

Cleft uvula

A

Lip

Primary palate

Alveolar process

Nasal cavity

Nasal septum

B

C

Lip

Primary palate

Site of incisive foramen

Alveolar process

Secondary palate

D

E

FIGURE 5-6 Various degrees of cleft palate. **A,** Cleft uvula. **B,** Bilateral cleft of the posterior palate. **C,** Complete unilateral cleft of the lip and alveolar process of the maxilla with a unilateral cleft of the primary palate. **D,** Complete bilateral cleft of the lip and alveolar process with bilateral cleft of the primary palate. **E,** Complete bilateral cleft of the lip and alveolar process with complete bilateral cleft of both the primary and secondary palates.

FIGURE 5-7 Complete bilateral cleft of the lip and alveolar process with complete bilateral cleft of both the primary and secondary palates. (Courtesy of Margaret J. Fehrenbach, RDH, MS.)

FIGURE 5-8 Cleft uvula, which is the least complicated form of cleft palate. (Courtesy of Margaret J. Fehrenbach, RDH, MS.)

TABLE 5-2	Tongue Development
TIME PERIOD	**TONGUE STRUCTURES INVOLVED**
Fourth to eighth weeks	Body: Tuberculum impar and lateral lingual swellings appear
	Base: Copula overgrowing second branchial arches
Eighth week	Completed tongue: Merging of anterior swellings of body and copula of base

COMPLETION OF TONGUE FORMATION

As the tongue develops still further, the copula of the tongue base, after overgrowing the second branchial arch, merges with the anterior swellings of the first branchial arch of the tongue body during the eighth week of prenatal development (see Figure 5-9, *C*). This fusion is superficially demarcated by the sulcus terminalis in the mature dorsal surface of the tongue, which is an inverted V-shaped groove marking the border between the base of the tongue and its body (see Figure 2-14).

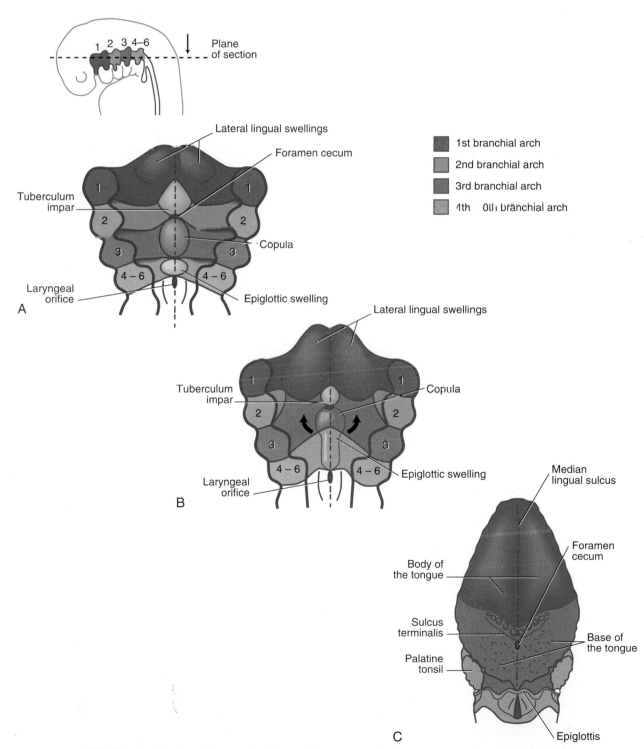

FIGURE 5-9 Diagram of the development of the tongue with derivations from the branchial arches highlighted. **A,** Tuberculum impar and lateral lingual swellings forming the body of the tongue. **B,** Copula and its involvement forming the base of the tongue *(arrows)*. **C,** Final fusion of the anterior swellings and the posterior swellings to complete the tongue.

The sulcus terminalis points backward toward the oropharynx at a small pit-like depression, the foramen cecum, which is the beginning of the thyroglossal duct. This duct shows the origin of the thyroid gland and the migration pathway of the thyroid gland into the neck region. It forms an open connection between the initial area of thyroid gland development and its final location. This duct later closes off and becomes obliterated before birth unless it undergoes cystic transformation (see Figure 11-14). However, no similar anatomic landmark is found between the base of the tongue and the epiglottic region after development.

By the end of the eighth week, the tongue has completed the fusion of these swellings. The tongue then contracts and moves anteriorly and inferiorly to avoid becoming an obstacle to the developing palatal shelves. However, the entire tongue is in the oral cavity proper at birth; its base and epiglottic region descend into the oropharynx by 4 years of age, while the body remains in the oral cavity proper. Thus, the tongue moves out of the pharynx into its proper place in the oral cavity proper. The tongue usually doubles in length, breadth, and thickness between birth and puberty, which is when it reaches its maximum size.

The intrinsic muscles of the tongue are believed to originate from the mesoderm of the occipital somites and not from the branchial arches (see Figure 3-13). Primitive muscle cells from these somites migrate into the developing tongue, taking their motor nerve supply from the hypoglossal nerve or twelfth cranial nerve. Reviewing the discussion in this part of the chapter explains how the single structure of the tongue is innervated by various cranial nerves (V, VII, IX, XII). This is because the tongue develops from the first four pairs of branchial arches, each with its own cranial nerve, and the occipital somites.

The lingual papillae, small elevated structures of specialized mucosa on the dorsal surface, appear toward the end of the eighth week (see Figures 2-14 and 9-16 to 9-20). The circumvallate and foliate lingual papillae appear first, close to the terminal branches of the glossopharyngeal nerve or ninth cranial nerve. The fungiform lingual papillae appear later, near the terminations of the chorda tympani branches of the facial nerve or seventh cranial nerve. Finally, the filiform lingual papillae develop during the early fetal period, which comprises the tenth to eleventh weeks.

Dorsal surface of the tongue

Mandibular teeth

Short attachment of the lingual frenum

FIGURE 5-10 Ankyloglossia resulting from a short attachment of the lingual frenum that extends to the tongue apex. (Courtesy of Margaret J. Fehrenbach, RDH, MS.)

The taste buds involved in taste sensation and that are associated with certain lingual papillae (circumvallate, foliate, and fungiform) develop during the eleventh to thirteenth weeks by inductive interaction between the epithelial cells of the tongue and invading nerve cells from the chorda tympani of the facial nerve or seventh cranial nerve as well as the glossopharyngeal nerve or ninth cranial nerve.

Clinical Considerations for Tongue Development

Abnormalities of the tongue are uncommon. However, one type that is more common than others is **ankyloglossia** (ang-ke-lo-**gloss**-ee-ah), sometimes described as "tongue-tied," which results from a short attachment of the lingual frenum that extends to the tongue apex (Figure 5-10). This restricts the movement of the tongue to varying degrees and may be associated with other craniofacial abnormalities. However, the tight lingual frenum usually stretches with time and use (see Figure 2-17). However, if it has not adjusted over time and movement is still not functional, orofacial myofunctional therapy (OMT) may be attempted before surgically cutting the lingual frenum is considered (see **Chapter 20**).

CHAPTER 6

Tooth Development and Eruption

Additional resources and practice exercises are provided on the companion Evolve website for this book:
http://evolve.elsevier.com/Fehrenbach/illustrated

●●● LEARNING OBJECTIVES

1. Define and pronounce the key terms in this chapter.
2. Outline the five stages of tooth development.
3. Integrate the study of tooth development into understanding the present tooth anatomy and the clinical considerations due to developmental disturbances.
4. Outline the process of root development.
5. Integrate the study of root development into understanding the present tooth anatomy and the clinical considerations due to developmental disturbances.
6. Discuss periodontal ligament and alveolar process development.

7. Identify the structures present during tooth crown and root development as well as the periodontal ligament and alveolar process development on a diagram.
8. Outline the events that occur during tooth eruption.
9. Integrate the study of tooth eruption into understanding the present tooth anatomy and the clinical considerations due to developmental disturbances.
10. Identify the structures present during tooth eruption on a diagram.

TOOTH DEVELOPMENT

Odontogenesis (oh-don-to-jen-eh-sis) is the process of tooth development. Dental professionals must have a clear understanding of the stages of odontogenesis, and the physiologic basis of each stage. Developmental disturbances can occur within each stage of odontogenesis, affecting the physiologic processes taking place. These developmental disturbances can have ramifications that may affect the dental care of a patient.

The term **dentition** (den-tish-in) is used to describe the natural teeth in the jaws (see **Chapter 15**). There are two dentitions: primary dentition and permanent dentition. The **primary dentition** of a child develops during the prenatal period and consists of 20 teeth, which erupt and are later shed (or exfoliated) (see **Chapter 18**). As the primary teeth are shed and the jaws grow and mature, the **permanent dentition**, consisting of as many as 32 teeth, gradually erupts and replaces the primary dentition (see **Chapters 16 and 17**). Overlapping between the primary and permanent dentition, a preteen has a mixed dentition, having some teeth from both dentitions (see Figures 15-4 and 18-17).

This chapter initially focuses on the development of the primary dentition, and then its eruption and shedding. The final discussion centers on the eruption of the permanent dentition. The process of development for both dentitions is similar; only the associated time frame for each is different. The overall general dental anatomy associated with both these dentitions as well as dentition periods is discussed further in **Chapter 15**.

Odontogenesis takes place in stages, which occur in a sequential fashion for both dentitions (Table 6-1). Odontogenesis is a continuous process until completed, and there is no clear-cut beginning or end point between stages. However, these stages are used to help focus on the different events in odontogenesis and are based mainly on the shape of the developing structures. After initiation of odontogenesis, the initial identifiable stages in tooth development include the bud stage, the cap stage, and the bell stage. Odontogenesis then progresses to the apposition stage with the formation of the partially mineralized dental tissue types, such as enamel, dentin, and cementum, and then finally to the maturation stage for these structures through continued mineralization (Table 6-2).

During these stages of odontogenesis, many physiologic processes occur. In many ways, these parallel the processes that occur in the formation of other embryonic structures, such as the face. These physiologic processes include induction, proliferation, differentiation, morphogenesis, and maturation (see Table 3-3). Except for the induction processes between cells, many of these processes overlap and are somewhat continuous during odontogenesis. However, one individual process does tend to be predominant, marking each stage of odontogenesis (see Table 6-1).

In the past, the study of odontogenesis included a discussion of *developmental lobes* that were thought to be growth centers during tooth development. These parts of the crown of the tooth are both microscopically and clinically visible by the presence of associated

TABLE 6-1	Tooth Development Stages		
STAGE AND TIME SPAN*	**MICROSCOPIC STRUCTURE**	**MAIN PROCESSES**	**HISTOLOGIC FEATURES**
Initiation stage at sixth to seventh week		Induction	Ectoderm lining stomodeum gives rise to oral epithelium and then to dental lamina; adjacent to deeper ectomesenchyme, which is derived from the neural crest cells. Both tissue types are separated by a basement membrane.
Bud stage at eighth week		Proliferation	Growth of dental lamina into bud shape that penetrates growing ectomesenchyme.
Cap stage at ninth to tenth week		Proliferation, differentiation, morphogenesis	Formation of tooth germ as enamel organ forms into cap shape that surrounds inside mass of dental papilla, with an outside mass of dental sac, both from the ectomesenchyme.
Bell stage at eleventh to twelfth week		Proliferation, differentiation, morphogenesis	Differentiation of enamel organ into bell shape with four cell types and dental papilla into two cell types.
Apposition stage at various times		Induction, proliferation	Dental tissue types secreted in successive layers as matrix.
Maturation stage at various times		Maturation	Dental tissue types fully mineralize to mature form.

*Note that these are approximate prenatal time spans for the development of the primary dentition.

depressions. Whether there may be any justification for including them in a discussion of tooth formation remains controversial; developmental lobes may simply be evidence of the tooth form only, but for completeness, information concerning developmental lobes is included in this textbook in **Unit IV**.

Not all the teeth in each dentition begin to develop at the same time across each arch of the jaws. The initial teeth for both dentitions develop in the mandibular anterior region, followed later by the maxillary anterior region, and then development progresses posteriorly in both jaws. This posterior progression of odontogenesis allows time for both the jaws to

TABLE 6-2	Dental Hard Tissue			
	ENAMEL	**DENTIN**	**CEMENTUM**	**ALVEOLAR PROCESS**
Embryologic background	Enamel organ	Dental papilla	Dental sac	Dental sac
Tissue source or type	Epithelium	Connective tissue	Connective tissue	Connective tissue
Formative cells	Ameloblasts	Odontoblasts	Cementoblasts	Osteoblasts
Incremental lines	Lines of Retzius	Imbrication lines of von Ebner	Arrest and reversal lines	Arrest and reversal lines
Mature cells	None, lost within reduced enamel epithelium with eruption	None within, only dentinal tubules with processes found instead in pulp	Cementocytes	Osteocytes
Resorptive cells	None per se; cells secrete proteinases	Odontoclasts	Odontoclasts or cementoclasts	Osteoclasts
Inorganic material levels (approximate)	96%	70%	65%	60%
Organic material and water levels (approximate)	1% organic, 3% water	20% organic, 10% water	23% organic, 12% water	25% organic, 15% water
Regeneration after eruption	None; only may undergo remineralization	Possible	Possible	Possible
Vascularity	None	None	None	Present
Innervation	None	Possibly present within dentinal tubule, found instead in pulp	None	Present

grow to accommodate the increased number of primary teeth, the larger primary molars, and then finally the overall larger permanent teeth.

The primary dentition develops during both the embryonic period and fetal period of prenatal development. Most of the permanent dentition is formed during the fetal period. Tooth development continues for years after birth, however, especially considering the formation of the permanent second and third molars (see **Unit IV** and **Appendix D** for tooth development timelines). Thus, teeth have the longest developmental period of any set of organs in the body.

INITIATION STAGE

Odontogenesis of the primary dentition begins between the sixth and seventh week of prenatal development, during the embryonic period (Figure 6-1). This first stage of tooth development, known as the initiation stage, involves the physiologic process of induction, which is an active interaction between the embryologic tissue types. Studies show that ectodermal tissue must influence the mesenchymal tissue in order to initiate odontogenesis, but the exact mechanisms are unknown at this time. Tooth initiation involves an initial signal from the ectoderm to the mesenchyme. The mesenchyme responds by reciprocally inducing the ectoderm to continue the developmental progression.

At the beginning of the sixth week, the stomodeum of the embryo (or primitive mouth) is lined by ectoderm (see **Chapter 4**). The outer part of the ectoderm gives rise to oral epithelium (ep-ee-thee-lee-um). The oral epithelium initially consists of two horseshoe-shaped bands of tissue at the surface of the stomodeum, one band for each future dental arch. At the same time, deep to the forming oral epithelium there is a type of mesenchyme known as ectomesenchyme (ek-toe-mes-eng-kime), which is derived from neural crest cells (NCCs) that have migrated to the region (see Figure 6-1).

Dental professionals need to consider the importance of NCCs. In addition to assisting in the formation of the cranial sensory ganglia, they also differentiate to form most of the connective tissue of the head.

FIGURE 6-1 Initiation stage of odontogenesis of the primary teeth on cross section within the developing mandibular arch. The stomodeum is now lined by oral epithelium, with the deeper ectomesenchyme derived from neural crest cells. A similar situation is occurring in the maxillary arch.

Embryonic connective tissue for most of the rest of the body is derived from mesoderm and is known as *mesenchyme,* whereas in the head it is known as *ectomesenchyme,* reflecting its origin from neuroectoderm (see **Chapters 3 and 4**). The proper migration of NCCs is essential for the development of the head and neck as well as the teeth. All the tissue of the mature tooth (except enamel and certain types of cementum) and its supporting periodontium are directly derived from NCCs, and any complication in their formation prevents proper dental development (see Figure 3-16 of Treacher Collins syndrome [TCS]).

An important acellular structure that separates the oral epithelium and the ectomesenchyme within the stomodeum is the basement membrane. The basement membrane involved here is similar to the one separating all epithelium and connective tissue (see Figure 8-4).

Developing tongue

Oral epithelium

Dental lamina

Ectomesenchyme of
developing mandible

FIGURE 6-2 Development of the dental lamina from the oral epithelium lining the mandibular arch where primary teeth will later form during the initiation stage, which is surrounded by ectomesenchyme. A similar situation is also occurring in the maxillary arch.

During the latter part of the seventh week, the oral epithelium grows deeper into the ectomesenchyme and is induced to produce a layer, the dental lamina (lam-i-nah) (Figure 6-2). This growth occurs in the developing jaws where the two future curved dental arches of the primary dentition will form. The dental lamina begins to form initially in the midline for both arches and progresses posteriorly. The underlying ecotomesenchyme also begins to undergo changes.

Clinical Considerations with Initiation
Stage Disturbances

Lack of initiation within the dental lamina results in the absence of a single tooth or multiple teeth (partial) or an entire dentition (complete), producing anodontia (an-ah-don-she-ah) (Box 6-1, *A-B*). However, partial anodontia is more common and most commonly occurs with the permanent third molar, maxillary lateral incisor, and mandibular second premolar (listed in order of occurrence). Anodontia can be associated with the syndrome of ectodermal dysplasia because many components of the tooth germ are indirectly or directly of ectodermal origin (see Figure 3-15.)

Anodontia (or hypodontia) can also result from endocrine dysfunction, systemic disease, and exposure to excess radiation, such as that in radiation therapy used with cancer treatment, and may cause disruption of occlusion and esthetic complications. Patients may need tooth replacement in the form of partial or full dentures, bridges, and/or implants. If severe, it can result in disruption of the complete development of the jaws.

In contrast, abnormal initiation may result in the development of one or more extra teeth, which are considered supernumerary (soo-per-nu-mer-air-ee) teeth (or hyperdontia) (see Box 6-1, *C-D*). These extra teeth are initiated from persisting clusters of the dental lamina and have a hereditary etiology. Certain regions of both dentitions commonly have supernumerary teeth, such as between the maxillary central incisors (mesiodens, see **Chapter 16**), distal to the maxillary third molars (distomolar or "fourth molar"), and in the premolar region (perimolar) of both dental arches (see **Chapter 17**) (listed in order of occurrence). They are smaller than usual, and most are accidentally discovered on radiographic examination. These extra teeth may be either erupted or nonerupted, and in both cases may cause dentition displacement, crowding, and delayed eruption to the adjacent teeth, as well as occlusal disruption; thus, removal by surgery is often necessary and/or orthodontic therapy.

BUD STAGE

The second stage of odontogenesis is considered the bud stage and occurs at the beginning of the eighth week of prenatal development for the primary dentition (Figures 6-3 and 6-4). This stage is named for an extensive proliferation of the dental lamina into buds, with these three-dimensional oval masses penetrating into the surrounding ectomesenchyme. At the end of the proliferation process involving the dental lamina of the primary dentition, both the future maxillary arch and the future mandibular arch will each have 10 buds. The underlying ectomesenchyme also undergoes adjacent proliferation. However, a basement membrane remains between the dental lamina bud and the surrounding growing and condensing ectomesenchyme.

Each of these buds from the dental lamina, together with the surrounding ectomesenchyme, will develop into a tooth germ with its associated supporting tissue during the next stage. Thus, all the teeth and their associated tissue types develop from both ectoderm and the mesenchymal tissue, ectomesenchyme, which is derived from NCCs. These two distinct tissue types interact at all stages of odontogenesis, supporting the concept of induction.

However, only proliferation of these two tissue types occurs during this stage; no structural change occurs in the cells of either the dental lamina or ectomesenchyme, as later occurs with differentiation and morphogenesis of these tissue types. In regions where teeth will not be developing, the dental lamina only remains thickened because it lines the stomodeum but does not produce buds. Later, this non–tooth-producing part of the dental lamina disintegrates as the developing oral mucosa comes to line the maturing oral cavity.

Clinical Considerations with Bud Stage Disturbances

Abnormal proliferation of the tooth bud can cause a single tooth or multiple teeth (partial) or an entire dentition (complete) to be larger or smaller than usual. Abnormally large teeth result in macrodontia (mak-roe-don-she-ah); abnormally small teeth result in microdontia (mi-kro-don-she-ah) (see Box 6-1, *E-F*). Individual teeth can sometimes appear larger than usual as a result of splitting of the enamel organ or fusion of two adjacent tooth germs; however, this is not a true case of partial macrodontia (discussed later in this chapter). In contrast, the dentition can appear smaller by being within a large set of jaws (considered relative). With true partial microdontia, hereditary factors are involved, and teeth commonly affected are the permanent maxillary lateral incisor (peg lateral; see **Chapter 16**) and permanent third molar (peg molar; see Figure 17-50). This can lead to esthetic and spacing complications that are treated with full restorative crowns on partial microdontic teeth (lateral incisor) and/or possibly extraction (third molar).

Complete microdontia of either dentition rarely occurs but can be associated with hypopituitarism or Down syndrome (see Figure 3-5). In contrast, systemic conditions such as childhood hyperpituitarism (gigantism) can produce complete macrodontia. However, some population groups have larger teeth overall than other groups; one of these is the Inuit people of arctic regions of North America.

CAP STAGE

The third stage of odontogenesis is considered the cap stage and occurs for the primary dentition between the ninth and tenth week of prenatal development, during the fetal period (Figures 6-5 and 6-6). The physiologic process of proliferation continues during this

BOX 6-1	**Common Dental Developmental Disturbances with Involved Developmental Stage**

Initiation Stage

Disturbance: Anodontia, partial or complete

Description: Absence of permanent or primary teeth that commonly include permanent third molar, maxillary lateral incisor **(A),** and second premolar **(B)** with partial anodontia

Etiologic factors: Hereditary, endocrine dysfunction, systemic disease, excess radiation exposure that prevent tooth germ(s) formation

Clinical ramifications: Disruption of occlusion and esthetic complications that are treated by prosthetic replacement with partial or full dentures, bridges, and/or implants

Absent permanent maxillary lateral incisor

Absent permanent mandibular second premolar

Disturbance: Supernumerary tooth or teeth

Description: Development of one or more extra teeth that are commonly found between the permanent maxillary central incisors (mesiodens—**C, D**), distal to third molars (distomolar), and premolar region (perimolar)

Etiologic factors: Hereditary with extra tooth germ(s) formation from persisting dental lamina cluster(s)

Clinical ramifications: Crowding, failure of eruption, and disruption of occlusion that are treated by surgical removal if needed and/or orthodontic therapy

Mesiodens between maxillary central incisors

Bud Stage

Disturbance: Microdontia or macrodontia, partial or complete

Description: Abnormally small or large teeth that commonly affects permanent maxillary lateral incisor **(E)** and third molar with partial microdontia **(F)**

Etiologic factors: Hereditary with partial; endocrine dysfunction with complete

Clinical ramifications: Esthetic and spacing complications that are treated with full restorative crown on microdontic tooth (lateral incisor) and/or possibly extraction (third molar)

Peg lateral

Peg molar

Continued

BOX 6-1 Common Dental Developmental Disturbances with Involved Developmental Stage—cont'd

Cap Stage
Disturbance: Dens in dente **(G, H)**
Description: Enamel organ invaginates into the dental papilla that commonly affects the permanent maxillary lateral incisor
Etiologic factors: Hereditary
Clinical ramifications: Deep lingual pit that may need endodontic therapy

Disturbance: Gemination **(I, J)**
Description: Tooth germ tries to divide and develops large single-rooted tooth with one pulp cavity and "twinning" commonly in crown of anteriors with correct number in the permanent or primary dentition
Etiologic factors: Hereditary
Clinical ramifications: Esthetic and spacing complications that can be treated by orthodontic therapy

Disturbance: Fusion **(K, L)**
Description: Union of two adjacent tooth germs that result in large tooth with two pulp cavities with one fewer tooth in dentition and is more common in anteriors in primary dentition *(arrow)*
Etiologic factors: Pressure
Clinical ramifications: Esthetic and spacing complications that can be treated by orthodontic therapy

Continued

BOX 6-1   Common Dental Developmental Disturbances with Involved Developmental Stage—cont'd

Disturbance: Tubercle **(M, N)**
Description: Small, rounded enamel extensions forming extra cusps that is commonly found on permanent posteriors occlusal surface or anteriors lingual surface
Etiologic factors: Trauma, pressure, or metabolic disease that affects enamel organ
Clinical ramifications: Occlusal complications

Apposition and Maturation Stage
Disturbance: Enamel dysplasia
Description: Faulty enamel development from interference involving ameloblasts that results in enamel pitting (enamel hypoplasia, **O**) and/or intrinsic color changes (enamel hypocalcification, **P**) with possible changes in enamel thickness
Etiologic factors: Local or systemic from traumatic birth, systemic infections, nutritional deficiencies, or dental fluorosis
Clinical ramifications: Esthetic and function complications

Enamel hypoplasia (with disclosing solution)

Enamel hypocalcification *(arrows)*

Disturbance: Concrescence **(Q)**
Description: Union of root structure of two or more teeth by cementum that commonly affects permanent maxillary molars
Etiologic factors: Traumatic injury or crowding of teeth
Clinical ramifications: Extraction or endodontic complications

Disturbance: Enamel pearl **(R, S)**
Description: Enamel sphere on root *(arrow)*
Etiologic factors: Displacement of ameloblasts to root surface
Clinical ramifications: Confused as calculus deposit on root and may prevent effective homecare

(Courtesy of Margaret J. Fehrenbach, RDH, MS.)

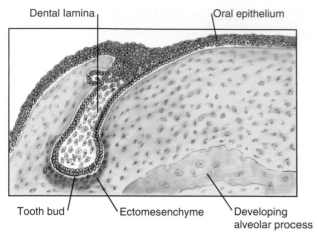

FIGURE 6-3 Bud stage, which involves extensive proliferation of the dental lamina into the ectomesenchyme in the form of buds—together creating the future tooth germs.

stage, but the tooth bud of the dental lamina does *not* grow into a large sphere surrounded by ectomesenchyme. Instead, there is unequal growth in different parts of the tooth bud, leading to formation of a three-dimensional cap shape overlying the ectomesenchyme that is still attached superiorly to the dental lamina.

Thus, not only does proliferation characterize this stage, but various levels of differentiation are also occurring, including the more specific processes of cytodifferentiation, histodifferentiation, and morphodifferentiation. Additionally during this stage, a primordium of the tooth (tooth germ) forms, containing each of the primordial types of tissue necessary to develop the future tooth. Therefore, the predominant physiologic process during the cap stage is one of morphogenesis.

From these combined physiologic processes, a depression results in the deepest part of each tooth bud of dental lamina, forming the cap shape of the enamel (ih-nam-l) organ(see Figures 6-5 and 6-6). It is important to note that the enamel organ was originally derived from ectoderm, making enamel an ectodermal product. In future development, the enamel organ will produce enamel on

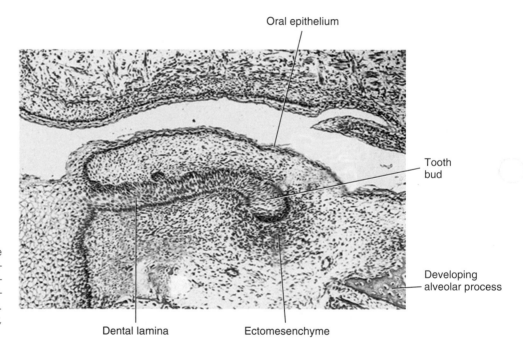

FIGURE 6-4 Photomicrograph of the bud stage, which involves extensive proliferation of the dental lamina into the ectomesenchyme in the form of buds—together creating the future tooth germs. (From Nanci A: *Ten Cate's oral histology,* ed 8, St Louis, 2013, Mosby.)

FIGURE 6-5 Cap stage, which involves proliferation and differentiation to form the tooth germ—the primordium of a primary tooth. The tooth germ at this time consists of the enamel organ, dental papilla, and dental sac. The primordium of the permanent succedaneous tooth from the growth of the successional dental lamina *(circle)* is located lingual to the primary tooth germ and is in the bud stage.

FIGURE 6-6 Photomicrograph of the cap stage with the formation of the enamel organ from the dental lamina, as well as the adjacent dental papilla and dental sac from the ectomesenchyme. The oral epithelium is lining the outer part of the stomodeum, and intramembranous bone development of the jaw is also occurring. (From Nanci A: *Ten Cate's oral histology,* ed 8, St Louis, 2013, Mosby.)

the outer surface of the crown of the tooth. The innermost margin of the cap shape of the enamel organ orchestrates the future crown form of the tooth, such as cusps; specifically, this may occur through nondividing cells in the **enamel knot** present in the region of the developing posterior teeth.

A part of the ectomesenchyme deep to the buds has now condensed into a mass within the concavity of the cap of the enamel organ. This inner mass of ectomesenchyme is now considered the **dental papilla** (pah-**pil**-ah)(see Figures 6-5 and 6-6). The dental papilla will produce the future dentin and pulp for the inner part of the tooth. Note that the dental papilla is originally derived from ectomesenchyme, which is derived from NCCs. Thus, dentin and pulp are of mesenchymal origin. However, a basement membrane still exists as before, but now it is between the enamel organ and the dental papilla, being the site of the future dentinoenamel junction.

The remaining ectomesenchyme surrounding the outside of the cap of the enamel organ condenses into the **dental sac** (or dental follicle). In future development, the capsule-like dental sac will produce the periodontium, the supporting tissue types of the tooth, including cementum, periodontal ligament, and alveolar process. It is important to note that the dental sac is originally derived from ectomesenchyme; thus, this supporting dental tissue is of mesenchymal origin. A similar basement membrane also separates the enamel organ and dental sac.

At the end of the cap stage, these three embryologic structures—the enamel organ, dental papilla, and dental sac—are now considered together to be the **tooth germ**, which is the primordium of the tooth (Table 6-3). These initial 10 tooth germs housed within each of the two developing dental arches develop into the primary dentition after each tissue type undergoes differentiation.

Already at the tenth week of prenatal development, during the cap stage for each primary tooth, initiation is occurring for the anterior teeth of the permanent dentition and then later for the premolars of the permanent dentition. Each primordium for these initially-formed permanent teeth appears as an extension of the dental lamina into the

TABLE 6-3	**Tooth Germ during Cap Stage**	
COMPONENT	**HISTOLOGIC FEATURES**	**FUTURE DENTAL TISSUE**
Enamel organ	Formation of tooth bud in a cap shape with deep central depression	Enamel
Dental papilla	Condensed mass of ectomesenchyme within the concavity of the enamel organ	Dentin and pulp
Dental sac	Condensed mass of ectomesenchyme surrounding outside of the enamel organ	Cementum, periodontal ligament, alveolar process

ectomesenchyme lingual to the developing primary tooth germs. Its site of origin is the **successional** (suk-**sesh**-shun-al) **dental lamina** (see Figure 6-26).

Permanent teeth formed with primary predecessors are considered to be **succedaneous** (suk-seh-**dane**-ee-us) and include the anterior teeth and premolars, which replace each primary anterior teeth and molars, respectively. The crown of each permanent succedaneous tooth will erupt lingual to the root(s) of its primary predecessor if the primary tooth has not been fully shed.

In contrast, the permanent molars are **nonsuccedaneous** (non-suk-seh-**dane**-ee-us) and have no primary predecessors. Instead, the six permanent molars per dental arch develop from a posterior extension of the dental lamina distal to the dental lamina of the primary second molar and its associated ectomesenchyme for each of the four quadrants of the oral cavity (see Figure 6-26).

FIGURE 6-7 Transitioning from the cap stage to the bell stage, the latter of which will exhibit differentiation of the tooth germ to its furthest extent. Both the enamel organ and dental papilla have begun to be differentiated into various layers in preparation for the appositional growth of enamel and dentin, respectively.

Clinical Considerations with Cap Stage Disturbances

During the cap stage, the enamel organ may abnormally invaginate by growth into the dental papilla, resulting in dens in dente (denz in den-tay) (or dens invaginatus) (see Box 6-1, *G-H*). The teeth most commonly affected are the permanent maxillary incisors, especially the lateral incisor, and may be associated with hereditary factors (see **Chapter 16**). The invagination produces an enamel-lined pocket extending from the lingual surface. This usually leaves the tooth with a deep lingual pit where the invagination occurs and may appear as a "tooth within a tooth" on radiographic examination. This lingual pit may lead to pulpal exposure and pathology and subsequent endodontic therapy; therefore, early detection is important.

Another disturbance that can occur during the cap stage is gemination (jem-i-nay-shin) (see Box 6-1, *I-J*). This disturbance occurs as the single tooth germ tries unsuccessfully to divide into two tooth germs, which then results in a large single-rooted tooth with a common enlarged pulp cavity. The tooth exhibits "twinning" in the crown, resulting in a broader, falsely macrodontic tooth, similar to fusion (discussed next). However, when this is verified by radiographic examination, it shows only one pulp cavity, with the correct number of teeth in either dentition with this disturbance. The appearance of splitting can be detected as a cleft with varying depths in the incisal surface, or it may manifest as two crowns. It usually occurs in the anteriors in either dentition, may be due to hereditary factors, and can create complications in esthetics and spacing that can be treated by orthodontic therapy in the permanent dentition.

Another disturbance that can occur during the cap stage is fusion (fu-zhin) (see Box 6-1, *K-L*). This results from the union of two adjacent tooth germs, possibly resulting from pressure in the region which leads to a broader, falsely macrodontic tooth similar to gemination. However, when it is verified by radiographic examination, it shows two distinct pulp cavities with the enamel, dentin, and pulp united. Fusion usually occurs only in the crown of the tooth, but it can involve both the crown and root, and each arch of the dentition with this disturbance has one less tooth. It occurs more commonly with the anteriors of the primary dentition and can present complications in esthetics and spacing that can be treated by orthodontic therapy.

Teeth may also have tubercles (tu-ber-kls) that appear as small rounded enamel extensions forming extra cusps (see Box 6-1, *M-N*; also **Chapters 16 and 17**). They are noted mainly on the occlusal surface of permanent molars, especially the third molars, and may also be present as a lingual extension on the cingulum on permanent maxillary anteriors, especially lateral incisors and canines, but can be found on any tooth in both dentitions. This disturbance may be due to trauma, pressure, or metabolic disease that affects the enamel organ as it forms the crown and may present occlusal complications.

BELL STAGE

The fourth stage of odontogenesis is considered the bell stage (Figures 6-7 and 6-8), which occurs for the primary dentition between the eleventh and twelfth week of prenatal development. It is characterized by continuation of the ongoing processes of proliferation, differentiation, and morphogenesis. However, differentiation on all level occurs to its furthest extent, and as a result, four different types of cells are now found within the enamel organ (Table 6-4). These cell types include the outer enamel epithelium, stellate reticulum, stratum

Oral
epithelium

Dental
lamina

Permanent
tooth bud

Differentiated
enamel organ

Alveolar
process

Differentiated
dental papilla

Primary
tooth

FIGURE 6-8 Photomicrograph of the bell stage of the primary tooth which exhibits differentiation of the tooth germ to its furthest extent. Both enamel organ and dental papilla have differentiated into various layers in preparation for the appositional growth of enamel and dentin, respectively. (From Nanci A: *Ten Cate's oral histology,* ed 8, St Louis, 2013, Mosby.)

TABLE 6-4	Bell Stage Structures (from Outer to Inner)	
CELL LAYERS	**HISTOLOGIC FEATURES**	**ROLE IN TOOTH FORMATION**
Dental sac	Increasing amount of collagen fibers forming around the enamel organ	Will differentiate into cementum, periodontal ligament, and alveolar process
Outer enamel epithelium	Outer cuboidal cells of enamel organ	Serves as protective barrier for enamel organ
Stellate reticulum	More outer star-shaped cells in many layers, forming a network within the enamel organ	Supports the production of enamel matrix
Stratum intermedium	More inner compressed layer of flat to cuboidal cells	Supports the production of enamel matrix
Inner enamel epithelium	Innermost tall, columnar cells of enamel organ	Will differentiate into ameloblasts that form enamel matrix
Outer cells of dental papilla	Outer layer of cells of the dental papilla nearest the inner enamel epithelium of the enamel organ. A basement membrane is between this outer layer and the inner enamel epithelium.	Will differentiate into odontoblasts that form dentin matrix
Central cells of dental papilla	Central cell mass of the dental papilla	Will differentiate into pulp tissue

intermedium, and inner enamel epithelium (from outer to inner). Thus, the cap shape of the enamel organ, evident during the last stage, now assumes a three-dimensional bell shape as the undersurface of the cap deepens. During this stage, the tooth crown assumes its final shape through morphodifferentiation, and the cells that will be making the hard tissue of the crown (ameloblasts and odontoblasts) undergo further histodifferentiation.

The outer cuboidal cells of the enamel organ are the outer enamel epithelium (OEE). The OEE serves as a protective barrier for the rest of the enamel organ during enamel production. The innermost tall columnar cells of the enamel organ are the inner enamel

epithelium (IEE). In future development, the IEE will differentiate by phases into enamel-secreting cells (ameloblasts). However, a basement membrane still remains between the IEE and the adjacent dental papilla.

Between the OEE and IEE are the two innermost layers, the stellate reticulum (stel-ate reh-tik-u-lum) and stratum intermedium (stra-tum in-ter-mede-ee-um). The stellate reticulum consists of star-shaped cells in many layers, forming a network. The stratum intermedium is made up of a compressed layer of flat to cuboidal cells. Both of these two intermediately-placed layers of the enamel organ help support the future production of enamel.

FIGURE 6-9 Close-up view of inner enamel epithelium of the enamel organ differentiating into the preameloblasts—the future cells that will form into ameloblasts and secrete enamel matrix. **A,** Inner enamel epithelium, with the central nuclei, line up along the basement membrane. **B,** Inner enamel epithelium that have elongated and repolarized the nuclei to become preameloblasts. The outer cells of the dental papilla are also lined up on the opposite side of the basement membrane.

At the same time, the dental papilla within the concavity of the enamel organ also undergoes extensive histodifferentiation so that it now consists of two types of tissue in layers: **outer cells of the dental papilla** and **central cells of the dental papilla** (see Table 6-4). In future development, the outer cells of the dental papilla will differentiate into dentin-secreting cells (odontoblasts), whereas the central cells of the dental papilla become the primordium of the pulp. The outermost placed dental sac increases only its amount of collagen fibers at this time and thus undergoes histodifferentiation into its mature dental tissue types of cementum, periodontal ligament, and alveolar process later than that of both the enamel organ and dental papilla.

APPOSITION AND MATURATION STAGES

The final stages of odontogenesis include the **apposition** (ap-oh-**zish**-in) **stage** (or secretory stage) during which the enamel, dentin, and cementum are secreted in successive layers. These hard dental tissue types are initially secreted as a **matrix** (**may**-triks), which is an extracellular substance or surrounding medium that in this case is partially mineralized. However the matrix serves as a framework for later full mineralization to the tissue type's expected level. This level of mineralization varies between enamel being the hardest, with dentin the next hardest, and finally to cementum, which has a similar hardness to bone tissue.

During the apposition stage, the process of induction continues to occur between the ectodermal tissue of the enamel organ and mesenchymal tissue of the dental papilla and dental sac; specifically, these are examples of the biologic concept known as *reciprocal induction.* Acting not only as a boundary between the two tissue types, the basement membrane conveys communications between the cells of the enamel organ, the dental papilla, and the dental sac, allowing for these important tissue interactions. Studies show that these interactions are necessary for the production of enamel, dentin, and cementum by the proliferation of cellular byproducts.

The final stage of odontogenesis, the **maturation stage**, is reached when the matrices of the hard dental tissue types subsequently fully mineralize to their correct levels. It is important to note that the period of time for these two final stages varies according to the tooth involved but overall involves the same chronology as the initiation of odontogenesis. The results of the maturation of each hard dental tissue are noted in Table 6-2; importantly, this table should be again consulted during the histologic study of each hard dental tissue in **Unit III**.

This part of the chapter mainly focuses first on the production of enamel and coronal dentin with the development of the crown of the tooth discussed (maturation of each tooth tissue and its histology are discussed in **Chapters 12 and 13**, respectively). This follows the same timeline as tooth development, given that development begins in the crown and then proceeds to the root, which is evident on most periapical or panoramic radiographs of a mixed dentition (see Figure 6-27, *A*). Root development with root dentin and cementum formation is discussed later in this chapter.

PREAMELOBLAST FORMATION

The events in the production of enamel and coronal dentin include the formation of preameloblasts, odontoblasts and dentin matrix, ameloblast and enamel matrix as well as the dentinoenamel junction from the basement membrane (see Table 6-4). The process is a complicated dance between these cells and their respective matrices.

After the formation of the IEE in the bell-shaped enamel organ, these innermost cells grow even more columnar as they elongate and differentiate into **preameloblasts** (pre-ah-**mel**-oh-blasts) (Figure 6-9), lining up alongside the basement membrane. During this differentiation process, the nucleus in each cell moves away from the center of the cell to the position farthest away from the basement membrane that separates the enamel organ from the dental papilla. This movement of the nuclei in each IEE cell occurs during cellular **repolarization** (re po-ler-i-**za**-shun), and studies show its importance in the change of the IEE cells into preameloblasts. In addition, the majority of the each cell's organelles become situated in the cell body distal to the nucleus.

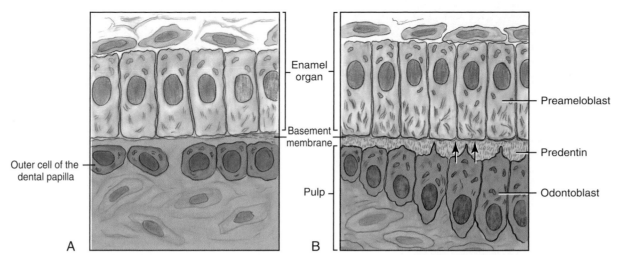

FIGURE 6-10 Close-up view of the outer cells of the dental papilla, which are induced to differentiate into the odontoblasts and form predentin upon the formation of preameloblasts from the inner enamel epithelium. **A,** Outer cells of the dental papilla line up along the basement membrane with repolarization of the nuclei to become odontoblasts. **B,** Odontoblasts start dentinogenesis—the appositional growth of predentin on their side of the basement membrane *(arrows)*.

In future development, the preameloblasts will induce dental papilla cells to differentiate into dentin-forming cells (odontoblasts), and then will themselves differentiate into cells that secrete enamel (ameloblasts). Thus, these initial changes to the cells occur within a presecretory stage with distinct phases where IEE is formed during the bell stage of tooth development (morphogenic phase) and then become preameloblasts (differentiation phase), which much later become ameloblasts (secretory stage, discussed later). These changes reflect the overall life cycle events of these complex cells involved in enamel production.

ODONTOBLAST AND DENTIN MATRIX FORMATION

After the IEE differentiates into preameloblasts, the outer cells of the dental papilla are induced to differentiate into odontoblasts (oh-**don**-toe-blasts) by the newly stepped up preameloblasts (Figures 6-10 and 6-11). During this time, these cells also undergo repolarization, which results in their nuclei moving from the center of the cell to a position in the cell farthest from the separating basement membrane. These repolarized cells also line up adjacent to the basement membrane in a mirror-image orientation on the opposite side from the already orderly preameloblasts.

After the differentiation and repolarization, the odontoblasts begin dentinogenesis (den-tin-oh-jen-i-sis), the appositional growth of dentin matrix, or predentin, laying it down on their side of the now disintegrating basement membrane. Thus, the odontoblasts start their synthetic and secretory activity for the most part some time before enamel matrix production begins. This timing difference in production explains why the dentin layer in any location in a developing tooth is slightly thicker than the corresponding layer of enamel matrix.

AMELOBLAST, ENAMEL MATRIX, AND DENTINOENAMEL JUNCTION FORMATION

After the differentiation of odontoblasts from the outer cells of the dental papilla and their formation of predentin, the basement membrane between the preameloblasts and the odontoblasts disintegrates.

FIGURE 6-11 Photomicrograph of the formation of predentin from the odontoblasts that then encloses the forming pulp from the central cells of the dental papilla. The enamel organ has its layers on the other side of the basement membrane that includes only the ameloblasts, stratum intermedium, and stellate reticulum in this view. (From Nanci A: *Ten Cate's oral histology,* ed 8, St Louis, 2013, Mosby.)

This disintegration of the basement membrane allows the preameloblasts to contact the newly formed predentin, which induces the preameloblasts to differentiate into ameloblasts (ah-**mel**-oh-blasts). The cellular changes in these cells show extensive Golgi complex surrounded by increased levels of rough endoplasmic reticulum, reflecting the intense synthetic and secretory activity going on.

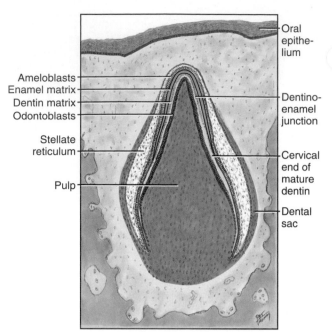

FIGURE 6-13 Apposition stage demonstrating both enamel and dentin matrix formation.

FIGURE 6-12 Preameloblasts being induced to differentiate into ameloblasts and beginning amelogenesis from Tomes process *(under large arrow)* with the appositional growth of enamel matrix on their side of the basement membrane. Later, this membrane will disintegrate and mineralize to form the dentinoenamel junction. The predentin is thicker than the enamel matrix because the odontoblasts differentiate and start matrix production for the most part earlier than the ameloblasts. The predentin also forms around the dentinal tubules that contain the odontoblastic process attached to the odontoblasts.

After differentiation, the ameloblasts begin **amelogenesis** (ah-mel-oh-**jen**-i-sis), the appositional growth of **enamel matrix**, laying it down on their side of the now disintegrating basement membrane (Figures 6-12, 6-13, 6-14, and 6-15). The enamel matrix is directly secreted from **Tomes** (tomes) **process**, an angled distal part of each ameloblast that faces the fully disintegrated basement membrane, formed from the group movement of the ameloblasts away from the basement membrane.

With the newly formed enamel matrix in contact with the predentin, mineralization of the disintegrated basement membrane now occurs, forming the **dentinoenamel** (**den**-tih-no-ih-nam-l) **junction** (**DEJ**), the inner junction between the dentin and enamel tissue. Continued appositional growth of both types of dental matrix becomes regular and rhythmic, as the cellular bodies of both the odontoblasts and ameloblasts initially retreat away from the DEJ, forming their perspective tissue types.

However, the odontoblasts (unlike the ameloblasts) will leave attached cellular extensions in the length of the predentin, the **odontoblastic** (oh-**don**-toe-blast-ik) **process**, as they move away from the DEJ. Each odontoblastic process is contained in a mineralized cylinder, the **dentinal tubule**. The maturation through mineralization of each type of matrix occurs later and is a different process for both enamel and dentin. However, the cell bodies of odontoblasts will remain within adjoining pulp attached by the odontoblastic processes. In contrast, the cell bodies of the ameloblasts (now in the maturation stage) will be involved first in the final phases of the mineralization process and active tooth eruption but will later be lost after tooth eruption (see later discussion).

FIGURE 6-14 Photomicrograph during the apposition stage demonstrating enamel and dentin matrix formation. (From Nanci A: *Ten Cate's oral histology*, ed 8, St Louis, 2013, Mosby.)

Clinical Considerations with Apposition Stage and Maturation Stage Disturbances

Certain factors may interfere with the metabolic processes of the ameloblasts, resulting in **enamel dysplasia** (dis-**play**-ze-ah), which is the faulty development of enamel (see Box 6-1, *O-P*). Many different types are possible and have either a local or a systemic etiology. Local enamel dysplasia may result from trauma or infection occurring to a small group of ameloblasts. Systemic enamel dysplasia involves larger numbers of ameloblasts and may result from traumatic birth, systemic infections, nutritional deficiencies, or dental fluorosis (from an excess systemic fluoride level).

Any tooth in which amelogenesis is active during the metabolic interference may be affected and changes in either local regions or the

Dentin   Ameloblasts   Enamel   Odontoblasts

Ameloblasts —

— Odontoblasts

Enamel —

— Dentin

B

FIGURE 6-15 Photomicrographs of enamel formation from ameloblasts and dentin formation from odontoblasts **(A** and **B)**. The stratum intermedium and stellate reticulum both cover the ameloblasts. **(A,** From Nanci A: *Ten Cate's oral histology,* ed 8, St Louis, 2013, Mosby. **B,** From the Dr Bernhard Gottlieb Collection, courtesy of James McIntosh, PhD, Assistant Professor Emeritus, Department of Biomedical Sciences, Baylor College of Dentistry, Dallas, TX.)

FIGURE 6-16 Amelogenesis imperfecta in the permanent dentition. A hereditary type of enamel dysplasia where the teeth have either no enamel or very thin enamel that chips off, leaving the yellow crowns of dentin, which undergo extreme attrition. **A,** Clinical view. **B,** Radiograph. (Courtesy of Margaret J. Fehrenbach, RDH, MS.)

entire tooth, or even an entire dentition, may occur. A type of enamel dysplasia, enamel hypoplasia, results from a reduction in the *quantity* of enamel matrix. As a result, the teeth appear with pitting and grooves in the enamel surface.

Enamel hypoplasia can be noted in the presence of Hutchinson incisors and mulberry molars, which is caused by the teratogen of syphilis (see Figure 3-17 and **Chapters 16 and 17**). From the labial iew, Hutchinson incisors have a crown with a screwdriver shape that .s wide cervically and narrow incisally with a notched incisal edge. Mulberry molars have enamel tubercles or extra extensions from the cusps on the occlusal surface.

Enamel dysplasia may also involve enamel hypocalcification. This disturbance results in reduction in the *quality* of the enamel maturation. The teeth appear more opaque, yellower, or even browner because of an intrinsic staining of enamel. A single affected area or white "sparkle spot" is called a *Turner spot,* and if the entire permanent crown is affected, it is called a *Turner tooth.* Enamel hypoplasia and hypocalcification may occur together and affect entire dentitions, which is a common finding in dental fluorosis (see Figure 12-5).

A certain type of enamel dysplasia, amelogenesis imperfecta (im-per-**fek**-tah), has a hereditary etiology and can affect all teeth of both dentitions (Figure 6-16). With this disturbance, the teeth have very thin enamel that chips off or have no enamel at all. Thus, the crowns are yellow because they are composed of mainly softer dentin and undergo extreme attrition, the mechanical loss of tooth material resulting from mastication; full-coverage crowns are needed for esthetic appearance, as well as to prevent further attrition.

In addition, dentin dysplasia, which is the faulty development of dentin, can result from an interference with the metabolic processes of the odontoblasts during dentinogenesis. This condition is much more rare than enamel dysplasia but can also be due to local or systemic factors (similar to enamel dysplasia) and can involve either dentin hypoplasia or hypocalcification, or both disturbances at the same time.

One type of dentin dysplasia is dentinogenesis imperfecta, which has a hereditary basis (Figure 6-17). This disturbance results in blue-gray or brown teeth with an opalescent sheen. The enamel appears as usual but chips off because of a lack of support by the abnormal underlying dentin, leaving crowns of dentin; the dentin has an irregular maturation quality (having increased amounts of interglobular dentin) (see Figure 13-4). The result is severe attrition because the dentin is less mineralized overall; full-coverage crowns are needed for esthetic appearance, as well as to prevent further attrition. Several types of the condition are recognized; most are Type II, whereas Type I is associated with osteogenesis imperfecta.

ROOT DEVELOPMENT

The process of root development takes place long after the crown is completely shaped and the tooth is starting to erupt into the oral cavity (see Figure 6-22 noting the root development over time). Most find it unbelievable that the tooth is formed starting with the crown and then moving to the apex of the root (unlike rooted plant life), unless they have studied dentistry or looked closely at their dental office radiographs (see Figure 6-27, *A*). The structure responsible for root development is the cervical (ser-vi-kal) loop (Figure 6-18, *A*). The cervical loop is the most cervical part of the enamel organ, a bilayer rim that consists of only IEE and OEE.

To form the root region, the cervical loop begins to grow deeper into the surrounding ectomesenchyme of the dental sac, elongating and moving away from the newly completed crown to enclose more of the dental papilla, forming the Hertwig (hirt-wig) epithelial (ep-ee-thee-lee-al) root sheath (HERS) (see Figure 6-18, *B-C*). The function of this membrane is to shape the root(s) by inducing dentin formation in the root so that it is continuous with coronal dentin. Thus, HERS will determine if the root will be curved or straight, short

FIGURE 6-17 Dentinogenesis imperfecta in the permanent dentition. A hereditary type of dentin dysplasia that results in blue-gray teeth with an opalescent sheen, chipped enamel, and crowns of dentin with severe attrition. (Courtesy of Margaret J. Fehrenbach, RDH, MS.)

or long, as well as single or multiple. This chapter first discusses root development in a single-rooted tooth and then later in a multirooted tooth.

ROOT DENTIN FORMATION

Root dentin forms when the outer cells of the dental papilla in the root area undergo induction and then differentiation and become odontoblasts (Figure 6-19). This induction occurs similarly to the process that happens in the crown area to produce coronal dentin, under the influence of the IEE of HERS. Lacking the intermediate layers of the stellate reticulum and stratum intermedium, HERS induces odontoblastic differentiation but fails to have IEE differentiate into enamel-forming ameloblasts. This accounts for the usual absence of enamel in the roots.

After the differentiation of odontoblasts in the root area, these cells undergo dentinogenesis and begin to secrete predentin. As in the crown area, a basement membrane is located between the IEE of the sheath and the odontoblasts in the root area.

When root dentin formation is completed, this part of the basement membrane also disintegrates, as does the entire HERS. After this disintegration of the root sheath, its cells may become the epithelial rests of Malassez (mal-ah-say) (ERM). These groups of cells of epithelium are then located in the mature periodontal ligament but can become cystic, presenting future periodontal infections; in addition, these cells are also demonstrating an involvement in periodontal ligament repair and regeneration (see Figure 14-26).

CEMENTUM AND PULP FORMATION

The process of cementogenesis (see-men-toe-jen-i-sis) from appositional growth of cementum in the root area also occurs when the HERS disintegrates (Figure 6-20). This disintegration of the sheath allows the undifferentiated cells of the dental sac to contact the newly formed surface of root dentin. This contact of the dental sac cells with the dentin surface induces these cells to become immature cementoblasts (see-men-tah-blasts).

The cementoblasts move to cover the root dentin and undergo cementogenesis, laying down cementum matrix, or cementoid (see-men-toyd). Unlike ameloblasts and odontoblasts, which leave no cellular bodies in their secreted products, many cementoblasts become entrapped by the cementum they produce and become mature cementocytes (see-men-toe-sites) in the later stages of appositional growth. As the cementoid surrounding the cementocytes becomes mineralized, or matured, it is then considered cementum (see Figure 14-2).

As a result of the appositional growth of cementum over the dentin, the dentinocemental (den-tih-no-see-men-tal) junction (DCJ) is formed where the disintegrating basement membrane between the two tissue types was located. Also at this time, the central cells of the dental papilla are forming into the pulp, which later becomes surrounded by the newly formed dentin (see Figure 13-9).

Clinical Considerations with Cementum Formation Disturbances

Excess cementum formation can occur rarely with concrescence (kahn-kres-ens) (see Box 6-1, *Q*). This is the union of the root structure of two or more teeth through the cementum only, mainly occurring with permanent maxillary molars (see **Chapter 17**). The teeth involved are originally separate but join because of the excessive cementum deposition on one or more teeth after eruption.

Traumatic injury or crowding of the teeth during the apposition and maturation stage of tooth development may be the cause. This may present complications during extraction and endodontic therapy, and thus preoperative radiographs are important in the detection of this disturbance.

MULTIROOTED TOOTH DEVELOPMENT

Like anterior teeth, multirooted premolars and molars originate as a single root on the base of the crown. This part of posterior teeth is considered the root trunk. The cervical cross section of the root trunk initially follows the form of the crown. However, the root of a

FIGURE 6-18 Root development. **A,** Cervical loop of a primary tooth, which is composed of the most cervical part of the enamel organ, with only the inner and outer enamel epithelium. **B,** Hertwig epithelial root sheath is formed from elongation of the cervical loop *(circle)*, which is responsible for the shape of the root (or roots) and the induction of root dentin. **C,** Microscopic section of the root sheath *(circle)*. Odontoblasts *(O)* are within the pulp *(P)* after forming dentin *(D)*. (From the Dr. Bernhard Gottlieb Collection, courtesy of James McIntosh, PhD, Assistant Professor Emeritus, Department of Biomedical Sciences, Baylor College of Dentistry, Dallas, TX.)

FIGURE 6-19 Appositional growth of dentin in the root area resulting from the induction of the outer cells of the dental papilla to differentiate into odontoblasts. Hertwig epithelial root sheath is disintegrating to produce the epithelial rests of Malassez.

FIGURE 6-20 Appositional growth of cementum in the root area after Hertwig epithelial root sheath disintegration and the induction of dental sac cells to differentiate into cementoblasts. The cementoblasts produce cementoid, entrapping the cells to become cementocytes. Nearby both the alveolar process and periodontal ligament are also beginning to develop further.

posterior tooth divides from the root trunk into the correct number of root branches for its tooth type (see Figure 17-7).

To produce multiple roots, there is differential growth of HERS that causes the root trunk of each multirooted tooth to divide into two or three roots (Figure 6-21). During the formation of the enamel organ on a multirooted tooth, elongation of its cervical loop occurs, which allows the development of long, tongue-like horizontal extensions or flaps within it. Two or three such extensions can be present on multirooted teeth, depending on the similar number of roots of the mature tooth.

The usually single cervical opening of the coronal enamel organ is then divided into two or three openings by openings horizontal extensions. On the pulpal surfaces of these openings, dentin formation starts after the induction of the odontoblasts and disintegration of HERS and the associated basement membrane. Cementoblasts are induced to form cementum on the newly formed dentin only at the periphery of each opening. Root development then proceeds in the same way as described for a single-rooted tooth.

Clinical Considerations with Root Formation Disturbances

In some cases, misplaced ameloblasts can migrate to the surface of root, causing enamel to be abnormally formed over the cemental root surface, which produces an **enamel pearl** (see Box 6-1, *R-S*). It appears as a small, spherical, enamel projection on the root surface, especially at the cementoenamel junction (CEJ), or in the furcations on molars where the roots divide. It may have a tiny dentin and pulp core and appear radiopaque (light) on radiographs. An enamel pearl may be confused with a calculus deposit upon exploration of the root surface but cannot be removed by scaling alone and may interfere with homecare. In many cases, the enamel pearl needs to be removed by a dental bur.

Another disturbance that can occur during root development is **dilaceration** (die-**lass**-er-ay-shun), resulting in either distorted root(s) or severe associated crown angulation in a formed tooth (see **Chapter 16** and Figure 17-36). Dilaceration is caused by a distortion of HERS due to an injury or pressure; it can occur in any tooth or group of teeth during tooth development. It can cause complications during extraction and endodontic therapy and underlines the importance of preoperative radiographic examination; sometimes the bend is pronounced enough to prevent eruption. This is in contrast to the disturbance of *flexion*, which is a deviation or

bend restricted just to the root; usually the bend is less than 90° to the crown.

Teeth may also have **accessory roots** (or supernumerary roots). These extra roots may be due to trauma, pressure, or metabolic disease that affects HERS. Any tooth may be affected, but it occurs mainly with the permanent third molars and is rare in incisors. These accessory roots can present complications in extraction and endodontic therapy; thus, preoperative radiographic examination is again necessary to rule out this disturbance.

PERIODONTAL LIGAMENT AND ALVEOLAR PROCESS DEVELOPMENT

As the crown and root develop, the surrounding supporting tissue types of the tooth also develop from the dental sac (see Figure 6-20). The ectomesenchyme from the dental sac begins to form the periodontal ligament (PDL) adjacent to the newly formed cementum. This process involves forming collagen fibers that are immediately organized into the fiber bundles of the PDL (see Figure 14-27). The ends of these fibers insert into the outer layers of the cementum and the surrounding alveolar process to support the tooth and are considered Sharpey fibers. The ectomesenchyme of the dental sac also begins to mineralize to form the tooth sockets, which are now considered the alveoli of each alveolar process surrounding the PDL (see Figure 14-14).

PRIMARY TOOTH ERUPTION AND SHEDDING

Eruption of the primary dentition takes place in chronologic order, as does the permanent dentition (Figure 6-22). This process involves **active eruption**, which is the actual vertical movement of the tooth. This is not the same as **passive eruption**, which occurs with aging, when the gingival tissue recedes but no actual tooth movement takes place. Passive eruption is usually completed by age 24 ± 6½ years, and only 12% of patients exhibited any amount of delayed passive eruption. In a fully erupted tooth, the gingival margin becomes located on the enamel

FIGURE 6-21 Apical view of multirooted tooth development from horizontal extensions *(arrows)* of the cervical loop for **(A)** a two-rooted tooth and **(B)** a three-rooted tooth. The detailed cross-section that shows the division that produces three roots **(C)** on a permanent maxillary molar.

0.5 to 2.0 mm coronal to the CEJ. The timelines for active eruption and root completion using approximate ages are useful for the clinician (for primary dentition with shedding, see Table 18-1 and Figure 20-5 for sequence; for permanent dentition, see Table 15-2, **Appendix D**, and Figure 20-6 for sequence).

How active eruption occurs is understood but *why* can only be theorized. No one can certify what forces "push" teeth through the oral soft tissue or can identify the timing mechanism that coincides with these eruptions; each theory for eruption presents a challenge in its conception. The processes of root growth, existence of a temporary ligament, vascular pressure, contractile collagen, and hormonal signals to genetic targets all have been used to explain eruption.

Active eruption of a primary tooth has many stages in the movement of the tooth. After enamel appositional growth ceases in the crown of each primary or permanent tooth, the ameloblasts place an acellular dental cuticle on the newly formed outer enamel surface. In addition, the layers of the enamel organ become compressed, forming the reduced enamel epithelium (REE) (Figures 6-23 and 6-24). The REE appears as a few layers of flattened cells overlying the enamel surface. When this formation of the REE occurs for a primary tooth, it can then begin to erupt into the oral cavity.

The external cells of the REE are mostly from the stratum intermedium cells but possibly also include cellular remnants of the stellate reticulum and OEE; thus, these undifferentiated epithelial cells will divide and multiply and eventually give rise to the junctional epithelium.

To allow for the eruption process, the REE first has to fuse with the oral epithelium lining the oral cavity (Figure 6-25). Second, enzymes from the REE then disintegrate the central part of the fused tissue, leaving a protective epithelial-lined eruption tunnel for the tooth to erupt through the surrounding oral epithelium into the oral cavity. This tissue disintegration causes the usually present inflammatory response known as "teething," which may be accompanied by tenderness and edema of the local tissue. Instituting proper homecare can reduce the amount of inflammation and, thus, most of the discomfort associated with these oral changes in infants as

their first teeth erupt, as well as in young adults when their third molars erupt.

As a primary tooth actively erupts, the coronal part of the fused epithelial tissue peels off the crown, leaving the cervical part still attached to the neck of the tooth like a banana being peeled. This fused tissue that remains near the CEJ after the tooth erupts then serves as the initial junctional epithelium of the tooth, creating a seal between the tissue and the tooth surface. This tissue is later replaced by a definitive junctional epithelium as the root becomes completely formed (see Figure 10-1).

The primary tooth is then shed as the succedaneous permanent tooth develops lingual to it. The process involving shedding of the primary tooth consists of differentiation of multinucleated osteoclasts from fused macrophages of the surrounding area, which absorb the alveolar process between the two teeth from their *ruffled borders* (see Figure 8-15). The fibrocellular follicle surrounding a succedaneous permanent tooth retains its connection with the lamina propria of the oral mucosa by means of a strand of fibrous tissue containing remnants of the dental lamina, known as the *gubernacular canal*. As a succedaneous permanent tooth erupts, its gubernacular canal is widened rapidly by local osteoclastic activity, delineating the eruptive pathway for the tooth.

In addition, **odontoclasts** (oh-**don**-toe-klasts) are formed from undifferentiated mesenchyme. These cells cause mainly primary tooth root resorption with the removal of dentin and cementum. Special fibroblasts, now considered fibroclasts, destroy any remaining connecting collagen fibers holding the primary tooth within its surrounding PDL.

The PDL develops only after root formation has been initiated; when established, the PDL must be remodeled to accommodate continued eruptive tooth movement. The remodeling of PDL fiber bundles is achieved by the fibroblasts and fibroclasts, which simultaneously create and breakdown the collagen fibrils as required across the entire extent of the ligament.

The process of shedding the primary tooth is intermittent ("on again/off again"), because at the same time that osteoclasts differentiate to resorb bone and odontoclasts differentiate to resorb dental tissue, the always-ready odontoblasts and cementoblasts work to replace the resorbed parts of the root as well as the fibroblasts to repair the PDL. Thus, a loose primary tooth may become tightened just when the supervising adult takes a child to the dental office to have it checked (perhaps because the child playing with it is driving the supervising adults crazy). When the primary tooth is finally shed, the mythological tooth fairy (and helpers) goes into action with rates of return now approaching very high levels.

PERMANENT TOOTH ERUPTION

The succedaneous permanent tooth usually erupts into the oral cavity in a position lingual to the roots of the shedding primary tooth, just as it develops that way (Figures 6-26, 6-27, and 6-28). The only exception to this is the permanent maxillary incisors, which move to a more facially placed position as they erupt into the oral cavity.

FIGURE 6-22 Chronologic order of the eruption of **(A)** the primary *(blue)* dentition and **(B)** the permanent *(white)* dentition (continued on next page). (Adapted with permission from Schour I, Massler M: The development of the human dentition, *J Am Dent Assoc* 28:1153-1160, 1941.)

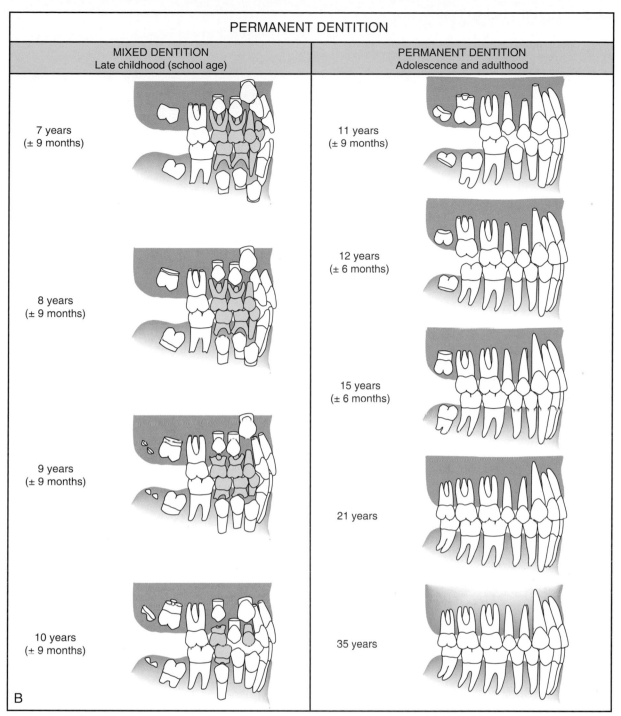

PERMANENT DENTITION	
MIXED DENTITION Late childhood (school age)	PERMANENT DENTITION Adolescence and adulthood
7 years (± 9 months)	11 years (± 9 months)
8 years (± 9 months)	12 years (± 6 months)
9 years (± 9 months)	15 years (± 6 months)
10 years (± 9 months)	21 years
	35 years

B

FIGURE 6-22, cont'd Chronologic order of the eruption of **(A)** the primary *(blue)* dentition and **(B)** the permanent *(white)* dentition.

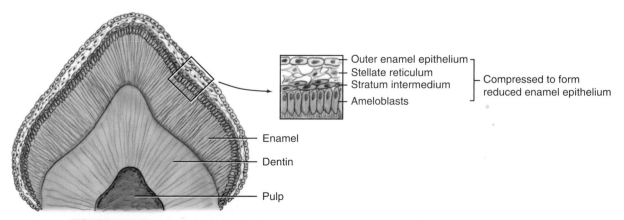

Outer enamel epithelium
Stellate reticulum
Stratum intermedium ⎤ Compressed to form reduced enamel epithelium
Ameloblasts

Enamel
Dentin
Pulp

FIGURE 6-23 Reduced enamel epithelium produced after the completion of enamel appositional growth when the enamel organ undergoes compression of its many layers on the enamel surface.

FIGURE 6-24 Photomicrograph of reduced enamel epithelium after the completion of enamel appositional growth when the enamel organ undergoes compression of its many layers on the enamel surface (noted as enamel space). (From Nanci A: *Ten Cate's oral histology,* ed 8, St Louis, 2013, Mosby.)

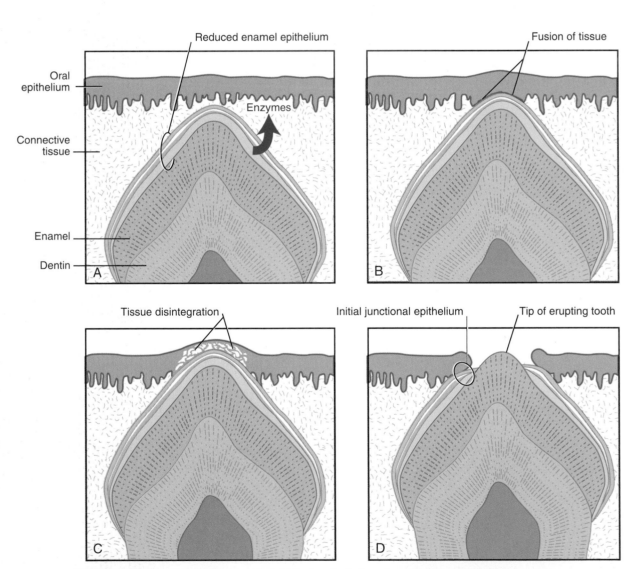

FIGURE 6-25 Process of tooth eruption. **A,** Oral cavity before the eruption process begins with reduced enamel epithelium (*circle*) covering the newly formed enamel; enzymes from the reduced enamel epithelium are present for tissue disintegration (*arrow*). **B,** Fusion of the reduced enamel epithelium with the oral epithelium. **C,** Disintegration of the central fused tissue, leaving an epithelial-lined eruption tunnel for tooth movement. **D,** Coronal fused epithelial tissue peels back from the crown during eruption, leaving the initial junctional epithelium (*circle*).

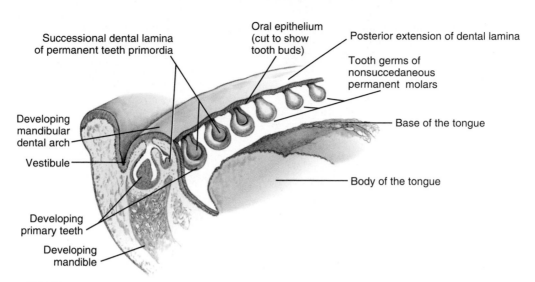

Successional dental lamina
of permanent teeth primordia

Oral epithelium
(cut to show
tooth buds)

Posterior extension of dental lamina

Tooth germs of
nonsuccedaneous
permanent molars

Developing
mandibular
dental arch

Vestibule

Base of the tongue

Body of the tongue

Developing
primary teeth

Developing
mandible

FIGURE 6-26 Development of the succedaneous permanent teeth in a lingual position to the primary teeth on a section of a fetal mandible.

The process of eruption for a succedaneous permanent tooth is the same as for the primary tooth after the widening of the *gubernacular canal:* The REE fuses with the oral epithelium and then degenerates, leaving an epithelial-lined eruption tunnel. The process of the nonsuccedaneous eruption of the permanent teeth is similar also, but no primary tooth is shed to allow for the process as with the succedaneous permanent teeth. Both succedaneous and nonsuccedaneous permanent teeth erupt in chronologic order (see Figure 6-22).

Clinical Considerations with Eruption Process

A permanent tooth often starts to erupt before the primary tooth is fully shed, possibly creating complications in spacing. Interceptive orthodontic therapy can prevent some of these situations. Thus, it is important for children with prolonged retention of any primary teeth to seek early dental consultation. Root fragments from primary molars may be left from the eruption process and create periodontal complications for the permanent dentition; panoramic radiographs of the mixed dentition are important in order to monitor tooth development (see Figure 6-27, *A*).

A residue may form on newly erupted teeth of both dentitions that may leave the teeth extrinsically stained. This green-gray residue, Nasmyth (nas-mith) membrane, consists of the fused tissue of the REE and oral epithelium, as well as the dental cuticle placed by the ameloblasts on the newly-formed outer enamel surface (Figure 6-29).

Nasmyth membrane then easily picks up extrinsic stain from food debris but can be removed by selective polishing; the child's supervising adults may need reassurance as to its background.

In addition, because the crown forms before the root, prevention of traumatic injury to the permanent teeth before they are fully anchored into the jaws is very important. Mouthguards, which consist of individually formed plastic coverings for the teeth, are recommended for children active in all types of sports. Any injury to dentition of children (such as, avulsion) must be promptly cared for to prevent injury to the forming teeth and supporting tissue types.

An odontogenic cyst that forms from the REE after the crown has completely formed and matured is considered a dentigerous (den-ti-jer-os) cyst (or follicular cyst) (Figure 6-30). This initially asymptomatic cyst forms around the crown of a nonerupted impacted or developing tooth—most commonly the permanent third molars. When this cyst becomes larger within the bone of the jaws, it may cause displaced teeth, jaw fracture, and pain; it must be completely removed surgically because it may become neoplastic otherwise.

If a dentigerous cyst appears on a partially erupted tooth, it is considered an *eruption cyst* and appears as fluctuant, blue, vesicle-like gingival lesion (Figure 6-31). Unlike the other types of dentigerous cysts, the eruption cyst disintegrates with eruption of the tooth and no further treatment is needed. Because it appears to enlarge as the tooth erupts, the child's supervising adults may need reassurance as to its background.

Unexfoliated primary teeth

Newly erupted permanent first molar

Forming unerupted permanent teeth

Unerupted permanent premolars

Unerupted permanent second molar

Erupted permanent first molar

B

Unerupted permanent canine

Maxillary arch

Erupted permanent incisors

Unexfoliated primary molars

Unexfoliated primary canine

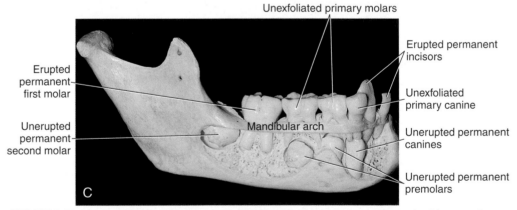

Unexfoliated primary molars

Erupted permanent incisors

Unexfoliated primary canine

Unerupted permanent canines

Unerupted permanent premolars

Erupted permanent first molar

Unerupted permanent second molar

Mandibular arch

C

FIGURE 6-27 Mixed dentition with primary teeth being shed and the permanent dentition erupting within the jaws of each arch. **A,** Panoramic radiograph. **B** and **C,** Maxilla and mandible with a section of facial cortical plate removed. (Courtesy of Margaret J. Fehrenbach, RDH, MS.)

FIGURE 6-28 Eruption process. **A,** Photomicrograph of mandibular sagittal section showing a mixed dentition of posterior teeth, primary and permanent. The primary molars are undergoing root resorption due to the nearby succedaneous permanent premolars and also present is the nearby formation of the roots of the nonsuccedaneous permanent first molar that needs to erupt into the oral cavity. **B** and **C,** Close-up microscopic sections of process: primary tooth resorption of root *(R)*, periodontal ligament *(PDL)* with its odontoclasts *(arrows)*, enamel space of permanent tooth undergoing eruption. (**A,** From Nanci A: *Ten Cate's oral histology,* ed 8, St Louis, 2013, Mosby; **B** and **C,** From the Dr. Bernhard Gottlieb Collection, courtesy of James McIntosh, PhD, Assistant Professor Emeritus, Department of Biomedical Sciences, Baylor College of Dentistry, Dallas, TX.)

FIGURE 6-29 Extrinsic staining of Nasmyth membrane after eruption of the teeth. Entire crowns of the primary dentition may be affected, as well as those of the permanent dentition. (Courtesy of Margaret J. Fehrenbach, RDH, MS.)

FIGURE 6-31 Eruption cyst *(arrow)* in a child. This less serious type of dentigerous cyst has formed over the crown of an erupting primary mandibular incisor. (Courtesy of Margaret J. Fehrenbach, RDH, MS.)

FIGURE 6-30 Radiograph of a dentigerous cyst *(dashed lines)* that is formed around the crown of an unerupted permanent mandibular third molar as a result of impaction. (Courtesy of Margaret J. Fehrenbach, RDH, MS.)

CHAPTER 7

Cells

Additional resources and practice exercises are provided on the companion Evolve website for this book: ⓔ
http://evolve.elsevier.com/Fehrenbach/illustrated.

●●● LEARNING OBJECTIVES

1. Define and pronounce the key terms in this chapter.
2. Discuss cell properties and components, including the cell membrane, cytoplasm, organelles, and inclusions.
3. Identify the components of the cell on a diagram.
4. Outline the cell cycle, describing the phases of mitosis that are involved.
5. Describe the extracellular materials surrounding the cell and its intercellular junctions.
6. Integrate the study of cell anatomy into the further study of dental histology.

CELL PROPERTIES

As an introduction to **Unit III**, the microscopic organization of the body is discussed in this chapter. **Histology** (his-tol-oh-jee) is the study of the microscopic structure and function of cells and the associated tissue. Another term for histology is *microanatomy* because the dimensions of the anatomic structures studied are on a microscopic scale; see **Appendix B** for information on the units of measurement used. A dental professional must have a clear understanding of the basic structural unit of the body, the cell and its components, as well as understanding the larger concepts involved in the histology of tissue, such as those found in the oral cavity. This chapter gives an overview of the cell and its various components, and then **Chapter 8** presents a review of basic tissue types in the body. A discussion of the histology of each of the tissue types within the oral cavity follows in later chapters of **Unit III** along with clinical considerations related to histology.

The smallest living unit of organization in the body is the **cell**, because each cell is capable of performing any necessary functions without the aid of other cells (Figures 7-1 and 7-2, Table 7-1). Each cell has a cell membrane, cytoplasm, organelles, and inclusions. Thus, every cell is a world unto itself (like a small gated city) surrounded by a boundary, having "factories" and other "industries" that make it almost self-sufficient.

Cells also interact with one another similar to how a city interacts with other cities. Cells with similar characteristics of form and function are grouped together to form a **tissue**, analogous to how states are then formed from cities having a common goal (see Table 7-1). Thus, a tissue is a collection of similarly specialized cells, which are most often surrounded by extracellular materials. Various tissue types are then bonded together to form an **organ**, a somewhat independent body part that performs a specific function or functions, similar to

countries formed from like-minded states. Organs can further function together globally as a **system**.

Cells in a tissue undergo cell division to reproduce and replace the dead tissue cells. As a result of the division process, two daughter cells that are identical to each other and to the original parent cell are formed. This process consists of different phases, which are discussed later in this chapter in regard to the different components of the cell.

However, cells also interact with the extracellular environment in many ways. Cells can perform **exocytosis** (ek-so-sigh-toe-sis), which is an active transport of material from a vesicle within the cell out into the extracellular environment. Exocytosis occurs when there is fusion of a vesicle membrane with the cell membrane and subsequent expulsion of the contained material.

The uptake of materials from the extracellular environment into the cell is **endocytosis** (en-do-sigh-toe-sis). Endocytosis can take place as an invagination of the cell membrane. Endocytosis can also take the form of **phagocytosis** (fag-oh-sigh-toe-sis), which is the engulfing and then digesting of solid waste and foreign material by the cell through enzymatic breakdown of the material (discussed later in this chapter).

CELL ANATOMY

The **cell membrane** (or plasma membrane) surrounds the cell (see Figures 7-1 and 7-2). Despite its fragile microscopic structure, it is a tough and resourceful "gatekeeper" for the cell's interior. The usual cell membrane is an intricate bilayer, consisting predominantly of phospholipids and proteins. The phospholipids serve largely as a diffusion regulator. The proteins of the cell membrane serve as structural reinforcements, as well as receptors for specific hormones, neurotransmitters, and immunoglobulins (or antibodies). The cell membrane

FIGURE 7-1 Electron micrograph of the cell and its most visible contents, such as its cell membrane and nucleus.

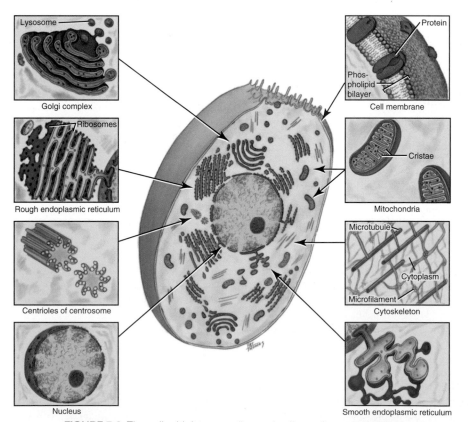

FIGURE 7-2 The cell with its organelles and cell membrane examined.

TABLE 7-1	Body Components
BODY COMPONENTS	**FEATURES**
Cell	Smallest living unit of organization: epithelial cell, neuron, myofiber, chondrocyte, osteocyte, fibroblast, erythrocyte, macrophage, sperm
Tissue	Collection of similarly specialized cells: epithelium, nervous tissue, muscle, cartilage, bone, connective tissue, blood
Organ	Independent body part formed from tissue: skin, brain, heart, liver
System	Organs functioning together: central nervous system, respiratory system, immune system, cardiovascular system

FIGURE 7-3 Nucleus and its various components: chromatin, nucleoplasm, nuclear envelope, nuclear pore, and nucleolus.

is associated with many of the mechanisms of intercellular junctions and other functions of the cell.

The **cytoplasm** (cy-to-plazm) includes the semifluid part contained within the cell membrane boundary, as well as the skeletal system of support or cytoskeleton (discussed later in this chapter). The cytoplasm contains not only a number of structures but also cavities or **vacuoles** (vak-you-oles).

ORGANELLES

The **organelles** (or-gan-eels) are metabolically active specialized structures within the cell (see Figures 7-1 and 7-2). The organelles allow each cell to function according to its genetic code. Organelles also subdivide the cell into compartments. The major organelles of the cell include the nucleus, mitochondria, ribosomes, endoplasmic reticulum, Golgi complex, lysosomes, and the cytoskeleton.

NUCLEUS

The **nucleus** (noo-kle-is) (plural, **nuclei** [noo-kle-eye]) is the largest, densest, and most conspicuous organelle in the cell when it is examined microscopically (Figure 7-3; see Figures 7-1 and 7-2). A nucleus is found in all cells of the body except mature red blood cells, and most cells have a single nucleus. However, some cells are multinucleated, such as osteoclasts or skeletal muscles (see Figures 8-15 and 8-18).

The chief nucleic acid in the nucleoplasm is deoxyribonucleic acid (DNA), in the form of **chromatin** (kro-mah-tin), which looks like diffuse stippling when the cell is viewed at lower-power microscopically. In an actively dividing cell, the chromatin condenses into visible, discrete, rodlike **chromosomes** (kro-mah-somes) (see Table 7-2). Each chromosome has a **centromere** (sen-tro-mere), a clear, constricted area near the middle. Chromosomes then become two filamentous, or threadlike, **chromatids** (kro-mah-tids) (or daughter chromosomes) joined by a centromere during cell division. After cell division, major segments of the chromosomes again become uncoiled and dispersed among the other components of the nucleoplasm as before.

The nucleus is the cell's "data bank" because it stores the genetic code. From its sequence of nucleotides in the chromatin, the DNA and ribonucleic acid (RNA) contain instructions for everything the cell is and will become. Thus, they control all functions the cell performs. The nucleus is also the "command center" of the cell, controlling the other organelles in the cell; it is influenced by what occurs inside the cell as well as outside the cell. Only certain genes are "turned on" to participate in the production of specific proteins at any particular time.

The chemical messages that result in genes switching on or off in the nucleus come from the cytoplasm, where, in turn, they are generated as a result of interaction between the surface membrane and the environment. Although genes contain the total range of the cell's possibilities, the cellular environment dictates which of these possibilities for differentiation, growth, development, and specialization will be expressed.

As would be expected, the nucleus is constantly active. Before cell division, new DNA must be synthesized and every single gene must be replicated. These genes, linked into chromosomes, are then separated into duplicate sets during cell division. In the nucleus, three very important types of RNA are produced: messenger RNA (mRNA) molecules, which are complementary copies of distinct segments of DNA; transfer RNA (tRNA) molecules, which are capable of specifically binding to and transporting amino acid units for protein synthesis; and ribosomal RNA (rRNA) molecules, which will be discussed later.

In addition to all the activity associated with cell division, the genes on the DNA selectively direct the synthesis of thousands of enzymes and other integral and cytoplasmic proteins, as well as any secretory products. This process involves transcription of information from various parts of the DNA molecules into new strands of mRNA, which carry the encoded instructions into the cytoplasm for processing through the process of translation, which involves tRNA, rRNA, and amino acids.

The fluid part within the nucleus is the **nucleoplasm** (noo-kle-ah-plazm), which contains important molecules used in the construction of ribosomes, nucleic acids, and other nuclear materials. The nucleus is surrounded by the **nuclear** (noo-kle-er) **envelope**, a membrane similar to the cell membrane, except that it is double-layered. The nuclear envelope is associated with many other organelles of the cell. The nuclear envelope may be pierced by **nuclear pores**, which act as avenues of communication between the inner nucleoplasm and the outer cytoplasm. The number and distribution of these nuclear pores vary with the cell type, with the level of cell activity, and with states of differentiation level of the same cell type.

Contained in the nucleus is the **nucleolus** (noo-kle-oh-lis), a prominent, rounded nuclear organelle that is centrally placed in the nucleoplasm when the cell is examined microscopically (see Figure 7-3). The nucleolus mainly produces rRNA and the nucleotides of the two other types of RNA. Without a nucleolus, no protein synthetic activity would occur within the cell; the nucleolus acts almost like a "city hall" in managing the activity within the cell. The roles of the nucleolus and ribosomes with rRNA in protein synthesis are discussed later.

MITOCHONDRIA

The mitochondria (mite-ah-kon-dree-ah) are the most numerous organelles in the cell. They are associated with energy conversion, and thus are the "power stations" for the cell (see Figures 7-1 and 7-2). They are a major source of adenosine triphosphate (ATP) and thus are the site of many metabolic reactions. Microscopically, mitochondria resemble small bags with a larger bag fitted inside because each bag is folded back on itself. These inner folds exist to increase the surface area for more dense packing of the particular proteins and enzyme molecules involved in aerobic cellular respiration. Internal to the folds, mitochondrial DNA, calcium and magnesium granules, enzymes, electrolytes, and water are present in a matrix. A matrix is a surrounding medium to a structure as discussed in **Chapter 6.**

Most of a cell's energy comes from mitochondria, produced by two of the pathways of aerobic cellular respiration. These involve both the Krebs cycle (or citric acid cycle) with its multienzyme system as well as the hydrogen pathway, which uses the electron transport chain of enzymes. Besides supplying energy, mitochondria help balance the concentration of water, calcium, and other ions in the cytoplasm. Cells with high levels of mitochondria are also known for high levels of activity, such as with "young" fibroblasts in healthy oral mucosa; the reverse is noted with the cellular changes encountered with inflammatory periodontal disease having lower levels of mitochondria in the "older" fibroblasts (see **Chapter 8**). This may also explain the possible interrelationship between two prominent inflammatory diseases: periodontal disease and cardiovascular disease (CVD).

RIBOSOMES

The ribosomes (ry-bo-somes) are the tiny sphere-shaped organelles in the cell (see Figure 7-2). The ribosomes are produced in the nucleolus from rRNA and protein molecules and are assembled in the cytoplasm. They function as mobile "protein factories" for the cell; their location changes based on the type of protein being made for the cell. They can be within mitochondria, free in the cytoplasm, or bound to membranes, either to the outer nuclear membrane or onto the surface of the rough endoplasmic reticulum (discussed next).

Ribosomes can also be found singly or in clusters within the cell. As many as 30 separate ribosomes may be attached sequentially to a single molecule of mRNA, with each ribosome making its own protein copy as it works its way along the length of the mRNA transcript. Within these ribosomes, free amino acids are being joined together according to the particular order specified by the mRNA transcript corresponding to the sequence of the required protein chain.

ENDOPLASMIC RETICULUM

The endoplasmic reticulum (en-do-plas-mik rey-tik-u-lum) (ER) is so called because it is more concentrated in the cell's inner or endoplasmic region as compared to the peripheral or ectoplasmic region (see Figures 7-1 and 7-2). The ER consists of parallel membrane-bound channels. All the membranes of the ER interconnect, forming a system of channels and folds microscopically, and are continuous with the nuclear envelope, like a "highway" system for the cell.

The ER can be classified as either smooth or rough, which is determined by the absence or presence of ribosomes, giving each a differing outer microscopic texture structure, as well as differing in function. The smooth ER (SER), which is free of ribosomes, appears microscopically smooth in surface texture. The rough ER (RER), as discussed earlier, is dotted with ribosomes on its outer surface, which makes it appear microscopically rough.

The outer layer of the nuclear envelope connects with all the ER in the cell, both smooth and rough. The ER's primary functions are modification, storage, segregation, and finally transport of proteins that the cell manufactures (on the ribosomes) for use in other sections of the cell or even outside the cell.

GOLGI COMPLEX

Once the ER has modified a new protein, it is then transferred to the Golgi (gol-jee) complex (or Golgi apparatus) for subsequent segregation, packaging, and transport of protein compounds just like a "distribution center" for the cell (see Figures 7-1 and 7-2). The Golgi complex is the second largest organelle after the nucleus and is composed of stacks of 3 to 20 flattened smooth-membrane vesicular sacs arranged parallel to one another.

Vesicles of protein molecules from the RER fuse with the Golgi complex, transferring protein molecules to be further modified, concentrated, and packaged by the Golgi complex. After this modification and packaging, the Golgi complex wraps up large numbers of these molecules into a single membranous vesicle and then sends it on its way to the cell's surface to be released by the process of exocytosis. These protein molecules, which include hormones, enzymes, and other secretory products, are released into the extracellular space or into capillaries as these vesicles fuse with the cell membrane. These products that are put together in the Golgi complex can include such substances as mucus secretory product for the salivary glands or insulin for the pancreas.

The modifications by the Golgi complex to the protein molecules include adding carbohydrates, thus forming glycoproteins, as it does in the production of mucus. The Golgi complex also may remove part of a polypeptide chain, as it does in the case of insulin. The Golgi complex not only prepares proteins for export by exocytosis but also produces a separate organelle, lysosomes (discussed next).

LYSOSOMES

The lysosomes (li-sah-somes) are organelles produced by the Golgi complex and function in both intracellular and extracellular digestion by the cell (see Figure 7-2). This digestive function is due to their ability to lyse, or digest, various waste and foreign materials in or around the cell, which occurs during phagocytosis, like a "sewer system" for the cell (Figure 7-4). Lysosomes break down many kinds of molecules using the powerful hydrolytic and digestive enzymes contained within them (see Figure 8-15). The main hydrolytic enzyme in lysosomes is hyaluronidase. Lysosomes are membrane-bound vesicles that develop as a bud that pinches off the end of one of the Golgi complex's flattened sacs. The enzymes of the lysosomes originally are produced on the RER and then are transported for packaging in the Golgi complex, where the lysosomes originate.

As the substances are broken down into sufficiently small and simple products, the usable material diffuses out of the lysosome into the cell's cytoplasm to be incorporated into new molecules being synthesized, a kind of cellular "recycling." Indigestible material remains in the lysosome and becomes a residual body. It either migrates to the cell surface to be released by exocytosis or remains as a remnant in the lysosome and becomes an inclusion (discussed later in this chapter). Although all cells, except red blood cells, are capable of some digestive activity, other cells, such as certain white blood cells (for example, neutrophils), have differentiated to specialize in digestive processes, especially during phagocytosis (see Figure 8-17). Phagocytosis is very active even at the junction between healthy gingival tissue and the tooth surface (see **Chapter 10**).

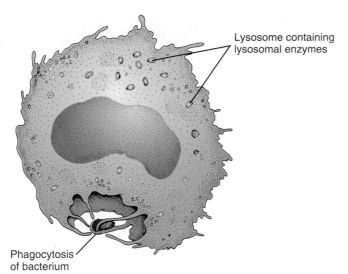

Lysosome containing lysosomal enzymes

Phagocytosis of bacterium

FIGURE 7-4 Phagocytosis, which is the engulfing and digesting of solid waste and foreign material (such as with the bacterium shown here) by a white blood cell (monocyte) through enzymatic breakdown of the matter from its enclosed lysosomes. (From Fehrenbach MJ: Inflammation and repair. In Ibsen OAC, Phelan JA, editors: *Oral pathology for dental hygienists*, ed 6, St Louis, 2014, Saunders.)

CENTROSOME

The **centrosome** (**sen**-tro-some) is a dense, somewhat oval-shaped organelle that contains a pair of cylindrical structures, the **centrioles** (**sen**-tree-ols) (see Figure 7-2). The centrosome is always located near the nucleus, which is important because it plays a significant role in forming the mitotic spindle apparatus during cell division. There are two centrioles within the centrosome, and each is composed of triplets of microtubules arranged in a cartwheel pattern. Without this self-replicating centriole-centrosome unit, a cell from the body cannot reproduce (discussed later in this chapter).

CYTOSKELETON

The interior of the cell is neither liquid nor gel in nature but somewhat between the two. Within the cell there is a three-dimensional system of support using cellular scaffolding, the **cytoskeleton** (sigh-toh-**skel**-eh-ton) (**CSK**) (see Figure 7-2). The components of the CSK include microfilaments, intermediate filaments, and microtubules as a shifting lattice arrangement of structural and contractile components distributed throughout the cell cytoplasm. This design lends basic stability to the cell as a whole, functioning like reinforced girders. It also acts to compartmentalize the cytoplasm, creating preferred "freeways" for the movement of molecules formed by cellular processes.

Both **microfilaments** (my-kroh-**fil**-ah-ments) and **microtubules** (my-kroh-**too**-bules) consist of specialized proteins. Microfilaments are delicate, threadlike microscopic structures. Microtubules are slender, hollow, tubular microscopic structures that may appear individually, doubly, or as triplets. Microtubules assist microfilaments in the maintenance of overall cell shape and in the transport of intracellular materials. Additionally, microtubules form the internal framework of cilia and flagella, centrioles, and the mitotic spindle for cell division (discussed later in this chapter).

Certain cells exhibit projections that help move substances along the surface of the cell or are for moving the entire cell in the extracellular environment. If the projections on the cell are shorter and more numerous, they are considered *cilia;* if the projections are fewer and longer, they are considered *flagella.*

Both the projections of cilia and flagella are useful in human reproduction. An ovum is propelled within the fallopian tube by cilia, and sperm are propelled by their own flagella (see Figure 3-1). Structurally, there is no major difference between cilia and flagella except for their relative lengths. Both consist of pairs of multiple microtubules that form a ring around two single microtubules. Cilia are also noted in the respiratory mucosa lining the nasal cavity and paranasal sinuses as they move the mucous coating of these tissue types along the surface (see Figure 11-20).

The **intermediate filaments** (**fil**-ah-ments) are of various types of thicker, threadlike microscopic structures within the cell. One type of intermediate filament, the **tonofilament** (**ton**-oh-fil-ah-ment), has a major role in intercellular junctions (discussed later in this chapter). Another type of intermediate filament is one that forms keratin, which is found in a calloused-type of epithelium located in the oral cavity on the attached gingiva as well as the dorsal surface of the tongue (see Figure 9-4).

INCLUSIONS

The cell also contains **inclusions** (in-**kloo**-zhins), which are metabolically inert substances that are also considered transient over time in the cell (see Figure 7-2). These include masses of organic chemicals and often are recognizable microscopically. These inclusions are released from storage by the cell and used as demand dictates. Lipids and glycogen can be decomposed for energy from inclusions in the cell. Melanin is stored as inclusions in certain cells of the skin and oral mucosa and is responsible for the pigmentation of these tissue types (see Figures 9-23 and 9-24). Inclusions also include residual bodies, which are spent lysosomes and their digested material.

CELL DIVISION

Cell division or **mitosis** (my-**toe**-sis) is a complex process involving many of the organelles of the cell (Table 7-2). Mitosis functions during tissue growth or regeneration, and its activity is dependent on the length of the individual cell's lifespan. Before cell division, the DNA is replicated during **interphase** (**in**-ter-faze) as part of the cell cycle, which is the cell's "living" time. Interphase has three phases: Gap 1, or G1 (initial resting phase: cell growth and functioning); synthesis, or S (cell DNA synthesis by duplication); and Gap 2, or G2 (second resting phase: resuming cell growth and functioning).

Following interphase, mitosis occurs with the cell's nuclear material dividing so that the resulting production is of two daughter cells that are identical to the parent cell as well as to each other (see **Chapter 3**). Then, at the same time, the other cytoplasmic components of the cell also are divided. The cell division that takes place during mitosis consists of four phases: **prophase** (**pro**-faze), **metaphase** (**met**-ah-faze), **anaphase** (**an**-ah-faze), and **telophase** (**tel**-oh-faze); cell division is followed again by interphase continuing the cell cycle.

EXTRACELLULAR MATERIALS

The cells in each tissue type are surrounded by extracellular materials, which include both tissue fluid and intercellular substance. **Tissue fluid** (or interstitial fluid) provides a medium or matrix for dissolving, mixing, and transporting substances and for carrying out chemical reactions. Similar to blood plasma in its content of ions and diffusible substances, tissue fluid contains a small amount of plasma proteins.

Tissue fluid enters the tissue to surround the cells by diffusing through the capillary walls as a filtrate from the plasma of the blood.

TABLE 7-2	Cell Cycle

CELL CYCLE PHASES	**MICROSCOPIC STRUCTURES**

Interphase: G1, S, G2 Phases

Cells between divisions engage in growth, metabolism, organelle replacement, and substance production, including chromatin and centrosome replication.

 Chromatin

Mitosis Phases

Prophase

Chromatin condenses into chromosomes in cell. Replicated centrioles migrate to opposite poles. Nuclear membrane and nucleolus disintegrate.

Centrosome with centrioles — Spindle fibers

Chromosomes — Centromere

Metaphase

Chromosomes move so that their centromeres are aligned in the equatorial plane. Mitotic spindle forms.

Spindle fibers

Centromere

Anaphase

Centromeres split, and each chromosome separates into two chromatids. Chromatids migrate to opposite poles by the mitotic spindle.

Telophase

Division into two daughter cells occurs. Nuclear membrane reappears.

(Electron micrographs from Stevens A, Lowe J: *Human histology,* ed 4, St Louis, 2015, Mosby.)

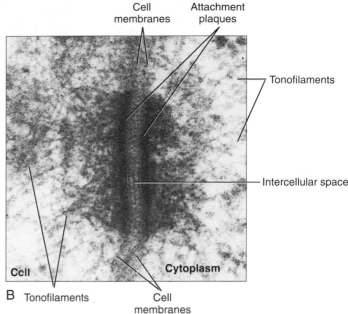

FIGURE 7-5 Intercellular junction between cells via a desmosome. **A,** Diagram. **B,** Electron micrograph. The cell adhesion between cell membranes is mediated by transmembrane proteins. This type occurs in the superficial layers of the skin (shown here), as well as in the oral mucosa. Note the attachment plaque, which is an attachment device involving tonofilaments. (**B,** From Lowe JS, Anderson PG: *Stevens and Lowe's Human Histology,* ed 4, St Louis, 2015, Elsevier/Mosby.)

Tissue fluid then drains back into the blood as lymph through osmosis, via the lymphatics (see **Chapter 8**). The amount of tissue fluid varies from tissue to tissue, with smaller variations occurring over time within any one tissue. An excess amount can accumulate when an injured tissue undergoes an inflammatory response, leading to edema with its tissue enlargement (see Figure 10-8).

Intercellular substance (or ground substance) is shapeless, colorless, and transparent material in which the cells of a tissue are imbedded; it also fills the spaces between the cells in a tissue. The intercellular substance serves as a barrier to the penetration of foreign materials into the tissue as well as a medium for the exchange of gases and metabolic substances. The surrounding cells produce the intercellular substance, and one of its most common elements is hyaluronic acid.

INTERCELLULAR JUNCTIONS

Certain cells in varying tissue are joined by the mechanism of intercellular junctions. These are mechanical attachments formed between cells, and also between cells and adjacent noncellular surfaces. With the formation of these intercellular junctions, the cell membranes of different cells come close together but do not completely attach. Higher-power magnification is needed to visualize these attachments, which appear as dense bodies. All intercellular junctions involve some sort of intricate attachment device. The attachment device includes an attachment plaque that is located within the cell as well as adjacent tonofilaments.

An intercellular junction between cells is formed by a desmosome (des-mo-some), such as that present in the superficial layers of the skin or oral mucosa (Figure 7-5). The desmosome appears to be disc-shaped, and can be likened to a "spot weld" within the structure of a tissue. The desmosomal junctions are also released during tissue turnover and then become reattached in new locations as the cells migrate, such as during repair after an injury to the skin or oral mucosa (see Figure 8-3).

Desmosomes can create an artifact when cells in the stratified squamous epithelium are fixed for prolonged microscopic study. The regularly plump cells appear prickly or spikey at their outer edges as they still maintain their junctional stronghold from the desmosomes. The individual dehydrated cells shrink from the drying fixation chemicals as a result of cytoplasm loss (see Figure 9-8).

Another type of intercellular junction is formed by a hemidesmosome (hem-eye-des-mo-some), which involves an attachment of a cell to an adjacent noncellular surface (Figure 7-6). This type of attachment is used for attaching the epithelium to connective tissue, such as with the basement membrane in the skin and oral mucosa (see Figure 8-4). The attachment device of a hemidesmosome represents half of a desmosome because it involves a smaller attachment plaque and has tonofilaments from only the cellular side. Thus, it appears as a thinner disc because the noncellular surface cannot produce the other half of the attachment mechanism. Hemidesmosomes are also involved as a mechanism allowing gingival tissue to be secured to the tooth surface by the epithelial attachment (see Figures 10-6 and 10-7), which is similar to the attachment between the nails and adjoining nail beds.

FIGURE 7-6 Intercellular junction between a cell with its cytoplasm and noncellular surface via a hemidesmosome. **A,** Diagram. **B,** Electron micrograph. The attachment of cells is to an adjacent noncellular surface is by the adhesion of the noncellular surface mediated by transmembrane protein. This type occurs at the basement membrane between epithelial and connective tissue (as shown here), as well as at the attachment of gingival tissue to the tooth surface. Note the smaller attachment plaques of the hemidesmosomal junction and tonofilaments on the cellular side. (**B,** From Lowe JS, Anderson PG: *Stevens and Lowe's Human Histology*, ed 4, St. Louis, 2015, Elsevier/Mosby.)

CHAPTER 8

Basic Tissue

Additional resources and practice exercises are provided on the companion Evolve website for this book: ⓔ
http://evolve.elsevier.com/Fehrenbach/illustrated.

●●● LEARNING OBJECTIVES

1. Define and pronounce the key terms in this chapter.
2. Discuss basic tissue properties.
3. Describe epithelium properties, including its histology, classification, regeneration, and repair.
4. Describe basement membrane properties, including its histology.
5. Integrate the study of the histology of both epithelium and the basement membrane into the further study of dental histology.
6. Discuss connective tissue properties, including its histology, classification, turnover, and repair.
7. Describe specialized connective tissue properties.
8. Describe cartilage properties, histology, development, repair, and aging.
9. Describe bone properties, histology, development, remodeling, repair, and aging.

10. Describe blood properties, plasma, and blood components.
11 Integrate the study of the basic histology of connective tissue into understanding the clinical considerations of the orofacial region.
12. Describe muscle properties, classifications, and histology.
13. Describe nerve tissue properties and histology as well as the nervous system divisions.
14. Integrate the study of the histology of both muscle and nerve tissue into the further study of dental histology.
15. Identify the components of each basic tissue on a diagram.

BASIC TISSUE PROPERTIES

Dental professionals must have a clear understanding of the histology of the basic tissue types before studying the distinct tissue types present in the oral cavity and associated regions of the face and neck. This information will help dental professionals fully understand the processes involving tissue renewal and repair and the process of aging during clinical care to promote orofacial health, as well as the underlying pathologic processes that can occur.

As was discussed in **Chapter 7**, the smallest living unit of organization in the body is the cell because each cell is capable of performing any necessary functions without the aid of other cells (see Figures 7-1 and 7-2). It was also noted that a group of cells with similar characteristics of form and function together form a tissue (see Table 7-1). A tissue is a collection of similarly specialized cells that will then form into organs.

Tissue types are categorized according to four basic histologic types. These basic histologic tissue types include epithelial, connective, muscle, and nerve tissue (Table 8-1). In addition, these basic tissue types have subcategories that serve specialized functions. It is during prenatal development that embryonic cell layers differentiate

into the various basic embryologic tissue types, including ectoderm, mesoderm, and endoderm, that will later form in some manner into these basic histologic tissue types of the body (see Table 3-4).

Most tissue of the body undergoes regeneration as the individual cells die and are removed from the tissue and new ones take their place. Regeneration is the natural renewal of a tissue and thus an organ; it is produced by growth and differentiation of new cells and intercellular substances. Regeneration occurs through growth from the same type of tissue that has been destroyed or from its precursor. Regeneration is a continuous physiologic process that occurs with most tissue types and in most organs; it even occurs with injury and disease. However, tooth enamel is an example of a tissue type that sadly does not undergo regeneration.

The turnover time is the time it takes for the newly divided cells to be completely replaced throughout the tissue. The turnover time differs for each of the basic tissue types in the orofacial region, as well as for specific regions of the oral cavity. A more complete understanding of turnover time may be the future basis for how the aging process as well as disease processes in the body are delayed or prevented, including those occurring in the oral cavity (see **Chapter 9**).

TABLE 8-1	Basic Tissue Classification
TISSUE	**TYPES**
Epithelium	Simple: Squamous, cuboidal, columnar, pseudostratified
	Stratified: Squamous (keratinized, nonkeratinized), cuboidal, columnar, transitional
Connective tissue	Solid soft: Connective tissue proper, specialized (adipose, fibrous, elastic, reticular)
	Solid firm: Cartilage
	Solid rigid: Bone
	Fluid: Blood, lymph
Muscle	Involuntary: Smooth, cardiac
	Voluntary: Skeletal
Nerve	Afferent: Sensory
	Efferent: Motor

EPITHELIUM PROPERTIES

Epithelium (plural, **epithelia**) (ep-ee-**thee**-lee-um, ep-ee-**thee**-lee-uh) is the tissue that covers and lines both the external and internal body surfaces, including vessels and small cavities. Epithelium not only serves as a protective covering or lining but is also involved in tissue absorption, secretion, sensory, and other specialized functions. It serves to protect the more complex inner structures from physical, chemical, and pathogenic attack, as well as dehydration and heat loss by its formation as an epithelial barrier.

Depending on individual classification, epithelial tissue can be derived from any of the three embryonic cell layers based on the location when developing. Importantly, for dental professionals, both the epithelium of the skin and oral mucosa are of similar ectodermal origin. In comparison, those lining the respiratory and digestive tract are of endodermal origin, and those lining the urinary tract are derived from mesoderm.

EPITHELIUM HISTOLOGY

Epithelium generally consists of closely grouped polyhedral cells surrounded by very little or no intercellular substance or tissue fluid (Figure 8-1). Epithelium is avascular, having no blood supply of its own. Cellular nutrition consisting of oxygen and metabolites is obtained by diffusion from the adjoining connective tissue, which is usually highly vascularized, sharing its source of nutrition.

This tissue is capable of rapid cellular turnover. In fact, epithelium is highly regenerative because its deeper germinal cells are capable of reproduction by mitosis (see Table 7-2). Epithelial cells usually undergo cellular differentiation as they move from the deeper germinal layers to the surface of the tissue to be shed or lost. An exception to the process of cellular maturation is the junctional epithelium of the gingival sulcular region that is attached to the tooth surface.

Epithelial cells are usually tightly joined to each another by intercellular junctions provided for by the desmosomes except in the more superficial layers (see Figure 7-5). The epithelial cells are also tightly joined in some cases to adjacent noncellular surfaces by hemidesmosomes, as is the case with its relationship to the basement membrane (see Figure 7-6) as well as the junctional epithelium of the gingival

sulcular region that is attached to the tooth surface (see Figures 10-6 and 10-7).

A basement membrane is located between most epithelium and deeper connective tissue, such as with both the skin and oral mucosa. Components of basement membrane are produced by both the overlying epithelium as well as the adjoining connective tissue (discussed later in this chapter).

EPITHELIUM CLASSIFICATION

Epithelium can be classified into two main categories based on the arrangement into layers of cells: simple and stratified (see Table 8-1). **Simple epithelium** consists of a single layer of epithelial cells. The further classification of the tissue involves different types of epithelial cells according to cellular structure; they can be classified as either simple squamous, simple cuboidal, or simple columnar (Table 8-2).

Simple squamous epithelium consists of flattened platelike epithelial cells, or **squames** (skwaymz), lining blood and lymphatic vessels, heart, and serous cavities, as well as interfaces in the lungs and kidneys. The term **endothelium** (en-do-**thee**-lee-um) is used to refer to the simple squamous epithelium lining of these vessels and serous cavities.

Simple cuboidal epithelium consists of cube-shaped cells that line the ducts of various glands, such as certain ducts of the salivary glands (see Figure 1-6). Simple columnar epithelium consists of rectangular cells, such as in the lining of other salivary gland ducts, as well as the inner enamel epithelium of a maturing tooth germ, whose cells become enamel-forming ameloblasts (see Figures 6-9 to 6-12).

Epithelium can also be considered **pseudostratified** (soo-doh-strat-i-fide) **columnar epithelium**, which is named as such since it falsely appears as multiple cell layers when viewed with lower power magnification due to the cells' nuclei appearing at different levels (Figure 8-2). However, in reality, as viewed with higher-power magnification, only cells of different heights are seen. Thus, this is a type of simple epithelium because all the cells line up to contact the inner surface of the basement membrane even if not all the cells reach the outer surface of the tissue. Pseudostratified columnar epithelium lines the upper respiratory tract, including the nasal cavity and paranasal sinuses (see Figure 11-20). This type of epithelium may have cilia or be nonciliated at the tissue surface (see **Chapter 7**).

In contrast to simple epithelium, **stratified** (strat-i-fide) **epithelium** consists of two or more layers of cells, with only the deepest layer lining up to contact the basement membrane (see Table 8-1). It is important to note that only the cellular shape of the surface layer is used to determine the classification of stratified epithelium. Thus, stratified epithelium can consist of cuboidal, columnar, or squamous epithelial cells, or a combination of cell types, as seen in a transitional epithelium.

Most epithelium in the body consists of **stratified squamous epithelium** (skway-mus), which includes the superficial layer of both the skin and oral mucosa (see Figures 8-1 and 8-7 and **Chapter 9**). Only the most superficial layers of this tissue are flat cells, or squames; the deeper cells vary from the deeper cuboidal to the more superficial polyhedral. Interdigitation of the outer epithelium with the deeper connective tissue occurs with the epithelial tissue forming **rete** (ree-tee) **ridges** (or rete pegs); however, there is always a basement membrane located between these two tissue types.

Stratified squamous epithelium can be nonkeratinized or keratinized. Nonkeratinized tissue can be found in certain regions of the oral mucosa as well as keratinized tissue. The keratin found within the the keratinized tissue is a tough, fibrous, opaque, waterproof protein that

FIGURE 8-1 Microscopic sections of the skin **(A** and **B),** which demonstrates the epidermis and dermis or epithelium and connective tissue, respectively. A basement membrane is located between these two tissue types. (**A,** From Stevens A, Lowe J: *Human histology,* ed 4, St Louis, 2015, Mosby. **B,** From the Dr. Bernhard Gottlieb Collection, courtesy of James McIntosh, PhD, Assistant Professor Emeritus, Department of Biomedical Sciences, Baylor College of Dentistry, Dallas, TX.)

is impervious to pathogenic invasion and resistant to friction (see **Chapter 9**). Keratin is produced during the maturation of the keratinocyte epithelial cells as they migrate from near the basement membrane to the surface of the keratinized tissue (see Figure 9-4).

Another example of keratinized stratified squamous epithelium is epidermis (ep-i-der-mis), which is the superficial layer of the skin (see Figures 8-1 and 8-7). The epidermis overlies a basement membrane and the adjoining deeper layers of connective tissue (dermis and hypodermis, respectively, which is discussed later). The skin has varying degrees of keratinization depending on the region of the body. Areas such as the palms of the hands and bottom of the feet have thicker layers of keratin, which form calluses. However, the keratin is

less densely packed in both the skin and oral cavity, as compared with the densely packed hard keratin of the nails and hair.

EPITHELIUM REGENERATION, TURNOVER, AND REPAIR

Turnover of both the epithelium in skin or oral mucosa occurs as a result of the cell division during the regeneration process. Cellular turnover of epithelium occurs as the newly formed deepest cells migrate superficially from their formation near the basement membrane. Thus, the turnover time is the time needed for a cell to divide

TABLE 8-2	Epithelial Cell Types

CELL TYPES AND FEATURES	MICROSCOPIC STRUCTURE*
Squamous cells Flattened cells with cell height much less than cell width (i.e., endothelium)	
Cuboidal cells Cube-shaped cells with approximately equal cell height and cell width (i.e., salivary gland duct lining)	
Columnar cells Rectangular cells in which cell height exceeds cell width (i.e., salivary gland duct lining)	

*Note that these epithelial cells are shown *only* within simple epithelium.
Microscopic sections from Stevens A, Lowe J: *Human histology*, ed 4, St Louis, 2015, Mosby.

FIGURE 8-2 Pseudostratified columnar epithelium. **A,** Photomicrograph. **B,** Diagram. This type of epithelium can line the respiratory system. The tissue falsely appears as multiple cell layers when viewed under lower-power magnification because the cells' nuclei appear at different levels. However, in reality, cells of different heights are present. And because all have a direct relationship with the basement membrane, it is considered simple epithelium. (**A,** From Stevens A, Lowe J: *Human histology*, ed 4, St Louis, 2015, Mosby.)

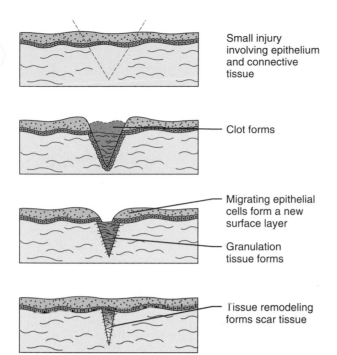

Small injury involving epithelium and connective tissue

Clot forms

Migrating epithelial cells form a new surface layer

Granulation tissue forms

Tissue remodeling forms scar tissue

FIGURE 8-3 Repair process of the skin or oral mucosa after an injury. Note the initial formation of the clot and migrating epithelial cells from the surrounding intact tissue and formation of granulation tissue in the later days of repair. Later, the tissue will remodel and form scar tissue. (From Fehrenbach MJ: Inflammation and repair. In Ibsen OAC, Phelan JA: *Oral pathology for dental hygienists,* ed 6, St Louis, 2014, Saunders.)

during mitosis and pass through the entire thickness of tissue. In order to migrate, the cells release and then regain their desmosomal connections at the intercellular junctions in the more superficial location.

The turnover time is faster for all types of epithelium, as compared to connective tissue. This faster turnover time is a result of the higher level of mitosis in those deepest dividing cells near the basement membrane. Thus, the older, superficial epithelial cells are being shed or lost at the same rate as the deeper germinal cells are dividing into more cells during turnover time.

These overall faster turnover times vary only slightly but sometimes importantly for the different types of epithelium. The epithelium of the oral mucosa generally has a faster turnover time than the epidermis of the skin (see Table 9-6). More specifically within the oral cavity, the epithelium of the buccal mucosa that lines the cheek tissue has a faster turnover time (14 days) than the epithelium that covers the skin (27 days). This difference becomes apparent when dental professionals sadly note a traumatic superficial injury to the facial skin lasting for weeks from a tight overlying rubber dam, and, at the same time, happily observe the quicker healing after the patient accidentally bites down on the superficial surface of the inner cheeks when taking dental radiographs.

The differences of turnover time are especially noted during repair or healing of the tissue after injury. Immediately after an injury to either the skin or oral mucosa, a clot from blood products forms in the area, and the inflammatory response is triggered by the white blood cells from the blood supply as they migrate into the tissue (Figure 8-3). If the source of injury is removed, tissue repair can begin within the next few days. The epithelial cells at the periphery of the injury lose their desmosomal intercellular junctions and then are able to migrate to form a new epithelial surface layer beneath the clot.

Thus, a clot is very important in repair of the epithelium and must be retained in the first days of repair because it acts as a guide to form a new surface. A clot stays moist in the oral cavity but dries out on the skin (called a *scab* when on the skin). Later, after the epithelial surface is repaired, the clot is then broken down by enzymes because it is no longer needed for healing. Repair of the epithelium is a process that is also tied to repair in the deeper connective tissue (discussed later in this chapter).

BASEMENT MEMBRANE PROPERTIES

As discussed earlier, the **basement membrane** is a thin, acellular structure always located between any form of epithelium and the underlying connective tissue, as noted in both the skin and oral mucosa (Figure 8-4, see Figures 7-6 and 8-7). This type of structure is even present between the components of the tooth germ during tooth development (see Figure 6-7).

BASEMENT MEMBRANE HISTOLOGY

The details of the basement membrane are not seen when it is viewed by scanning or lower-power magnification; only its location can be indicated. A higher-power magnification, such as that afforded by an electron microscope, is needed to see the intricacies of the basement membrane. The basement membrane consists of two layers: basal lamina and reticular lamina. The terms *basement membrane* and *basal lamina* are sometimes used interchangeably, but the basal lamina is, in fact, only a part of the basement membrane. The term "basal lamina" is usually used with electron microscopy, whereas the term "basement membrane" is usually used with lower-power light microscopy.

The superficial layer of the basement membrane is the **basal lamina** (**bay**-sal **lam**-i-nah), which is produced by the epithelium, and it is about 40 to 50 nm thick. Microscopically, the basal lamina consists of two sublayers: The *lamina lucida* is a clear layer that is closer to the epithelium, and the *lamina densa* is a dense layer that is closer to the connective tissue. The deeper layer of the basement membrane is usually the **reticular** (re-**tik**-u-ler) **lamina** (the exception is lung alveoli and kidney, with fusion of basal laminae). The reticular lamina consists of collagen fibers and reticular fibers produced and secreted by the underlying connective tissue (discussed later).

Attachment mechanisms are also part of the basement membrane. These involve hemidesmosomes with the attachment plaque as well as tonofilaments from the epithelium and the **anchoring collagen** (**kol**-ah-jen) **fibers** from the connective tissue (see Figure 7-6). The tonofilaments from the epithelium loop through the attachment plaque, whereas the collagen fibers of the reticular lamina loop into the lamina densa of the basal lamina, forming a flexible attachment between the two tissue types.

It is important to note that the interface between the epithelium and connective tissue of both the skin and oral mucosa where the basement membrane is located is not two-dimensional, as seen in microscopic cross sections of the tissue with its epithelial rete ridges and connective tissue papillae (discussed next). Instead, in reality, the interface consists of three-dimensional interdigitation of the two tissue types. This complex arrangement increases the amount of surface area for the interface, thus increasing the mechanical strength of the interface, as well as the nutrition potential for the avascular epithelium from the vascularized connective tissue.

CONNECTIVE TISSUE PROPERTIES

All of the **connective tissue** of the body when taken together represents, by weight, the most abundant type of basic tissue in the body—even if it is epithelium that is mainly seen when clinically examining

FIGURE 8-4 Basement membrane with its basal lamina and reticular lamina. Close-up view shows the attachment devices from an epithelial cell by way of hemidesmosomes and tonofilaments with attachment plaques connecting to the connective tissue by way of anchoring collagen fibers.

the body. Connective tissue is derived from the somites during prenatal development (see Figure 3-13). The functions of connective tissue are as varied as its types; connective tissue is involved in support, attachment, packing, insulation, storage, transport, repair, and defense.

CONNECTIVE TISSUE HISTOLOGY

Compared with epithelium, connective tissue is usually composed of fewer cells spaced farther apart and containing larger amounts of matrix between the cells (except for adipose connective tissue) (see Figure 8-1). Within connective tissue, the matrix is composed of intercellular substance and fibers.

Most connective tissue is renewable because its cells are capable of mitosis, and because most of its cells can even produce their own matrix of intercellular substance and fibers. In most cases, connective tissue is vascularized (except cartilage), each having its own blood supply.

Differing cells are found within the various types of connective tissue. The most common cell in all types of connective tissue is the fibroblast (fi-bro-blast) (Figure 8-5). Fibroblasts synthesize certain types of protein fibers and intercellular substances needed to sustain the connective tissue. They are flat, elongated spindle-shaped cells with

cytoplasmic processes at each end. Subpopulations of fibroblasts may be possible within connective tissue. Fibroblasts are considered fixed cells in connective tissue because they do not leave the tissue to enter the blood as compared to cells with mobility, such as white blood cells.

Young fibroblasts that are actively engaged in the production of fibers and intercellular substance appear to have large amounts of cytoplasm, mitochondria, and rough endoplasmic reticulum. Fibroblasts can show aging and inactivity, with a reduction in cytoplasm, mitochondria, and rough endoplasmic reticulum, which is evident in the later stages of chronic advanced periodontal disease (see **Chapter 10**). If adequately stimulated during repair, however, fibroblasts may revert to a more active state.

Other cells found in connective tissue include migrated white blood cells from the blood supply, such as monocytes (macrophages), basophils (mast cells), lymphocytes (including plasma cells), and neutrophils (discussed later in this chapter). Certain other transient cell types are found in specific classifications of connective tissue and are discussed later in this chapter.

Differing types of protein fibers are found in various types of connective tissue. The main connective tissue fiber type found in the body is the collagen fibers (Figure 8-6). Tissue containing a large amount of collagen fibers is considered a *collagenous connective tissue*, but all connective tissue (except blood) contain some collagen

FIGURE 8-5 Fibroblasts. **A,** Diagram. **B,** Photomicrograph. The fibroblasts are within loose connective tissue, showing their spindle or fusiform shape. The cell forms the fibers of the connective tissue, as well as the intercellular substance between the tissue components. (**B,** From Stevens A, Lowe J: *Human histology,* ed 4, St Louis, 2015, Mosby.)

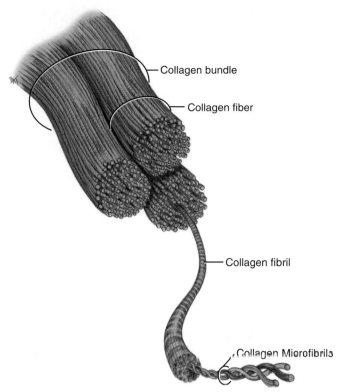

FIGURE 8-6 Collagen bundle that is composed of fibers, and smaller subunits—fibrils and microfibrils.

TABLE 8-3	Collagen Types
MAIN TYPES OF COLLAGEN	**FEATURES**
Type I	Most common type in dermis of skin, skeletal bone, tendons, and virtually all connective tissue of the body as well as lamina propria of oral mucosa, dentin, pulp, periodontium, and the jawbones
Type II	In hyaline and elastic cartilage
Type III	In granulation tissue, produced quickly by young fibroblasts before tougher Type I synthesized, thus commonly found alongside Type I; main component of reticular fibers but also found in artery walls, skin, intestines, and uterus
Type IV	In basal laminae of basement membrane, eye lens, and filtration system of capillaries and kidney's nephron glomeruli

fibers. Collagen fibers are composed of the protein collagen, including distinct types that have been shown by immunologic study to have great tensile strength. All collagen fibers are composed of smaller subunits, or *fibrils,* which are composed of *microfibrils*—similar to a strong, intact rope that is composed of smaller entwined strands of roping material.

Over 29 types of collagen have been identified and described; however, over 90% of the collagen in the body or in fetal tissue is composed of only Types I-IV collagen (Table 8-3). The most common type of collagen protein is Type I collagen, which is found in the teeth, lamina propria of the oral mucosa, dermis of the skin, bone, tendons, and virtually all other types of connective tissue. Cells responsible for the synthesis of Type I collagen include fibroblasts and osteoblasts, which produce fibers and intercellular substance as well as bone, respectively, and odontoblasts, which produce dentin (see Figure 6-11).

The **elastic** (e-las-tik) **fibers** are another type of fiber, composed of microfilaments embedded in the protein elastin, which results in a very elastic type of tissue. Thus, this tissue has the ability to stretch and then to return to its original shape after contraction or extension. Certain regions in the oral cavity, such as the soft palate, contain elastic fibers in the connective tissue of lamina propria to allow this type of tissue movement (see Figure 9-10).

The **reticular fibers** can be found in relationship to an evolving embryonic tissue and thus are found more rarely in the adult body. Reticular fibers are composed of the protein reticulin and are very fine, hairlike fibers that branch, forming a network in the tissue that contains them. However, reticular connective tissue still predominates in the lymph nodes and spleen in an adult.

CONNECTIVE TISSUE CLASSIFICATION

One method of classifying connective tissue is according to texture, which can be soft, firm, rigid, or fluid in nature (see Table 8-1). Soft connective tissue includes the tissue found in the deeper layers of both the skin and oral mucosa, such as a connective tissue proper. Firm

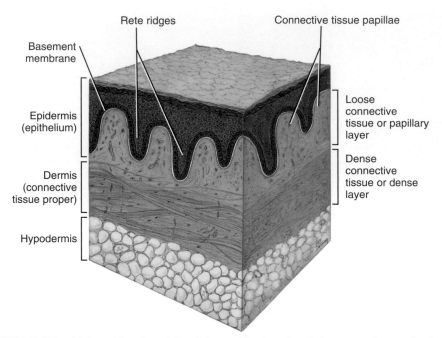

FIGURE 8-7 Skin with its epidermis and dermis layers. The hypodermis is present deep to the dermis. Note the interdigitating rete ridges of the epidermis with the connective tissue papillae of the dermis.

connective tissue consists of different types of cartilage. Rigid, hard form of connective tissue consists of bone. Fluid connective tissue consists of blood with all its components and lymph.

CONNECTIVE TISSUE PROPER

Soft connective tissue can be classified as loose, dense, or specialized. Both loose and dense types of connective tissue are found together in two adjoining layers as the **connective tissue proper**. The connective tissue proper is found deep to the epithelium and basement membrane, in the deeper layers of both the skin and oral mucosa.

The connective tissue proper in the skin is the **dermis** (der-mis) and is found deep to the epidermis (discussed earlier; see Figures 8-1 and Figure 8-7). Even deeper to the dermis is the **hypodermis** (hi-poh-der-mis), a subcutaneous tissue that is composed of loose connective tissue and adipose connective tissue, which is a specialized connective tissue, as well as glandular tissue, large blood vessels, and nerves. Cartilage, bone, and muscle can be present deep to the hypodermis of the skin, depending on the region of the body. In oral mucosa, the connective tissue proper is considered the lamina propria, and the deeper connective tissue sometimes present is the submucosa, similar to the hypodermis in the skin (see Figures 9-1 and 9-6).

Loose Connective Tissue The superficial layer of both the dermis of the skin and lamina propria of the oral mucosa is composed of **loose connective tissue** (see Figure 8-7). In both the dermis or lamina propria of oral mucosa, this layer of loose connective tissue is also considered the **papillary** (pap-i-lar-ee) **layer**. The papillary layer forms **connective tissue papillae** (pah-pil-ay), which is interdigitated with the epithelial rete ridges discussed earlier. This papillary layer has no overly prominent connective tissue element; all of the components of the papillary layer are present in equal amounts. Thus, equal amounts of cells, intercellular substance, fibers, and tissue fluid are in an irregular and loose arrangement. This loose layer of the connective tissue proper serves as protective padding for the deeper structures of the body.

Dense Connective Tissue Deep to the loose connective tissue is **dense connective tissue**, such as that found in the deepest layers of

both the dermis or lamina propria (see Figure 8-7). Similar to loose connective tissue, all of the same components of connective tissue are still present. However in contrast to loose connective tissue, dense connective tissue is tightly packed with a regular arrangement, and it also consists mainly of protein fibers, which give this tissue its strength.

The dense connective tissue in both the dermis and lamina propria is also considered the **dense layer** (or reticular layer). Thus, the dense layer is deep to the papillary layer in the connective tissue proper. In contrast, tendons, aponeuroses, and ligaments are a type of dense connective tissue that has a regular arrangement of strong, parallel collagen fibers with few fibroblasts or cells.

CONNECTIVE TISSUE PROPER REGENERATION, TURNOVER, AND REPAIR

Turnover of both the connective tissue proper in skin or oral mucosa occurs as a result of the production of fibers and intercellular substance by the fibroblasts during regeneration (see Figure 8-5). Other types of cells can also undergo mitosis and create additional cells, such as certain white blood cells and endothelial cells. The overall turnover time for a connective tissue proper is slower than its adjoining epithelium; it also demonstrates individual variance from region to region.

When injured, the connective tissue proper in both the skin or oral mucosa goes through stages of repair that are related to the events in the more superficial epithelium (see Figure 8-3). After a clot forms and an inflammatory response is triggered with white blood cells, fibroblasts migrate to produce an immature connective tissue deep to the clot and newly forming epithelial surface.

This immature connective tissue is considered **granulation** (gran-yoo-lay-shin) **tissue** and has few fibers and an increased amount of blood vessels. Granulation tissue can clinically appear as a redder, soft tissue that bleeds easily after injury or surgery, such as in the oral cavity after a tooth extraction. In addition, this tissue may become abundant, interfering with the repair process. Surgical removal of excess granulation tissue may be necessary to allow for optimum repair; this sometimes occurs after chronic advanced periodontal disease.

Later, during the repair process, this temporary granulation tissue is replaced by paler and firmer scar tissue in the area. It is paler because scar tissue contains an increased amount of fibers and fewer blood vessels. The amount of scar tissue varies, depending on the type and size of the injury, amount of granulation tissue, and movement of tissue after injury. Interestingly, the skin shows more scar tissue production both clinically and microscopically after repair than does the oral mucosa. This difference may be based on differing developmental origins of the tissue producing differing types of fibroblasts and thus different types of fibers.

The repair process can also be affected by hormones such as noted with systemic glucocorticoids (for example, cortisone) hinder repair by depressing the inflammatory reaction or by inhibiting the growth of fibroblasts, the production of collagen, and the formation of endothelial cells. Systemic stress, thyroidectomy, testosterone, adrenocorticotropic hormone, and large doses of estrogen suppress the formation of granulation tissue and impair healing. Progesterone increases and accelerates the vascularization of granulation tissue and appears to increase the susceptibility of the gingival tissue to mechanical injury by causing dilation of the marginal vessels.

At birth, the skin has not developed a sufficient protective layer or facilitated the synthesis of immune cells. It often looks to be transparent and therefore is sensitive to damage, and it must be protected by extra clothing and kept away from environmental stress. At puberty, glandular and hair development, as well as the immune system, begins to function at an increased rate, giving extra protection to the skin against the coming adult world. During this time, the skin is in a very active metabolic state but still vulnerable to sensitization by allergens.

By age 20, however, the skin begins to deteriorate, and by the age of 50 is in a rapid state of degradation due to the aging process. Collagen fibers begin to fall apart; elastic fibers stiffen and thicken, wrinkling the skin. Oil glands in skin cease production, and melanin production decreases, leading to more pallid color and grey hairs. Keratin cells cease production and already produced keratin becomes thin and stiff.

Most importantly to dental professionals, the skin with aging begins to heal poorly after injury (see earlier discussion) with fibroblasts now having less replication activity (considered replicative senescence). The skin also becomes susceptible to disease states that include inflammation (such as with dermatitis), infection (such as with herpes zoster), and cancer (such as with basal cell carcinoma and melanoma). Solar damage will accelerate the aging process in skin, as does increased environmental toxicity (chronic alcohol and tobacco use) (see Figure 1-8 for solar damage of the lips). The aging of the oral mucosa will be discussed in **Chapters 9 and 10**.

SPECIALIZED CONNECTIVE TISSUE PROPERTIES

Specialized connective tissue includes adipose, elastic, or reticular. **Adipose** (ad-i-pose) **connective tissue** is a fatty tissue that is found beneath the skin, around organs and various joints, and in regions of the oral cavity. Unlike most connective tissue, this type of connective tissue has cells packed tightly together with little or no matrix. After fibroblasts, the predominant type of cell found in this tissue is the adipocyte, which stores fat intracellularly.

Elastic connective tissue has a large number of elastic fibers in its matrix, which combine strength with elasticity, such as in the tissue of

FIGURE 8-8 Cartilage, including its cells—chondroblasts and chondrocytes, as well as the outer layer of perichondrium, which is a formative connective tissue sheath.

Labels: Perichondrium · Chondroblast · Daughter chondrocytes in lacuna · Cartilage matrix · Singular chondrocyte in lacuna

the vocal cords. **Reticular connective tissue** is a delicate network of interwoven reticular fibers forming a supportive framework for blood vessels and internal organs.

CARTILAGE PROPERTIES

The firm but flexible, nonmineralized connective tissue in the body is **cartilage** (kar-ti-lij) (Figure 8-8). Cartilage forms most of the temporary skeleton of the embryo and then serves as structural support for certain soft tissue after birth. Additionally, cartilage serves as a model or template in which certain bones of the body subsequently develop. Cartilage is also present at articular surfaces of most freely movable joints, such as the temporomandibular joint (see Figure 19-3).

CARTILAGE HISTOLOGY

Cartilage is composed of cells and matrix. Its matrix or surrounding medium is composed of fibers, mainly collagen, and intercellular substance. Thus, this matrix is similar to soft connective tissue in composition, except that the matrix of cartilage is firmer. The connective tissue surrounding most cartilage (except at joints) is the **perichondrium** (per-ee-kon-dre-um), a fibrous connective tissue sheath containing blood vessels. Since cartilage itself is avascular (having no blood vessels), it receives its nutrition from this associated surrounding tissue.

Two types of cells found in cartilage are the immature **chondroblasts** (kon-dro-blasts), which lie internal to the perichondrium and produce cartilage matrix, and the **chondrocytes** (kon-dro-sites), which are mature chondroblasts that maintain the cartilage matrix (see Figure 8-8). After the production of cartilage matrix, the chondrocyte becomes surrounded and enclosed by the matrix. Only a small space surrounds the chondrocyte within the cartilage matrix, the **lacuna** (lah-ku-nah) (plural, **lacunae** [lah-ku-nay]).

The three types of cartilage—hyaline, elastic, and fibrocartilage—have slightly differing histologic features. Histologists believe that this distinction between types of cartilage is not to be stressed and that most cartilage contains a combination of the different types.

Hyaline (hi-ah-line) **cartilage** is the most common type found in the body and contains only collagen fibers as part of its matrix. The associated collagen fibers of hyaline cartilage are much finer in substance than those within dense connective tissue, thus it is the weakest type. Hyaline cartilage can be found in the embryonic skeleton and in subsequent growth centers, such as within the mandibular condyle (see Figure 19-4). All cartilage starts as hyaline cartilage and are then modified into the other two types of cartilage according to need.

Elastic cartilage is similar to hyaline, except that it has numerous elastic fibers in its matrix, in addition to its numerous collagen fibers. Elastic cartilage is found in the external ear, auditory tube, epiglottis, and parts of the larynx that need its elastic nature.

Fibrocartilage (fi-bro-**kar**-ti-lij) is never found alone and merges gradually with its neighboring hyaline cartilage, such as in the outer part of the of the bones of the temporomandibular joint (see Figure 19-3). Unlike elastic cartilage, fibrocartilage is not merely a modification of hyaline. Rather, it is a transitional type of cartilage between hyaline cartilage and dense connective tissue of tendons and ligaments. The cells of the tissue are enclosed in capsules of matrix, giving it great tensile strength. Unlike both elastic and hyaline cartilage, fibrocartilage has no true layer of perichondrium overlying it.

CARTILAGE DEVELOPMENT

Cartilage can develop or grow in size in two different ways, interstitial growth and appositional growth, as does other tissue such as bone (see **Chapter 3**). Interstitial growth is growth from deep within the tissue by the mitosis of each chondrocyte, thus producing larger numbers of daughter cells within a single lacuna (each of which secretes more matrix) and expanding the tissue (see Figure 8-8). This interstitial growth is important in the development of bone that uses cartilage as a model for its own formation during endochondral ossification (discussed next).

Appositional growth is layered growth on the outside of the tissue from an outer layer of chondroblasts within the perichondrium. This layer of chondroblasts is always present on the external surface of cartilage to allow appositional growth of cartilage after an injury or remodeling.

CARTILAGE REPAIR AND AGING

Unlike rigid bone which is discussed next, cartilage has some flexibility resulting from its fibers in the matrix; however, it has no inorganic or mineralized materials. Cartilage, unlike most connective tissue, is also avascular. Much like epithelium, this tissue depends on its surrounding connective tissue for its cellular nutrition, such as oxygen and metabolites. Because it has no vascularity of its own, cartilage takes longer to repair than vascularized bone. Cartilage also has no nerve supply within its tissue. Thus, cartilage even when subjected to trauma or surgery does not produce overly painful symptoms.

During repair, avascular cartilage is dependent on neighboring connective tissue from the perichondrium for nutrition to transform it slowly into cartilage. With this transformation, the newly formed cartilage slowly proliferates and fills in the defect by appositional growth. In contrast, fractured mature cartilage is often united by dense connective tissue, and if vascularization is initiated, then healing cartilage may eventually be replaced by bone.

As cartilage ages, it becomes less cellular with its chondrocytes dying. It may start to contain firm fibers in parallel groups, or it may even form areas of scattered mineralization. These tend to coalesce over time with the tissue becoming hard and brittle and losing flexibility. Furthermore, in regard to the temporomandibular joint, cartilage may form abnormally within an aging joint disc that is usually only composed of dense fibrous connective tissue, possibly causing clinical difficulties.

FIGURE 8-9 Anatomy of bone showing close-up views of its periosteum, compact bone, and cancellous bone. Note also the endosteum and bone marrow of the bone.

BONE PROPERTIES

The hard, rigid form connective tissue that constitutes most of the mature skeleton is the **bone** (Figure 8-9). Thus, bone serves as protective and structural support for soft tissue and as an attachment mechanism. It also aids in movement, manufactures blood cells through its red bone marrow, and is a storehouse for calcium and other minerals. Bone also surrounds the root(s) of a tooth, creating the alveolus as the alveolar bone proper (see Figure 14-14).

Because bone is vascularized with its own blood supply, it repairs quickly compared with avascular cartilage. Even though bone is rigid, it is important to remember that it does not consist of an inanimate inner rod being moved by the skeletal muscles. Instead, it is a living and functioning tissue in the body. Bone has also undergone the most developmental differentiation of all the connective tissue.

When bone is examined grossly, the outer part of bone is covered by **periosteum** (per-ee-**os**-te-im) (see Figure 8-9). Periosteum is a double-layered, dense connective tissue sheath. The outer layer contains blood vessels and nerves. The inner layer contains a single layer of cells that give rise to bone-forming cells, the osteoblasts.

Deep to the periosteum is a dense layer of **compact** (**kom**-pak) **bone**. Deep to the compact bone is a spongy bone, or **cancellous** (kan-**sel**-us) **bone**. Both compact bone and cancellous bone have the same cellular components, but each has a different arrangement of those components (discussed next).

It is important to understand that the differences between these two types of bone include the relative amount of solid bone and also

FIGURE 8-10 Histology of compact bone. Note the cells of bone, osteoblasts, and osteocytes, as well as the periosteum, the outer formative sheath of connective tissue. The initial bone matrix or osteoid will mineralize later into primary bone first and then secondary bone.

the size and number of soft tissue spaces in each; however, no sharp boundary exists between these two types of bone within an individual bone. Each bone type is located where it best serves the needs for either strength or lightness of weight. Compact bone is strong because it has fewer soft tissue spaces, but it is heavy. In contrast, cancellous bone is light because it is formed by pieces of solid bone that join to form a lattice; it is not as strong because it has more soft tissue spaces.

Lining the medullary cavity of bone on the inside of the layers of compact bone and cancellous bone is the endosteum (en-dos-te-um) (see Figure 8-9). The endosteum has the same composition as the periosteum but is thinner. On the innermost part of bone in the medullary cavity is the bone marrow (mar-oh). This gelatinous substance is where the stem cells of the blood are located, lymphocytes are created, and B-cells mature (discussed later). These stem cells can continue to produce most of the components of the blood.

BONE HISTOLOGY

Bone consists of cells and a partially mineralized matrix that is 60% inorganic or mineralized material (Figure 8-10). It is this inorganic substance in a crystalline formation of mainly calcium hydroxyapatite (hy-drox-see-ap-ah-tite), having the chemical formula $Ca_{10}(PO_4)_6(OH)_2$ that gives bone its hardness. This same type of inorganic crystal is found in differing percentages in the hard dental tissue, such as enamel, dentin, and cementum (see Table 6-2 for comparison of dental hard tissue types). Smaller amounts of other minerals (such as magnesium, potassium, calcium carbonate, and fluoride) are also present. This inorganic material has matrix packed between its bone cells. The matrix is composed of organic collagen fibers and intercellular substance.

Bone matrix is initially formed as osteoid (os-te-oid), which later undergoes mineralization. The osteoid is produced by osteoblasts (os-te-oh-blasts), which are cuboidal cells that arise from fibroblasts. Osteoblasts are also involved in the later mineralization of osteoid to form bone. Always present in the periosteum is a layer of osteoblasts at the external surface of the compact bone; it allows remodeling of bone and repair of injured bone.

Within fully mineralized bone are osteocytes (os-tee-oh-sites), which are entrapped mature osteoblasts. Similar to the chondrocyte, the cell body of the osteocyte is surrounded by bone, except for the space immediately around it, the lacunae. The cytoplasmic processes of the osteocyte radiate outward in all directions in the bone and are located in tubular canals of matrix, or canaliculi (kan-ah-lik-u-lie).

A

B

FIGURE 8-11 Haversian system in compact bone. A, Lamellae creating osteons. Note the Volkmann canal and its communication with larger blood vessels external to the bone. B, Close-up view highlighting osteons with the central Haversian canals, osteocytes, and canaliculi. (A, From Applegate EJ: The anatomy and physiology learning system, ed 4, St Louis, 2011, Saunders.)

These canals provide for interaction between the osteocytes. However, unlike chondrocytes, osteoblasts never undergo mitosis during tissue formation, and thus only one osteocyte is ever found in a lacuna.

Bone matrix in compact bone is formed into closely apposed sheets, or lamellae (lah-mel-ay). Within and between the lamellae are embedded osteocytes with their cytoplasmic processes in the canals. This highly organized arrangement of concentric lamellae in compact bone is the Haversian (hah-ver-zi-an) system.

In the Haversian system, these lamellae form concentric layers of matrix into cylinders or osteons (os-te-onz) (Figure 8-11). The osteon

FIGURE 8-12 Intramembranous ossification, which is the formation of osteoid within two dense connective tissue sheets that will eventually replace the initially formed connective tissue. During intramembranous ossification, mesenchyme differentiates into osteoblasts to form osteoid, which later matures into bone.

is the unit of structure in compact bone and consists of 5 to 20 lamellae. This arrangement in the osteon is like the growth rings in a cross section of a tree trunk. However, unlike tree rings that form at a rate of around one per year, an entire Haversian system is produced all at the same time, no matter the number of concentric lamellae that may be involved.

The Haversian canal (or central canal) is a central vascular canal within each osteon surrounded by the lamellae. It contains longitudinally running blood vessels, nerves, and a small amount of connective tissue and is lined by endosteum. The Haversian canals communicate not only with each other but also with the osteocytic processes in the canaliculi, providing cellular nutrition for the surrounding bone. This organized system of bone is noted within the structure of the alveolar bone proper (see Figure 14-15).

Located on the outer part of the Haversian system in compact bone are Volkmann (volk-man) canals, or similar nutrient canals that contain the same vascular and nerve components as the Haversian canals, being also lined by endosteum. Volkmann canals pass obliquely or at 90° to the Haversian canals of the osteons and communicate with them, as well as with the larger blood supply external to the bone. These more perpendicular canals are noted within the alveolus or tooth socket so that it is sometimes referred to as the *cribriform plate* because they appear grossly as perforating holes (see Figure 14-14, *B*).

In contrast to the highly organized compact bone, cancellous bone has its bone matrix formed into trabeculae (trah-bek-u-lay), or joined matrix pieces forming a lattice (see Figure 8-9). Lamellae of the matrix of cancellous bone are not arranged into concentric layers around a central blood vessel as with the compact bone, but rather their concentric rings are formed into cone-shaped spicules. Osteocytes in lacunae with their cytoplasmic processes are located between the lamellae of the trabeculae. Surrounding the trabeculae are soft tissue spaces that consist of vascular canals with blood vessels, nerves, and varying amounts of connective tissue. These spaces also serve as a nutritional source for the lattice structure of bone.

BONE DEVELOPMENT

Bone development is termed ossification (os-i-fi-kay-shun) and has two methods for development: intramembranous and endochondral ossification. The bone produced by both these developmental methods is microscopically the same; only the process of formation is different. Intramembranous (in-trah-mem-bran-us) ossification is formation of osteoid between two dense connective tissue sheets, which then eventually replaces the outer connective

tissue (Figure 8-12). During intramembranous ossification, mesenchymal cells differentiate into osteoblasts to form the osteoid.

Intramembranous ossification uses a method of appositional growth similar to that of cartilage with layers of osteoid being produced. The osteoid later becomes mineralized to form bone. Certain bones in the body (such as the flat bones and clavicle) can form this way, enlarging over time as the appositional growth of bone occurs. The maxilla and the majority of the mandible are formed by intramembranous ossification (see Figure 6-6 and **Chapter 14**).

Endochondral (en-do-kon-dril) ossification is the formation of the osteoid within a hyaline cartilage model that subsequently becomes mineralized and dies (Figure 8-13). Osteoblasts penetrate the disintegrating cartilage and form primary ossification centers that continue forming osteoid toward the ends of the bone during prenatal development. Thus, bone matrix eventually replaces the earlier cartilage model. This type of ossification first uses the method of interstitial growth of the initial cartilage tissue to form the model, or pattern, of the future bone's shape. Later, appositional growth of osteoid, with layers laid down on the outer perimeter, occurs to complete the final bone mass within the model.

Most long bones of the body are formed this way because it allows bone to grow in length from deep within the tissue. Later after birth, secondary ossification centers, which allow further growth of the bones until puberty end, are also formed. In particular, the head of the mandibular condyle is formed by endochondral ossification that has a multidirectional growth capacity (see **Chapter 14** and Figure 19-4).

Regardless of its method of development, bone also goes through similar specific stages of development (Figure 8-14). The first bone to be produced by either method of ossification is an immature bone, the primary bone (or woven bone). Within primary bone, the lamellae are indistinct because of the irregular arrangement of the collagen fibers and lamellae, whether located within the Haversian system or trabeculae.

Primary bone is a temporary tissue that is replaced by the more mature secondary bone. In contrast to primary bone, secondary bone has a well-organized arrangement of collagen fibers and distinct lamellae. Depending on the specific needs of the bone in any given area, secondary bone can be compact or cancellous.

BONE REMODELING, REPAIR, AND AGING

It is important to keep in mind that a bone's overall structure is not static and, therefore, never remains the same. Throughout life, bone in the body is constantly being remodeled or regenerated. Bone

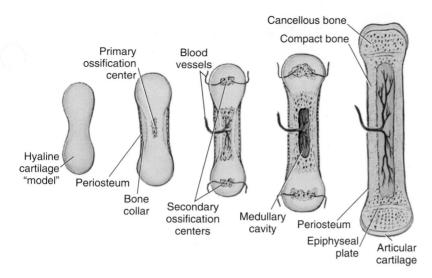

FIGURE 8-13 Endochondral ossification over time, which is the formation of the osteoid within a cartilage model that subsequently becomes mineralized and dies. Osteoblasts penetrate the disintegrating cartilage and form a primary ossification center that continues forming osteoid toward the ends of the bone during prenatal development. Later, after birth, secondary ossification centers form, which allows further growth of bones. (From Applegate EJ: *The anatomy and physiology learning system*, ed 4, St Louis, 2011, Saunders.)

FIGURE 8-14 Stages of bone development, in this case that of compact bone, from primary bone **(A)** to secondary bone **(B)**. These two stages occur during both methods of ossification, as well as during the repair of bone.

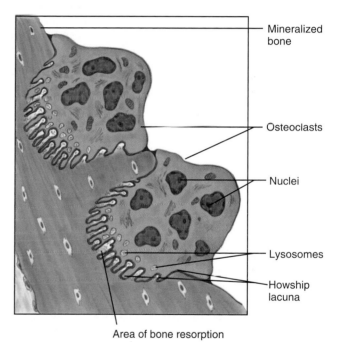

Area of bone resorption

FIGURE 8-15 Osteoclasts within Howship lacunae resorbing bone from their ruffled borders. Note the multiple nuclei within their cytoplasm, which contain lysosomes that break down the bone when discharged into the surrounding tissue.

undergoes removal in certain areas and new bone formation in other areas with the two processes balancing each other within a healthy body. Appositional growth with layered formation of bone along its periphery is accomplished by the osteoblasts, which later become entrapped as osteocytes (see Figure 8-10).

After bone fracture and during the repair of bone, bone also goes through the stages of bone formation, no matter how the bone initially developed. In the area to be repaired, bone forms initially as primary bone, which matures into secondary bone to complete the repair (see Figure 8-14). The repair of bone depends on adequate blood supply, the presence of periosteum with active osteoblasts, and adequate mineral and vitamin levels.

Resorption of bone involves the removal of bone (Figure 8-15). The cell that causes resorption of bone is the osteoclast (os-te-oh-klast). The osteoclast is a large multinucleated cell located on the surface of secondary bone in a large, shallow pit created by this resorption, a **Howship lacuna** (how-ship). The osteoclast is formed from the fusion of numbers of macrophage blood cells (discussed later in this chapter). Each osteoclast contains a large number of lysosomes in its cytoplasm, and these are discharged into the surrounding tissue. The enzymes of the lysosomes then break down the bone when the osteoclast attaches by way of its ruffled border.

TABLE 8-4	Blood Components		
TYPE	**MICROSCOPIC STRUCTURE**	**HISTOLOGIC FEATURES**	**FUNCTION**
Red blood cell (or erythrocyte)		Biconcave disc without nucleus	Binds and transports oxygen and carbon dioxide
Platelets (or thrombocytes)		Discs without nucleus; cell fragments derived from special line of blood cell	Clotting mechanism
White blood cell (or leukocyte)	See Table 8-5	Rounded cells with nucleus, many variations possible (see Table 8-5)	Inflammatory response and immune response

Localized resorption (re-sorp-shun) occurs in a specific area of a bone as a result of infection, altered mechanical stress, or pressure on the bone so that it adapts by removing bone tissue. In contrast, generalized resorption occurs over the entire skeleton in varying amounts because of endocrine activity to increase blood levels of calcium and phosphate needed by the body.

Microscopically, a cross section of bone demonstrates layers related to its development that look like growth rings in a tree, similar to those noted in cementum (see Figures 14-10 and 14-13). The arrest lines, or resting lines, appear as smooth lines between the layers of bone because of osteoblasts having rested, formed bone, and then rested again after appositional growth. Thus, arrest lines show the incremental or layered nature of appositional growth. In contrast, reversal lines appear as scalloped lines between the layers of bone. Reversal lines represent areas where bone resorption has first taken place, followed quickly by appositional growth of new bone.

As a person grows from fetal life through childhood, puberty, and finishes growth as a young adult, the bones of the skeleton change in size and shape; these can be noted on radiographs. The "bone age" of a child is the average age at which children reach this stage of bone maturation, and a child's current height and bone age can be used to predict adult height. With aging, the generalized loss of bone mass or density is increased.

Clinical Considerations with Bone Tissue

Resorption of bone can occur in an uncontrolled manner during active advanced periodontal disease (considered periodontitis), which is in contrast to that occurring in a controlled manner with orthodontic therapy (see **Chapters 14 and 20,** respectively). At the same time as resorption, regeneration of bone occurs even in the presence of injury and disease. Excess generalized bone resorption, as well as excess bone appositional growth, can occur in certain systemic bone disorders when the two processes are no longer balanced, such as Paget disease.

Bone mass or density can increasingly be lost in women after menopause with the bones losing calcium and other minerals. This can become accelerated with the systemic bone disease of osteoporosis, especially for older women. The spinal column also becomes curved, compressed, and shorter; bone spurs may also form on the vertebrae that have become thinner with mineral and fluid loss; now bones become more brittle and may break more easily, especially those involved with the hip. This tissue degeneration can also affect the bones involved with the temporomandibular joint.

BLOOD PROPERTIES

The blood is a fluid connective tissue that serves as a transport medium for cellular nutrients, such as respiratory gases like oxygen and carbon dioxide, as well as metabolites for the entire body. Blood is carried in endothelium-lined blood vessels, and its medium consists of plasma and blood components (Table 8-4).

PLASMA

The plasma (plaz-mah) is the fluid substance in the blood vessels that carries the plasma proteins, blood cells, and metabolites. It is more consistent in composition than tissue fluid and lymph, yet it contain most of the same materials with the addition of red blood cells (se Chapter 7). Serum, another fluid product, is distinguished from the plasma from which it is derived due to the removal of clotting proteins. If a sample of blood is treated with an agent to prevent clotting and is spun in a centrifuge, the plasma fraction is the least dense and will float as the top layer.

BLOOD COMPONENTS

Blood cells and associated derivatives are also called the *formed elements* of the blood. Most blood cells develop from a common stem cell in the bone marrow (Figure 8-16). The formed elements of the blood include the numerous red blood cells. Not only are these cells present in the blood and its vessels, but also certain related components are also present in surrounding connective tissue.

Thus the most common cell in the blood is the red blood cell (RBC) (or erythrocyte) (see Table 8-4). An RBC is a biconcave disc that contains hemoglobin, which binds and then transports the oxygen and carbon dioxide. It has no nucleus and does not undergo mitosis because it is directly formed from the bone marrow's stem cells. There are 5 to 6 million per cubic milliliter of blood and are more common than other blood cells. In centrifuged blood, the RBCs settle to the bottom because they are also denser than the rest; this fraction is the *hematocrit.*

The blood also contains platelets (plate-lits) (or thrombocytes), which are smaller than RBCs, disc shaped, and also have no nucleus. However, these formed elements are not considered true blood cells but instead fragments of bone marrow cells (or megakaryocyte and platelets are also found in much lesser numbers than RBCs ... 250,000 to 400,000 per cubic milliliter. Platelets function in the clotting mechanism.

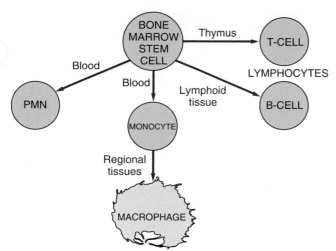

FIGURE 8-16 Flowchart demonstrating that most blood cells develop from a common stem cell type in the bone marrow. B-cell lymphocytes stay and mature in the bone marrow, and T-cell lymphocytes travel to mature in other glands or tissue in the body, such as the thymus. Later, both types of lymphocytes will engage in immune responses throughout the body. Note also the polymorphonuclear leukocyte (PMN; or neutrophil) and monocyte (or macrophage). (From Fehrenbach MJ: Immunity and immunologic oral lesions. In Ibsen OAC, Phelan JA: *Oral pathology for dental hygienists*, ed 6, St Louis 2014, Saunders.)

In even smaller numbers in the blood is the white blood cell (WBC) (or leukocyte) (see Tables 8-4 and 8-5). Like RBCs, WBCs form from bone marrow stem cells. The WBCs later mature in the bone marrow or in various lymphatic organs. They are involved in the defense mechanisms of the body, including the inflammatory and immune responses. Thus, WBCs are also usually found in both epithelium and connective tissue after they migrate from the blood by moving through openings between the cell junctions of the endothelial lining of the vessel to participate in defense mechanisms.

The WBCs differ from RBCs because they possess a nucleus, have more cytoplasm, and have the power of active amoeboid movement in order to migrate from the blood to the tissue; thus, unlike RBCs, WBCs perform their functions not only in the blood but also in other tissue. They are also even less numerous than platelets (only 5,000 to 10,000 per cubic milliliter). There are five main types based on their microscopic structure: neutrophils, lymphocytes, monocytes, eosinophils, and basophils. The fraction of centrifuged blood that settles on the surface of the hematocrit consists of the WBCs along with platelets, forming the intermediately-placed buffy coat with the plasma fraction superior to it.

The most common WBC in the blood is the polymorphonuclear leukocyte (pol-ee-mor fah-**noo**-klee-er **loo**-ko-site) (PMN; or neutrophil) (Figure 8-17). These are the first cells to appear at an injury site when the inflammatory response is triggered; thus, large numbers of the PMNs can be present in the suppuration, or pus, which in certain cases forms locally at the injury site. PMNs constitute 54% to 62% of the total blood WBC count. They have a short life span, contain lysosomal enzymes, are active in phagocytosis, and respond to chemotactic factors (see **Chapter 7**).

The second most common WBC in the blood is the lymphocyte (**lim**-fo-site), which makes up 25% to 33% of the count. There are three functional types of lymphocytes: B cell, T cell, and natural killer (NK) cell. B- cells mature in the bone marrow and gut-associated lymphoid tissue such as lymph nodes (see Figure 11-16), whereas T cells mature in the thymus (see Figure 8-16). NK cells also mature in the bone marrow. NK cells are large cells that are involved in the first

line of defense against tumor- or virally-infected cells by killing them and thus are not considered part of the immune response.

Cytokines are produced by B and T cells and are chemical mediators of the immune response (see the discussion in **Chapter 14** related to periodontal disease). Thus, both of these types of lymphocytes are involved in the immune response (see Table 8-5). In the past, the immune response was broken into two strict divisions: humoral with B-cells and cell-mediated with T-cells. However, the distinction between the two divisions is now considered less important because they are strongly related.

One important difference between the two divisions remains: The B-cell lymphocytes divide during the immune response to form plasma cells. Once mature, plasma cells produce an immunoglobulin (im-u-nah-**glob**-ul-in) (Ig), which is also considered an antibody and one of the blood proteins. There are five distinct classes of immunoglobulins: IgA (serum or secretory types), IgD, IgE, IgG, and IgM (Table 8-6). Each plasma cell produces only one specific class of immunoglobulin in response to a specific immunogen (im-un-ah-jen) (or antigen). Immunogens are mainly proteins that are seen by the body as foreign and are capable of triggering an immune response.

Although immunoglobulin structure overall is very similar, a small region at the tip of the protein (hypervariable region) is extremely variable, allowing generation of an infinite number with slightly different tip structures, or antigen binding sites, to exist. An immunoglobulin, along with its specific immunogen (with epitope variable region), often forms an immune complex in an effort to render the immunogen unable to cause disease. Immunoglobulins can be extracted from the blood of recovering patients and used for passive immunization against certain infectious diseases.

However, the most common WBC in the connective tissue proper is the macrophage (mak-rah-faje), which is considered a monocyte (mon-ah-site) before it migrates from the blood into the tissue. They have a longer lifespan than PMNs but constitute only 2% to 10% of the WBC count. After migration, macrophages arrive at the site of injury later and in fewer numbers than PMNs when the inflammatory response is triggered. Macrophages contain lysosomal enzymes, are involved in phagocytosis (as are PMNs), are actively mobile, and have the ability to respond to chemotactic factors and cytokines (see Figure 7-4). Macrophages also assist in the immune response to facilitate immunoglobulin production. In certain disease states, numbers of macrophages may fuse together, forming giant cells with multiple nuclei. In bone connective tissue, these are then considered osteoclasts that will resorb bone (discussed earlier).

The eosinophil (e-ah-**sin**-ah-fil) is usually only 6% of the WBC count, but its percentage is increased during a hypersensitivity response (allergy) and in parasitic diseases because its primary function seems to be the phagocytosis of immune complexes.

The basophil (bay-sah-fil) is usually found to be less than 1% of the WBC count and is also involved in the hypersensitivity response. Other WBCs located in the connective tissue include the mast cell, which is similar in structure to the basophil. As with basophils, mast cells are also involved in the hypersensitivity response. However, even though both cells are derived from the bone marrow, they probably originate from different stem cells.

Clinical Considerations with Blood-Related Situations

Dental professionals must understand certain laboratory procedures that patients may have undergone, when viewing the medical record. These procedures include a complete blood count (CBC), which is an evaluation of both RBC and WBC types to detect infections, anemia, or leukemia. A platelet count can also be performed to determine

TABLE 8-5	Blood Cells and Related Tissue Cells		
CELLS	**MICROSCOPIC STRUCTURE**	**FEATURES**	**FUNCTIONS**
Polymorphonuclear leukocyte (or neutrophil)		Multilobed nucleus with granules	Inflammatory response: Phagocytosis
Lymphocyte		Eccentric round nucleus without granules: B, T, and natural killer cells	B and T cell immune response: Humoral and cell-mediated. Natural killer cells; defense against tumor- and virally infected cells
Plasma cell		Round cartwheel nucleus derived from B-cell lymphocytes	Humoral immune response: Produces immunoglobulins (or antibodies)
Monocyte (in blood)/ macrophage (in tissue)		Bean-shaped nucleus with poorly staining granules	Inflammatory and immune response: Phagocytosis, as well as process and present immunogens (or antigens)
Eosinophil		Bilobed nucleus with granules	Hypersensitivity response
Basophil		Irregularly shaped bilobed/trilobed nucleus with granules	Hypersensitivity response
Mast cell (in tissue)		Irregularly shaped bilobed nucleus with granules	Hypersensitivity response

the platelet number if bleeding problems are a consideration due to past medical history, and a coagulation (bleeding) test can also be performed to test platelet function. These procedures may also be recommended to the patient if there is clinical evidence of unusual periodontal diseases, such as an aggressive periodontitis with its uncontrolled loss of periodontal support.

The latest clinical use of a blood product in dental procedures, which is already well known in medicine, is platelet-rich plasma (PRP)—an autogenous blood clot taken from one's own blood system, which is then used later to support both soft and hard tissue healing (i.e., osteoid, blood vessels, and even collagen). This increase in healing level occurs because the PRP contains vast amount of growth factors as well as having other various healing mechanisms along with the high concentration of platelets. The PRP is used to coat implants and is placed in soft tissue flaps following periodontal surgery to promote repair of bony defects, as well as with graft placement.

With postexposure prophylaxis of dental healthcare personnel (DHCP), a passive injection of hepatitis B immunoglobulin (HBIG) is given if there is evidence that they are without seroconversion after the usually required vaccination for the infection. It is made from human plasma containing immunoglobulins made in response to the type B form of hepatitis.

MUSCLE PROPERTIES

The muscle in the body is part of the muscular system, and similar to connective tissue, most muscles are derived from somites (see Figure 3-13). Each muscle shortens under neural control, causing soft tissue and bony structures of the body to move. The three types of muscle are classified according to structure, function, and innervation: skeletal, smooth, and cardiac (see Table 8-1).

MUSCLE CLASSIFICATION

Each type of muscle has its own type of action, which is the movement accomplished when the muscle cells contract. Smooth muscle and

FIGURE 8-17 Electron micrograph of a polymorphonuclear leukocyte (or neutrophil), which is the most common white blood cell. (Courtesy of Jan Cope, RDH, MS, Associate Professor, Oregon Institute of Technology, Klamath Falls, OR.)

TABLE 8-6	Known Immunoglobulins (Antibodies) from Plasma Cells
IMMUNOGLOBULIN	**FEATURES AND FUNCTIONS**
IgA	Has two subgroups: serous in blood; secretory in saliva, tears, and breast milk; both aid in defense against pathogens in body fluids
IgD	Functions in activation of B-cell lymphocytes as antigen receptor; has been shown to activate basophils and mast cells to produce antimicrobial factors
IgE	Involved in hypersensitivity response; binds to mast cells and basophils and releases bioactive substances such as histamine
IgG	Has four subgroups; major immunoglobulin in blood serum and can pass placental barrier to form first passive immunity for newborn
IgM	Involved in early immune responses against pathogens because of involvement with IgD in activation of B-cell lymphocytes before sufficient immunoglobulin production

cardiac muscle are considered involuntary muscles because they are under autonomic nervous system control (discussed next). Smooth muscles are located in organs, glands, and the linings of blood vessels. Cardiac muscle is in the wall of the heart (myocardium).

Skeletal muscles are considered voluntary muscles because they are under voluntary control, involving the somatic nervous system (Figure 8-18). All the major muscles of the body's appendages and trunk are skeletal muscles. Thus, skeletal muscles are usually attached to bones of the skeleton. Skeletal muscles also include the muscles of the facial expression, tongue, pharynx, and upper esophagus, as well as the muscles of mastication that assist the temporomandibular joint in the actions involved in mastication (see Figure 19-8).

SKELETAL MUSCLE HISTOLOGY

Skeletal muscles are also called *striated muscles* because the muscle cells appear striped microscopically. Each muscle is composed of numerous muscle bundles, or fascicles, which then are composed of numerous muscle cells, or *myofibers*. Each myofiber extends the entire length of the muscle and is composed of smaller myofibrils surrounded by the other organelles of the cell. Each myofibril is composed of even smaller myofilaments.

NERVE TISSUE PROPERTIES

Nerve tissue forms the nervous system in the body, being derived from the neuroectoderm within the embryo (see Figure 3-10). Nerves function to carry messages or impulses based on electrical potentials. Nerve tissue in the body causes muscles to contract, resulting in facial expressions and joint movements, such as those associated with mastication and speech. The tissue stimulates glands to secrete hormones

and regulates many other systems of the body, such as the cardiovascular system. It also allows for the perception of sensations, such as pain, touch, taste, and smell.

NERVE TISSUE HISTOLOGY

A **neuron** (noor-on) is the functional cellular component of the nervous system and is composed of three parts: one neural cell body with two different types of neural cytoplasmic processes (Figure 8-19). The neural cell body is not involved in the process of impulse transmission but provides the metabolic support for the entire neuron.

One type of process associated with the cell body is an **axon** (ax-on), a long, thin, singular, cable-like process that conducts impulses away from the cell body. An axon is encased in its own cell membrane, having nerve excitability and conduction due to changes that develop in the nerve membrane. Certain axons can also be additionally covered by a myelin sheath.

The myelin sheath consists of tightly wrapped layers of phospholipid-rich membrane surrounding the Schwann cell cytoplasm; there is very little cytoplasm sandwiched between them. It is only in the outermost layer of the myelin sheath where the Schwann cell and its nucleus are located. Along a myelinated axon are the nodes of Ranvier, which form a gap between the adjacent Schwann cells. The insulating properties of the myelin sheath and its gaps allow the axon to conduct impulses more quickly. The other type of process associated with the cell body is the dendrite—a threadlike process that usually contains multiple branches, which functions to receive and conduct impulses toward the cell body.

A **nerve** is a bundle of neural processes outside the central nervous system (CNS) and in the peripheral nervous system (PNS). A **synapse** (sin-aps) is the junction between two neurons or between a neuron and an effector organ (such as a muscle or gland) where neural impulses are transmitted by chemical means (neurotransmitter substance). To function, most tissue or organs have innervation, a supply of nerves. A nerve allows information to be carried to and from the

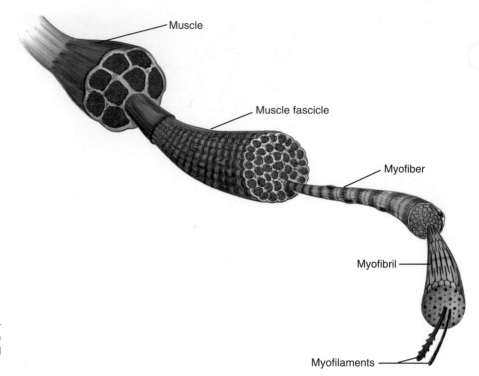

FIGURE 8-18 Skeletal muscle with its striations and which is composed of smaller muscle bundles, fascicles, myofibers, myofibrils, and myofilaments.

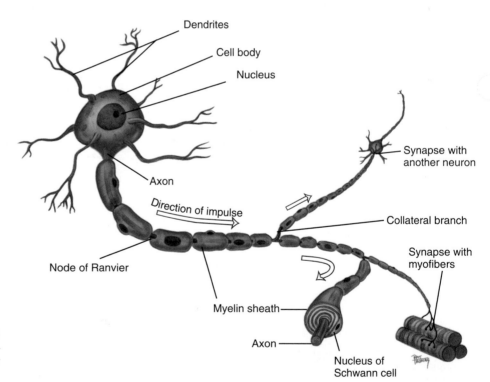

FIGURE 8-19 Neuron with its dendrites, cell body, and axon, showing a synaptic relationship with the muscle, as well as with another neuron.

brain, which is the central information center. An aggregation of neuron cell bodies outside the CNS is termed a *ganglion* (plural, *ganglia*).

The two functional types of nerves are afferent and efferent nerves. An afferent nerve, or sensory nerve, carries information or relays impulses from the periphery of the body to the brain (or spinal cord). Thus, an afferent nerve carries sensory information (such as taste, pain, or proprioception) to the brain. Proprioception is information concerning the movement and position of the body. This sensory information is sent on to the brain to be analyzed, acted upon, associated with other information, and stored as memory.

An efferent nerve, or motor nerve, carries information away from the brain to the periphery of the body. Thus, an efferent nerve carries information to the muscles or glands in order to activate them, often in response to information received by the afferent nerve pathway. One motor neuron with its branching fibers may control hundreds of muscle fibers. Autonomic nerves are (by definition) always efferent.

Within the pulp, the nerves include sensory types. In addition, the afferent axons of these sensory pulp nerves are also located in the dentinal tubules that make up the dentin. Thus, when the either dentin or pulp is injured or restored, the sensation of pain is perceived by the brain.

TABLE 8-7	Nervous System Divisions
DIVISIONS	**COMPONENTS**
Central nervous system	Brain and spinal cord
Peripheral nervous system	Spinal and cranial nerves of the somatic nervous system and autonomic nervous system (includes sympathetic and parasympathetic systems)

NERVOUS SYSTEM

The nervous system has two main divisions: the CNS and the PNS (Table 8-7). These two systems are not separate but rely on each other and thus constantly interact. The CNS consists of the brain and spinal cord. The PNS consists of the spinal and cranial nerves and includes both the somatic nervous system and the autonomic nervous system (ANS). The spinal nerves extend from the spinal cord to the periphery of the body. The cranial nerves are initially attached to the brain, which then pass through openings in the skull. Certain cranial nerves are associated with the oral cavity, especially the fifth cranial nerve or trigeminal nerve. The somatic nervous system operates with conscious control of the individual to move the skeletal muscles.

The ANS is a part of the PNS and operates without conscious control as the caretaker of the body. Autonomic nerves are efferent processes, and they are always in two-neuron circuits. The first neuron carries autonomic impulses to a ganglion, where they are transmitted to the body of the second neuron. The ANS itself has two divisions: a sympathetic system and parasympathetic system (see Table 8-7). Most tissue or organ systems are supplied by both divisions of the ANS.

The sympathetic nervous system is involved in fight-or-flight responses, such as in the inhibition of salivary gland secretion (hyposalivation). Such a response by the sympathetic system leads to a dry mouth (xerostomia) (see Figure 11-9). Sympathetic neurons arise in the spinal cord and synapse in ganglia arranged in a chain extending nearly the length of the vertebral column on both sides. Therefore, all the sympathetic neurons in the head have already synapsed in a ganglion. Sympathetic fibers reach the cranial tissue that they supply by traveling with the arteries.

The parasympathetic nervous system is involved in rest-or-digest responses, such as the stimulation of salivary gland secretion. Such a response leads to salivary flow to aid in digestion. Parasympathetic fibers associated with glands of the head and neck region are carried in various cranial nerves, and their ganglia are located in the head. Therefore, parasympathetic neurons in this region may be either preganglionic neurons (before synapsing in the ganglion) or postganglionic neurons (after synapsing in the ganglion).

CHAPTER 9

Oral Mucosa

ⓔ Additional resources and practice exercises are provided on the companion Evolve website for this book: http://evolve.elsevier.com/Fehrenbach/illustrated.

●●●LEARNING OBJECTIVES

1. Define and pronounce the key terms in this chapter.
2. List and describe the types of oral mucosa, characterizing each type of epithelium associated with the oral cavity.
3. Discuss the clinical considerations for oral mucosa pathology, integrating it into patient care.
4. Identify the components of each type of oral mucosa on a diagram.
5. List and discuss the clinical correlations associated with the regional differences in the oral mucosa, integrating it into patient care.
6. Discuss tongue and lingual papillae properties as well as oral mucosa pigmentation and the clinical considerations for both.
7. Discuss the turnover times for regions of the oral cavity and associated clinical correlations, as well as repair and aging considerations, integrating it into patient care.

ORAL MUCOSA PROPERTIES

Dental professionals must have a clear understanding of the basic histology of the oral mucosa, its regional differences, and any related clinical considerations. Only then will they be able to further understand the clinical considerations involved with the process of aging, as well as injury to the oral mucosa. This injury to the oral mucosa can include that which occurs with trauma, inflammation, infection, and cancer as discussed later in this chapter. With this information, they then can promote the health of the oral mucosa.

Oral mucosa almost continuously lines the oral cavity. Microscopically oral mucosa is composed of stratified squamous epithelium overlying a connective tissue proper, or lamina propria, with possibly a deeper submucosa (Figure 9-1). In the skin, these two similar tissue types are known as the *epidermis* and *dermis* (see **Chapter 8**).

Even though the entire oral cavity has an epithelial covering with connective tissue making up the bulk of lamina propria, regional differences are noted throughout in the oral mucosa. For example, the oral mucosa is perforated in various regions by the ducts of salivary glands (see Figure 11-6). Other areas have thinner or thicker epithelium and some areas of the lamina propria contain specialized fibers. This chapter also discusses these regional differences; however, the gingival sulcular region is discussed in more detail in **Chapter 10**.

As always, a basement membrane lies between the epithelium and connective tissue of the oral mucosa (see Figures 7-6 and 8-4). It serves not as a separation between the two tissue types but as a continuous structure linking the two. Studies are focusing on trying to understand the interactions between these two tissue types, and the basement membrane may hold these answers.

Three main types of oral mucosa are found in the oral cavity: lining, masticatory, and specialized mucosa (Table 9-1). This classification of oral mucosa is based on the general histologic features of the tissue. As noted before, the specific histologic features of each oral region are discussed later in this chapter. Overall, the clinical appearance of the tissue reflects the underlying histology, both in health and disease.

Thus, the oral cavity has correctly been described as a mirror that reflects the health of the individual. Changes indicative of disease are seen as alterations in the oral mucosa lining the mouth, which can reveal systemic conditions such as diabetes or vitamin deficiency or the local effects of chronic tobacco or alcohol use.

LINING MUCOSA

The **lining mucosa** (mu-ko-sah) is a type of oral mucosa noted for its softer surface texture, moist surface, and ability to stretch and be compressed, acting as a cushion for the underlying structures. Lining mucosa includes that of the buccal mucosa, labial mucosa, alveolar mucosa, as well as the oral mucosa lining the ventral surface of the tongue, floor of the mouth, and soft palate.

Microscopically lining mucosa is a type that is associated with non-keratinized stratified squamous epithelium (Figure 9-2). In contrast to masticatory mucosa, which is discussed next, the interface between the epithelium and the lamina propria is generally smoother with fewer and less-pronounced rete ridges and connective tissue papillae. In addition to these factors, the presence of elastic fibers in the lamina propria also provides the tissue with a movable base.

A submucosa deep to the lamina propria is usually present in lining mucosa, overlying muscle and allowing compression of the superficial tissue. These general histologic features allow this type of mucosa to serve in regions of the oral cavity where a movable base is needed, such as during speech, mastication, and swallowing. Thus, surgical incisions in this tissue frequently require sutures for closure due to tissue movement. Local anesthetic injections into lining mucosa are also easier to accomplish than in masticatory mucosa with less discomfort and easy dispersion of the agent, but infections also spread rapidly. And dental medications have less difficulty being absorbed since this type is the most permeable to liquid.

MASTICATORY MUCOSA

The **masticatory (mass-ti-ka-tor-ee) mucosa** is a type of oral mucosa noted for its rubbery surface texture and resiliency. Masticatory mucosa includes that of the hard palate, attached gingiva, and dorsal surface of the tongue. Microscopically masticatory mucosa is associated with orthokeratinized stratified squamous epithelium as well as parakeratinized stratified squamous epithelium, which will both be discussed later in this chapter (Figures 9-3, 9-4, and 9-5). Unlike lining mucosa discussed earlier, the interface between the epithelium and lamina propria in masticatory mucosa is highly interdigitated with numerous and more-pronounced rete ridges and connective tissue papillae, giving it a firm base. In addition, the deeper submucosa is an extremely thin layer or is absent. When masticatory mucosa overlies bone, with or without submucosa, it increases the firmness of the tissue.

These general histologic features allow masticatory mucosa to function in the regions that need a firm base, such as during mastication and speech. Thus, sutures are rarely needed for this tissue after surgery because it has less tissue movement. However, local anesthetic injections are more difficult and cause greater discomfort in masticatory mucosa than those in lining mucosa due to its firmness, as well as when any swelling from an infectious source occurs in the tissue. And dental medications have more difficulty being absorbed because this type is least permeable to liquid.

SPECIALIZED MUCOSA

The **specialized mucosa** is a type of oral mucosa found on the dorsal surface of the tongue, as well as the lateral surface of the tongue, in the

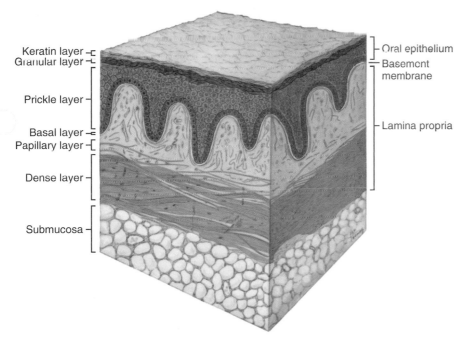

Keratin layer
Granular layer
Prickle layer
Basal layer
Papillary layer
Dense layer
Submucosa

Oral epithelium
Basement membrane
Lamina propria

Oral Mucosa
(and underlying tissue)

FIGURE 9-1 General histologic features of an oral mucosa composed of stratified squamous epithelium overlying lamina propria with a deeper submucosa present.

TABLE 9-1	Oral Mucosa Types		
TYPES	**REGIONS**	**GENERAL CLINICAL APPEARANCE**	**GENERAL HISTOLOGIC FEATURES**
Lining mucosa	Buccal mucosa, labial mucosa, alveolar mucosa, ventral surface of the tongue, floor of the mouth, and soft palate	Softer surface texture, moist surface, and ability to stretch and be compressed, acting as a cushion	Nonkeratinized epithelium with smooth interface, few rete ridges and connective tissue papillae, with elastic fibers in lamina propria and submucosa
Masticatory mucosa	Attached gingiva, hard palate, and dorsal surface of the tongue	Rubbery surface texture and resiliency, serving as firm base	Keratinized epithelium and interdigitated interface with many rete ridges and connective tissue papillae with thin layer of submucosa or none
Specialized mucosa	Dorsal and lateral surface of the tongue	Associated with lingual papillae	Discrete structures of epithelium and lamina propria; many with taste buds (see Table 9-5)

form of the lingual papillae (see Figures 2-14 and 2-15). Microscopically lingual papillae are discrete structures composed of keratinized epithelium and lamina propria (discussed later in this chapter).

EPITHELIUM OF ORAL MUCOSA

Three types of stratified squamous epithelium are found within the oral cavity: nonkeratinized, orthokeratinized, and parakeratinized (Table 9-2). Although all three types of epithelium are similar in many ways, they are also different, primarily in the surface layers of the epithelium as will be discussed in this chapter.

Nonkeratinized epithelium is associated with lining mucosa. Orthokeratinized and parakeratinized epithelium are both associated with masticatory mucosa as well as specialized mucosa. All types of epithelium usually act as an environmental barrier to pathogenic invasion and mechanical irritation as well as offering protection against dryness. These

protective features are accentuated in the types of epithelium that contain keratin (ker-ah-tin). Histologists use the term *keratinocytes* for the epithelial cells in oral mucosa that can produce keratin either at the usual levels if it is a keratinized tissue, or at higher levels when the tissue becomes traumatized, even in previously nonkeratinized tissue (Table 9-3).

The nonkeratinocytes, those cells that do not produce keratin in epithelium, are present in much smaller numbers in oral mucosa (see Table 9-3). These cells include melanocytes (discussed later in this chapter) along with the associated production of melanin pigmentation. Also present in epithelium of oral mucosa are Granstein and Langerhans cells, both of which arise from the bone marrow and help the tissue's immune responses, as well as Merkel cells, which are involved in tactile sensory information. White blood

FIGURE 9-4 Electron micrograph of keratinized epithelium showing both the granular and keratin layers. Small keratohyaline granules are visible in the granular layer; the cells of the keratin layer are flattened and contain keratin. However, it is hard to discern at this lower-power magnification whether this tissue is orthokeratinized or parakeratinized based on the presence of nuclei of the keratin layer. (From Nanci A: *Ten Cate's oral histology*, ed 8, St Louis, 2013, Mosby.)

Nonkeratinized Stratified Squamous Epithelium
(and deeper tissue)

FIGURE 9-2 General histologic features of a lining mucosa composed of nonkeratinized stratified squamous epithelium (with three layers) overlying lamina propria. A deeper submucosa is usually present overlying muscle.

FIGURE 9-3 General histologic features of masticatory mucosa composed of orthokeratinized stratified squamous epithelium (with four layers) overlying lamina propria. A deeper thin submucosa may or may not be present and may overlay bone (as shown here). Note that the cells in the keratin layer have lost their nuclei and are filled with keratin. However, the artifact of the spiky look of the prickle layer has not been shown.

Orthokeratinized Stratified Squamous Epithelium
(and deeper tissue)

Keratin layer
Granular layer
Prickle layer
Basal layer
Lamina propria
Alveolar process

Squames with keratin and nuclei

Parakeratinized Stratified Squamous Epithelium
(and deeper tissue)

FIGURE 9-5 General histologic features of masticatory mucosa, which is composed of parakeratinized stratified squamous epithelium (with three to four layers) overlying lamina propria. Note that the cells in the keratin layer have retained their nuclei and are filled with keratin. However, the artifact of the spiky look of the prickle layer that can occur with microscopic fixation is not demonstrated. A deeper thin submucosa may or may not be present. If the submucosa is not present (as shown here), the oral mucosa and periosteum of the bone combine and are then considered a mucoperiosteum that is directly attached to the underlying bone of the alveolar process.

TABLE 9-2	Epithelium of Oral Mucosa	
TYPES OF EPITHELIUM	**ASSOCIATED ORAL MUCOSA**	**GENERAL HISTOLOGIC FEATURES**
Nonkeratinized epithelium	Lining mucosa	Basal, intermediate, superficial layers
Orthokeratinized epithelium	Masticatory mucosa	Basal, prickle, granular, keratin layers (cells contain only keratin and no nuclei)
Parakeratinized epithelium	Masticatory mucosa	Basal, prickle, granular, keratin layers (cells contain keratin and nuclei)

TABLE 9-3	Cells Types in Epithelium*	
TYPES	**FEATURES**	**FUNCTIONS**
Epithelial cell	Rapidly renewing cell that usually undergoes pathway of differentiation with desmosomes; can be derived from all three embryonic cell layers	Forms cohesive sheet that resists physical forces and usually serves as barrier to infection
Granstein cell	Similar to Langerhans cell	Same as Langerhans cell
Langerhans cell	Dendritic bone marrow–derived cell with Langerhans granule; predominately suprabasal	Immune response with T-cell lymphocytes; antigen trapping and processing
Melanocyte	Dendritic cell of neural crest cell origin; premelanosomes and melanosomes present; forms a continuous network in basal layers	Synthesis of melanin pigmentation inclusion granules (melanosomes) with transfer to adjacent keratinocytes by injection
Merkel cell	Nondendritic neural cell noted in basal layers; characteristic electron-dense vesicles and associated nerve axon	Tactile sensory information

*White blood cells are not included in this table.

cells are also present, with the polymorphonuclear leukocyte being the most commonly occurring one in all forms of oral mucosa (see Figure 8-17).

Using recent ultrastructural studies, the superficial surface layer of most types of epithelium in oral mucosa has now been shown to contain cellular ridge-like folds, **microplicae** (my-kro-**plee**-kay) (MPL). These are known to be typical of the surfaces of the body covered with protective mucus, or in the case of the oral cavity, saliva. The role of MPL present on the superficial layer of oral epithelial cells is still unknown, but it may form a protective structure along with the saliva.

NONKERATINIZED STRATIFIED SQUAMOUS EPITHELIUM

The **nonkeratinized stratified squamous epithelium** (non-ker-ah-tin-izd strat-i-fide skway-mus ep-ee-thee-lee-um) is located in the superficial layers of lining mucosa, such as in the labial mucosa, buccal mucosa, and alveolar mucosa, as well as in the oral mucosa lining the floor of the mouth, the ventral surface of the tongue, and the soft palate (see Figure 9-2). Lining mucosa has similar epithelial histologic features, even though it has its own regional differences. Nonkeratinized epithelium is the most common form of epithelium in the oral cavity.

Each area of lining mucosa has at least three layers within the epithelium. A **basal** (bay-sal) **layer,** or *stratum basale,* is the deepest of

the three layers. The basal layer is a single layer of cuboidal epithelial cells overlying the basement membrane, which, in turn, is situated superior to the lamina propria. The basal layer produces the basal lamina of the basement membrane.

The basal layer is also considered germinative because mitosis of the epithelial cells occurs within this layer; however, this cell division is seen only under higher-power magnification of the tissue (see Table 7-2). Future ultrastructural studies may show the existence of an epithelial stem cell in the basal layer that produces other stem and daughter cells, similar to the situation for blood cells in the bone marrow.

The layer of epithelium superficial to the basal layer in nonkeratinized epithelium is the intermediate layer, or *stratum intermedium*. The intermediate layer is composed of larger, stacked, polyhedral-shaped cells. These cells appear larger and plumper than the basal layer cells because they have larger amounts cytoplasm. However, as they migrate superficially, the cells of the intermediate layer have lost the ability to undergo mitosis. The intermediate layer makes up the bulk of nonkeratinized stratified squamous epithelium.

At the most superficial level in nonkeratinized epithelium is the superficial layer, or *stratum superficiale*. It is hard to discern the exact division between the superficial layer and the deeper intermediate layers in lining mucosa when viewing microscopic sections. The superficial layer shows even larger, similarly stacked polyhedral epithelial cells but with the outer cells flattening into squames. The squames in these layers show shedding or loss as they age and die during the turnover of the tissue. In summary, maturation within this nonkeratinized tissue is at a lesser level than keratinized tissue, seeing only the increase in the size of cells as they migrate superficially, unlike the more complex changes that occur in the most superficial layers of keratinized tissue.

ORTHOKERATINIZED STRATIFIED SQUAMOUS EPITHELIUM

In contrast to nonkeratinized tissue, the orthokeratinized (or-tho-ker-ah-tin-izd) stratified squamous epithelium demonstrates a keratinization of the epithelial cells throughout its most superficial layers (see Figures 9-3 and 9-4). Orthokeratinized epithelium is the least common form of epithelium found in the oral cavity. It is associated with the masticatory mucosa of the hard palate and the attached gingiva. It is also associated with the specialized mucosa of the lingual papillae on the dorsal surface of the tongue. As this tissue matures, it forms keratin within its most superficial cells, as well as showing a visible and physiologic difference in the cells as they migrate superficially.

Like nonkeratinized epithelium, orthokeratinized epithelium has a single basal layer, or *stratum basale*, undergoing mitosis. This layer also produces the basal lamina of the adjacent basement membrane. Unlike nonkeratinized epithelium, however, orthokeratinized epithelium has more layers superficial to the basal layer—four separate layers with somewhat distinct divisions.

Superficial to the basal layer is the prickle layer, or the *stratum spinosum*. This is named for an artifact that occurs when the regularly plump epithelial cells of this layer are fixed for prolonged microscopic study; the cells shrink as a result of cytoplasm loss from the drying fixation chemicals (see Figure 7-5). Thus, a prickly or spiky look results when the individual dehydrated cells are still joined at their outer edges by desmosomes. In live tissue, they migrate to this superior level in the tissue, and also lose the ability to undergo mitosis, such as noted in the deeper basal layer. The prickle layer makes up the bulk of orthokeratinized epithelium.

Superficial to the prickle layer is the granular layer, or *stratum granulosum*. The epithelial cells in this layer are flat and stacked in a layer three to five cells thick. In their cytoplasm, each of the cells has a nucleus with prominent keratohyaline (ker-ah-toe-hi-ah-lene) granules, which appear microscopically as dark spots. The keratohyaline granules form a chemical precursor for the keratin (keratohyalin) that is found in the more superficial layers.

The most superficial layer in orthokeratinized epithelium is the keratin layer, or *stratum corneum*, which shows variable thickness depending on the oral cavity region. The cells in the keratin layer are flat and have no nuclei, and their cytoplasm is filled with keratin. The soft, opaque, waterproof keratin is formed from a complex of keratohyaline granules and intermediate filaments from the cells, and it appears microscopically as a translucent dense material. The outer cells of the keratin layer, or squames, show increased flattening and also shedding or loss because they are no longer viable.

In addition, parts of the keratin material are also shed as a result of the turnover of the tissue. However, these squames and their cornified cell envelope make up a major part of the epithelial barrier discussed earlier and are continuously being renewed as cells mature from the deeper layers. The epithelial barrier serves as protection from physical, chemical, and pathogenic attack, as well as dehydration and heat loss that sometimes can occur in the oral cavity environment.

PARAKERATINIZED STRATIFIED SQUAMOUS EPITHELIUM

The parakeratinized (pare-ah-ker-ah-tin-izd) stratified squamous epithelium is associated with the masticatory mucosa of the attached gingiva in higher levels than the presence of orthokeratinization (see Figures 9-4 and 9-5). Most histologists believe that parakeratinized epithelium is an immature form of orthokeratinized epithelium. The presence of this form of keratinization on the skin is considered a disease state; therefore, parakeratinization is one of the unique histologic features of the healthy oral cavity. Parakeratinized epithelium along with orthokeratinized epithelium is also associated with the specialized mucosa of the lingual papillae on the dorsal surface of the tongue.

Parakeratinized epithelium may have all the same layers of epithelium as orthokeratinized epithelium (such as the basal layer, prickle layer, granular layer, and keratin layer), although the granular layer may be indistinct or absent altogether.

The main difference between parakeratinized epithelium and orthokeratinized epithelium is in the cells of the keratin layer. In parakeratinized epithelium, the most superficial layer is still being shed and lost similar to orthokeratinized epithelium. However, these cells of the keratin layer contain not only keratin but also nuclei, unlike those of orthokeratinized epithelium. This distinction is sometimes difficult to discern under lower-power magnification in microscopic sections. Studies have shown that even though the epithelial cells have nuclei in the parakeratinized epithelium, they possibly are no longer viable, which is similar to the orthokeratinized epithelium. Further ultrastructural studies need to be done to see if this main difference in the cells of the keratin layers between the two types of tissue plays out in their functioning.

LAMINA PROPRIA OF ORAL MUCOSA

All forms of epithelium, whether associated with lining, masticatory, or specialized mucosa, have an adjoining connective tissue proper located deep to the basement membrane. In the case of oral mucosa, it is considered the lamina propria (lam-i-nah pro-pree-ah) (see Figure 9-1). The main fiber group in the lamina propria is Type I collagen fibers, but elastic fibers are present in certain regions of the oral cavity (see Table 8-3). The lamina propria, like all forms of connective tissue proper, has two layers: papillary and dense (Figure 9-6).

The papillary layer is the more superficial layer of the lamina propria. It consists of loose connective tissue within the connective tissue papillae, along with blood vessels and nerve tissue. The tissue has an equal amount of fibers, cells, and intercellular substance. The dense layer is the deeper layer of the lamina propria. It consists of dense connective tissue with a large amount of fibers. Between the papillary layer and the deeper layers of the lamina propria is a capillary (cap-ih-lary) plexus, which provides nutrition for the all layers of the oral mucosa by way of the adjacent basement membrane, sending capillaries into the surrounding connective tissue papillae.

A submucosa (sub-mu-ko-sah) may or may not be present deep to the dense layer of the lamina propria, depending on the region of the oral cavity (see Figures 9-1 and 9-11). If present, the submucosa usually contains loose connective tissue and may also contain adipose connective tissue or salivary glands, as well as overlying the bone or muscle within the oral cavity.

Lining mucosa does not have prominent connective tissue papillae that alternate with the rete ridges present in masticatory mucosa. In addition, elastic fibers are present in the papillary layer, thus allowing the lining mucosa to stretch and recoil during speech, mastication, and swallowing. In contrast to lining mucosa, masticatory mucosa has numerous and prominent connective tissue papillae, giving the oral mucosa a firm base, which is needed for speech and mastication.

The most common cell in the lamina propria of all types of oral mucosa, similar to differing locations of connective tissue proper, is the fibroblast (see Figure 8-5). Fibroblasts synthesize different types of protein fibers and intercellular substance. Histologists believe that subpopulations of the fibroblast may exist and that controlling the beneficial productive groups may be the answer to periodontal disease and age-related changes that occur in the lamina propria and other components of the periodontium. Other cells present in the lamina propria

FIGURE 9-6 General histologic features of the lamina propria (with two layers) of the oral mucosa and its relationship to the adjoining basement membrane and overlying epithelium.

Labels on figure: Basal layer of epithelium; Basement membrane; Collagen fibers; Fibroblast; Nerve; Capillary branch to papilla; Papillary layer; Capillary plexus; Dense layer

in smaller numbers are white blood cells, such as polymorphonuclear leukocytes, macrophages, lymphocytes, and mast cells (see Table 8-5).

Clinical Considerations for Oral Mucosa Pathology

Unlike keratinized epithelium, nonkeratinized epithelium usually has no superficial layers showing keratinization. Nonkeratinized epithelium may, however, readily transform into a keratinizing type in response to frictional or chemical trauma, in which case it undergoes **hyperkeratinization** (hi-per-ker-ah-tin-**zay**-shun).

This change to hyperkeratinization commonly occurs on the usually nonkeratinized buccal mucosa when the linea alba forms a white ridge of calloused tissue that extends horizontally at the level where the maxillary and mandibular teeth come together and occlude (see Figure 2-3, *B*). Microscopically an excess amount of keratin is noted at the linea alba, and the tissue has all the layers of an orthokeratinized tissue, including its granular and keratin layers.

In patients who have habits such as clenching or grinding (with bruxism) their teeth, a larger area of the buccal mucosa than just the nearby linea alba becomes hyperkeratinized (Figure 9-7). This larger white, rough, raised lesion needs to be recorded so that changes may be made in the dental treatment plan regarding the patient's parafunctional habits (see **Chapter 20**). Even keratinized tissue can undergo a further level of hyperkeratinization; an increase in the amount of keratin is produced as a result of chronic trauma to the region. This occurs to attached gingiva in the form of fibrosis during the later stages of advanced periodontal disease.

Changes such as hyperkeratinization are reversible if the source of the injury is removed, but it takes time for the keratin to be shed by the tissue. Thus it is important to rule out malignant changes, and a baseline biopsy and microscopic study of any whitened tissue may be indicated. This is especially true if the patient is within a high-risk cancer category, such as those with a history of chronic tobacco or alcohol use or those who are human papillomavirus (HPV) positive. Hyperkeratinized tissue is also associated with the chronic heat production from smoking or hot fluids on the hard palate in the form of nicotinic stomatitis, as well as with the chronic use of spit tobacco in the oral vestibules (see Figure 11-12).

ORAL MUCOSA REGIONAL DIFFERENCES

Specific histologic features are noted in the different regions of the oral cavity (Table 9-4). These specific histologic features are the basis for the differences observed clinically when these regions are examined.

Labels on figure: Hyperkeratosis; Buccal mucosa; Mandibular posterior teeth

FIGURE 9-7 Hyperkeratinization of the buccal mucosa shown by larger white, rough, raised calloused lesion than that of the nearby linea alba. Buccal mucosa usually has nonkeratinized epithelium, but this tissue has undergone chronic physical injury to the area as a result of grinding, or bruxism, of the teeth. Thus, the epithelium has become keratinized in response. Other more serious lesions of the oral cavity must be ruled out when considering this lesion. (Courtesy of Margaret J. Fehrenbach, RDH, MS.)

TABLE 9-4	Regional Differences in Oral Mucosa		
REGION AND CLINICAL APPEARANCE	**EPITHELIUM**	**LAMINA PROPRIA**	**SUBMUCOSA**
Lining Mucosa			
Labial mucosa and buccal mucosa: Opaque pink, shiny, moist with possible areas of melanin pigmentation and Fordyce spots	Thick nonkeratinized	Irregular and blunt connective tissue papillae, some elastic fibers, extensive vascular supply	Present with adipose connective tissue and minor salivary glands with firm attachment to muscle
Alveolar mucosa: Reddish-pink, shiny, moist, extremely mobile	Thin nonkeratinized	Connective tissue papillae sometimes absent, many elastic fibers, with extensive vascular supply	Present with minor salivary glands and many elastic fibers with loose attachment to muscle or bone
Ventral surface of the tongue and floor of the mouth: Reddish pink, moist, shiny, compressible with vascular blue areas; mobility varies	Extremely thin nonkeratinized	Extensive vascular supply **Ventral surface of the tongue:** Numerous connective tissue papillae, some elastic fibers, minor salivary glands **Floor of the mouth:** Broad connective tissue papillae	Present **Ventral surface of the tongue:** Extremely thin and firmly attached to muscle **Floor of the mouth:** Adipose connective tissue with submandibular and sublingual salivary glands, loosely attached to bone or muscles
Soft palate: Deep pink with yellow hue and moist surface; compressible and extremely elastic	Thin nonkeratinized	Thick lamina propria with numerous connective tissue papillae and distinct elastic layer	Extremely thin with adipose connective tissue and minor salivary glands with a firm attachment to underlying muscle
Masticatory Mucosa			
Hard palate: Pink, immobile, and firm medial zone along with palatal rugae and median palatine raphe; cushioned lateral zones	Thick orthokeratinized; medial zone considered part of the mucoperiosteum to the underlying bone	Medial zone considered part of the mucoperiosteum to underlying bone, along with the features of palatal rugae and median palatine raphe	Present only in lateral zones with anterior part having adipose connective tissue and posterior part having minor salivary glands; absent in medial zone along with palatal rugae and median palatine raphe
Attached gingiva: Opaque pink, dull, firm, immobile with areas of melanin pigmentation possible and varying amounts of stippling	Thick keratinized (mainly parakeratinized, some orthokeratinized); part of the mucoperiosteum to the underlying bone	Tall, narrow connective tissue papillae, extensive vascular supply; part of the mucoperiosteum to the underlying bone	Not present

One way to integrate these two interrelated concepts is to review the clinical appearance of the different regions of oral mucosa when armed with the new knowledge of the specific underlying histologic features.

Thus, the novice dental professional must first look closely at the clinical photographs of the different regions of the oral cavity, as well as in the descriptions of their clinical appearances presented in **Chapter 2,** and compare these with the histologic features discussed in this chapter. Next, practice finding these regional differences in the oral cavity using a mirror and this textbook for review in order to improve skills of examination. Later, locate them on peers and then on patients in a clinical setting during an intraoral examination.

LABIAL MUCOSA AND BUCCAL MUCOSA
CLINICAL APPEARANCE
The labial mucosa and buccal mucosa line the inner lips and cheeks (see Figures 2-2 and 2-3). Both of these regions appear clinically as an opaque pink, shiny, moist, compressible tissue that stretches easily. Areas of melanin pigmentation may be noted (discussed later in this chapter). A variable number of Fordyce spots (or granules) are

scattered throughout the tissue. These are a variant usually present in the oral cavity, which are visible as small, yellowish bumps on the surface of the oral mucosa. They correspond to deposits of sebum from misplaced sebaceous glands in the submucosa. The oral mucosa of the inner lips and cheeks is classified as a lining mucosa.

HISTOLOGIC FEATURES
The nonkeratinized stratified squamous epithelium of the labial mucosa and buccal mucosa is extremely thick and overlies and obscures a lamina propria with an extensive vascular supply, giving the overall mucosa an opaque and pinkish clinical appearance (Figure 9-8 and see Figure 11-8). The lamina propria has irregular and blunt connective tissue papillae but contains elastic fibers in addition to its collagen fibers, giving the tissue the ability to stretch and return to its original shape.

The lamina propria overlies a submucosa that contains adipose connective tissue and minor salivary glands, giving the tissue its compressibility and moisture, respectively. The submucosa is firmly attached to the underlying muscle in the region of the labial and buccal mucosa, thus preventing any of the nearby tissue from interfering during mastication or speech because the oral mucosa and muscle function as one unit.

FIGURE 9-8 Photomicrograph of the buccal mucosa with extremely thick nonkeratinized stratified squamous epithelium *(E)* overlying an extensively vascular lamina propria *(LP)*. However, the deeper submucosa usually overlying muscle is not shown. Note the prickly or spikey look to the cells of the prickle cell layer due to microscopic fixation causing the individual dehydrated cells to shrink; the desmosomes create this artifact due to the maintenance of their junctional stronghold. (From Young B, Heath JW: *Wheater's functional histology,* ed 6, Edinburgh, 2014, Churchill Livingstone.)

ALVEOLAR MUCOSA
CLINICAL APPEARANCE

The alveolar mucosa is a reddish-pink tissue with blue vascular areas (see Figures 2-2, 2-9, and 2-10). This shiny, moist region is extremely mobile and lines the vestibules of the oral cavity. The alveolar mucosa is classified as a lining mucosa.

HISTOLOGIC FEATURES

The epithelium of the alveolar mucosa is extremely thin nonkeratinized stratified squamous epithelium that overlies, but does not obscure, an extensive vascular supply in the lamina propria, making the alveolar mucosa redder than the labial mucosa or buccal mucosa (see Figures 9-12 and 9-13). Connective tissue papillae are sometimes absent and numerous elastic fibers are present in the lamina propria, thus allowing mobility of the tissue. Where the alveolar mucosa meets the attached gingiva is the anatomic feature of the mucogingival junction (discussed in more detail with the attached gingiva).

The submucosa associated with the alveolar mucosa has minor salivary glands and, again, numerous elastic fibers in a loose connective tissue, thus giving the tissue its moisture and additional mobility, respectively. The submucosa is loosely attached to the underlying muscle or bone, increasing the ability of the tissue to move because the alveolar mucosa is located between the moving lips and the stationary attached gingiva. Local anesthetic injections placed in the height or depth of vestibule within the alveolar mucosa (such as the posterior superior alveolar nerve block or incisive nerve block) have less discomfort levels noted than those involving the bones of the palate or bony jaws.

VENTRAL SURFACE OF THE TONGUE AND FLOOR OF THE MOUTH
CLINICAL APPEARANCE

Both the ventral surface of the tongue and floor of the mouth appear as a reddish-pink tissue with vascular blue areas of veins (see Figures 2-16 and 2-17). The tissue is also moist, shiny, and compressible. Although the floor of the mouth has some mobility, the ventral surface of the tongue is firmly attached, yet it allows some stretching along with the tongue muscles. Both the ventral surface of the tongue and the floor of the mouth are classified as a lining mucosa.

FIGURE 9-9 Photomicrograph of the ventral surface of the tongue that demonstrates the extremely thin nonkeratinized stratified squamous epithelium overlying (but not obscuring) a lamina propria with an extensive vascular supply and numerous connective tissue papillae. The deeper submucosa is also extremely thin but firmly attached to the underlying tongue muscle. (From Nanci A: *Ten Cate's oral histology,* ed 8, St Louis, 2013 Mosby.)

HISTOLOGIC FEATURES

Both the ventral surface of the tongue and the floor of the mouth have an extremely thin nonkeratinized stratified squamous epithelium overlying, but not obscuring, a lamina propria with an extensive vascular supply, thus making both regions redder and the veins (such as the deep lingual veins) more apparent (Figure 9-9).

The connective tissue papillae of the lamina propria of the ventral surface of the tongue are numerous. Some elastic fibers and a few minor salivary glands provide the ability to stretch and supply moisture. The submucosa associated with the ventral surface of the tongue is extremely thin and firmly attached to the underlying tongue muscle. This arrangement allows the oral mucosa and muscles to function as one unit, thus reducing mobility during mastication and speech.

The connective tissue papillae of the lamina propria are also broad in the floor of the mouth. The submucosa deep to the lamina propria consists of loose connective tissue with adipose connective tissue and includes the submandibular salivary gland and sublingual salivary gland, giving the tissue its compressibility and moisture, respectively. The submucosa associated with the floor of the mouth is loosely attached to the underlying bone and muscles, thus giving

FIGURE 9-10 Photomicrograph of the junction of the soft palate and hard palate *(arrow with dotted line),* which is also a junction between a lining mucosa and a masticatory mucosa, as well as a junction between nonkeratinized epithelium and keratinized epithelium. (From Nanci A: *Ten Cate's oral histology,* ed 8, St Louis, 2013, Mosby.)

the tissue its mobility when the attached tongue moves during mastication and speech.

SOFT PALATE
CLINICAL APPEARANCE

The posterior part of the palate, the soft palate, is deep pink with a yellowish hue and a moist surface (see Figures 2-11 and 2-12). The tissue is compressible and extremely elastic to allow speech and swallowing. The soft palate is classified as a lining mucosa.

HISTOLOGIC FEATURES

The soft palate has a thin nonkeratinized stratified squamous epithelium overlying a thick lamina propria (Figure 9-10). The lamina propria has numerous connective tissue papillae and a distinct elastic connective tissue layer for increased mobility with its elastic fibers.

The submucosa associated with the oral mucosa of the soft palate is extremely thin and has a firm attachment to the underlying muscle to allow the mechanisms of speech and swallowing. Again, this arrangement allows the oral mucosa and muscles to function as one unit. The submucosa contains adipose connective tissue, which gives the tissue its yellow hue and compressibility, and minor salivary glands, which give the tissue its moisture.

HARD PALATE
CLINICAL APPEARANCE

The anterior part of the palate, the hard palate, appears as a whiter pink tissue that is immobile and firm (see Figures 2-11 and 2-12). However, a cushioned feeling is noted when the hard palate is palpated in the posterior lateral zones and a firmer feeling in the adjacent medial zone. The palatine rugae and the median palatine raphe are also firm to the touch. Palatine rugae are permanent and unique to each person and can be used to establish identity through discrimination, like fingerprints. The mucogingival junction is absent between the tissue of the hard palate and the lingual surfaces of attached gingiva of the maxillary teeth; instead the two types of tissue blend into each other. The hard palate is classified as a masticatory mucosa.

HISTOLOGIC FEATURES

The hard palate has a thick layer of orthokeratinized stratified squamous epithelium overlying a thick lamina propria (Figure 9-11). This palatal epithelium is continuous with the nearby lingual surfaces of the attached gingiva of the maxillary teeth. Because the palate is devoid of freely moveable alveolar mucosa, there is no mucogingival junction present between the two types of tissue. In addition, only the lateral zones of the hard palate have a submucosa overlying the bones of the palate, giving the tissue here a cushioned feeling when palpated (see Figures 9-1 and 9-11, *A*).

The submucosa in the anterior part of the lateral zone (from the canines to the premolars) contains adipose connective tissue. The submucosa in the posterior part of the lateral zone of the hard palate (around the molars) contains minor salivary glands. However, the submucosa in these areas of the hard palate is thinner than that associated with lining mucosa, which becomes apparent when injections of local anesthetic are placed in the lateral zones of the hard palate (such as the anterior middle superior alveolar nerve block or the greater palatine nerve block) because they can produce more discomfort; these levels can be modified with pressure anesthesia methods.

Submucosa is absent in the medial zone of the hard palate; thus, the tissue has a firmer feeling when palpated (see Figure 9-11, *B*). This firm feeling is enhanced because the oral mucosa is directly attached to the periosteum of the underlying bones of the palate by way of the lamina propria. Thus the overlying oral mucosa when combined with the periosteum of the bones of the palate in this situation is considered a mucoperiosteum (see Figure 9-4). A **mucoperiosteum** (mu-ko-per-ee-**os**-te-um) is a structure consisting of a mucous membrane combined with the periosteum of the adjacent bone. Here, the mucoperiosteum attaches directly to the underlying bones of the palate without the usual intervening submucosa, providing a firm, inelastic attachment. The oral mucosa and periosteum are so intimately united as to form nearly a single membrane.

Because there is no submucosa present, local anesthetic injections placed in the medial zone of the hard palate (such as the nasopalatine nerve block) can be discomforting unless pressure anesthesia methods are also used. Both landmarks on the hard palate, the palatine rugae and the median palatine raphe, have histologic features similar to those of the medial zone of the hard palate.

ATTACHED GINGIVA
CLINICAL APPEARANCE

Healthy attached gingiva is opaque pink, and areas of melanin pigmentation may be present (discussed later in this chapter) (see Figures 2-9 and 2-10). When dried, the tissue is dull, firm, and immobile. **Stippling** is observed clinically as small pinpoint depressions, which give the surface of the attached gingiva an orange-peel appearance; this is analogous to the button tufting on upholstery, as will be demonstrated with the discussion of its histologic features. The amount of stippling varies even within healthy oral cavities. The attached gingiva that covers the alveolar process of each of the dental arches is classified as a masticatory mucosa.

Also noted is the mucogingival junction, which is a sharply defined scalloped junction between the pinker attached gingiva and the redder alveolar mucosa. Thus, there are three areas where this anatomic landmark of the mucogingival junction can be noted in the oral cavity: on the facial of the maxillary arch and on both the facial and lingual of the mandibular arch; however, this landmark is not present on the palate of the maxillary arch. The clinical importance of the mucogingival junction is in measuring the width of attached gingiva by demarcating its apical border; the amount of attached gingiva determines

Epithelium

Lamina propria

Submucosa

Bone of the palate

Epithelium

Lamina propria

Bone of the palate

FIGURE 9-11 Photomicrographs of the hard palate with orthokeratinized epithelium overlying lamina propria. **A,** The cushioned lateral zone of the hard palate that has a deeper thin submucosa overlying bones of the palate, which can contain either adipose tissue (anterior part) or salivary glands (posterior part). **B,** The firmer medial zone of the hard palate that has no submucosa present, so the oral mucosa combines with the periosteum of the underlying bones of the palate to form a mucoperiosteum. (**A,** From Nanci A: *Ten Cate's oral histology,* ed 8, St Louis, 2013, Mosby. **B,** From Berkowitz B, Moxham B: *Oral anatomy, histology, and embryology,* ed 4, St Louis, 2009, Mosby.)

the support level that the tooth has by way of both the periodontal ligament and alveolar process. The attached gingiva, as well as other types of gingival tissue such as those that line the gingival sulcus and attach deep to the tooth surface, are discussed further in **Chapter 10.**

HISTOLOGIC FEATURES

The attached gingiva has a thick layer of mainly parakeratinized stratified squamous epithelium that obscures the extensive vascular supply in the lamina propria, making the tissue appear opaque and pinkish (Figure 9-12). Again, the cells of the keratin layer that have nuclei along with keratin may be difficult to see under lower-power magnification in microscopic sections. However, minor amounts of orthokeratinized stratified squamous epithelium without nuclei may still be present in the keratin layer (see Figure 9-12, *A*).

The lamina propria of the attached gingiva also has tall, narrow connective tissue papillae; its clinically noted stippling is due to a strong attachment or pull of the epithelium toward the lamina propria in these areas (see Figure 9-12, *B*). No submucosa is present, which is similar to the medial zone of the hard palate and palatal landmarks. The lamina propria is directly attached to the underlying alveolar process of the jaws, making the attached gingiva firm and immobile. Thus, the overlying oral mucosa when combined with the periosteum of the alveolar process in this situation is considered a mucoperiosteum (see Figures 9-5 and 9-12, *B*). A mucoperiosteum is a structure consisting of a mucous membrane combined with the periosteum of bone. Here the mucoperiosteum attaches directly to the underlying alveolar

process of the jaws without the usual intervening submucosa, providing a firm, inelastic attachment. The oral mucosa and periosteum are so intimately united as to form nearly a single membrane.

Microscopically the mucogingival junction can be seen as a dividing zone between the keratinized attached gingiva and the nonkeratinized alveolar mucosa and thus is between a masticatory mucosa and a lining mucosa (Figures 9-13 and 9-14). It is also a junction between a tissue with a thick epithelial layer in the pinkish attached gingiva and a tissue with a thin epithelial layer in the redder alveolar mucosa, even though both tissue types have a similar extensive vascular supply in the lamina propria.

TONGUE AND LINGUAL PAPILLAE PROPERTIES

Microscopically the tongue is a mass of striated muscle in its core, covered by oral mucosa (Figure 9-15). In the mobile anterior part of the tongue, the striated muscle bundles are tightly packed with relatively little intervening adipose connective tissue in the core. In the bulkier, less-mobile posterior part of the tongue, the adipose connective tissue is more abundant in the core. Collections of minor salivary glands are numerous in the submucosa and muscular core of the posterior part of the tongue, particularly close to the junction between the posterior and anterior parts.

The V-shaped line, the sulcus terminalis, divides the dorsal surface of the tongue into the anterior two-thirds, or body, of the tongue, and the posterior one-third, which is the base of the tongue (see Figure 2-14).

FIGURE 9-12 Photomicrographs of the attached gingiva. **A,** The attached gingiva has a thick layer of mainly parakeratinized epithelium *(E)* overlying an extensively vascular lamina propria *(LP).* Note that the cells in the keratin layer have retained their nuclei and are filled with keratin *(arrows),* although it is hard to see at this lower-power magnification. The deeper alveolar process with its periosteum is not shown. **B,** The stippling on surface *(arrows)* is due to a strong attachment or pull of the epithelium toward the lamina propria in these areas. The oral mucosa when combined with the periosteum of the underlying alveolar process *(AP)* forms a mucoperiosteum; there is no intervening submucosa present. (**A,** From Nanci A: *Ten Cate's oral histology,* ed 8, St Louis, 2013, Mosby. **B,** From Berkowitz B, Moxham B: *Oral anatomy, histology, and embryology,* ed 4, St Louis, 2009, Mosby.)

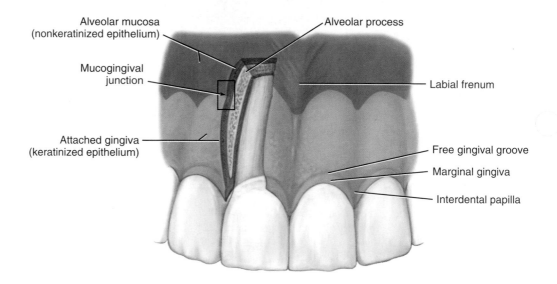

Alveolar mucosa (nonkeratinized epithelium)

Mucogingival junction

Attached gingiva (keratinized epithelium)

Alveolar process

Labial frenum

Free gingival groove

Marginal gingiva

Interdental papilla

Lining mucosa (nonkeratinized)

Mucogingival junction

Masticatory mucosa (keratinized)

FIGURE 9-13 Histologic features of the mucogingival junction *(arrow),* which is a junction between the alveolar mucosa and attached gingiva, as well as between a lining mucosa (nonkeratinized) and masticatory mucosa (keratinized).

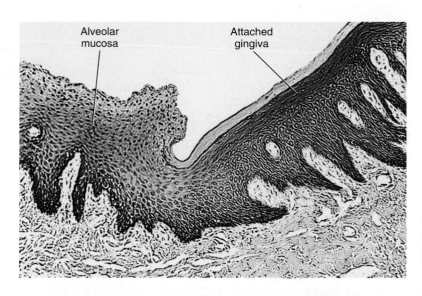

FIGURE 9-14 Photomicrograph of the mucogingival junction, which is a junction between the nonkeratinized alveolar mucosa and the keratinized attached gingiva, as well as between a lining mucosa and a masticatory mucosa. (From Nanci A: *Ten Cate's oral histology,* ed 8, St Louis, 2013, Mosby.)

FIGURE 9-15 Photomicrographs of the muscular core of the tongue. **A,** In the mobile anterior tongue, the striated muscle bundles *(M)* are tightly packed with relatively little intervening adipose connective tissue *(A)*, unlike the less mobile posterior. **B,** Collections of salivary glands *(S)* are numerous in the submucosa and muscular core of the posterior tongue. (From Stevens A, Lowe J: *Human histology,* ed 4, St Louis, 2015, Mosby.)

The dorsal surface of the tongue has both a masticatory mucosa and specialized mucosa present. A masticatory mucosa of orthokeratinized stratified squamous epithelium generally covers the surface of the muscle associated with the tongue.

The specialized mucosa found on the dorsal surface is associated with the lingual papillae, which are small discrete structures or appendages of keratinized epithelium with both orthokeratinized and parakeratinized epithelium present overlying a lamina propria (see Figures 2-14 and 2-15). Lingual papillae are also found on the lateral surface of the tongue. There are four types of lingual papillae: filiform, fungiform, foliate, and circumvallate (Table 9-5). The development of the lingual papillae and the tongue is discussed in **Chapter 5.**

Three types of lingual papillae are associated with taste buds: fungiform, foliate, and circumvallate. A taste bud is a barrel-shaped organ of taste derived from the epithelium (Figure 9-16). Each taste bud is composed of 30 to 80 spindle-shaped cells that extend from the basement membrane of the oral mucosa to the epithelial surface of the lingual papilla. The turnover time of the taste bud cells is a fairly rapid process of about 10 days.

The two types of taste bud cells are the supporting cells and the taste cells. However, the difference between the two is hard to discern under lower-power magnification of most microscopic sections, and indifferent immature forms are also noted. The *supporting cells* maintain the taste bud and are usually located on the outer part of the taste bud. The *taste cells* are usually located in the central part of the taste bud and produce taste sensations (see Figures 9-15 and 9-16).

To produce a taste sensation, dissolved molecules of food in the oral cavity contact the taste receptors of the taste cells at the taste pore, which is an opening in the most superficial part of the taste bud (Figure 9-17). Taste cells are also associated with sensory neuron processes among the cells in the inferior part of the taste bud. These sensory neuron processes receive messages of taste sensation through the taste receptors. The message generated is then sent to the central nervous system by the connecting nerves where it is identified as a certain type of taste.

Evidence suggests that the four fundamental taste sensations—sweet, sour, salty, and bitter—are different because of four slightly differentiated taste cells. However, the tastes experienced are the result of the blending of the four fundamental taste sensations and the addition of other sensations by the tongue as well as the interplay of smell and taste. In the past, the tongue was thought to have a specific mapping of taste sensations, but studies have proved this assumption false. Other

TABLE 9-5	Comparison of Lingual Papillae			
COMPARISONS	**FILIFORM**	**FUNGIFORM**	**FOLIATE**	**CIRCUMVALLATE**
Clinical appearance	Most common on body; fine-pointed cones giving the tongue velvety texture	Lesser numbers on body; mushroom-shaped, small, red dots	About 4 to 11 vertical ridges on lateral surface of posterior tongue	About 7 to 15 large, raised, mushroom-shaped structures anterior to sulcus terminalis
Histologic features	Pointed structure with thick layer of keratinized epithelium, overlying core of lamina propria; no taste buds	Mushroom-shaped structure with thin layer of keratinized epithelium overlying core of lamina propria with taste buds in most superficial part	Leaf-shaped structure of keratinized epithelium overlying core of lamina propria with taste buds in superficial lateral part	Mushroom-shaped structure with similar histology to fungiform but also sunken deep to tongue surface, taste buds in papilla base, and surrounded by a trough with von Ebner minor salivary glands in submucosa
Function	Possibly mechanical	Taste	Taste	Taste

FIGURE 9-16 Microscopic sections **(A** and **B)** of taste buds *(TB)* with supporting cells *(SC)* and taste cells *(TC)*; immature forms are also present. However, it is hard to discern the associated nerves and differences between the two cell types at this lower-power magnification. Note taste pores *(TP)* at most superficial parts. (From Stevens A, Lowe J: *Human histology,* ed 4, St Louis, 2015, Mosby.)

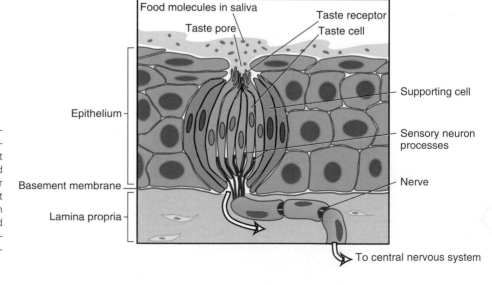

FIGURE 9-17 Events involved in taste sensation with a taste bud. Dissolved food contacts the taste receptors of the taste cells at the taste pore. Taste cells are also associated with sensory neuron processes in the inferior part of the taste bud, among the cells that receive messages of taste sensation from the taste receptors. The message produced is then sent by the nerve to the central nervous system, where it is identified as a certain type of taste.

taste sensations through current studies have now branched out to include umami (or savory) and fatty acid tastes.

FILIFORM LINGUAL PAPILLAE
CLINICAL APPEARANCE

The filiform lingual papillae are the most common lingual papillae located on the body of the dorsal surface of the tongue (see Figure 2-14). They are shaped like fine-pointed cones of 2 to 3 mm with the tips naturally turned toward the pharynx, giving the dorsal surface of the tongue its velvety texture. Filiform are sensitive to changes in the body and thus are associated with certain clinical considerations (discussed later in this chapter).

HISTOLOGIC FEATURES

A filiform is a pointed structure with a thick layer of orthokeratinized or parakeratinized epithelium overlying a core of lamina propria (Figure 9-18). An increased amount of keratin is noted also at the surface of each filiform, forming a flocked "Christmas tree" arrangement and whiter color noted for this lingual papilla. No taste buds are present in the epithelium. The filiform possibly have a rudimentary mechanical function as a result of their rougher surface texture, which is related to the increased amount of surface keratinization present and thus may aid in guiding food back to the pharynx for swallowing.

FUNGIFORM LINGUAL PAPILLAE
CLINICAL APPEARANCE

The fungiform lingual papillae are found in lesser numbers than are the filiform on the body of the dorsal surface of the tongue (see Figure 2-14). They appear as smaller reddish dots, which on closer inspection are slightly raised and mushroom-shaped with a 1 mm diameter. Fungiform are not found near the sulcus terminalis.

HISTOLOGIC FEATURES

A fungiform is a smaller mushroom-shaped structure with a thin layer of orthokeratinized or parakeratinized epithelium overlying a highly vascularized core of lamina propria, thus producing the redder clinical appearance of this lingual papilla (see Figure 9-18). A variable number of taste buds are located in the most superficial part of the epithelial layer; however, taste buds are not located near the base of the structure. Thus, the function of the fungiform is taste sensation.

FOLIATE LINGUAL PAPILLAE
CLINICAL APPEARANCE

The foliate lingual papillae appear as 4 to 11 vertical ridges parallel to one another on the lateral surface of the tongue in its most posterior part (see Figure 2-15).

HISTOLOGIC FEATURES

The foliate are leaf-shaped structures with a layer of orthokeratinized or parakeratinized epithelium overlying a core of lamina propria (Figure 9-19). Taste buds are located in the epithelial layer on the lateral parts of the leaf-shaped structure. Thus, the function of the foliate is taste sensation. Some histologists believe that the foliate are not true lingual papillae because of their rudimentary clinical appearance, developmental background, and location.

FIGURE 9-18 Microscopic section of the dorsal surface of the tongue showing a fungiform lingual papilla *(Fg)* and filiform lingual papillae *(Fi)*. Note the mushroom shape of the fungiform and the tree shape of the filiform. However, the taste buds at the superficial surface of fungiform are difficult to discern at this low level of magnification. (From Young B, Heath JW: *Wheater's functional histology,* ed 6, Edinburgh, 2014, Churchill Livingstone.)

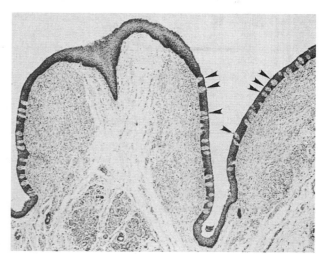

FIGURE 9-19 Microscopic section of the lateral surface of the tongue with foliate lingual papillae. Taste buds *(arrows)* are located in the epithelial layer on the lateral parts of the leaf-shaped structure. (From Nanci A: *Ten Cate's oral histology,* ed 8, St Louis, 2013, Mosby.)

CIRCUMVALLATE LINGUAL PAPILLAE
CLINICAL FEATURES

The circumvallate lingual papillae are lined up in an inverted V-shaped row on the dorsal surface of the tongue facing the pharynx, just anterior to the sulcus terminalis. When the tongue is arched and extended, the circumvallate lingual papillae appear as 7 to 15 raised, large, mushroom-shaped structures, mimicking the outline of the sulcus terminalis (see Figure 2-14, *A*). With the tongue in a more relaxed and natural position, the circumvallate are sunken as deep as the tongue surface because they are surrounded by a circular trough or trench. The circumvallate have a larger diameter than the fungiform, measuring from 3 to 5 mm.

FIGURE 9-20 Microscopic section of the posterior part of the dorsal surface of the tongue showing a circumvallate lingual papilla *(Cv)*, with taste buds *(arrows)* within the epithelial layer and surrounded by a circular trough *(Tr)*. Note von Ebner salivary glands *(VE)*, which flush the trough between tastes. (From Young B, Heath JW: *Wheater's functional histology,* ed 6, Edinburgh, 2014, Churchill Livingstone.)

HISTOLOGIC FEATURES

The circumvallate are larger mushroom-shaped structures with orthokeratinized or parakeratinized epithelium overlying a core of lamina propria (Figure 9-20). Hundreds of taste buds are located in the epithelium surrounding the entire base of each lingual papilla, opposite the circular trough lined by the surrounding tongue surface tissue.

It is important to note that von Ebner salivary glands are also present in the submucosa deep to the lamina propria of the circumvallate. These are minor salivary glands with only serous cells present (see **Chapter 11**). With ducts that open into the trough, they flush the area near the taste pores so as to introduce new taste sensations from several sequential food molecules. Thus, the function of the circumvallate is taste sensation.

Clinical Considerations for Tongue Pathology

Two more commonly found lesions are associated with the dorsal surface of the tongue, and involve the filiform lingual papillae. Neither lesion is serious, but both should be recorded on the patient record if present. One of these tongue lesions is geographic tongue, which appears as red and then paler pink to white patches on the body of the tongue (Figure 9-21). These patches change shape with time, resembling a geographic map. The lesion is found in all age groups and shows the sensitivity of the filiform lingual papillae to changes in their environment.

These red and white surface patches of geographic tongue correspond to groups of filiform undergoing changes from parakeratinized epithelium, which appears redder, to orthokeratinized epithelium, which appears whiter. This lesion is sometimes associated with soreness or slight burning on the surface of the tongue. However, no treatment is needed for geographic tongue, although dental professionals should reassure the patient and rule out any other more serious tongue lesions.

A less common lesion noted on the dorsal tongue surface is black hairy tongue (Figure 9-22). With this lesion, the usual level of shedding of epithelium of the filiform lingual papillae does not occur. As a result, a thick layer of dead cells and keratin builds up on the tongue surface, which becomes extrinsically stained by tobacco, medications, or chromogenic (colored) oral bacteria. Studies show that this condition, in some cases, might be an effect of fungal overgrowth, possibly as a result of high doses of antibiotics or radiation therapy. Brushing the tongue is recommended in this case to promote tissue shedding and remove debris.

FIGURE 9-21 Geographic tongue showing its sensitivity of the filiform lingual papillae. This results in redder to paler pink and white patches appearing on the dorsal surface of the body of the tongue over time. (Courtesy of Margaret J. Fehrenbach, RDH, MS.)

Generally, brushing the dorsal surface of the tongue is important for overall homecare of the oral cavity and to reduce bad breath (or malodor, halitosis) because microbial colonization by dental biofilm on the tongue's surface is a contributing factor.

ORAL MUCOSA PIGMENTATION

The oral mucosa can range in color from pink to reddish pink (se **Chapter 2**). The presence of melanin pigmentation within the epithelium may give rise to localized flat areas of the oral mucosa that range in color from brown to brownish black (Figure 9-23).

FIGURE 9-22 Black hairy tongue on the dorsal surface of the tongue where the usual level of shedding of epithelium of the filiform lingual papillae is lacking. This results in the formation of a thick layer of dead cells and keratin, which becomes stained. (Courtesy of Margaret J. Fehrenbach, RDH, MS.)

FIGURE 9-23 Pigmentation of the attached gingiva associated with the permanent dentition that is most abundant at the base of the interdental gingiva. (Courtesy of Margaret J. Fehrenbach, RDH, MS.)

Melanin is a pigment formed by melanocytes (meh-lah-no-sites), which are epidermal cells derived from the neural crest cells. Melanocytes are clear cells that occupy a position in the basal layer of the stratified squamous epithelium between the dividing epithelial cells (Figure 9-24). The melanocytes have small cytoplasmic granules as inclusions called *melanosomes,* which store the melanin pigment. They inject these granules into the neighboring newly formed epithelial cells of the basal layer.

As the tissue undergoes regeneration during its turnover time, the injected cells migrate to the surface of the oral mucosa and appear clinically as a group of localized, flat, pigmented areas or macules. Because melanocytes are evenly distributed throughout the oral mucosa, clinical levels of pigmentation are based on the degree of melanin-producing activity of the melanocytes, which is controlled by genetic programming. Thus, this is a variation that can be present in the oral cavity; it appears most abundant in the attached gingiva at the base of the interdental gingiva with both dentitions (see Figure 9-23).

Clinical Considerations with Oral Mucosa Pigmentation

The pathology involved in a nevus (or mole) is different from that of a variation of melanin pigmentation levels within a tissue. The nevus is a benign tumor of melanin; in further contrast is the melanoma, which is a cancer involving melanin. Both lesions can appear in the oral cavity usually as one distinct small flat macule or raised papule. The melanoma may or may not appear at the site of an existing nevus.

The pigmentation of both the oral mucosa and skin may increase with certain endocrine diseases. Additionally, if dramatic localized pigment changes are recently noted in the oral cavity, biopsy and microscopic study are recommended to rule out any malignancies. Many oral pathologists also recommend the removal of any nevus within the oral cavity to reduce the risk of carcinomatous change.

ORAL MUCOSA TURNOVER, REPAIR, AND AGING

Overall, the turnover time for the oral mucosa is faster than that for the skin as the tissue undergoes the regeneration process (see Chapter 8). Regional differences in the turnover times, however, do exist within the oral cavity (Table 9-6). The gingival epithelium in the gingival sulcular region that attaches deep to the tooth surface, the junctional epithelium, has the fastest turnover time of all the oral tissue at 4 to 6 days (see Chapter 10). One of the lowest turnover times is for the hard palate at 24 days. The turnover times of all other oral mucosa regions fall between these two end points—between 4 and 24 days. Regional differences in the pattern of epithelial maturation or keratinization appear to be associated with different turnover times; nonkeratinized buccal mucosa turns over faster than keratinized attached gingiva, around 1.5 times faster; thus, lining mucosa turns over faster than masticatory mucosa.

Generally, the epithelium of any region of oral mucosa has a faster turnover time than cells of the lamina propria, although the turnover time of its matrix, both fibers and intercellular substance, is quite rapid in response. As stated before, all regions of the oral cavity have a faster turnover time than the skin, which has a turnover time of 27 days. Such differences noted in turnover times for oral mucosa regions can have important implications for healing and rate of recovery time from injury such as periodontal disease or tooth extraction. Skin regions also have varying levels of turnover times; for example, the face is faster than the legs.

The repair process of the oral mucosa is similar to that of the skin, except that it involves a moist clot and not a dried scab like the skin (see Figure 8-3). After an injury to the oral mucosa, the clot from blood products forms in the area, and the inflammatory response is triggered with its white blood cells. In the next days, as tissue repair begins, the epithelial cells at the periphery of the injury will lose their desmosomal junctions and migrate to form a new epithelial surface layer beneath the clot. Thus, the clot is highly important in repair of the epithelium and must be retained in the first days of repair because it acts as a guide to form a new surface. Instructions must be given to patients before tooth extractions outlining behaviors to avoid in order not to disturb the clot, thus preventing *dry socket,* a postextraction infection. Later, after the epithelial surface is repaired, the clot breaks down through enzymatic activity because it is no longer needed.

At the same time, fibroblasts migrate to produce an immature connective tissue in the injured lamina propria deep to the clot and newly

FIGURE 9-24 Pigmentation process. **A,** Electron micrograph of a melanocyte in the basal layer of pigmented oral epithelium where the dense melanosomes are abundant near the basement membrane *(arrowheads). Inset:* Photomicrograph showing a melanocyte, which appears dark because it has been stained to reveal the presence of melanin. **B,** Photomicrograph of the attached gingiva, showing the pigmentation process within the oral mucosa. Note the granular layer *(arrows)* and the deposits of melanin, particularly in the basal layer. (**A** and inset, From Nanci A: *Ten Cate's oral histology,* ed 8, St Louis, 2013, Mosby. **B,** Courtesy of TS Leeson, Professor Emeritus, Cell Biology and Anatomy, Medicine and Oral Health, University of Alberta, Alberta, Canada.)

TABLE 9-6	Oral Tissue Mean Turnover Time*
ORAL TISSUE	**MEAN TURNOVER TIME**
Hard palate	24 days
Floor of mouth	20 days
Buccal and labial mucosa	14 days
Attached gingiva	10 days
Taste buds	10 days
Junctional epithelium (attached to tooth)	4 to 6 days

*Note that for comparison, the turnover time for the skin is 27 days.

forming epithelial surface (see Figure 8-5). This immature connective tissue is considered *granulation tissue* and has fewer fibers and an increased number of blood vessels. Granulation tissue appears as a soft, bright red tissue that bleeds easily.

This temporary granulation tissue is later replaced by firmer and paler scar tissue in the affected area. Replacement tissue is characterized by an increased amount of fibers and fewer blood vessels. The amount of scar tissue varies depending on the type and size of the wound, amount of granulation tissue, and movement of tissue after injury. The oral mucosa shows less scar tissue, either clinically or microscopically after repair than does the skin, because fewer fibers are located in this area than in the skin when it undergoes a similar injury. Studies show that the minimal scar tissue formation in oral mucosa after repair is similar to fetal tissue repair.

The formation of a lesser amount of scar tissue in the oral mucosa is useful both esthetically and functionally when oral or periodontal surgery is performed. Histologists believe it may be linked to the differing embryologic origins of the fibroblasts from the two tissue types; skin fibroblasts are derived from the mesoderm, and oral mucosa fibroblasts are derived from neural crest cells. Recent studies have found distinct differences in the aging profiles of cells (oral mucosa and patient-matched skin fibroblasts) isolated from these tissue types; thus, increased replicative potential of oral mucosa fibroblasts may confer upon them preferential wound-healing capacities.

After the source of injury is removed, the repair of the oral mucosa generally follows a time frame similar to its turnover time. Studies show that epithelial cells possess receptors for growth factors and respond also to chemical mediators of the inflammatory process. Future studies may show a way to speed repair and even prevent aging in the oral mucosa.

The process of aging of the oral mucosa mirrors some of the changes observed in the skin and lips (Figure 9-25). Unlike skin and lips, the deeper oral mucosa is protected from changes due to solar damage (see Figure 1-8). However, similar to skin, it is important to remember that it is sometimes difficult to distinguish changes caused by the aging process in the oral mucosa from those changes caused by chronic disease (discussed next).

Aging of the oral mucosa is seen clinically as a reduction of stippling on the attached gingiva, an increase of Fordyce spots in the labial and buccal mucosa, and an enlargement of the lingual veins to form lingual varicosities on the ventral surface of the tongue. The number of lingual papillae and associated taste buds, especially the foliate lingual papillae, is also reduced and may be related to changes noted in taste perception as a person ages. Many of the changes in the oral cavity may be due to changes in the salivary glands that result in less production of saliva (hyposalivation); these changes make the oral mucosa drier (xerostomia) and thus less protective. However these changes in saliva are not directly due to the aging process but mainly due to medications taken by older individuals or concurrent disease processes (see Figure 11-9).

FIGURE 9-25 Various changes resulting from the aging process in the oral cavity. **A,** Loss of stippling of the attached gingiva. **B,** Lingual varicosities on the ventral surface of the tongue. (Courtesy of Margaret J. Fehrenbach, RDH, MS.)

Microscopically the thickness and number of rete ridges in the epithelium diminish as the oral mucosa ages, showing the overall sagging and lack of firmness of the tissue. In addition, the degree of keratinization of the masticatory mucosa declines, especially in the attached gingiva. Cell division at the basal layer of the epithelium does not slow down, but studies show that the turnover times do slow down for all regions of the oral cavity.

Microscopically changes also occur in the composition of the matrix of the lamina propria and in a less-defined division between the papillary and dense layers in older oral mucosa. Collagen fibers appear thickened and are arranged into dense bundles resembling those found in tendons or ligaments. Elastic fibers, if present in the lamina propria, appear changed, even though more of them are present. This change in elastic fibers may explain the loss of resiliency found in aged oral mucosa. The fibroblasts decrease in quantity, appear smaller, and are less active in older oral mucosa. The entire lamina propria has a slower collagen turnover time. Overall, with the aging process, the ability of the oral mucosa to repair itself is reduced and the length of the repair time is increased, just as turnover time is increased.

With increasing aging of the patient base, dental professionals must consider the associated effects of aging on the oral mucosa during dental treatment—one being longer times for healing. Age-associated changes (such as loss of stippling and lingual varicosities) should be distinguished from conditions resulting from oral or systemic disease.

In the future, many changes associated with the aging process may be delayed or prevented. With present knowledge, some cases of gingival recession might be prevented by appropriate toothbrushing techniques, placement of a protective mouthguard against occlusal forces, or institution of crown-lengthening procedures. Other changes, such as a drier mouth (hyposalivation with xerostomia) and loss of resiliency, should be considered and complications prevented when treatment is performed on older patients.

Recent tissue engineering of oral mucosa combines cells and materials to produce a three-dimensional reconstruction of the tissue type so as to simulate its anatomic structure and function. This shows promise for clinical use, such as the replacement of soft tissue defects in the oral cavity occurring with gingival recession and tissue trauma occurring with oral cancer. This also impacts the approaches to biocompatibility evaluation of dental materials and oral homecare products as well as therapies associated with implant-soft tissue interfaces. Newer approaches used today for replacing injured oral mucosa are the use of autologous grafts and cultured epithelial sheets.

Clinical Considerations with Oral Mucosa Pathology

Granulation tissue may become abundant and may actually interfere with the repair process in oral mucosa. Surgical removal of excess granulation tissue may be necessary to allow for optimal repair, such as after a tooth extraction or certain periodontal surgical techniques with advanced chronic periodontal or pulpal disease (Figure 9-26).

Dental professionals must also consider the faster turnover time and faster repair times for oral regions as compared to the skin, when diagnosing lesions of the oral mucosa. Should the lesion be traumatic, complete healing takes up to approximately 2 weeks, depending on the region involved and if the source of the injury is first removed. Possible sources of injury to the oral mucosa may be physical, chemical, or infectious; assumptions should never be made about the source of any lesion of the oral mucosa. Biopsy followed with microscopic study is the only way to effectively diagnose any lesion.

A delay of approximately 2 weeks to allow a lesion to undergo healing before obtaining a referral or instigating a more serious clinical treatment plan does not adversely affect a patient's health. However, a longer delay (e.g., until the next maintenance visit) before the lesion is checked is not in the best interest of a patient. This is because malignant changes involved with cancer in a worst-case scenario do not heal but grow in size and may metastasize. The larger lesion that has metastasized gives the patient a poorer prognosis if the lesion is later determined to be malignant after microscopic study.

Turnover times also have implications during the treatment of cancer by surgical, chemical, and radiologic means because these methods can injure the oral mucosa while they are used to halt or reduce the cancerous growth. Healing that is required also varies according to the original turnover times of the tissue, even if it takes longer due to the trauma of therapy. Thus, the buccal mucosa heals faster than the hard palate when subjected to cancer therapy methods.

As was stated before, it is important to remember that it is sometimes difficult to distinguish changes caused by the aging process in the oral

FIGURE 9-26 Postoperative excessive granulation tissue, in this case after endodontic therapy, that may interfere with the repair process and need to be surgically removed. (From Gutmann JL, Dumsha TC, Lovdahl PE: *Problem solving in endodontics,* ed 5, St Louis, 2011, Mosby.)

mucosa from those changes caused by chronic disease. Exposure of the dental tissue from gingival recession of attached gingiva in the aged population is argued to be more a sign of disease than of age (see Figure 10-10). Also thought to be a sign of disease in the aged is creasing and then cracking at the labial commissures, which possibly results from a loss of vertical dimension of the dentition and jaws (see Figure 14-22 and **Chapter 20**).

CHAPTER 10

Gingival and Dentogingival Junctional Tissue

Additional resources and practice exercises are provided on the companion Evolve website for this book: ℮
http://evolve.elsevier.com/Fehrenbach/illustrated.

●●●● LEARNING OBJECTIVES

1. Define and pronounce the key terms in this chapter.
2. List and describe each type of gingival tissue.
3. Describe the histologic features of each type of gingival tissue and the clinical considerations for gingival tissue esthetics, integrating it into patient care.
4. Identify the components of each type of gingival tissue on a diagram.

5. Describe dentogingival junctional properties, histology, and development.
6. Identify the structure of the dentogingival junctional tissue on a diagram.
7. Discuss the clinical considerations for gingival tissue pathology, integrating it into patient care.
8. Discuss turnover of the dentogingival junctional tissue and its clinical implications.

GINGIVAL TISSUE PROPERTIES

Gingival tissue in the oral cavity is the most important tissue of the orofacial region for dental professionals to know and understand, and the most challenging as well. All of the periodontal therapy performed and homecare instruction given are for the purpose of creating a healthy environment for the gingival tissue. Even with restorative treatment, the impact on the gingival tissue must be considered. When healthy, it presents an effective barrier to the barrage of insults to deeper periodontal tissue. When the gingival tissue is not healthy, it can provide a gateway for periodontal disease to advance into the deeper tissue of the periodontium, leading to a poorer prognosis for long-term retention of the teeth. Thus, the dental professional must have a clear understanding of the histology of the healthy gingival tissue. This helps in understanding the pathologic changes that occur during the disease states involving the gingival tissue. It is important to keep in mind that the clinical appearance of the tissue reflects the underlying histology, both in health and disease.

GINGIVAL TISSUE ANATOMY

Gingival tissue surrounds the maxillary and mandibular teeth in each alveolus and also covers each alveolar process (Figure 10-1; see Figures 2-9 and 2-10). When examining the gingival tissue in a clinical setting, different types are present in the oral cavity. The gingival tissue that tightly adheres to the alveolar process that surrounds the roots of the teeth is the attached gingiva. The gingival tissue between adjacent teeth adjoining the attached gingiva is the interdental gingiva, forming the individual extensions of the interdental papillae. The interdental papillae fill in the area between the teeth apical to their contact areas to prevent food impaction

(see **Chapter 15**). The interdental papillae assume a conical shape for the anterior teeth and a blunted shape buccolingually for the posterior teeth.

Apical to the contact area, the interdental gingiva assumes a nonvisible concave shape between the facial and lingual gingival surfaces forming the gingival col (kohl) (Figure 10-2). The col varies in depth and width, depending on the expanse of the contacting tooth surfaces. It is mainly present in the broad interdental gingiva of the posterior teeth and is visible clinically only when teeth are extracted. In comparison, it is generally not present with the interproximal tissue associated with anterior teeth because the latter tissue is narrower. In the absence of contact between adjacent teeth, the attached gingiva extends uninterrupted from the facial to the lingual aspect.

The attached gingiva is considered a masticatory mucosa (see **Chapter 9**). Healthy attached gingiva is pink in color with some areas of melanin pigmentation possible (see Figures 2-9 and 9-23). The tissue when dried is dull, firm, and immobile, with varying amounts of stippling.

The width of the attached gingiva is measured by the distance between the mucogingival junction that remains stationary after the permanent dentition eruption and the projection on the external surface of the apex of the gingival sulcus (see Figure 2-9 and discussion in **Chapter 9**). The width of the attached gingiva on the facial aspect varies according to its location and is an important clinical parameter of periodontal health. It is generally greatest in the incisor region at 3.5 to 4.5 mm for maxillary arch, 3.3 to 3.9 mm for mandibular arch to narrowest in the posterior quadrants at 1.9 mm for maxillary arch, and 1.8 mm in mandibular first premolars.

The palatal surface of the attached gingiva in the maxillary arch blends with the equally firm and resilient oral mucosa of the hard palate. On the lingual aspect of the mandibular arch, the attached

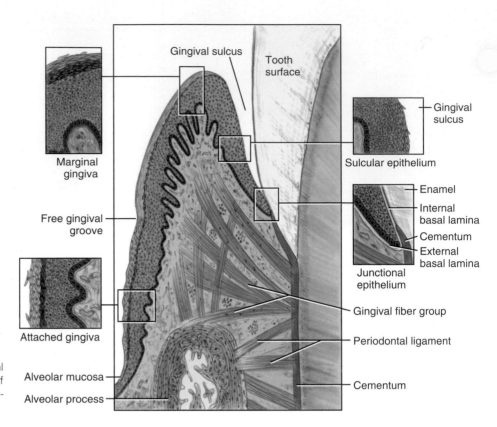

Gingival sulcus

Tooth surface

Gingival sulcus

Sulcular epithelium

Enamel

Internal basal lamina

Cementum

External basal lamina

Junctional epithelium

Gingival fiber group

Periodontal ligament

Cementum

Marginal gingiva

Free gingival groove

Attached gingiva

Alveolar mucosa

Alveolar process

FIGURE 10-1 Gingival and dentogingival junctional tissue highlighting the histology of the marginal gingiva, attached gingiva, sulcular epithelium, and junctional epithelium.

FIGURE 10-2 Faciolingual microscopic section showing the col between the facial and lingual interdental papillae inferior to the cervix of the tooth. The col is covered with nonkeratinized stratified squamous epithelium with the surrounding marginal gingiva demonstrating keratinization. (From Newman MG, Takei HH, Klokkevold, PR: *Carranza's Clinical periodontology,* ed 12, Philadelphia, 2014, Saunders/Elsevier.)

gingiva terminates at the junction of the lingual alveolar mucosa, which is continuous with the oral mucosa lining the floor of the mouth.

At the gingival margin of each tooth is the marginal gingiva (or free gingiva), which is continuous with the attached gingiva. The gingival tissue that faces the tooth, the dentogingival junctional tissue, which is not easily examined within the oral cavity, is discussed later. Both the attached gingiva and the marginal gingiva are more easily examined within the oral cavity, whether the gingival tissue is healthy or not.

The marginal gingiva varies in width from 0.5 to 2.0 mm from the free gingival crest to the attached gingiva (see Figure 2-10).

The marginal gingiva follows the scalloped pattern established by the contour of the cementoenamel junction (CEJ) of the teeth. When dried the marginal tissue is similar in clinical appearance to the attached gingiva, including pinkness, dullness, and firmness, because the marginal gingiva is also considered a masticatory mucosa. However, the marginal gingiva lacks the presence of stippling, and the tissue is mobile or free from the underlying tooth surface, which can be demonstrated with a periodontal probe or blowing air into the gingival sulcus. In addition, the marginal gingiva is more translucent than the attached gingiva—so much so that the darker subgingival calculus and even the dark margins of poorly executed prosthetic crowns can show through if present.

GINGIVAL TISSUE HISTOLOGY

The attached gingiva and the marginal gingiva share similar histology because both are considered masticatory mucosa; however, each has histologic features specific to the tissue (Figure 10-3). The attached gingiva has an overlying thick layer of mainly parakeratinized stratified squamous epithelium, which obscures its extensive vascular supply in the underlying lamina propria, making the tissue appear pinkish instead of the vascularized reddish or bluish (see Figure 9-12). The lamina propria also has tall, narrow connective tissue papillae alternating with the rete ridges, giving the tissue its varying amounts of stippling. Thus, the interface between the epithelium and lamina propria is highly interdigitated. The lamina propria is directly attached to the underlying bony jaws, making the attached gingiva firm and immobile. The lamina propria thus serves as a mucoperiosteum along with the periosteum of the alveolar process.

In contrast, the marginal gingiva has an overlying surface layer of only orthokeratinized stratified squamous epithelium. The associated underlying lamina propria also has tall, narrow papillae, but this lamina propria is continuous with the lamina propria of the gingival tissue that faces the tooth. And unlike the attached gingiva, the marginal gingiva is not attached to the underlying bony alveolar process, making

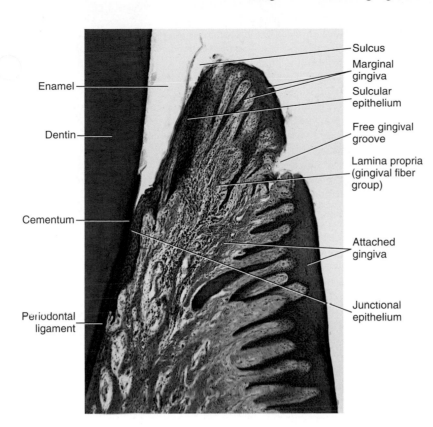

Enamel

Dentin

Cementum

Periodontal
ligament

Sulcus

Marginal
gingiva

Sulcular
epithelium

Free gingival
groove

Lamina propria
(gingival fiber
group)

Attached
gingiva

Junctional
epithelium

FIGURE 10-3 Photomicrograph of both the gingival and dentogingival junctional tissue demonstrating the epithelium and lamina propria of these two types of tissue, which is continuous with the periodontal ligament that is adjacent to the hard tissue of the tooth that includes the enamel (space), dentin, and cementum. Decalcification of the specimen has removed the tooth enamel, leaving an enamel space. (From the Dr. Bernhard Gottlieb Collection, courtesy of James McIntosh, PhD, Assistant Professor Emeritus, Department of Biomedical Sciences, Baylor College of Dentistry, Dallas, TX.)

this tissue firm but mobile. Further, the epithelium covering the col consists of the marginal gingiva of the adjacent teeth, except that in this small area it is nonkeratinized. The lack of keratinization of the col tissue may be important in the formation of periodontal disease along with its thinness and apically-inclined form (see later discussion).

It is important to note that the gingival fiber group is located in the lamina propria of the marginal gingiva (see Figure 14-32). Some histologists consider the gingival fiber group part of the periodontal ligament, but this fiber group supports only the gingival tissue and not the tooth in relationship to the jaws as does the other periodontal ligament fiber groups. The lamina propria of the marginal gingiva is also continuous with the adjacent connective tissue, which includes the lamina propria of the attached gingiva, as well as the periodontal ligament.

Clinical Considerations for Gingival Tissue Esthetics

In a healthy situation, gingival contours form a silhouette around the cervical section of a tooth, a fact that should be acknowledged when considering overall esthetics of smile design (see Figure 2-9). The cervical peak of the individual gingival contour is referred to as the *gingival apex of the contour.* The apex of maxillary central incisors and canines is distal to a line drawn through the midline or long axis of the tooth. The apex of a maxillary lateral incisor is equal to the midline or long axis of the tooth. The apex of a lateral incisor is also 1 mm short of the central incisor and canine's apex heights. The canine and central incisor apices are equal in height.

The gingival contour is also related to its position in regard to the lip line with continued consideration of smile design. The optimal smile line clinical appearance should reveal the least amount of maxillary facial gingival tissue as possible under the lip line. The lateral incisor may touch the lip line or be 1 to 2 mm coronal to the lip line, revealing some maxillary facial gingival tissue.

However, cases of a "gummy smile" with an excessive display of maxillary facial gingival tissue are not ideal, such as when the maxillary central incisors and canines barely touch the lip line or border of the upper lip. This can result from the abnormal eruption of the teeth; the teeth are covered by excessive tissue and appear short, even though they may actually be the proper length. The muscles that control the movement of the upper lip could be hyperactive, causing the lip to rise up higher than usual so that more tissue is exposed when smiling. In addition, the excessive bulging protrusion of the maxilla may also be involved.

In most cases, orthodontic therapy, possibly with orofacial myofunctional therapy (OMT), and in conjunction with orthognathic surgical intervention as well as esthetic periodontal surgery, can alter the clinical appearance of the gingival contours for a more pleasing smile (see **Chapter 20** for more discussion).

DENTOGINGIVAL JUNCTIONAL TISSUE PROPERTIES

The **dentogingival** (den-to-jin-ji-val) **junction** is the junction between the tooth surface and the gingival tissue (see Figures 10-1 and 10-3). The sulcular epithelium and junctional epithelium together form the **dentogingival junctional** (jungk-shun-al) **tissue**. Both the sulcular epithelium and junctional epithelium are difficult to examine within healthy gingival tissue in a clinical setting due to their location in relationship to the gingival sulcus.

The **sulcular epithelium** (sul-ku-lar ep-ee-thee-lee-um) **(SE)** (or crevicular epithelium) stands away from the tooth, creating a gingival sulcus. The gingival sulcus is filled with **gingival crevicular** (jin-ji-val kre-**vik**-koo-ler) **fluid (GCF)** from the adjacent blood supply in the lamina propria. The usual GCF flow rate is quite slow, calculated at 1 to 2 microliters per tooth per hour. Thus, the amount of GCF is minimal at one time in the healthy state.

The GCF from the lamina propria seeps between the epithelial cells and then into the gingival sulcus. This fluid allows the components of the blood system to reach the tooth surface through the junctional epithelium from the blood vessels of the adjacent lamina propria. The GCF contains both the immunologic components and cells of the blood, although in lower amounts and in different proportions. It also contains sticky plasma proteins in the sulcus that serve as adhesive for its lining tissue, keeping it intact.

Thus the GCF includes white blood cells (WBCs), especially the polymorphonuclear leukocytes (PMNs), as well as the immunoglobulins of IgG, IgM, and serum IgA produced by plasma cells, which all have a role in the specific defense mechanism against disease. Any immunologic reactions in the blood system are directly relevant to those found in the GCF and may affect the periodontal health of the tooth and associated gingival tissue. It also supplies complement factors that serve to initiate both vascular and cellular inflammatory responses that can possibly damage the periodontium. Later, the GCF passes from the gingival sulcus into the oral cavity, where it mixes with saliva.

A deeper extension of the SE is the junctional epithelium (JE), which lines the floor of the gingival sulcus and is attached to the tooth surface. The JE is attached to the tooth surface by way of an **epithelial** (ep-ee-**thee**-lee-al) **attachment (EA)**. The attachment of the JE to the tooth surface can occur either on enamel, cementum, or dentin. The position of the EA on the tooth surface is initially on the cervical half of the anatomic crown when the tooth first becomes functional after eruption (discussed later). The slight depression of the free gingival

groove on the outer surface of the gingiva corresponds to the apical border of the inner JE and not to the depth of the gingival sulcus.

Instead, the probing depth of the gingival sulcus is measured by the use of a calibrated periodontal probe. The depth of the healthy gingival sulcus varies from 0.5 to 3 mm, with an average of 1.8 mm. However, the clinical probing depth of the gingival sulcus may be considerably different from the true microscopic gingival sulcus depth. In a healthy-case scenario and taking a more microscopic perspective of what occurs with probing: the instrument is gently inserted, slides by the SE, and is stopped by the EA of the JE.

Probing measurements of the gingival sulcus are also subject to variations depending on the clinician's insertion pressure, the accuracy of the readings, and the ability of the probe tip to easily penetrate tissue that is ulcerated or inflamed; digital probes are available for more consistent results between clinicians. Studies show that probing the gingival sulcus surrounding both teeth and implants does not seem to cause irreversible damage to the soft tissue because it quickly heals itself (discussed later in this chapter).

DENTOGINGIVAL JUNCTIONAL TISSUE HISTOLOGY

Microscopically the SE consists of stratified squamous epithelium similar to the deeper epithelium of the attached gingiva and adjacent outer marginal gingiva, making it a transition tissue between the gingival epithelium and JE (Figures 10-4 and 10-5). However, the

FIGURE 10-4 Photomicrographs of the sulcular epithelium. **A,** Deep to the sulcular epithelium is the lamina propria of both the marginal gingiva and the attached gingiva, as well as the alveolar crest of the alveolar bone proper. **B,** Close-up view showing the nonkeratinized epithelium of the inner sulcular epithelium. Note that the interface between the sulcular epithelium and the lamina propria that it shares with the marginal and attached outer gingival tissue is relatively smooth compared to the strongly interdigitated interface of the gingival tissue. (From the Dr. Bernhard Gottlieb Collection, courtesy of James McIntosh, PhD, Assistant Professor Emeritus, Department of Biomedical Sciences, Baylor College of Dentistry, Dallas, TX.)

FIGURE 10-5 Photomicrograph of the initial junctional epithelium before eruption *(arrows)* overlying the enamel *(E, enamel space)*. Decalcification of the specimen has removed the tooth enamel, leaving an enamel space. Note the cementoenamel junction *(J)*, the cementum *C)*, and dentin *(D)*. Deep to the junctional epithelium is the underlying interconnecting connective tissue *(CT)* of the both lamina propria and adjacent periodontal ligament. (From the Dr. Bernhard Gottlieb Collection, courtesy of James McIntosh, PhD, Assistant Professor Emeritus, Department of Biomedical Sciences, Baylor College of Dentistry, Dallas, TX.)

thinner SE is nonkeratinized, unlike the keratinized marginal gingiva and attached gingiva. In addition, the interface between the SE and the lamina propria that it shares with the outer gingival tissue is relatively smooth compared to the strongly interdigitated interface of the outer gingival tissue. The deeper interface between the JE and the underlying lamina propria is also relatively smooth, without rete ridges or connective tissue papillae.

When looking microscopically at the JE itself, the JE cells are loosely packed, with fewer intercellular junctions using desmosomes between cells, as compared with other types of gingival tissue (Figures 10-6 and 10-7). The number of intercellular spaces between the epithelial cells of the JE is also at a higher level than other types of gingival tissue and all are filled with tissue fluid. Thus, overall the JE is more permeable than other gingival tissue due to its fewer desmosomal junctions and increased intercellular spaces.

This increased permeability allows for emigration of large numbers of mobile WBCs from the blood vessels in the deeper lamina propria into the JE, even in healthy tissue. This mainly involves the PMNs, with those cells actively undergoing phagocytosis (see Figure 8-17). The PMNs also enter the GCF in the gingival sulcus in healthy mouths. In the absence of clinical signs of inflammation, approximately 30,000 PMNs migrate per minute through the JE into the oral cavity. The increased presence of these WBCs may keep the tissue healthy by protecting it from microorganisms within the dental biofilm and also associated toxins that continually form on the exposed tooth surface in the vicinity. Antigen-presenting cells that are present may be involved as well (see **Chapter 8**).

In addition, the JE is also thinner than the SE, ranging coronally from only 15 to 30 cells thick at the floor of the gingival sulcus, and then tapering to a final thickness of 3 to 4 cells at its apical part. The suprabasal cells, which make up the most superficial layer of the JE, serve as part of the EA of the gingiva to the tooth surface. These more suprabasal epithelial cells of the JE provide the hemidesmosomes and an internal basal lamina (bay-sal lam-i-nah) that create the EA because this is a cell-to-noncellular type of intercellular junction (see Figure 7-6 and Figures 10-6 and 10-7). Furthermore, because the structure of the EA is similar to that of the junction between the epithelium and subadjacent connective tissue, this internal basal lamina also consists of a lamina lucida and lamina densa.

Basal layer

External basal lamina

Lamina propria

Suprabasal epithelial cell of the junctional epithelium

Tooth surface (enamel)

Hemidesmosome

Lamina densa ⎫ Internal
Lamina lucida ⎬ basal
⎭ lamina

Cementoenamel junction

Cementum

FIGURE 10-6 Epithelial attachment of the junctional epithelium with its intricate attachment mechanisms to the tooth surface. Note that the interface between the junctional epithelium and the lamina propria is relatively smooth when healthy.

FIGURE 10-7 Electron micrographs of junctional epithelium and its epithelial attachment. Decalcification of the specimen has removed the tooth enamel, leaving an enamel space. **A,** Attachment of the junctional epithelium *(JE)* to the enamel surface *(ES, enamel space)* at the internal basal lamina *(IBL)* and to the connective tissue *(CT)* of the lamina propria by the external basal lamina *(EBL)*. Note its wide intercellular spaces and the lack of cellular differentiation of the layers of epithelium that would denote maturation. **B,** Close-up showing the structure of the attachment of a single junctional epithelium cell *(Nu, nucleus)* to the enamel surface by the internal basal lamina and hemidesmosomes *(HD)* and tonofilaments *(Tf)*. (**A** and **B,** From Nanci A: *Ten Cate's oral histology,* ed 8, St Louis, 2013, Mosby/Elsevier.)

The internal basal lamina of the EA is also continuous with the **external basal lamina** between the JE and the lamina propria at the apical extent of the JE. The EA is very strong in a healthy state, acting as a type of protective seal between the soft gingival tissue and the hard tooth surface.

The deepest layer of the JE, or basal layer, undergoes constant and rapid cell division, or mitosis. This process allows a constant coronal migration of the cells as they die and are shed into the gingival sulcus. However, the few layers present in the JE—from its basal layer to the suprabasal layer—do not show any change in cellular structure related to maturation, unlike other types of gingival tissue. Thus, the JE does not mature like keratinized tissue, such as the marginal gingiva or attached gingiva, which fills its matured superficial cells with keratin. Nor does JE have cells like nonkeratinized tissue of the sulcular gingiva and throughout the rest of the oral cavity that enlarge and migrate superficially. Thus, the JE cells do not mature and form into either a granular layer or intermediate layer.

However, without a keratinizing superficial layer at the free surface of the JE, there is no physical barrier to microbial attack as with other oral keratinized tissue, such as the attached gingiva. Other structural and functional characteristics of the JE must compensate for the absence of this barrier. The JE fulfills this difficult task with its special structural framework and the collaboration of its epithelial and nonepithelial cells that provide very potent antimicrobial mechanisms, such as the WBCs. However, these defense mechanisms do not preclude the development of extensive inflammatory lesions in the gingival tissue, and, occasionally, the inflammatory lesion may eventually progress to the loss of the connective tissue attachment of the periodontal ligament to the tooth as well as the alveolar process (discussed later).

The JE cells have many organelles in their cytoplasm, such as rough endoplasmic reticulum, Golgi complex, and mitochondria, indicating a high metabolic activity. However, even with that heightened state, the JE cells remain immature or undifferentiated until they die and are shed or lost in the gingival sulcus. The key to this state of striking cellular immaturity of the JE may be found in future ultrastructural studies of the adjoining lamina propria; this lamina propria appears to be functionally different from the connective tissue underlying the other types of oral epithelium that do mature. Lysosomes are also found in large numbers in JE epithelial cells; enzymes contained within these lysosomes participate in the destruction of microorganisms contained in dental biofilm.

Clinical Considerations for Gingival Tissue Pathology

With active periodontal disease, both the marginal gingiva and attached gingiva can become enlarged, especially the interdental papillae (Figure 10-8). This spongy enlargement results from edema occurring in the lamina propria of the tissue caused by the inflammatory response. This is due to tissue fluid from the capillary plexus of the lamina propria flowing out to flush the area of its injurious agents with edema (see Figure 9-6). The gingival tissue can also become redder with active periodontal disease because hyperemia, or increased blood flow, also occurs in the capillaries of the lamina propria. Later, the color can change to magenta as the inflammation becomes chronic and the blood undergoes stasis. The stippling may also be lost because the inflammatory edema reduces the strong interdigitation between the epithelium and lamina propria. The location of the free gingival crest can also change with periodontal disease, such as when the gingival tissue becomes inflamed; the gingival margin can become more coronal.

With increased homecare and other methods of dental biofilm control, the edema from inflammation can lessen, and both the marginal and attached gingiva can shrink down to their previous levels. These are all signs of gingivitis, the inflammation of the gingiva, which can be either acute or chronic and may also overlay the deeper destruction of the periodontium (see more discussion of gingivitis in this chapter).

Another type of gingival enlargement, gingival hyperplasia, can affect both the epithelium and lamina propria, causing a permanent fibrous enlargement with the gingival margin becoming more

FIGURE 10-8 Edema of both the marginal gingiva and the attached gingiva with its tissue enlargement *(dashed lines)* as a result of acute inflammation with the active periodontal disease of gingivitis. (Courtesy of Margaret J. Fehrenbach, RDH, MS.)

FIGURE 10-9 Gingival hyperplasia caused by the intake of certain drugs and associated poor homecare. (Courtesy of Margaret J. Fehrenbach, RDH, MS.)

coronal (Figure 10-9). **Gingival hyperplasia** (hi-per-**play**-ze-ah) is an overgrowth of mainly the interproximal gingiva and results from the intake of drugs for seizure control (phenytoin sodium), certain antibiotics, and specific heart medications. These drugs may either increase the populations or production outputs of certain fibroblast populations. The amount of gingival overgrowth is related to the drug dosage, as well as the amount of inflammation present that is induced by dental biofilm levels.

The gingival overgrowth of gingival hyperplasia can interfere with proper homecare, increasing dental biofilm amounts, and

FIGURE 10-10 Gingival recession of a permanent mandibular anterior tooth, possibly due to an adjacent tight frenal attachment. (Courtesy of Margaret J. Fehrenbach, RDH, MS.)

thus may need to be periodically removed by surgery due to recurrence. Although gingivectomy was considered appropriate in the past, most cases of gingival enlargement are now treated by a flap approach that includes resection of hyperplastic tissue. The surgeon can then access alveolar process defects for management, ensure an adequate postsurgical band of keratinized gingiva, and minimize the risk of postsurgical bleeding. Hyperplasia of the dentogingival junctional tissue is also a hallmark of chronic advanced periodontal disease within the tissue (discussed later).

In contrast, **gingival recession** (re-**sesh**-un) results in the gingival margin becoming more apical (Figure 10-10). This change in the gingival margin can result from periodontal disease, tooth position, abrasion by incorrect toothbrushing methods, abfraction from occlusal stresses (such as parafunctional habits), aging process, and possibly tight frenal attachments. The width of the attached gingiva may also decrease with periodontal disease, reducing the underlying support for the tooth, and should be recorded in the patient's chart as well as should any changes present in the gingival tissue.

When a graft procedure is performed to reduce the amount of gingival recession on the root, keratinization is taken into consideration because the goal of grafting is to increase the amount of attached keratinized tissue. One type of graft, the free gingival graft (FGG), uses a thickness of both keratinized epithelium and lamina propria harvested from the hard palate and grafted to the root to form a new band of keratinized attached gingiva. This procedure generally is somewhat successful, but the graft tends to be lighter colored, and studies show that the epithelium does not survive the procedure, which means that the donor site requires extra time to heal and allow migration of the surrounding epithelium to cover the site.

In contrast, a subepithelial connective tissue graft (SECTG) consists of only lamina propria that is taken from the surrounding keratinized attached gingiva and then grafted directly to the root. Epithelial cells from the surrounding tissue migrate to cover the graft and heal the area. This procedure is consistently successful; the new keratinized attached gingiva blends with the surrounding tissue, and healing of the donor site is rapid. Thus, the induction to form keratin in the gingival tissue's superficial layers may come from the deeper lamina propria and does not involve only the epithelium. These two types of grafting are considered passive mucogingival repair procedures. In contrast, active tissue engineering for mucogingival repair looks promising for the future as they produce and study three-dimensional models of the oral mucosa that can be applied to patient care.

DENTOGINGIVAL JUNCTIONAL TISSUE DEVELOPMENT

Before the eruption of the tooth and after enamel maturation, the ameloblasts secrete a basal lamina on the tooth surface that serves as a part of the primary EA. As the tooth actively erupts, the coronal part of the fused tissue consisting of the reduced enamel epithelium (REE) and surrounding oral epithelium peels back off the crown (see Figure 6-25, D). The ameloblasts also develop hemidesmosomes for the primary EA and become firmly attached to the enamel surface (see Figure 10-5). However, the cervical part of the fused tissue remains attached to the neck of the tooth by the primary EA. This fused tissue, which remains near the CEJ after the tooth erupts, serves as the initial JE of the tooth, creating the first tissue attached to the tooth surface. This tissue is later replaced by a definitive JE as the root is formed (see Figures 10-6 and 10-7).

The definitive JE is formed from all the cell types present in the REE as a result of mitosis of the cells. This proliferating tissue now can provide both the basal lamina and hemidesmosomes for the secondary EA to the tooth surface. After eruption of the tooth, 3 or 4 years may pass before the initial tissue becomes the definitive JE, a multilayer nonkeratinizing squamous epithelium. Although initially controversial, studies now show that the ameloblasts undergo cellular changes that make them indistinguishable from the other newly formed JE cells, with the transformed ameloblasts eventually replaced by these new cells.

DENTOGINGIVAL JUNCTIONAL TISSUE TURNOVER

In both the SE and epithelium of the marginal gingiva, the turnover process insuring the regeneration of the tissue occurs in a manner similar to that of the epithelium of the attached gingiva; the basal cells migrate superficially after mitosis, undergo maturation, and take the place of the superficial cells, which are shed in the oral cavity as they die.

In the junctional epithelium, even though it does not undergo cellular maturation, its basal cells still migrate superficially upon dividing and continuously replace the dying suprabasal cells that are desquamated into the gingival sulcus at a fast pace. The migratory route of the cells as turnover takes place in the JE is in a coronal direction, parallel to the tooth surface. Such cells continuously dissolve and reestablish their attachments by hemidesmosomes on the tooth surface. Most interestingly, the JE has the fastest turnover time in the entire oral cavity, which is approximately 4 to 6 days (see Table 9-6).

Clinical Considerations for Dentogingival Junctional Epithelium Pathology

The increased permeability of the JE allows emigration of the PMN type of WBC and also allows microorganisms from the dental biofilm and associated toxins from the exposed tooth surface to enter this tissue from the deeper lamina propria. When these damaging agents can enter the JE, the gingival tissue undergoes the initial signs of active periodontal disease with gingivitis (jin-ji-vie-tis). These signs include acute or even chronic inflammation with the formation of edema (as was discussed earlier) as well as an increased number of WBCs and epithelial ulceration with tissue thinning (see Figure 10-8).

The process of gingivitis begins with the recognition of the invasion by microorganisms from the dental biofilm by the gingival epithelial cells. Embedded in the cell membrane of the gingival epithelial cells

FIGURE 10-11 Bleeding on probing of a periodontal pocket due to increased blood vessels in the deeper lamina propria, which are now closer to the surface because of ulceration of the junctional epithelium caused by periodontal inflammation. (Courtesy of Margaret J. Fehrenbach, RDH, MS.)

(and many others including the skin and gastrointestinal tract) are toll-like receptors (TLRs). These are transmembrane proteins that extend through the gingival epithelial cell membrane, having both internal and external parts; they recognize the presence of the bacterial endotoxins and then mobilize the inflammatory response.

The ulceration of the JE allows even more damaging agents to enter the deepest parts of periodontium, thus progressing the disease toward the bony jaw. The interface between the dentogingival junctional tissue and the lamina propria that is smooth in healthy tissue, with inflammation shows the formation of rete ridges and connective tissue papillae. The lamina propria also shows breakdown of the collagen fibers as the disease advances.

Bleeding on probing (BoP), even with a gentle touch, begins to occur even with early gingivitis are present (Figure 10-11). This is due to the periodontal probe damaging the increased blood vessels in the capillary plexus of the lamina propria, which are now closer to the surface because of the ulceration of the JE. Bleeding can also occur during patient homecare. The presence of bleeding is one of the first clinical signs of active periodontal disease in uncomplicated cases and should be recorded per individual tooth and tooth surface in the patient's chart. However, in patients who smoke tobacco, the gingival tissue rarely bleeds because of unknown factors that do not seem related to dental biofilm and calculus formation but to the incorporated nicotine that causes vasoconstriction, a narrowing of the blood vessels.

Periodontal inflammation is also accompanied by an increase in the amount of GCF in order to fight the microbial attack, either of a serous (clear) or suppurative nature, distending the already enlarged tissue even further. Thus, relatively large amounts of fluid now pass through the more permeable epithelial wall. This is noted clinically only when it involves the visible whiter suppuration, or pus, resulting from the presence of cellular debris and extensive populations of PMNs.

Current clinical practice does not usually allow measurement of these increased fluid levels in the gingival sulcus. In the future, however, this measurement may be possible in a dental office setting; it is now used mainly during dental research to show the level of activity of the disease. It is important to keep in mind that GCF also supplies the minerals for subgingival calculus formation, as well as a moist environment needed for dental biofilm growth.

Studies have shown that the JE cells themselves may play a much more active role in the innate defense system than previously assumed by synthesizing a variety of molecules involved in the combat against

FIGURE 10-12 Photomicrographs of periodontitis, a chronic advanced periodontal disease that progresses in an apical direction. **A,** Ulcerated junctional epithelium (*right*) that has become a lateral wall of pocket epithelium with its true apical migration of the epithelial attachment on the tooth (*left*) causing a deepened gingival sulcus or periodontal pocket. **B,** Slightly more apical view showing epithelial proliferative and atrophic changes and marked inflammatory infiltrate and destruction of collagen fibers of the pocket epithelium. **C,** Higher magnification of the newly formed pocket epithelium (*close-up view of B*) with migrated pocket epithelium giving it a long epithelial attachment (*EA*), increased numbers of blood vessels in the lamina propria, and formation of rete ridges (*RR*) and connective tissue papillae at the interface between the dentogingival junctional tissue and the lamina propria, as well as the breakdown of the collagen fibers (*CF*) of the lamina propria and adjacent periodontal ligament. (From Newman MG, Takei HH, Klokkevold, PR: *Carranza's Clinical Periodontology,* ed 12, Philadelphia, 2014, Saunders/Elsevier.)

microorganisms and their products. In addition, these JE cells may express molecules that mediate the migration of PMNs toward the apical part of the gingival sulcus.

When the deeper tissue of the periodontium is affected by periodontal disease, further damage can occur, and the disease can become chronic in nature; this condition is now considered to be **periodontitis** (pare-e-oh-don-**tic**-tis) (Figure 10-12). With the advancement of periodontal disease, the prognosis for retention of the tooth becomes risky, then guarded, as alveolar process is lost and the lamina propria and adjacent periodontal ligament become increasingly disorganized with the inherent collagen fibers breaking down (see **Chapter 14**). As the disease progresses apically, exposed furcations (areas between the roots) are now present around the posterior teeth, and the teeth become increasingly mobile (see Figure 17-35). Pathological migration may also be present due to a weakened periodontium; the occlusal forces need not be at an abnormal level if the periodontal support is already reduced by periodontal disease (see Figure 14-34).

True apical migration of the EA also occurs with advanced periodontal disease, causing a deepened gingival sulcus, which is now considered a **periodontal** (pare-ee-o-**don**-tal) **pocket**, lined by **pocket epithelium (PE)** instead of dentogingival junctional tissue (see Figure 10-11). The depth of the periodontal pockets must be recorded in the patient's chart to monitor periodontal disease. Unlike in clinically healthy situations, parts of the upper lining can sometimes be seen in periodontally involved gingival tissue if air is blown into the periodontal pocket, exposing the newly denuded roots of the tooth.

The most prominent histologic characteristics of PE are the presence of ulceration and gingival hyperplasia with the formation of rete ridges and connective tissue papillae at the once smooth tissue interface. In addition, the PE has a surface wrinkled papillary relief, increased levels of exfoliation of epithelial cells, WBC migration, and bacterial internalization, as well as internalization-induced programmed epithelial cell death.

Periodontopathogens within a periodontal pocket are believed to play an important role in periodontitis, such as *Aggregatibacter actinomycetemcomitans (Aa)* or *Porphyromonas gingivalis (Pg).* These pathogens have developed sophisticated methods to disturb the structural and functional integrity of the JE, including the production of gingipains or cysteine proteinases. These virulence factors may specifically degrade components of the cell-to-cell contacts of the JE, furthering the progression of disease. And an increased number of mononuclear WBCs, such as the T-cell and B-cell lymphocytes and monocytes/macrophages, together with PMNs, are also considered as factors that contribute to the focal disintegration of the JE as it forms into PE.

A periodontal pocket can become a localized infected fascial space and may result in an abscess formation with a papule appearing on the gingival surface. Incision and drainage of the abscess may be necessary, as well as systemic antibiotics if systemic signs of infection are present. The placement of local antimicrobial delivery systems within the periodontal pocket to reduce localized infections may also be considered.

Endoscopic evaluation of the periodontal pocket is also becoming available in dental settings outside of the research facilities; it can facilitate subgingival visual examination without reliance on tactile sense and without surgical flap access. The clinician views a video monitor that displays the magnified image transmitted by a fiberoptic bundle attached to a subgingival instrument. This direct real-time visualization of the gingival sulcular region may aid the clinician in periodontal disease diagnosis and therapy. Techniques for identification and interpretation of the hard and soft tissue images, as well as the location of root fractures or deposits, defective restorations, and caries, are being developed.

Given that the turnover time of the JE is approximately 1 week (unlike most oral tissue that have slower turnover times), evaluation of periodontal therapy must occur after this time to allow initial healing of the area. Therefore, follow-up scheduling of patients should occur after this biologic temporal factor of turnover time. In addition, patients must have the information and skills necessary to enact a change in their homecare to allow optimal initial healing during this healing period. The final outcome of periodontal pocket healing depends on the sequence of events during the repair stages as discussed earlier. If the epithelium proliferates along the tooth surface before the other more supportive tissue reaches the area, the result will be a long JE. This less than stellar pattern of healing does not promote any new periodontal ligament support or alveolar process attachment associated with the tooth; thus the tooth now has a more risky prognosis.

In regard to newly placed implants, the superior tissue present originates only from epithelial cells of the oral mucosa, as opposed to the JE located around natural teeth, which originates also from the REE (see earlier discussion and Figure 14-23). Structurally, the *periimplant tissue* closely resembles a long JE and is discussed as such by many clinicians, although dissimilarities have also been reported in some studies. It is unknown if the situation of a long JE has a risky prognosis for the implant as it does for a poorly healing periodontal case with natural teeth. However, such an adaptive potential is also observed in the regenerating JE around teeth following gingivectomy, which is performed to surgically reduce pocket depths by removal of the soft tissue pocket wall, with a completely new JE forming within 20 days.

It is hoped that someday a patient with extensive periodontal tissue damage could have treatment performed that would allow a more coronal reattachment of the EA of the JE and complete periodontium regeneration involving a sound periodontal ligament and alveolar process attachment. Corresponding changes would also then occur in the way periodontal therapy is performed and homecare instructions are given. Thus, practicing dental professionals must keep up with changes in this area to remain current in periodontal therapy and homecare instruction.

CHAPTER 11

Head and Neck Structures

Additional resources and practice exercises are provided on the companion Evolve website for this book: ⓔ
http://evolve.elsevier.com/Fehrenbach/illustrated.

●●●● LEARNING OBJECTIVES

1. Define and pronounce the key terms in this chapter.
2. Discuss gland properties.
3. Discuss salivary gland properties, including its histologic features and development, as well as the clinical considerations concerning salivary gland pathology, integrating it into patient care.
4. Discuss thyroid gland properties, including its histologic features and development, as well as the clinical considerations concerning thyroid gland pathology, integrating it into patient care.

5. Discuss properties of lymphatics, including the lymph nodes and intraoral tonsillar tissue, and the clinical considerations concerning lymphoid tissue pathology, integrating it into patient care.
6. Discuss the properties of the nasal cavity and paranasal sinuses, as well as clinical considerations concerning each of them, integrating it into patient care.
7. Identify the components of head and neck structures on a diagram.

HEAD AND NECK STRUCTURES

Dental professionals must have a clear understanding of the histology as well as the prenatal development concerning not only the oral cavity but also the associated head and neck structures. The clinical functioning of the head and neck structures is related to the their underlying histology. In addition, many pathologic lesions that are encountered in the oral cavity can be associated with changes in these associated structures of the head and neck, and thus are reflected in changes in their underlying histology. The head and neck structures to be discussed in this chapter include the salivary glands, thyroid gland, lymphatics, nasal cavity, and paranasal sinuses.

GLAND PROPERTIES

A **gland** is a structure that produces a secretion necessary for body functioning. An **exocrine** (ek-sah-krin) **gland** is a gland having a duct associated with it. A **duct** is a passageway that allows the glandular secretion to be emptied directly into the location where the secretion is to be used. An **endocrine gland** is a ductless gland with its secretions conveyed directly into the blood and then carried by the blood vessels to some distant location to be used. Motor nerves associated with both types of glands help regulate the flow of the secretion. Sensory nerves are also present in the gland.

SALIVARY GLAND PROPERTIES

The oral fluid contains not only saliva but also other components as well, such as food debris, microorganisms and their byproducts, serum components, and desquamated oral epithelial cells. The **salivary** (sal-i-ver-ee) **glands** produce **saliva** (sah-li-vah), or "spit." Saliva contains minerals, electrolytes, proteins, buffers, enzymes, immunoglobulins (secretory IgA), and metabolic wastes. The secretion by these glands is controlled by the autonomic nervous system (see **Chapter 8**).

Saliva lubricates and cleanses the oral mucosa, protecting it from dryness and potential carcinogens by way of its mucins and other glycoproteins. This secretory product also helps in digestion of food by enzymatic activity. Additionally, it serves as a buffer by its bicarbonate and phosphate ions as well as by salivary proteins and their byproducts, protecting the oral mucosa against acids from food products and dental biofilm and then later the stomach lining. Saliva is also involved in antibacterial activity through its lysozyme content as well as secretory IgA (see **Chapters 7 and 8,** respectively). The glycoprotein of lactoferrin content inhibits the growth of bacteria that need iron by chelating with the element.

Finally, saliva helps maintain tooth integrity because it is involved in the posteruptive maturation of enamel. It also helps continue the remineralization of the tooth surface because it is supersaturated with calcium and phosphate ions, which can be increased by having fluoride added to the saliva. However, because it contributes to the formation of the salivary pellicle on the tooth and oral mucosa surfaces, saliva is also involved in the first step in dental biofilm formation. It also supplies the minerals for supragingival calculus formation.

Salivary glands are classified as either major or minor, depending on their size, but both types have similar histologic features. Further, both the major and minor salivary glands are exocrine glands, and thus have associated ducts that help convey the saliva directly into the oral cavity so it can be used; in addition, the minor glands do not have named ducts as the major glands have (discussed later in this chapter).

SALIVARY GLAND HISTOLOGY

Both major and minor salivary glands are composed of both epithelium and connective tissue (Figure 11-1). Epithelial cells both line the ducts and produce the saliva. Connective tissue surrounds the epithelium, protecting and supporting the gland. The connective tissue of the gland is divided into the **capsule** (kap-sule), which surrounds the outer part of the entire gland, and the septa. Each **septum** (sep-tum) (plural, **septa** [sep-tah]) helps divide the inner part of the gland into the larger **lobes** and then smaller **lobules** (lob-ules). Both the capsule and septa carry nerves and blood vessels that serve the gland.

SECRETORY CELLS AND ACINI

Epithelial cells that produce the saliva are the **secretory** (sek-kre-tory) **cells** (Figure 11-2). The two types of secretory cells are classified as either mucous or serous cells, depending on the type of secretion produced. **Mucous** (mu-kis) **cells** produce a mucous secretory product with mainly mucins. Mucins in saliva lubricate and can form a surface barrier as well as aid in aggregating microorganisms. In contrast, **serous** (sere-us) **cells** produce a serous secretory product with proteins and glycoproteins. The serous cells also produce the enzyme amylase that catalyzes the hydrolysis of starch into sugars, which is the beginning of the chemical process of digestion.

A combination of secretory cells present in the gland can produce a mixed secretory product. However, in these mixed glands, one type of cell predominates so that the product is either mainly mucous or mainly serous even if it has a range of both cell types.

Secretory cells are found in a group, or **acinus** (as-i-nus) (plural, **acini** [as-i-ny]), which resembles a cluster of grapes. Each acinus is located at the terminal part of the gland connected to the ductal system with many acini within each lobule of the gland. Each acinus

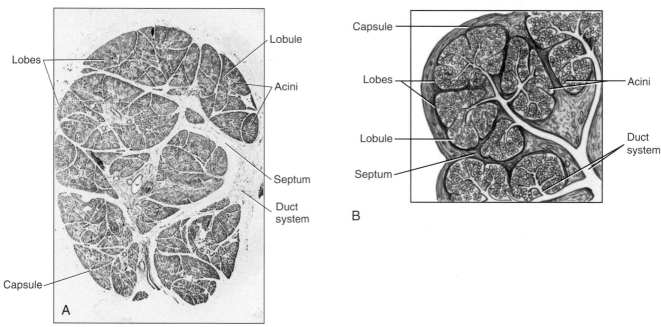

FIGURE 11-1 Salivary gland. **A,** Micrograph. **B,** Diagram. (**A,** From Nanci A: *Ten Cate's oral histology,* ed 8, St Louis, 2013, Mosby/Elsevier.)

FIGURE 11-2 Microscopic section of a lobule highlighting the two main types of acini: mucous acinus and serous acinus. (From Nanci A: *Ten Cate's oral histology,* ed 8, St Louis, 2013, Mosby/Elsevier.)

FIGURE 11-3 Photomicrograph of the parotid salivary gland showing connective tissue septa dividing the serous acini into lobules to produce a mainly serous secretory product. Note also the striated and excretory ducts. (From Nanci A: *Ten Cate's oral histology*, ed 8, St Louis, 2013, Mosby/Elsevier.)

FIGURE 11-4 Photomicrograph of the submandibular salivary gland highlighting a mucous acinus with its mucous cells and an attached serous demilune as well as a serous acinus, which means the gland produces a mixed salivary product. Note also the striated duct. (From Nanci A: *Ten Cate's oral histology*, ed 8, St Louis, 2013, Mosby/Elsevier.)

FIGURE 11-5 Photomicrograph of the sublingual salivary gland highlighting a serous demilune capping the mucous cells of a mucous acinus, which means it produces a mixed secretory product since it has mainly mucous acini but also some mucous acini with serous demilunes. (From Nanci A: *Ten Cate's oral histology*, ed 8, St Louis, 2013, Mosby/Elsevier.)

consists of a single layer of cuboidal epithelial cells surrounding a **lumen** (loo-men), which is a central opening where the saliva is deposited after being produced by the secretory cells.

The main two forms of acini are classified in terms of the type of epithelial cell present and the secretory product being produced. **Serous acini** are composed of serous cells producing a watery serous secretory product and have a narrow lumen (Figure 11-3). In contrast, **mucous acini** are composed of mucous cells producing a viscous mucous secretory product and their lumen is wider. Some mucous acini have a **serous demilune** (dem-ee-lune), which consists of a "bonnet" or cap of serous cells superficial to the group of mucous secretory cells and may be considered *mucoserous* or *seromucous* (Figures 11-4 and 11-5). Because the mucous acini with a serous demilune contain both types of secretory cells, they produce a mixed secretory product. However, the major distinctions between serous cells and mucous cells have become less important with additional studies of their cellular functioning.

Both the major and minor salivary glands have differing types of acini (Table 11-1). The major glands show a range of acini types: the parotid has only serous acini, the submandibular has both including mucous acini with serous demilunes but mainly has serous acini, and the sublingual has mainly mucous acini with some having serous demilunes. Most minor salivary glands have mainly mucous acini with a few having serous demilunes as well as also having a few serous acini. However, the minor salivary glands of von Ebner are an exception, having only serous acini (discussed later). However, the types of acini are often difficult to classify at lower-power magnification of microscopic sections of the glands and some of the features noted microscopically may be artifacts.

To facilitate the flow of saliva out of each lumen into the connecting ducts, **myoepithelial** (my-oh-epee-thee-lee-al) **cells** are located on the surface of some of the acini, as well as on their connection to the ductal system, the intercalated ducts (Figure 11-6). Each myoepithelial

TABLE 11-1	Comparison of Major Salivary Glands		
	PAROTID	**SUBMANDIBULAR**	**SUBLINGUAL**
Size and capsulation	Largest, capsule present	Intermediate, capsule present	Smallest, no capsule
Location	Behind mandibular ramus, anterior and inferior to ear	Beneath the mandible	Floor of the mouth
Excretory ducts	Parotid duct (Stenson): Opens opposite maxillary second molar on buccal mucosa	Submandibular duct (Wharton): Opens near lingual frenum on floor of mouth at sublingual caruncles	Sublingual duct (Bartholin): Opens in same area as submandibular duct; may have additional ducts at submandibular folds
Striated ducts	Short	Long	Rare or absent
Intercalated ducts	Long	Short	Absent
Acini	Only serous	Mainly serous but with some mucous with serous demilunes	Mainly mucous but with some serous demilunes
Secretory product	Only serous	Mixed and but mainly serous	Mixed but mainly mucous

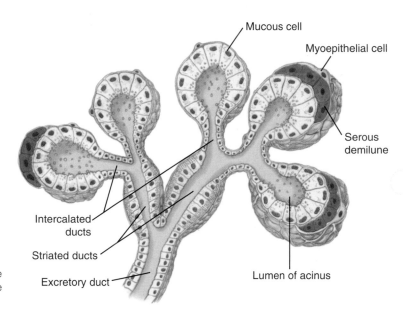

FIGURE 11-6 Salivary gland and its ductal epithelium. Note the serous demilunes on top of the mucous secretory cells of the mucous acini as well as the myoepithelial cells.

cell consists of a cell body with four to eight cytoplasmic processes radiating outward. They are specialized cells of epithelium that resemble an octopus on a rock; thus, they are situated on the surface of the acini and have a contractile nature.

When the myoepithelial cells contract, the acinus and its contents are squeezed, forcing the saliva out of the lumen and into the connecting duct; more than one myoepithelial cell can sometimes be found on a single acinus. When associated with the ducts of the salivary glands in this case, the cells orient themselves lengthwise and contract to shorten or widen the ducts to keep them open. Studies show additional functions of these cells, such as signaling the secretory cells and protecting the salivary gland tissue.

DUCTAL SYSTEM

The ductal system of salivary glands consists of hollow tubes connected initially with the acinus, and then with other ducts, as the ducts progressively grow larger from the inner to the outer parts of the gland (see Figure 11-6). Each type of duct is lined by different epithelium, depending on its location in the gland (see Table 8-2). In comparison, each major salivary gland displays differences in the length or types of ducts present (see Table 11-1); minor salivary glands do not show these differences due to the shortness of their ductal system. It is important to note that the ductal system does not serve just as a pipeline for the passageway of saliva; many of the parts of the duct system also actively participate in the production and modification of saliva.

The duct associated with an acinus or terminal part of the gland is the **intercalated** (in-**turk**-ah-lay-ted) **duct**. The intercalated duct is attached to the acinus, much as a stalk is attached to a cluster of grapes. The intercalated duct consists of a hollow tube lined with a single layer of cuboidal epithelial cells. Many are found in each lobule of the gland. These ducts not only serve as a passageway for saliva, but they also contribute many macromolecular components to the saliva. These include lysozyme and lactoferrin, which are stored in the secretory granules of ductal cells.

The **striated** (**stri**-ate-ed) **duct** is a part of the ductal system that is connected to the intercalated ducts in the lobules of the gland. The overall diameter of this duct is greater than that of each acinus, and its lumen is larger than those of both the acini and intercalated ducts. The striated duct consists of a hollow tube lined with a single layer of columnar epithelial cells characterized by what appear to be *basal striations*. Instead these visual vertical infranuclear striations are due to the presence of numerous elongated mitochondria in narrow cytoplasmic partitions separated by highly infolded and interdigitated cell membranes. Not only does the striated duct serve as a passageway for saliva, but it also is involved in the modification of saliva. Its ductal cells actively resorb and secrete electrolytes into the saliva from the adjacent blood vessels near the visually striated regions.

The final part of the salivary gland ductal system is the **excretory** (ex-**kreh**-tor-ee) **duct**, or secretory duct, which is located in the septum of the gland. These ducts are larger in diameter than the striated ducts. Saliva exits by this duct into the oral cavity. The excretory duct is a hollow tube lined with a variety of epithelial cells. The cells lining the excretory duct initially consist of pseudostratified columnar epithelium, which then undergoes a transition to stratified cuboidal epithelium as the duct moves to the outer part of the gland.

On the outer part of the ductal system that empties into the oral cavity, the excretory duct lining becomes stratified squamous epithelium, blending with surrounding oral mucosa at the ductal opening. Thus, the excretory duct serves as a passageway for saliva; however, it may have other functions with further research.

MAJOR SALIVARY GLANDS

The **major salivary glands** are three, large, paired glands that have ducts named for them (Figure 11-7; see Table 11-1 and Figure 1-5). These major salivary glands are the parotid, the submandibular, and the sublingual glands.

Although the capsulated parotid salivary gland is the largest major salivary gland, it provides only 25% of the total salivary volume. It is located in an area behind the mandibular ramus, anterior and inferior to the ear (see Figure 11-7, A). The parotid gland has only serous acini, making the gland secrete a watery serous secretory product as well as enzymes such as amylase (see Figure 11-3).

The duct associated with the parotid gland is the parotid duct (or Stenson duct). This long duct emerges from the gland and then opens up into the oral cavity on the inner surface of the buccal mucosa, usually opposite the maxillary second molar at the parotid papilla (see Figure 2-2).

The capsulated submandibular salivary gland is the second-largest major salivary gland, but it provides 60% to 65% of the total salivary volume. It lies beneath the mandible in the submandibular fossa, posterior to the sublingual salivary gland (see Figure 11-7, B). However, because the submandibular gland has both serous and mucous acini with serous demilunes, the gland secretes a more viscous mixed secretory product than the parotid, but it is mainly serous (see Figure 11-4).

The duct associated with the submandibular gland is the submandibular duct (or Wharton duct). This long duct travels anteriorly on the floor of the mouth and opens into the oral cavity at each sublingual caruncle (see Figure 2-17).

The sublingual salivary gland is the smallest, most diffuse, and the only major salivary gland without a capsule. It provides only 10% of the total salivary volume. It is located in the sublingual fossa, anterior to the submandibular salivary glands, on the floor of the mouth (see Figure 11-7, C). The sublingual gland has mainly mucous acini but with some mucous acini having serous demilunes. Thus, the gland secretes a mixed secretory product, but with a predominately viscous mucous component (see Figure 11-5).

The short ducts associated with the sublingual gland combine to form the sublingual duct (or Bartholin duct). The sublingual duct then opens into the oral cavity through the same opening as the submandibular duct, at each sublingual caruncle (see Figure 2-17). Other smaller ducts of Rivinus of the sublingual gland also open directly along the sublingual folds.

MINOR SALIVARY GLANDS

The **minor salivary glands** are much smaller than the major salivary glands but are more numerous. The minor salivary glands are also exocrine glands, but their unnamed ducts are shorter than those of any of the major salivary glands. The saliva secreted by minor salivary glands reaches the oral cavity through the short ducts that open directly onto oral mucosa surface. These glands are scattered in the tissue of the buccal, labial, and lingual mucosa, as well as the soft palate, lateral zones of the hard palate, and the floor of the mouth (Figure 11-8).

Most minor salivary glands have mainly mucous acini, with a few having serous demilunes as well as also having a few serous acini. As a result, most minor salivary glands secrete a mainly viscous mucous secretory product with slight serous influence. The minor salivary glands allow a continuous slow secretory flow and thus have an important role in protecting and moistening the oral mucosa, especially at night when the major salivary glands are mostly inactive.

The exception to minor salivary glands that mainly have mucous acini is the **von Ebner** (von **eeb**-ner) **salivary glands**, associated with the larger circumvallate lingual papillae on the posterior part of the dorsal surface of the tongue (see Figure 9-20). These glands contain only serous acini and thus secrete only a watery serous secretory product. The salivary flow of these glands flush the trough around the circumvallate allowing for new taste sensations.

SALIVARY GLAND DEVELOPMENT

Between the sixth and eighth weeks of prenatal development, the three major salivary glands begin as epithelial proliferations, or buds, from the ectoderm lining of the primitive mouth. The rounded terminal ends of these epithelial buds grow into the underlying mesenchyme, producing the secretory cells of the glandular acini and the ductal system.

The parts of the glands that contain supporting connective tissue, such as the outer capsule and inner septa, are produced from the mesenchyme, which is influenced by neural crest cells. It is important to note that interaction between the developing components of the epithelium, mesenchyme, nerves, and blood vessels is necessary for complete development of the salivary glands.

The parotid salivary glands appear early in the sixth week of prenatal development and are the first major salivary glands formed. The epithelial buds of these glands are located on the inner part of the cheek, near the labial commissures of the primitive mouth. These buds grow posteriorly toward the otic placodes of the ears and branch to form solid cords with rounded terminal ends near the developing facial nerve.

Later, at approximately 10 weeks of prenatal development, these cords are canalized and form ducts with the largest becoming the parotid duct for the parotid gland. The rounded terminal ends of the cords form the acini of the glands. Secretion by the parotid glands via the parotid duct begins at approximately 18 weeks of gestation. Again, the supporting connective tissue of the gland develops from the surrounding mesenchyme.

The submandibular salivary glands develop later than the parotid glands and appear late in the sixth week of prenatal development. They develop bilaterally from epithelial buds in the sulcus surrounding the sublingual folds on the floor of the primitive mouth. Solid cords branch from the buds and grow posteriorly, lateral to the developing tongue.

A

Parotid
salivary
gland

Parotid
duct
(Stenson duct)

B

Submandibular
duct (Wharton duct)

Submandibular
salivary gland
(deep lobe)

Submandibular salivary
gland (superficial lobe)

C

Sublingual fold

Sublingual duct
opening

Sublingual caruncle with
duct openings from the
submandibular and
sublingual glands

Submandibular duct
(Wharton duct)

Sublingual gland

Sublingual ducts

Sublingual duct
(Bartholin duct)

FIGURE 11-7 Major salivary glands. **A,** Parotid. **B,** Submandibular. **C,** Sublingual with the tongue elevated and the floor of mouth sectioned. (**A** and **B,** From Fehrenbach MJ, Herring SW: *Illustrated anatomy of the head and neck,* ed 4, Philadelphia, 2012, Saunders/Elsevier.)

The cords of the submandibular gland later branch further and then become canalized to form the ductal part. The submandibular gland acini develop from the cords' rounded terminal ends at 12 weeks, and secretory activity via the submandibular duct begins at 16 weeks. Growth of the submandibular gland continues after birth with the formation of more acini. Lateral to both sides of the tongue, a linear groove develops and closes over to form the submandibular duct.

The sublingual salivary glands appear in the eighth week of prenatal development, later than the other two major salivary glands. They develop from epithelial buds in the sulcus surrounding the sublingual

folds on the floor of the mouth, lateral to the developing submandibular gland. These buds branch and form into cords that canalize to form the sublingual ducts associated with the gland. The rounded terminal ends of the cords form acini.

Much like the major salivary glands, the minor salivary glands arise from both the ectoderm and endoderm associated with the primitive mouth. They then remain after development as small, isolated acini and ducts within the oral mucosa or submucosa lining the mouth.

The contractile myoepithelial cells, which are important in the secretion of saliva from each acinus, arise from neural crest cells, and

FIGURE 11-8 Photomicrograph of a minor salivary gland located in the submucosa deep to the epithelium and lamina propria of the labial mucosa. The gland has mucous acini; most minor salivary glands have mainly mucous acini. The saliva secreted by minor salivary glands reaches the oral cavity through unnamed short ducts that open directly onto oral mucosa surface. (From Nanci A: *Ten Cate's oral histology,* ed 8, St Louis, 2013, Mosby/Elsevier.)

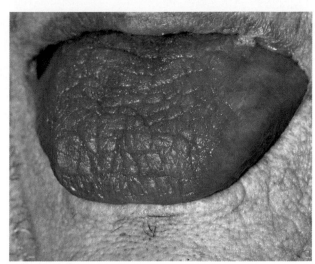

FIGURE 11-9 Xerostomia (dry mouth) due to hyposalivation (reduced saliva) in an aged oral cavity causing inflammation of the oral mucosa, including the tongue and lips. (Courtesy of Margaret J. Fehrenbach, RDH, MS.)

thus are ectodermal in origin. They surround the developing acini, as well as parts of the ductal system, and become active between the 24th and 25th week of prenatal development.

AGING SALIVARY GLANDS

With the aging process, there is a generalized loss of salivary gland tissue; up to 30% to 60% loss has been demonstrated. Changes of the duct system have been also noted. Although decreased production of saliva is often observed in older persons, whether this is related directly to the reduction in tissue has not been shown (discussed next). The process of aging does not seem to influence the production of resting saliva, or unstimulated saliva production, but studies show that stimulated saliva production may be less than usual in older individuals. The glands also contain occasional adipocytes (or fat cells), which increases with aging (see Figure 11-3).

Clinical Considerations for Salivary Gland Pathology

Certain medications, disease processes, or destruction of salivary tissue may result in decreased production of saliva by salivary glands. The decreased production of saliva is considered **hyposalivation** (hi-po-sal-i-**vay**-shen) and can result in **xerostomia** (zer-oh-**sto**-me-ah), or dry mouth (Figure 11-9). Xerostomia can result in increased trauma to a nonprotected oral mucosa, increased cervical caries, speech and mastication problems, and bad breath or halitosis. The disease processes causing hyposalivation can include diabetes, Sjögren syndrome, and rheumatoid arthritis. Destruction occurs after radiation therapy for head and neck cancer because the salivary glands often are in the radiation field, and its cells are highly sensitive. Series of chemotherapies for cancer or bone marrow transplantation also may cause reduced salivary function.

Thus, important changes must be made in the dental treatment plan of the patients with xerostomia due to hyposalivation after checking that the source of the disturbance is not related to any disease processes (such as diabetes) that must first be dealt with directly.

Such alterations in care include the recommendation of sipping water, artificial saliva use, remineralization products application such as fluoride and casein phosphopeptide-amorphous calcium phosphate (CPP-ACP), avoidance of alcohol-containing products, and increased recare visits. Medications that stimulate salivary production are available for nondrug-related hyposalivation. Transplanting lost salivary tissue is now being performed in some cases of extreme xerostomia with hyposalivation.

The salivary glands may also become blocked, stopping the drainage of saliva from the duct. This blockage can cause glandular enlargement and tenderness resulting from retention of saliva in the gland. The blockage of the duct can result from either stone (or sialolith) formation or trauma to the duct opening on the surface of the oral cavity, such as biting the tissue. The tortuous travel of the submandibular duct to its ductal opening for a considerable upward distance may be the reason why this gland is the one most commonly involved in stone formation.

This retention of saliva in the salivary gland can result in a **mucocele** (**mu**-kah-sele), if it involves a minor salivary gland, or in a **ranula** (**ran**-u-lah), if it involves the submandibular salivary gland (Figures 11-10 and 11-11). These two salivary gland lesions are treated by removal of the stone or surgical removal of the entire gland in the case of a minor gland with severed duct.

Another oral lesion associated with salivary glands is **nicotinic stomatitis** (nik-ah-**tin**-ik sto-mah-**ti**-tis) (Figure 11-12). With this lesion, the hard palate is whitened by hyperkeratinization caused by chronic heat production from smoking or hot liquid consumption (see **Chapter 9**). This chronic heat production also causes inflammation of the duct openings of the minor salivary glands of the palatal area, which become dilated in response. This inflammation of the ductal epithelium is seen clinically in the red macules scattered on the whiter background of the palatal oral mucosa.

Saliva is also being used, similarly to the secretions of urine and blood, to test for drug usage, systemic diseases, and changes in physiologic and psychological states, as well as oral cancer. Unlike the other bodily secretions, using saliva is very successful as a screening test because of the ease and low cost with which the sample can be obtained, removing the invasive nature of the diagnostic test.

THYROID GLAND PROPERTIES

The thyroid gland is the largest endocrine gland and is located in the anterior and lateral regions of the neck, inferior to the thyroid cartilage (see Figure 1-13). Because it is ductless, the thyroid gland produces and secretes its products or hormones directly into the blood, such as thyroxine. Thyroxine (thy-rok-sin) is a hormone that stimulates the metabolic rate. The gland consists of two lateral lobes connected anteriorly by an isthmus. In a healthy patient, the gland is not visible but can be palpated and should be mobile, moving superiorly when a person swallows.

THYROID GLAND HISTOLOGY

The thyroid gland is covered by a connective tissue capsule that then extends into the gland by way of septa (Figure 11-13). The septa divide the gland into larger lobes and then smaller lobules. Each lobule is composed of follicles (fol-i-kls), irregularly-shaped spheroidal masses that are embedded in a meshwork of reticular fibers. Each follicle consists of a layer of simple cuboidal epithelium enclosing a cavity that is usually filled with colloid (kol-oid), a stiff material, which is reserved for the future production of thyroxine.

The parathyroid glands typically consist of four to eight small endocrine glands, two on each side, usually close to the thyroid gland, or even inside it on its posterior surface. These glands are not visible or palpable during an extraoral examination of a patient. However, the parathyroid glands may alter the physiology of the thyroid gland because of their involvement in a disease process.

THYROID GLAND DEVELOPMENT

The thyroid gland is the first endocrine gland to appear in embryonic development and develops from endoderm invaded by mesenchyme. At approximately the 24th day of prenatal development, the thyroid gland develops. It forms from a median downgrowth at the base of the tongue, connected by a thyroglossal (thy-ro-gloss-al) duct, a narrow tube that later closes off and becomes obliterated (Figure 11-14).

The foramen cecum, which is the opening of the thyroglossal duct, is a small, pit-like depression located at the apex of the sulcus terminalis points where it points backward toward the oropharynx. This

FIGURE 11-10 Mucocele *(arrow)* on the lower lip involving the severance of the associated minor salivary gland duct and resulting in blockage of the gland resulting enlargement of the gland. (Courtesy of Margaret J. Fehrenbach, RDH, MS.)

FIGURE 11-12 Nicotinic stomatitis with hyperkeratinization of the palatal oral mucosa with its whiter clinical appearance and inflammation of the minor salivary glands ductal openings noted as redder areas *(arrows)*. This lesion can be from chronic heat production from smoking or hot liquid consumption. (Courtesy of Margaret J. Fehrenbach, RDH, MS.)

Floor of mouth

Lingual frenum

Ranula

Mandibular teeth

FIGURE 11-11 Ranula on one side of the floor of the mouth that involves the blockage of the submandibular salivary gland duct from stone formation resulting in enlargement of the gland. (Courtesy of Margaret J. Fehrenbach, RDH, MS.)

duct shows the origin of the thyroid and the migration pathway of the thyroid gland into the neck region.

During a disease process involving the thyroid gland (such as an endocrine disorder), the gland may become enlarged and possibly may be actually viewed during an extraoral examination. This enlarged thyroid gland is considered a goiter (goy-ter) (Figure 11-15). A goiter may be firm and tender when palpated and may contain hard masses. Any patient who has any undiagnosed changes noted in the thyroid gland or complains of related symptoms should have a medical referral.

LYMPHATICS PROPERTIES

The lymphatics (lim-fat-iks) are a part of the immune system and help fight disease processes. They also serve other functions in the body. The lymphatic system consists of a network of lymphatic vessels linking lymph nodes throughout most of the body. Tonsillar tissue

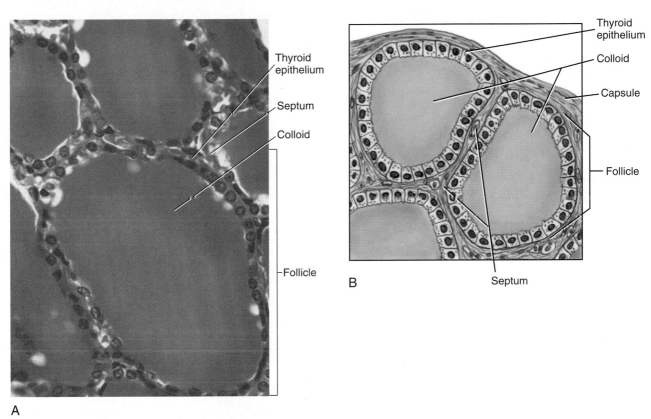

FIGURE 11-13 Histology of the thyroid gland. **A,** Photomicrograph. **B,** Diagram. (**A,** From Young B, Woodford P, O'Dowd G: *Wheater's functional histology,* ed 6, Edinburgh, 2014, Churchill Livingstone.)

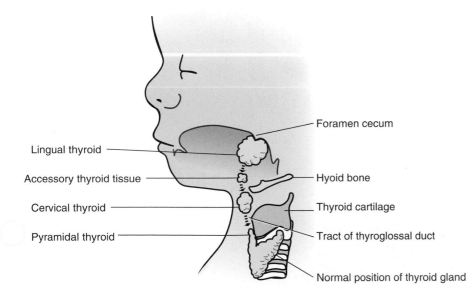

FIGURE 11-14 Development of the thyroid gland from a median downgrowth of the tongue *(broken line),* connected by a thyroglossal duct. Remnants of thyroid tissue can remain at these original sites and become cystic.

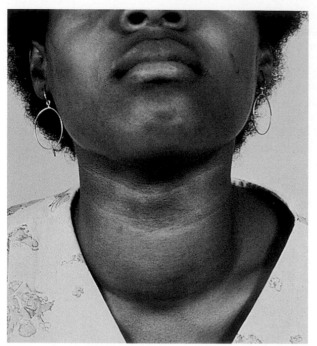

FIGURE 11-15 Goiter or enlarged thyroid gland caused by an endocrine disorder. (Courtesy of Margaret J. Fehrenbach, RDH, MS.)

located in the oral cavity and pharynx is part of the lymphatic system. This chapter describes only the intraoral tonsillar tissue in detail; the tubal tonsillar tissue is not discussed.

The **lymphatic vessels** are a system of endothelial-lined channels that are mostly parallel to the venous blood vessels in location but are more numerous. Tissue fluid drains from the surrounding region into the lymphatic vessels as **lymph** (limf). Lymph is similar in composition to tissue fluid and plasma (see **Chapters 7 and 8**).

Each lymphatic vessel drains its particular region, and all of these vessels communicate with one another. Lymphatic vessels are lined with endothelium similar to blood vessels, but the lymphatic vessels are larger and thicker in diameter than capillaries of the blood system. Lymphatic vessels are found within most of the oral tissue, even within the tooth's pulp.

Smaller lymphatic vessels containing lymph converge into the larger endothelial-lined **lymphatic ducts**, which empty into the venous system of the blood in the chest area. The drainage pattern of the lymphatic vessels into the lymphatic ducts depends on the side of the body involved, either the right or left, because the lymphatic ducts are different on each side.

LYMPH NODES

The lymph nodes are bean-shaped bodies grouped in clusters along the connecting lymphatic vessels, positioned to filter toxic products from the

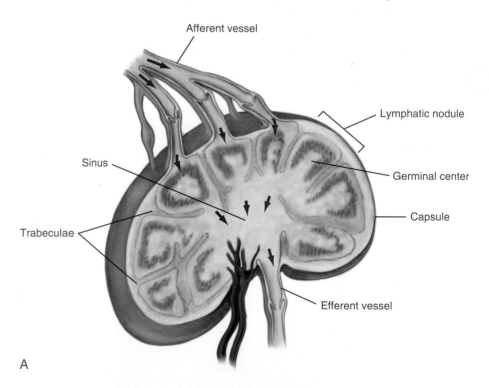

A

FIGURE 11-16 Lymph node and its structure. **A,** Diagram showing entering of lymph by the afferent vessels and exiting by way of the efferent vessel *(arrows).* **B,** Photomicrograph showing the lymphatic nodule with its germinal center *(GC)* and capsule *(C).* (**A,** From Fehrenbach MJ, Herring SW: *Illustrated anatomy of the head and neck,* ed 4, Philadelphia, 2012, Saunders/Elsevier. **B,** From Young B, Woodford P, O'Dowd G: *Wheater's functional histology,* ed 6, Edinburgh, 2014, Churchill Livingstone.)

lymph to prevent their entry into the blood system (Figure 11-16, *A*). They are located in various regions of the head and neck area (see Figures 1-2 and 1-12).

In healthy patients, lymph nodes are usually small, soft, and free or mobile in the surrounding tissue. They can be superficial in position with the smaller blood vessels, or deep in the tissue with the larger blood vessels. Usually, lymph nodes cannot be seen or palpated during an extraoral examination of a healthy patient.

The lymph flows into the lymph node through many **afferent** (af-er-int) **vessels**. On one side of the node is a depression, or **hilus** (hi-lus), where the lymph flows out of the node through fewer vessels, or even a single **efferent** (ef-er-ent) **vessel**. Lymph nodes can be classified as either primary or secondary nodes. Lymph from a particular tissue region drains into primary nodes (or regional nodes). Primary nodes, in turn, drain into secondary nodes (or central nodes).

LYMPH NODE HISTOLOGY

Each lymph node is composed of organized lymphoid tissue and contains lymphocytes that actively filter toxic products from the lymph (see Figure 8-16). The node itself is surrounded by a capsule with bands of connective tissue, the trabeculae, extending from the capsule into the node. The **trabeculae** (trah-**bek**-u-lay) separate the node into masses of lymphocytes, the **lymphatic nodules** (nah-**jools**) (or lymphatic follicles). The lymph flows between the lymphatic nodules and other tissue spaces or sinuses.

Each lymphatic nodule has a **germinal** (**jurm**-i-nil) **center** containing many immature lymphocytes (see Figure 11-16, *B*). As they mature, these lymphocytes enter either the area of the nodule surrounding the germinal center or the lymph. These mature lymphocytes are of the B-cell type and are mainly involved in the humoral immune response with immunoglobulin production by the plasma cells (see Figure 8-16).

LYMPH NODE DEVELOPMENT

Lymphatic vessels develop from the blood vessels by a process of budding and fusion of isolated cell groups of mesenchyme. Peripherally located mesenchymal cells form the lymphatic nodules in the connective tissue associated with the developing lymphatic vessels. The sinuses then surround nodules, which completes the development of a lymph node. Later, a capsule and trabeculae will form around the developing lymphatic nodules from the surrounding mesenchyme.

INTRAORAL TONSILLAR TISSUE PROPERTIES AND HISTOLOGY

Intraoral tonsillar tissue consists of nonencapsulated masses of lymphoid tissue located in the lamina propria of the oral mucosa. It is covered by stratified squamous epithelium that is continuous with the surrounding oral mucosa. Tonsils, like lymph nodes, contain lymphocytes that remove toxic products and then move to the epithelial surface as they mature. Unlike lymph nodes, tonsillar tissue is not located along lymphatic vessels but is situated near airway and food passages to protect the body against disease processes from the related toxins. Tonsillar development is described in **Chapter 4**. The palatine tonsils are two rounded masses of variable size located between the anterior faucial pillar and posterior faucial pillar (see Figure 2-11).

Microscopically, each mass of intraoral tonsillar tissue contains fused-together lymphatic nodules that generally have germinal centers (Figure 11-17). Each tonsil also has 10 to 20 epithelial invaginations,

or grooves, which penetrate deeply into the tonsil to form tonsillar crypts. These crypts usually contain shed epithelial cells, mature lymphocytes, and oral bacteria.

The lingual tonsil is an indistinct layer of diffuse lymphoid tissue located on the base of the dorsal surface of the tongue, posterior to the circumvallate lingual papillae (see Figure 2-14, *A*). The lymphoid tissue consists of many lymphatic nodules, usually each with a germinal center and only one associated tonsillar crypt.

Behind the uvula, on the superior and posterior walls of the nasopharynx, are the **pharyngeal** (fah-**rin**-je-il) **tonsils**, forming an incomplete ring of tissue, the Waldeyer ring. When they become enlarged, as is common in children, they are considered the *adenoids*.

Clinical Considerations for Lymphoid Tissue Pathology

When a patient has an active disease process (such as cancer or infection) in a specific region, the region's lymph nodes respond. The resultant enlarged lymph node with its change in the consistency of its lymphoid tissue is from the process of **lymphadenopathy** (lim-fad-uh-**nop**-ah-thee). Lymphadenopathy is due to both an increase in the size of each individual lymphocyte and the overall cell count in the lymphoid tissue. With more and larger lymphocytes within the lymph node itself, the lymphoid tissue is better able to fight the disease process.

The presence of lymphadenopathy allows the node to now be easily palpated during an extraoral examination. More important, changes in consistency from firm to bony hard may occur. Palpation of an involved node may be painful, and the node can become fixed and attached to the surrounding tissue.

Lymphadenopathy can also occur in the intraoral tonsillar tissue, causing tissue enlargement that can be viewed on an intraoral examination (Figure 11-18). The intraoral tonsils may also be tender when swallowing Severe lymphadenopathy may cause airway obstruction and complications from the infection of the tonsillar tissue. If any lymph nodes are palpable or if there is an enlargement or infection of intraoral tonsillar tissue, these findings should be recorded in the patient record and a medical referral should be made.

The immune system and the associated lymphatics are also triggered with the development or progression of periodontal disease (see **Chapters 10 and 14**). In addition, during the immune system's response, the liver releases *C* (*cross*)-*reactive protein* (CRP), which allows the recognition of periodontopathogens and damaged cells of the periodontium, attracting other inflammatory mediators to the damaged and infected site. CRP also marks the periodontopathogens for destruction by white blood cells; the primary white blood cells responsible for killing invading these pathogens are neutrophils (see **Chapter 8**).

NASAL CAVITY PROPERTIES

The **nasal cavity** (nay-zil **kav**-it-ee) is the inner space of the nose (Figure 11-19). It communicates with the exterior by two nares. The nares are separated by the midline nasal septum, which consists of both bone and cartilage (see Figure 1-4). The nasal septum also divides the internal nasal cavity into two parts.

Each lateral wall of the nasal cavity has three projecting structures, or **nasal conchae** (**kong**-kay), which extend inward. Beneath each concha are openings through which the paranasal sinuses or nasolacrimal ducts communicate with the nasal cavity. The posterior part of the nasal cavity communicates with the nasopharynx and then with the rest of the respiratory system. The development of the nasal cavity and septum is described in **Chapter 5**.

A

B

FIGURE 11-17 Histology of the palatine tonsils. **A,** Diagram. **B,** Photomicrograph showing lymphatic nodule *(LN)* and the crypt *(C)* lined by epithelium. Note that the crypt usually contains oral bacteria. (**B,** From Stevens A, Lowe J: *Human histology,* ed 4, St Louis, 2015, Mosby/Elsevier.)

NASAL CAVITY HISTOLOGY

The nasal cavity is lined by a respiratory mucosa like the rest of the respiratory system. Respiratory mucosa (mu-ko-sah) is different from oral mucosa lining the oral cavity but similar to that lining the trachea and bronchi (see Figure 8-2). It consists of ciliated pseudostratified columnar epithelium (Figure 11-20). Within the epithelium, and surrounded by mucous and serous glands, are goblet cells, which rest on the basement membrane. Fluids or mucus from the goblet cells and glands keep this mucosa moist, provide humidity, and trap any foreign materials from the inspired air.

The moist mucus forms a superficial coating on the respiratory mucosa. This coating is moved by ciliary action posteriorly to the nasopharynx, where it is either expectorated or swallowed. In this manner, foreign materials are trapped and removed. Because the lamina propria of the mucosa is extremely vascular, it also warms the incoming breathed air. In the roof of each part of the nasal cavity is a specialized region containing the olfactory (ol-fak-tor-e) mucosa, which carries the receptors for the sense of smell.

Overlying the conchae is an extensive, superficial plexus of large, thin-walled vessels termed erectile (e-rek-tile) tissue. This tissue is capable of considerable engorgement. This engorgement happens at periodic intervals of 30 to 60 minutes, thus closing off the involved side of the nasal cavity to enable the respiratory mucosa to recover from the effects of dryness during respiration. The deepest parts of the lamina propria are continuous with the periosteum of the nasal bone or perichondrium of the nasal cartilage.

The respiratory mucosa of the nasal cavity and septum is continuous and similar to that of the nasopharynx (see Figure 2-18). The respiratory mucosa of the nasopharynx gives way to the stratified squamous epithelium of the oropharynx. The stronger stratified squamous epithelium of the oropharynx, with its soft palate and posterior wall of the pharynx, allows the mechanical stress of swallowing.

PARANASAL SINUSES PROPERTIES

The **paranasal sinuses** (pare-ah-na-zil sy-nuses) are paired air-filled cavities in bone that include the frontal, sphenoidal, ethmoidal, and maxillary sinuses (Figure 11-21). The sinuses communicate with the nasal cavity through small openings in the lateral nasal wall. The openings mark the outpouchings from which the paranasal sinuses develop. The sinuses serve to lighten the skull bones, act as sound resonators, and provide mucus for the nasal cavity.

PARANASAL SINUSES HISTOLOGY

The sinuses are lined with respiratory mucosa consisting of ciliated pseudostratified columnar epithelium continuous with the epithelial lining of the nasal cavity (see Figures 8-2 and 11-20). The epithelium of the sinuses, although it is similar to that of the nasal cavity, is thinner and contains fewer goblet cells. The respiratory mucosa of the sinuses also shows a thinner underlying lamina propria that is continuous with the deeper periosteum of the bone. It also has fewer associated glands, and no erectile tissue is present in the sinuses.

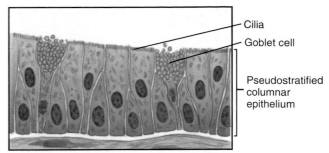

FIGURE 11-20 Histology of the respiratory mucosa lining the nasal cavity.

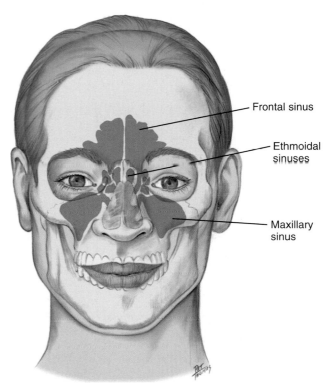

FIGURE 11-21 Paranasal sinuses: frontal, ethmoidal, maxillary. Sphenoidal sinus is not shown in this view because it is deep to the ethmoidal sinus. (From Fehrenbach MJ, Herring SW: *Illustrated anatomy of the head and neck*, ed 4, Philadelphia, 2012, Saunders/Elsevier.)

FIGURE 11-18 Lymphadenopathy of the palatine tonsils *(arrows)* showing enlargement. (From Fehrenbach MJ, Herring SW: *Illustrated anatomy of the head and neck*, ed 4, Philadelphia, 2012, Saunders/Elsevier.)

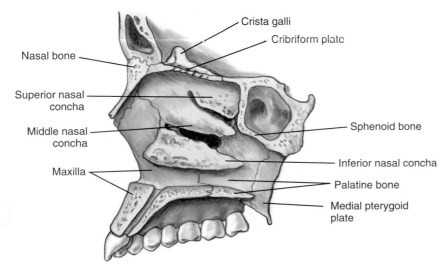

FIGURE 11-19 Nasal cavity and its nasal conchae. (From Fehrenbach MJ, Herring SW: *Illustrated anatomy of the head and neck*, ed 4, Philadelphia, 2012, Saunders/Elsevier.)

PARANASAL SINUSES DEVELOPMENT

Certain sinuses develop during late fetal life; the rest develop after birth. They form as outgrowths of the wall of the nasal cavity and become air-filled extensions in the adjacent bones. The original openings of the outgrowths persist as orifices of the adult sinuses.

The maxillary sinuses are small at birth, and only a few of the ethmoidal sinuses are present. The maxillary sinuses grow until puberty, and are not fully developed until all the permanent teeth have erupted in early adulthood. The ethmoidal sinuses do not start to grow until 6 to 8 years of age.

The frontal sinuses and sphenoidal sinuses are not present at birth. At approximately 2 years of age, the two anterior ethmoidal sinuses grow into the frontal bone, forming the frontal sinus on each side, and are visible on radiographs by the seventh year. At the same time, the two posterior ethmoidal sinuses grow into the sphenoid bone and form the sphenoidal sinuses. Growth of sinuses in the size and shape of the face is important during infancy and childhood and adds resonance to the voice during puberty.

Clinical Considerations for Nasal Cavity and Paranasal Sinus Pathology

The respiratory mucosa of the nasal cavity and paranasal sinuses can become inflamed and the space congested with mucus as a result of allergies or respiratory tract infection. This inflammation can lead to a stuffed-up feeling in the nasal cavity and sinusitis (sy-nu-si-tis) in the sinus. The symptoms for both are discomfort caused by the pressure of the increased mucus production with nasal or pharyngeal discharge.

With blocked nasal passages and with sinusitis, medications are used to produce vasoconstriction in the blood vessels while reducing the amount of mucus produced. In cases of chronic sinusitis, surgical treatment may be needed. Patients undergoing these respiratory difficulties may not be able to use nitrous oxide adequately, may feel uncomfortable with the use of a rubber dam, and may breathe through the mouth, causing chronic gingivitis of the maxillary anterior teeth.

Because the roots of the maxillary posterior teeth are in close proximity to the maxillary sinus, maxillary sinusitis can sometimes result as infection spreads from a periapical abscess associated with one of the roots of a maxillary posterior tooth (Figure 11-22). As the infection spreads, the sinus floor is perforated, and the mucosa of the sinus becomes involved in the infection. During an extraction, a contaminated tooth or root fragments can also be surgically displaced into the maxillary sinus. In addition, because of their close proximity, the pain from maxillary sinusitis can sometimes be mistakenly misinterpreted by the patient as involving the maxillary teeth instead of the sinus(es) (see Chapter 17). Differential diagnosis of the symptoms and radiographs can aid in determining the correct cause of this facial pain.

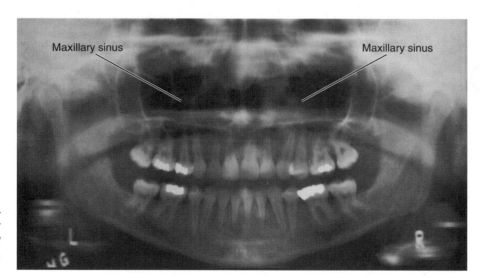

FIGURE 11-22 Panoramic radiograph demonstrating that the roots of the maxillary posterior teeth are in close proximity to the maxillary sinuses. (Courtesy of Margaret J. Fehrenbach, RDH, MS.)

CHAPTER 12

Enamel

Additional resources and practice exercises are provided on the companion Evolve website for this book: ⓔ
http://evolve.elsevier.com/Fehrenbach/illustrated.

●●● LEARNING OBJECTIVES

1. Define and pronounce the key terms in this chapter.
2. Describe the enamel properties and the clinical considerations concerned with enamel structure, integrating it into patient care.
3. Discuss the processes involved in the apposition and maturation stages of enamel, as well as the

clinical considerations concerned with enamel formation and pathology, integrating it into patient care.
4. Discuss the histology of enamel and the clinical considerations for dental procedures concerning enamel, integrating it into patient care.
5. Identify the components of the enamel on a diagram.

ENAMEL PROPERTIES

Preservation of the enamel of every tooth during a patient's lifetime is one of the goals of every dental professional because it is not a renewable tissue. Dental professionals must take into consideration the properties and histology of enamel when deciding the caries risk for patients, counseling patients and communities on fluoride use, applying enamel sealants as well as restorations, and using and recommending polishing or toothpaste agents (discussed later).

Mature enamel is a crystalline material that is the hardest mineralized tissue in the body (Table 12-1; see Table 6-2). Enamel can endure crushing pressure of around 100,000 pounds per square inch. A layering of the deeper dentin and surrounding periodontium, coupled with the hardness of the enamel, produces a cushioning effect of the tooth's differing structures enabling it to endure the pressures of mastication.

In its mature state, it is noted for its almost total absence of the softer organic matrix. Enamel in a healthy state, without trauma or disease, can be removed only by rotary cutting instruments or rough files, such as those used in dental practice. Enamel is avascular and has no nerve supply within it. Although enamel is the hardest mineralized tissue in the body, it can be lost forever because it is nonvital and therefore not a renewable tissue. However, it is not a static tissue, because it can undergo mineralization changes (discussed later).

Mature enamel is by weight 96% inorganic material or mineralized, 1% organic material, and 3% water. This crystalline formation of mature enamel consists mainly of calcium hydroxyapatite with the chemical formula of $Ca_{10}(PO_4)_6(OH)_2$. The calcium hydroxyapatite is similar to that found in lesser percentages in dentin, cementum, and the alveolar process. On radiographs, the differences in the mineralization of different parts of the tooth and surrounding periodontium can be noted (see Figure 2-5). Enamel appears more radiopaque

(or lighter) than either dentin or pulp because it is denser than the latter structures, both of which appear more radiolucent (or darker).

Other minerals, such as carbonate, magnesium, potassium, sodium, and fluoride, are also present in smaller amounts. Studies have challenged this composition of enamel, and, instead, maintain that it is mainly carbonated hydroxyapatite, because of its relationship with fluoride uptake. Whatever the true composition, the ribbon like crystals of enamel are set at different angles throughout the crown area, each 30% larger than those in dentin. The sheer size difference of enamel and dentinal crystals is a leading factor contributing to enamel's hardness over dentin. Discussion of the elegant crystalline nature of enamel is inadequate at best, but this chapter is an attempt to do justice to this beautiful jewel-like material.

Enamel is usually the only part of a tooth that is seen clinically in a healthy oral cavity because it covers the anatomic crown (see Figure 15-8). Enamel provides a hard surface for mastication and speech; it is able to withstand the masticatory impact of 20 to 30 pounds of pressure per tooth. Enamel shows a thinner layer in the cervical region and is thicker in masticatory surfaces, such as at the incisal ridge and cusps, where impact can be greater. Thickness can also range per tooth type—from 0 to 2 mm for incisors to 2.6 mm for molars.

Enamel also provides the pleasing whiteness of a healthy smile. Enamel alone is various shades of bluish white, which is seen on the incisal ridge of newly erupted incisors, but it turns various shades of yellow-white elsewhere because of the underlying dentin (see Figure 16-8, A). The enamel on primary teeth has a more opaque crystalline form, and thus appears whiter than on permanent teeth (see Figure 15-4).

Because the overall shade of enamel varies in each person and possibly within a dentition, a shade value is taken when integrating tooth-colored restorative materials or artificial teeth or crowns within an individual dentition. The goal is to match the color of the patient's surrounding natural teeth as closely as possible. This shade value is selected by comparing the patient's natural teeth to a shade guide of plastic model crowns that have been moistened and are viewed in natural light. New technology allows a digital read-out of the color of the enamel (vital whitening process or bleaching is discussed later.)

Clinical Considerations with Enamel Structure

One way that enamel and other hard tissue of the tooth are lost is through attrition (ah-**trish**-un), which is the wearing away of hard tissue as a result of tooth-to-tooth contact (Table 12-2). The wear on masticatory surfaces from attrition increases with aging. Permanent first molars wear more than seconds; seconds wear more than thirds. However, attrition can occur at severe levels, involving an excessive loss of enamel, and is discussed in **Chapter 20** with regard to parafunctional habits (see also Figures 16-8, *B*, 16-17, 16-24, and 20-8).

TABLE 12-1	Comparison of the Physical Properties of Enamel and Dentin	
PHYSICAL PROPERTY	**ENAMEL**	**DENTIN**
Specific gravity	2.9	2.14
Hardness (Knoop number)	296	64
Stiffness (Young modulus)	131 GN/m2	12 GN/m2
Compressive strength	76 MN/m2	262 MN/m2
Tensile strength	46 MN/m2	33 MN/m2

GN, Giganewtons (N × 109); *MN*, meganewtons (N × 106)
(From Nanci A: *Ten Cate's oral histology*, ed 8, St Louis, 2013, Mosby/Elsevier.)

The relationship between the loss of the vertical dimension of the face, attrition, and alveolar process loss is discussed in **Chapter 14**.

Enamel loss may also result from friction caused by excessive toothbrushing and abrasive toothpaste. This wear of enamel is considered **abrasion** (uh-**brey**-zhun). Dental personnel must keep this in mind when discussing homecare with patients and explain that there is no need to harshly treat the teeth in order to keep them healthy.

Enamel can also be lost by **erosion** (e-**ro**-zhun) through chemical means. Erosion is particularly apparent in patients with the eating disorder of bulimia, in which patients force themselves to vomit to remove their stomach contents in pursuit of weight loss (Figure 12-1, *A*). The lingual surface of the maxillary anterior teeth and the occlusal surface of maxillary posterior teeth are eroded by the acid content of the vomit. The yellow underlying dentin is thereby exposed and can undergo attrition, because it is less mineralized than enamel. Treatment of bulimia is multifactorial and includes behavior changes. Similar erosion can be caused by gastric reflux, as well as certain recreational drug use (for example, "meth mouth"). If facial enamel lesions of the anterior teeth are evident, the patient may be overusing acid-containing carbonated soft, sport, or health drinks (especially diet formulations and those containing citric acid).

Another way that enamel can be lost is by **enamel** (ih-**nam**-l) **caries**. Caries is a process through which a cavity is created by demineralization, or loss of minerals. This demineralization is due to acid production by cariogenic bacteria and occurs to enamel when the pH is less than 5.5 (see later discussion in this chapter).

Finally, enamel can be lost as a result of **abfraction** (ab-**frak**-shen) (see Figure 12-1, *B*). Abfraction is caused by increasing the tensile and compressive forces during tooth flexure, which possibly occurs during parafunctional habits with their occlusal loading (see **Chapter 20**). It consists of cervical lesions that cannot be attributed to any particular cause, such as erosion or toothbrush abrasion. Abfraction causes the

TABLE 12-2	Enamel Structure Loss	
.METHOD	**FEATURES**	**CLINICAL APPEARANCE**
Attrition	Loss through tooth-to-tooth contact from mastication with aging or more severely with parafunctional habits	• Matching wear on masticatory surfaces • Shiny facets on amalgam contacts • Enamel and dentin wear at the same rate • Possible fracture of cusps or restorations
Abrasion	Loss through friction from toothbrushing and/or toothpaste	• Usually located at facial cervical regions • Lesions more wide than deep • Canines commonly affected because of tooth position
Erosion	Loss through chemical means (via acid) not involving bacteria	• Broad concavities within smooth surface enamel • Cupping of occlusal surface (or incisal grooving) with dentin exposure (with possible dentinal hypersensitivity) • Increased incisal translucency • Wear on nonmasticatory surfaces (exact location depends on acid intake-type) • Raised and shiny amalgam restorations • Preservation of enamel cuff in gingival crevice • Pulp exposure and loss of surface characteristics of enamel in primary teeth
Caries	Loss through chemical means (via acid) from cariogenic bacteria by way of dental biofilm	• All surfaces can be affected • Occlusal surfaces more commonly affected, especially in pits and grooves • Possibly rapid progression of interproximal smooth surface lesions if progress goes unchecked • Cervical lesions sometimes secondary to other forms of hard tissue loss or gingival recession
Abfraction	Possible loss through tensile and compressive forces during tooth flexure with parafunctional habits	• Can affect both facial and lingual cervical regions • Deep, narrow V-shaped notch • Commonly affects single teeth that have occlusal loads

enamel to pop off, starting at the cervical region, thus exposing the lesion to possible further wear, dentinal hypersensitivity, or caries.

The type of tooth surface polishing agent used by dental professionals, as well as by patients at home, is also a very important consideration in retaining enamel structure. Older toothpastes and professional polishing agents abraded the enamel surface, removing valuable tooth layers to obtain temporary esthetic results (vital whitening of enamel is discussed later). Selective polishing methods are now used only to remove extrinsic stain on natural enamel surfaces; many clinicians use ultrasonic devices for removal instead, because it is faster and prevents overall enamel removal. However, the use of less abrasive professional and homecare polishing agents, such as with the newer air polishing agents (glycine), helps preserve the limited enamel on the crowns. It is also not necessary to polish the teeth to remove dental biofilm before topical fluoride application or, in many cases, before enamel sealant placement.

ENAMEL MATRIX FORMATION

Amelogenesis is formation of enamel matrix that occurs during the apposition stage of tooth development. The exact time of the apposition stage for each tooth varies according to the tooth that is undergoing development. Many factors can affect amelogenesis (see Figure 6-16).

Enamel matrix is produced by ameloblasts during its secretory phase (Figure 12-2). Each ameloblast is approximately 4 micrometers in diameter, 40 micrometers in length, and is hexagonal or six-sided in a cross section. The ameloblasts are columnar cells that differentiate

FIGURE 12-1 Enamel loss. **A,** Lingual erosion in a patient with a past history of bulimia. Note that the facial surface of the permanent maxillary central incisors has been restored using a veneer because of the amount of hard tissue loss, which caused the teeth to look more transparent and gray. **B,** Abfraction of the maxillary right quadrant, especially on the permanent maxillary lateral incisor. The permanent maxillary first premolar has been already been restored once but now has secondary enamel caries around the margins. (Courtesy of Margaret J. Fehrenbach, RDH, MS.)

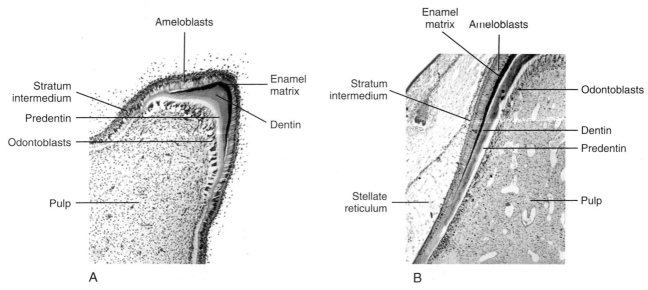

FIGURE 12-2 Photomicrographs of a tooth undergoing matrix formation of both enamel and dentin. **A,** Dentin already showing maturation. **B,** The close-up view shows ameloblasts producing enamel matrix from their Tomes processes. (From Nanci A: *Ten Cate's oral histology,* ed 8, St Louis, 2013, Mosby/Elsevier.)

during the apposition stage in the crown area. Ameloblasts are not differentiated in the root area; thus, the enamel is usually just confined to the anatomic crown.

The enamel matrix is secreted from each ameloblast from its own Tomes process with its "picket-fence" microscopic structure (see Figures 6-12 and 12-2, *B*). Tomes process is not a true process, but, instead, it is a projection of the basal or secretory end of each ameloblast that faces the dentinoenamel junction (DEJ). This is unlike the process associated with the odontoblast, which is a true cytoplasmic process from a cell body. However, like the odontoblasts on the other side of the DEJ, ameloblasts produce approximately 4 μm of enamel matrix daily during tooth development.

Tomes process is responsible for the way the enamel matrix is laid down; it is the guiding factor similar to a snowplow going through a snowy parking lot. First, the body of the cell between the processes deposits enamel matrix between the ameloblasts, which will become the periphery of the enamel rods, forming an outside mold for the enamel between the enamel rods (at the interrod enamel or interprismatic region), which is discussed later with the rods. Secondly, the Tomes process of individual ameloblasts will infill the future main body of the enamel rod. Thus there is a one-to-one relationship between the secretory face of Tomes process and each enamel rod produced. However, multiple ameloblasts contribute to the enamel between the enamel rods (at the interrod enamel or interprismatic region).

Enamel matrix is an ectodermal product, because ameloblasts are derived from the inner enamel epithelium of the enamel organ, which was originally derived from the ectoderm of the embryo. Initially, enamel matrix is composed of proteins, carbohydrates, and only a small amount of calcium hydroxyapatite crystals. Unlike dentin, cementum, and the alveolar process, which are mesodermal products, enamel does not contain collagen protein. Instead, it has two unique classes of proteins, amelogenins and ameloblastin, as well as enamelins, the latter being very similar to keratin.

Because it only has a small amount of calcium, the initial enamel matrix is therefore only partially mineralized, as compared with fully matured or mineralized enamel (discussed later). Ameloblasts are also responsible for this partially mineralized state of the enamel matrix, because they actively pump calcium hydroxyapatite into the forming enamel matrix as it is being secreted by each of the Tomes processes.

Enamel matrix is first formed in the incisal or occlusal part of the future crown nearer to the forming DEJ (Figure 12-3). This is the first wave of enamel appositional growth on the masticatory surface and

later moves to the nonmasticatory surface. The second wave of enamel appositional growth overlaps the first wave with the entire process moving cervically to the cementoenamel junction (CEJ). This is discussed in more detail under "Enamel Matrix Maturation." The morphology of the CEJ is discussed further in **Chapter 14**.

Certain developmental disturbances, such as an enamel pearl and enamel dysplasia, can occur in enamel during the apposition stage (see Box 6-1, *O-P*). Another common developmental disturbance is the deepened pit and groove patterns on the lingual surface of anterior teeth and on the occlusal surface of posterior teeth (see **Chapters 16 and 17**; Figures 16-10 and 17-8). These are created when ameloblasts back into one another during the apposition stage, cutting off their source of nutrition. This loss of nutritional support causes incomplete maturation of enamel matrix, making it weak or even absent in that area. These areas of incompletely matured enamel can lead to enamel caries with the presence of a supporting environment (discussed later in this chapter).

ENAMEL MATRIX MATURATION

During the maturation stage of tooth development, enamel matrix completes its mineralization process to its full level of 96% after the apposition stage when it is only partially mineralized at approximately 30%. Thus, mineralization of enamel matrix to a fully matured tissue actually covers two stages of tooth development—the apposition and maturation stages. Enamel mineralization also continues after eruption of the tooth (discussed next).

During the maturation of enamel matrix, ameloblasts move from production to actively transporting materials for mineralization by undergoing cellular modulation in cycles that correspond to mineralization waves that travel across the crown of a developing tooth from least mature regions to most mature regions of the enamel (discussed next). First the cells accomplish the removal of water and organic material from the enamel. This allows introduction of additional inorganic material next into the already partially mineralized enamel. Thus, ameloblasts are specifically responsible for maturation of enamel matrix into mature enamel.

Two waves of enamel mineralization during the maturation stage follow the same pattern as that of the apposition stage (see Figure 12-3). The first wave of enamel mineralization occurs in the incisal or occlusal part of the future crown nearer to the DEJ and moves to the nonmasticatory

Less mineralized More mineralized

Matrix formation   Maturation

FIGURE 12-3 Wave patterns in the crown from the time of enamel matrix formation to maturation of enamel.

surface. The second wave of enamel mineralization overlaps the first wave as the process moves cervically to the forming CEJ.

After the ameloblasts are finished with both enamel appositional growth and maturation, they become part of the reduced enamel epithelium (REE) along with the other tissue types of the compressed enamel organ (see Figures 6-23 and 6-24). They undergo a reduction in height and a decrease in their volume and organelle content. The REE will later fuse with the oral mucosa, creating a protective tunnel to allow the enamel cusp tip to erupt through the oral mucosa into the oral cavity (see Figure 6-25, *D*). Unfortunately, the ameloblasts are lost forever as the fused tissue disintegrates during tooth eruption, preventing any further enamel appositional growth. The entire tissue can later become part of Nasmyth membrane (see Figure 6-29).

Enamel is not a renewable tissue because there is no way to retrieve the lost ameloblasts and then have them become involved in tissue regeneration of enamel. Research now involves the study of amelogenins, which is the principal extracellular matrix protein component involved in this process of mineralizing enamel. Amelogenins may play a substantial role in controlling the growth and organization of enamel crystals, which may be able to be harnessed for enamel replacement after enamel loss through caries or other pathology (discussed next).

After the tooth erupts into the oral cavity, however, the mineralization of enamel continues. This posteruptive maturation is due to the deposition of minerals, such as fluoride and calcium, from saliva into hypomineralized areas of enamel (see discussion of fluoride next).

Clinical Considerations with Enamel Pathology

As discussed earlier, the weak areas of deepened pits and grooves are targets for enamel caries (Figure 12-4, *A*). Dental biofilm can become sheltered in these irregular areas or niches that cannot even be reached by careful homecare. The dental biofilm produces acids that slowly demineralize the weakened enamel areas, producing caries. There is a constant "tug-of-war" between demineralization and remineralization at the enamel surface; when demineralization outweighs remineralization, enamel caries results.

Remineralization is the deposition of minerals into mature enamel from salivary minerals and fluoride or other therapies (discussed later). However, with the cariogenic process, the surface enamel of the pit or groove remains intact as the subsurface zones become further demineralized. Thus, enamel caries remains in the subsurface, enlarging its pathway to the connected dentin and/or pulp area to form dentinal caries, or pulpitis, if the acidic and/or bacterial assault continues.

Protection against enamel caries is provided by the use of enamel sealants that cover the deepened pit and groove patterns on the teeth (see **Chapters 16 and 17**). Educating patients about the importance of enamel sealants in caries prevention is an important responsibility for dental professionals. Many clinicians are now recommending enamel sealants for adults because of the increased risk of future caries at these unrestored sites or nearby restored margins.

Similar to the enamel caries that occurs in deepened pits and grooves, smooth surface caries, which tends to occur interproximally, does not involve the breakdown or demineralization of the surface layers of enamel (see Figure 12-4, *B*). Zones are also present with smooth surface caries, as they are with caries of pits and grooves. In the past, enamel caries predominated on smooth surfaces interproximally on the teeth. However, with the widespread use of fluoride, the very nature of tooth decay has changed; the outer enamel surfaces of teeth are strengthened and more resistant, and thus pit and groove cavities are now more prevalent than smooth surface cavities.

Pit and groove caries are traditionally the most difficult to detect using radiographs due to the direction from which the images are taken. Instead, incipient enamel caries both in the pits and grooves and on smooth surfaces are first noted in many cases, clinically, as a white-spot lesion, with the involved enamel appearing whiter and rougher as a result of slight surface demineralization of the enamel. However, this initial lesion may also be detected through the use of a "sticky" explorer for both types of enamel caries. The enamel surface having been finally undermined, the explorer falls into the already destroyed subsurface.

It is important to remember that early subsurface lesions cannot be detected on radiographs until they spread at least 200 micrometers into the dentin, a process that can take more than 3 to 5 years, and

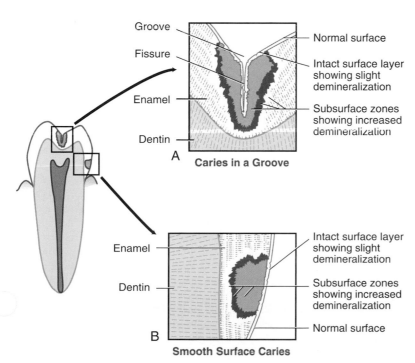

FIGURE 12-4 Process of enamel caries demonstrating the different zones for the two main types of caries. **A,** Caries in a groove. **B,** Smooth surface caries. Note that both types initially have an intact surface layer with slight demineralization and that the increased demineralization of caries occurs mainly in the subsurface zones.

usually only for smooth surface caries. Light-induced devices that measure changes in laser fluorescence of hard tissue allow dental professionals to better diagnose early carious lesions involving the enamel in a pit and groove before involving the deeper and more extensive dentin layers. However, clinicians should not rely on readings alone to determine the extension of incipient pit and groove caries.

If caries is only present in the enamel, it does not cause pain to the patient because the enamel has no nerves within it. For the same reason, initial cavity preparation is usually painless during removal of enamel only. Pain occurs only when the deeper layers of dentin, and then the associated pulpal tissue, are involved (see Figure 13-12). Thus, it is important to emphasize to patients the need for recall examinations for early detection of decay before pain is involved. Pain is a late finding in caries, and the risk of tooth loss increases while waiting for this symptom to appear.

A theory of systemic fluoride action proposes that fluoride enters the crystalline formation of enamel during tooth development. This action may produce differences in the morphology of the teeth, resulting in more caries-resistant teeth, which are slightly smaller in their occlusal surfaces and have shallower pit and groove patterns; further studies in this area are necessary for a more complete understanding. Fluoride can enter the enamel systemically through the blood supply of developing teeth by ingestion of fluoride in drops, tablets, or treated water, all of which are considered preeruptive methods.

In contrast, studies have shown that topical fluoride use (as opposed to systemic use) has a more important role in caries control than previously thought. Topical use results in an increased level of remineralization of any demineralized regions at the surface, which can actually reverse the carious process. Remineralization is the deposition of minerals into enamel in a way that resembles that of posteruptive maturation, although the minerals are now being deposited into previously demineralized enamel. This remineralization may produce an enamel crystal that is larger and thus more resistant to acid attack. Fluoride can also enter enamel topically by direct contact on exposed teeth surfaces by ingestion of fluoridated water or professional application, or by directed use of prescription or over-the-counter rinses, gels, foams, chewable tablets, and fluoridated toothpastes, all of which are considered posteruptive methods. Fluoride in prophylaxis pastes provided for use in the dental office provides only brief action and must not take the place of topical fluoride applications.

In addition to its direct mineralizing effect on enamel, fluoride may affect oral bacteria by interfering with the actual microbial acid production, reducing potential enamel destruction. Thus, the need for daily topical fluoride exposure, through a combination of fluoride therapies, has been demonstrated for all age groups. In addition, other noninvasive caries management system therapies such as casein phosphopeptide-amorphous calcium phosphate (CPP-ACP) are being used for tooth remineralization.

Just as important clinically to situations with reduced fluoride levels is that of excess systemic fluoride intake during tooth development, which can occur in areas where the water naturally has a higher than usual level of fluoride. This can cause a type of enamel dysplasia (dis-play-ze-ah), which is called *dental fluorosis* or *mottled enamel* (Figure 12-5; see **Chapter 6**). This type of dysplasia can involve both enamel hypoplasia with pitting and also enamel hypocalcification with intrinsic staining of the enamel, giving affected teeth a spotty discoloration. Dental fluorosis can also occur in lesser amounts in younger children who ingest too much flavored fluoridated toothpaste or inappropriate prescription of systemic fluoride. Vital whitening (or bleaching) may be able to even out the tooth color, or esthetic restorations can be placed (discussed later in this chapter).

FIGURE 12-5 Dental fluorosis with its intrinsic staining of the enamel caused by ingestion of excess amounts of fluoride that in this case occurred naturally in the water system. (From Ibsen OAC, Phelan JA: *Oral pathology for dental hygienists*, ed 6, Philadelphia, 2014, Saunders/Elsevier.)

ENAMEL HISTOLOGY

The enamel rod (or enamel prism) is the crystalline structural unit of enamel; thus, enamel is composed of millions of enamel rods (Figure 12-6). Enamel rods and associated structures should be viewed under a microscope to best understand them. The crystals that make up the rod are long ribbons of crystallites that start off thin and become thicker as enamel matures through mineralization. Each enamel rod becomes hexagonal in cross section with the enamel crystals in the rod being generally oriented parallel to its long axis. However, when fully matured, the enamel rods are no longer perfectly hexagonal but instead have an irregular outline because of crowding, flattening each other during the final part of their mineralization. In most areas of enamel, the mature rod is 4 micrometers in diameter and up to 2.5 mm in length. And each enamel rod is generally cylindrical in longitudinal section.

It is important to note that there are many variations in the structural arrangement of the enamel components, and the crystals within each enamel rod are highly complex as a result, with each ameloblast and their own Tomes process affecting the crystal pattern. Also the orientations of similar structured crystals in the adjacent area between the rods (the interrod enamel or interprismatic region, discussed next in this section) diverge slightly from the long axis of the rod core, which is noted as different planes in enamel sections because they have these different orientations.

In addition, the crystals in the rod groups bend sinusoidally to the right or left at a slightly different angle than do adjacent groups, increasing the enamel's strength (see Figure 12-6). This is shown in the Hunter-Schreger (hun-ter-shray-ger) bands (HSB), alternating light to dark lines noted in certain sections of enamel using reflected rather than transmitted light (see Figure 12-8, *D*).

The arrangement of enamel rods is understood more clearly than their internal structure. Enamel rods are found in rows along the tooth, and within each row the long axis of the enamel rod is generally perpendicular to the underlying dentin as well as the DEJ with a slight inclination toward the cusp as they pass outward, thus preventing enamel fracture. Near the cusp tip they run more vertically; and in cervical enamel, they run mainly horizontally. However, in permanent dentition, the enamel rods near the CEJ tilt slightly toward the root of the tooth.

FIGURE 12-6 A, Diagram of an enamel rod produced by an ameloblast with its surrounding region of interrod enamel (or interprismatic region) created by surrounding ameloblasts. Note the interdigitation of the rod with other adjacent rods in a block of enamel with varying crystal orientations *(B, C, D)* depending on the exposed facets of the rod. **B,** Electron micrograph in cross section. **C** and **D,** Crystal orientation along the other two cut facets of the block of enamel, all crystals showing the bending of adjacent crystals of the rod core in comparison to interrod enamel (or interprismatic region). (**B, C,** and **D,** From Nanci A: *Ten Cate's oral histology,* ed 8, St Louis, 2013, Mosby/Elsevier.)

Most rods extend the width of the enamel from the DEJ to the outer enamel surface. Thus, each rod varies in length because the width of enamel varies in different locations of the crown area. Those near the cusps or incisal ridges, where the enamel is the thickest, are quite long compared with those near the CEJ. However, the course of the rods from these two end points is not an overall straight course. Rather, the rods show varying degrees of curvature from the DEJ to the outer enamel surface. This curved course of the enamel rods reflects the movements of the ameloblasts during enamel production.

Enamel rods interdigitate at each cusp tip to form a complex known as *gnarled enamel.* This reduces the occlusal stress on enamel considerably, especially at the pronounced cusp tips of posterior teeth. If enamel was not stacked as a spiraling lattice of rod direction in these high-use areas, it would shatter with occlusal stress. The rods also interlock in other areas of the crown, and this contributes to the stiffness and hardness of enamel.

Surrounding the outer part of each enamel rod is the interrod enamel, creating an interprismatic region that has been secreted by surrounding ameloblasts (see Figure 12-6). Even though similar in structure to the enamel rod, this interrod enamel (or interprismatic region) appears different from the rod core on cross sections because of its divergent crystalline orientation. At these boundaries, the crystallites are oriented in different directions, and fractures form easily at this interface. Whether an organic rod sheath or lesser-mineralized interprismatic substance exists between the enamel rods remains controversial.

The DEJ between mature enamel and dentin appears scalloped on a cross section of a tooth (Figure 12-7). The convex side of the DEJ is toward the dentin, and the concave side is toward the enamel. This difference in the length of the enamel rods and corresponding dentinal tubules occurs during the appositional growth of the two tissue types (see **Chapter 6**). The DEJ was formerly the basement membrane between the enamel organ and the dental papilla. In reality, the DEJ is simply a ridge between the two tissue types that allows increased adherence between them, adding to the strength of the junction when the teeth are in function during mastication so as to prevent shearing of

FIGURE 12-7 Microscopic section of the dentinoenamel junction demonstrating its scalloped interface *(arrow)*, having its concave side toward the enamel *(E)* and its convex side toward the dentin *(D)*. (From the Dr. Bernhard Gottlieb Collection, courtesy of James McIntosh, PhD, Assistant Professor Emeritus, Department of Biomedical Sciences, Baylor College of Dentistry, Dallas, TX.)

the enamel during function. Thus, the presence of the DEJ is most pronounced in the coronal region, where occlusal forces are the greatest.

The **lines of Retzius** (ret-zee-us) are the incremental lines (or striae) that appear in a microscopic section of mature enamel (Figure 12-8, *A-C*). These lines are composed of bands or cross striations on the enamel rods that, when combined in longitudinal sections, seem to traverse the enamel rods. In contrast, the lines of Retzius appear as concentric rings on transverse sections of enamel, similar to the growth rings in a tree.

Associated with the lines of Retzius are the raised **imbrication** (im-bri-kay-shun) **lines** and grooves of **perikymata** (per-ee-ki-maht-ah) noted clinically on the nonmasticatory surfaces of teeth in the oral cavity (Figure 12-9). The imbrication lines and perikymata are usually lost through tooth wear, except on the protected cervical regions of some teeth. This is especially true for the permanent maxillary central incisors, canines, and first premolars; the surface texture of the enamel in these areas may be confused as calculus near the CEJ.

The exact mechanism that produces the imbrication lines in enamel is still being debated. Some researchers hypothesize that the lines are a result of the diurnal, or 24-hour, metabolic rhythm of the ameloblasts

FIGURE 12-8 Microscopic sections of the lines of Retzius that traverse the rods of the enamel *(E)*. **A,** Long section of rods demonstrating their direction *(arrow)* overlying dentin *(D)* and pulp *(P)* in the crown. **B,** Close-up view of long section of rods demonstrating their direction *(arrow)*. **C,** Cross section of rods overlying dentin *(D)* with the lines of Retzius resembling growth rings of a tree. **D,** Alternating light to dark Hunter-Schreger bands demonstrated using reflected rather than transmitted light (in this case polarized light) (From the Dr. Bernhard Gottlieb Collection, courtesy of James McIntosh, PhD, Assistant Professor Emeritus, Department of Biomedical Sciences, Baylor College of Dentistry, Dallas, TX.)

FIGURE 12-9 Raised imbrication lines and grooves of the perikymata. **A,** Labial view of the permanent maxillary canine. **B,** Scanning electron micrograph of the labial surface of the tooth. (From Nanci A: *Ten Cate's oral histology*, ed 8, St Louis, 2013, Mosby/Elsevier.)

FIGURE 12-10 Microscopic section of the neonatal line *(arrow)*, a pronounced line of Retzius that corresponds to the birth of the individual. Thus, it demarcates the enamel formed prenatally *(P)* and after birth *(B)*. (From the Dr. Bernhard Gottlieb Collection, courtesy of James McIntosh, PhD, Assistant Professor Emeritus, Department of Biomedical Sciences, Baylor College of Dentistry, Dallas, TX.)

producing the enamel matrix, which consists of an active secretory work period followed by an inactive rest period during tooth development. Thus, each band on the enamel rod demonstrates the work/rest pattern of the ameloblasts that generally occurs over a span of a week.

The **neonatal** (ne-oh-nate-l) **line** is a pronounced incremental line of Retzius (Figure 12-10). The neonatal line marks the trauma experienced by the ameloblasts during birth, again illustrating the sensitivity of the ameloblasts as they form enamel matrix. Even minor physiologic changes affect them and elicit changes in enamel structure that can be seen only microscopically such as these lines. The darker line marks the border between the enamel matrix formed before and after birth. As one would expect, the neonatal line is found in all the crown enamel of the primary dentition and in the larger cusps of the permanent first molars. They contain irregular structures of enamel crystals with disordered arrangements, basically formed by the abrupt bending of the crystals toward the root during enamel formation; usually, the crystals gradually bend back again to regain their previous orientation as they move to the crown. Accentuated incremental lines also are produced by systemic disturbances (e.g., fevers) that affect amelogenesis.

The **enamel spindles** are another microscopic feature of mature enamel and represent short dentinal tubules near the DEJ (Figure 12-11). Enamel spindles are especially noted beneath the cusps and incisal ridges or tips of the teeth. Enamel spindles result from odontoblasts that crossed the basement membrane before it mineralized into the DEJ. Thus, these dentinal tubules become trapped during the appositional growth of enamel matrix, which becomes mineralized around them. Clinical implications of enamel spindles are unknown at this time, and it is doubtful that these dentinal tubules contain any live odontoblastic processes, as does the other elongated tubules within dentin.

The **enamel tufts** are another microscopic feature and are noted as small, dark brushes with their bases near the DEJ (Figure 12-12). Enamel tufts are best seen on transverse sections of enamel in the inner one third of enamel. They represent areas of less mineralization from an anomaly of crystallization and seem to have no clinical importance.

FIGURE 12-11 Microscopic section of enamel spindles *(arrows)* within the enamel and near the dentinoenamel junction. (From the Dr. Bernhard Gottlieb Collection, courtesy of James McIntosh, PhD, Assistant Professor Emeritus, Department of Biomedical Sciences, Baylor College of Dentistry, Dallas, TX.)

FIGURE 12-12 Transverse section of enamel showing enamel tufts *(white arrow)* and enamel lamella *(black arrow)*. (From the Dr. Bernhard Gottlieb Collection, courtesy of James McIntosh, PhD, Assistant Professor Emeritus, Department of Biomedical Sciences, Baylor College of Dentistry, Dallas, TX.)

The enamel lamellae (lah-mel-ay) are partially mineralized vertical sheets of enamel matrix that extend from the DEJ near the tooth's cervix to the outer occlusal surface (see Figure 12-12). Enamel lamellae are best seen on transverse sections of enamel. Enamel lamellae are narrower and longer than enamel tufts. This is another anomaly of crystallization that has unknown clinical importance. Both enamel tufts and enamel lamellae may be likened to "geologic faults" within mature enamel.

Finally, microscopic images of primary teeth enamel show smooth enamel surface where few areas of irregularity or linear structures are apparent. In contrast, similar images of permanent enamel show a not perfectly smooth surface; there are furrows and irregularities of variable depth and width.

Clinical Considerations for Dental Procedures Involving Enamel

The microscopic features of enamel must be taken into consideration during clinical treatment involving enamel. Enamel resembles a steel product with a moderate level of hardness, which also makes it brittle;

FIGURE 12-13 Photomicrograph showing the enamel rods after acid etching, which demineralizes the interrod enamel (or interprismatic region) to allow the flow of the enamel sealant or other restorative materials into the enamel fsor greater strength. (From Nanci A: *Ten Cate's oral histology,* ed 8, St Louis, 2013, Mosby/Elsevier.)

therefore, an underlying layer of more break-resistant dentin must be present to preserve its integrity (see earlier discussion and Table 12-1). This property, along with the direction of the enamel rods, is taken into consideration during cavity preparation, as well as the dentinal tubule direction (discussed later).

First, the decay and adjacent parts of the enamel are removed in a way that allows all the enamel rods to remain supported by other rods and the underlying dentin. An isolated enamel rod is extremely brittle and breaks away easily. If enamel rods are undercut during cavity preparation, they may break, thus rendering the margin of restoration possibly leaky, and thus defective. This brittleness of unsupported enamel also is noted during the progression of caries: The enamel breaks away easily, as the dentin is undermined beneath it. In the case of an amalgam Class I cavity preparation, the walls of the cavity should be perpendicular or 90° to the cavosurface, which will then expose the rods with its crystals. However, when using a bonding resin it is important to prepare the same cavity prep with a 45° bevel to the cavosurface to expose the enamel rods and its crystal for subsequent acid etching in order to significantly increase the bond strength.

Acid etching is briefly used to remove some of the organic parts of the enamel crystals in the interrod enamel (or interprismatic region), increasing porosity, enabling a bonding resin or an enamel sealant to flow into the newly created gaps, and thus offer more surface area for better adherence (Figure 12-13). It also removes the smear layer of the adherent dental biofilm debris.

This demineralization by acid etching is clinically apparent as the surface of enamel whitens. The arrangement of enamelin (discussed earlier) between and around the crystallized rods contributes to enamel's permeability (microporosity) to these materials as well as fluids, bacteria, and the acid byproducts of dental biofilm. When placing certain enamel sealants (hydrophobic), dental professionals must be careful to protect the demineralized enamel surface from being contaminated and remineralized by saliva, thereby reducing sealant uptake; luckily, new sealants are more resistant to this situation. The difference in surface smoothness or roughness (as discussed earlier) between the primary and permanent dentitions will also have an impact on a clinician's approach when acid etching the tooth surface for restorations or sealants.

Vital whitening of the teeth, called *bleaching* by patients, is performed externally to remove the gross levels of intrinsic staining that has occurred due to the process of aging of enamel as well as lifestyle choices (e.g., ingestion of dark drinks and foods, as well as tobacco use; see **Chapter 13** about staining of dentin). Staining occurs in the interrod enamel (or interprismatic region) internally on the tooth, which causes the tooth to appear darker or less white overall. The shade of the tooth is taken and recorded (as discussed earlier with dental restorations and replacement) to gauge the changes in whiteness over time during the whitening procedure. Certain natural shades of teeth are more easily whitened than others (yellow is more

compliant than gray). This procedure can be a lifesaver for patients with intrinsic stains, such as with tetracycline and dental fluorosis, to even out the overall tooth color.

In a perfect state, enamel is colorless, but it does reflect underlying tooth structure with any gross stains because light reflection properties of the tooth are low. Oxygen radicals from the peroxide in the whitening agents contact the stains in the interrrod enamel within the enamel layer. When this occurs, stains will be removed, and the teeth now appear whiter in color. Teeth not only appear whiter but also reflect light in increased amounts, which makes the teeth appear brighter as well. Studies at this time show that whitening does not produce any ultrastructural or microhardness changes in the dental tissue. Additional studies show that patients who have whitened their teeth take better care of them.

CHAPTER 13

Dentin and Pulp

●●● LEARNING OBJECTIVES

1. Define and pronounce the key terms in this chapter.
2. Discuss the dentin-pulp complex.
3. Describe the properties of dentin and the clinical consideration for dentin structure, integrating it into patient care.
4. Describe the processes involved in the stages of apposition and the maturation of dentin.
5. Outline the types of dentin and discuss the clinical considerations for dentin pathology, integrating it into patient care.
6. Discuss the histology of dentin.
7. Describe pulp properties, including its anatomic components.
8. Discuss the histology of pulp and the clinical considerations for pulp pathology and repair, integrating it into patient care.
9. Identify the components of both the dentin and the pulp on a diagram.

DENTIN-PULP COMPLEX

Unlike enamel, both dentin and pulp cannot be viewed clinically if the teeth and associated periodontium are healthy. That is because both dentin and pulp make up the inner parts of the tooth and are not exposed to the oral environment except when certain dental pathology exists. In addition, because of the shared developmental background, close proximity, and interdependence, dentin and pulp form a dentin-pulp complex. This chapter discusses these two types of tissue together as one developmental and functioning unit.

Dental professionals must have a clear understanding of the histology of these two types of tissue. In the past, these two inner types of dental tissue were thought of as being analogous to a "black box" that was opened only during restorative treatment or endodontic therapy and hidden the rest of the time. With the advent of expanded responsibilities and increased preventive concerns for patients, all dental professionals must be able to know about these two interesting and challenging dental tissue types.

DENTIN PROPERTIES

Mature dentin is a crystalline material that is less hard than enamel but slightly harder than bone (see Tables 6-2 and 12-1). Mature dentin is by weight 70% inorganic or mineralized material, 20% organic material, and 10% water. This crystalline formation of mature dentin mainly consists of calcium hydroxyapatite with the chemical formula of $Ca_{10}(PO_4)_6(OH)_2$. The calcium hydroxyapatite found in dentin is similar to that found in a higher percentage in enamel and in lower percentages in both cementum and bone tissue, such as the alveolar process. In addition, the crystals in dentin are platelike in shape and 30% smaller in size than those in enamel.

Small amounts of other minerals, such as carbonate and fluoride, are also present. Dentin is covered by enamel in the crown and cementum in the root, as well as enclosing the innermost pulp. Thus, dentin makes up the bulk of the tooth and protects the pulp. Dentin also has great tensile strength, providing an elastic basis for the more brittle enamel.

Because of the translucency of overlying enamel, the dentin of the tooth gives the white enamel crown its underlying yellow hue, which is a deeper tone in permanent teeth. When the pulp undergoes infection or even dies, there is discoloration of the dentin, which causes darkening of the clinical crown. On a radiograph, the differences in the mineralization levels of different parts of the tooth can be noted (see Figure 2-5). Dentin appears more radiolucent (or darker) than enamel because it is less dense but more radiopaque (or lighter) than pulp, which has the least density of the three types of dental tissue.

Clinical Considerations for Dentin Structure

If the outer layers of enamel are lost with aging, such as with attrition from mastication, the newly exposed dentin on the crown is various shades of yellow-white and appears rougher in surface texture than enamel (see Figure 16-17). Attrition, which is the wearing away of a tooth surface through tooth-to-tooth contact, can also occur in the newly exposed dentin as well as enamel (see Figure 20-8). In contrast to hard enamel, this attrition can occur at a more rapid rate when dentin is exposed because its mineralized content is lower. Coronal dentin can be exposed after attrition of the enamel and also with certain enamel dysplasias. Coronal dentin can also become exposed on the incisal ridge of anteriors when trauma causes it to become chipped or worn (see Figure 16-9, *C*).

Root dentin can be exposed when the thin layer of cementum is lost due to gingival recession with its lower margin of the free gingival crest (Figure 13-1) (see **Chapter 10**). It also appears various shades of yellow-white and appears rougher in surface texture than enamel. When hand instruments are used on the root to remove deposits such as calculus, there can be improper removal of dentin changing the overall root shape and function. Dentin that is lost externally on either the crown or root is not fully replaced by the possible addition of secondary dentin on the inside of the tooth along the outer pulpal wall (discussed later in this chapter).

Another way that dentin can become exposed and then lost is through dentinal caries, the demineralization resulting from cariogenic bacteria (discussed later in this chapter). Dentin demineralizes when the pH is less than 6.8. Finally, cavity preparation during restorative treatment exposes and then removes any carious dentin in order to prevent further decay.

Dentinal hypersensitivity can occur when instruments expose dentin, such as on root surfaces; this can be prevented with certain mineralizing products or temporarily reduced with the use of local anesthetic injections during dental procedures (discussed later in this chapter).

Removal of extrinsic stains by hand instrumentation can also remove even more dentin; thus ultrasonic devices or air polishing with glycine, which remove no hard tooth tissue when used correctly, may be better choices for extrinsic stain removal.

When dentin remains exposed, it can also pick up intrinsic beverage, food, and tobacco stains over time, becoming more yellow or even brown to black (see Figures 13-1 and 16-17). It absorbs these stains because it is more permeable, or porous, than intact enamel. Dentin is permeable due to both its high organic content and the presence of dentinal tubules, acting as a sponge to contain these staining products and causing esthetic concerns for patients. Vital whitening, called *bleaching* by patients, can be performed either at the office or in the home to remove some of the intrinsic stains within dentin, including those related to tooth development such as tetracycline stain, to even out the overall tooth color (see Figure 3-19). However, whitening at home must be done with appropriate supervision because it may also lead to dentinal hypersensitivity. Vital whitening is discussed further in **Chapter 12**. Studies at this time show that tooth whitening does not produce ultrastructural changes in the dental tissue.

DENTIN MATRIX FORMATION

Dentinogenesis is the formation of the initial dentin matrix or predentin during the apposition stage of tooth development (Figure 13-2). The exact time of the apposition stage varies according to the tooth that is undergoing development. Many factors can affect dentinogenesis when it is occurring (see **Chapter 6**).

Predentin is a mesenchymal product consisting of nonmineralized collagen fibers produced by the odontoblasts; mainly Type I collagen and also small amounts of Type III and V, along with dentin phosphoprotein. The latter acidic protein is important in the regulation of mineralization of dentin because it is highly attractable to calcium.

Originally, odontoblasts were the outer cells of the dental papilla before the apposition stage of tooth development. Thus, dentin and pulp have similar developmental backgrounds because both are originally derived from the dental papilla of the tooth germ. These newly formed odontoblasts are induced by the equally newly formed ameloblasts to produce predentin in layers, moving away from the dentinoenamel junction (DEJ). Unlike cartilage and bone as well as cementum, the odontoblast's cell body does not become entrapped in the product; rather, one long, cytoplasmic attached extension remains behind within the formed dentin. Odontoblasts produce approximately 4 µm of predentin daily during tooth development, similar to the amount of

FIGURE 13-2 Microscopic section of odontoblasts *(arrows)* producing predentin *(PD)* that will mature into dentin *(D)*. (From the Dr. Bernhard Gottlieb Collection, courtesy of James McIntosh, PhD, Assistant Professor Emeritus, Department of Biomedical Sciences, Baylor College of Dentistry, Dallas, TX.)

FIGURE 13-1 Clinical facial view of gingival recession exposing root dentin. Note the difference in color between the whitish enamel and the more yellowish dentin, which has also undergone additional staining of the root surfaces due to exposure. (Courtesy of Margaret J. Fehrenbach, RDH, MS.)

enamel matrix produced daily by the ameloblasts on the other side of the DEJ.

However, the appositional growth of dentin, unlike enamel, occurs throughout the life of the tooth, filling in the pulp chamber of both the crown and root (discussed later in this chapter). The wave pattern of dentin development follows the same format as that of enamel but on the opposite side of the DEJ (see Figures 12-2 and 12-3). It starts at the incisal or occlusal part of the future crown and then spreads down as far as the adjacent cervical loop of the enamel organ. Although ameloblasts are lost after the eruption of the tooth and enamel production ceases, production of dentin continues because of the retention of the odontoblasts. These tall, bowling pin–shaped cells remain within the tooth, lined up along the outer pulpal wall.

DENTIN MATRIX MATURATION

Maturation of dentin or mineralization of predentin occurs soon after its appositional growth. The process of dentin maturation takes place in two phases: primary and secondary (Figure 13-3). Initially, the calcium hydroxyapatite crystals form as globules, or calcospherules, in the collagen fibers of the predentin, which allows both the expansion and fusion during the primary mineralization phase. This process is analogous to the wash of watercolor paint placed on wet paper for a background, as the blobs of color run into each other—although, within dentin, it is a three-dimensional process.

Later, new areas of mineralization occur as globules form in the partially mineralized predentin during the secondary mineralization phase. These new areas of crystal formation are more or less regularly layered on the initial crystals, allowing them to expand, although they fuse incompletely. This process is analogous to additional blobs of paint placed in specific areas over a fuzzy painted background, but

the colors of this additional layer do not run into each other to cover the page because the paper is no longer wet.

This incomplete fusion during the secondary mineralization phase results in differences noted in the microscopic appearance of the crystalline form of dentin. In areas where both primary and secondary mineralization have occurred with complete crystalline fusion, these appear as lighter rounded areas on a microscopic section of dentin and are considered **globular** (**glob**-u-lar) **dentin** (Figure 13-4).

In contrast, the darker arclike areas in a microscopic section of dentin are considered **interglobular** (in-ter-**glob**-u-lar) **dentin**. In these areas, only primary mineralization has occurred within the predentin, and the globules of dentin do not fuse completely. Thus, interglobular dentin is slightly less mineralized than globular dentin. Interglobular dentin is especially evident in coronal dentin, near the DEJ, and in certain dental anomalies, such as in dentin dysplasia (see Figure 6-17).

MATURE DENTIN COMPONENTS

Within mature dentin, certain components (such as dentinal tubules and their contents) are present (Figures 13-5 and 13-6). Dentinal tubules are long tubes in the dentin that extend from the DEJ in the crown area, or dentinocemental junction (DCJ) in the root area, to the outer wall of the pulp. After appositional growth of predentin and maturation into dentin, the cell bodies of the odontoblasts remain in the pulp inside the tooth, along its outer wall (discussed later). The tubules are also tapered with their width being thinner near the DEJ or DCJ and then wider as they near the pulp.

Like enamel, dentin is avascular. Instead of its own blood vessels supplying its nutrition, odontoblasts within the dentin receive it by way of tissue fluid in the dentinal tubules that originally traveled from the blood vessels located in the adjacent pulp. Within each dentinal tubule is a space of variable size containing dentinal fluid, an odontoblastic process, and possibly part of an afferent axon.

The **dentinal** (den-tin-al) **fluid** in the tubule presumably also includes the tissue fluid surrounding the cell membrane of the odontoblast, which is continuous from the cell body in the pulp. The odontoblastic process is a long cellular extension located within the dentinal tubule that is still attached to the cell body of the odontoblast within the pulp. In a microscopic section of a tooth, odontoblastic processes within the dentinal tubule sometimes are not found at the periphery of dentin near the DEJ or DCJ. This absence may or may not be an artifact, given that live cell structures are difficult to preserve in dead mineralized tissue.

Studies suggest that the process occupies the full length of the tubule from the DEJ or DCJ to the pulp during only the early stages of odontogenesis. In mature dentin, however, the process may or may not run the full length of the dentinal tubule to extend near either the outlying DEJ or DCJ.

A sensory axon, or afferent axon, is associated with part of the odontoblastic process in some dentinal tubules. The myelinated axon may not extend farther than the process, and thus may not be located along either the DEJ or DCJ. Yet, the nerve cell body associated with the axon is located in the pulp along with the odontoblastic cell body. This axon is involved in registration of the sensation of pain, predominantly, and not usually any other sensations, even when triggered by other sensations such as heat (discussed later).

The direction of the tubule reflects the pathway of the odontoblast during appositional growth of predentin. There are two types of curvature established by the direction of the dentinal tubules, primary and secondary (Figure 13-7). The *primary curvature* of the dentinal tubules reflects the overall tubule course over time,

Mantle dentin

Odontoblastic process

Odontoblasts

Globules

Ameloblasts

Predentin

FIGURE 13-3 Photomicrograph of dentin maturation showing the odontoblasts producing predentin that contains odontoblastic processes with the ameloblasts located on the opposite side of the dentinoenamel junction. The predentin matures by forming globules, which undergo mineralization into mantle dentin because it is near the dentinoenamel junction. (From Nanci A: *Ten Cate's oral histology,* ed 8, St Louis, 2013, Mosby/Elsevier.)

which resembles a large S-shaped curve. The *secondary curvature* of the tubule consists of small, delicate curves noted in the primary curvature, reflecting the smaller daily changes in odontoblast direction during the appositional growth of dentin.

Dentinal tubules are not interrupted by the formation of the interglobular areas of dentin but pass right through them. Tubules can branch at any point along the way from the DEJ or DCJ to the pulp. Dentinal tubules are also crowded near the pulp because of the narrowing of this region (see Figure 13-5). Finally, dentin tubules are responsible for permeability of material across the dentinal surface if exposed. The quantity and diameter of these dentinal tubules affects

the permeability of dentin and may enhance the carious process (see later discussion in this chapter).

DENTIN TYPES

Dentin is not a uniform tissue within the tooth but differs from region to region (Table 13-1). Different types of dentin can be designated by their relationship to the dentinal tubules (Figure 13-8; see also Figure 13-5). Dentin that creates the wall of the dentinal tubule is **peritubular** (pare-i-**tube**-u-lar) **dentin** (or intratubular dentin). Peritubular dentin is highly mineralized after dentin maturation.

- Dentin
- Globular mineralization front
- Predentin
- Odontoblasts
- Pulp

A

- Enamel
- Dentinoenamel junction
- Dentin
- Globular dentin
- Interglobular dentin

B

C   25 μm

FIGURE 13-4 Photomicrographs of globular and interglobular dentin. **A,** Section of the globular mineralized front near the outer pulpal wall during primary mineralization. **B,** Ground section near the dentinoenamel junction with its highly mineralized globular dentin (lighter) and less mineralized interglobular dentin (darker) after both primary and secondary mineralization. **C,** Scanning electron micrograph of globular dentin. (From Nanci A: *Ten Cate's oral histology,* ed 8, St Louis, 2013, Mosby/Elsevier.)

FIGURE 13-5 Photomicrograph of the dentinal tubules in dentin with the odontoblastic processes entering the tubules from the pulp. The pulp contains an outer layer of the cell bodies of odontoblasts to which the odontoblastic processes are still attached. (From Nanci A: *Ten Cate's oral histology*, ed 8, St Louis, 2013, Mosby/Elsevier.)

FIGURE 13-6 Microscopic section of the components of the dentinal tubule. The dentinal tubules contain odontoblastic processes *(arrows)*, as well as dentinal fluid. (From Nanci A: *Ten Cate's oral histology*, ed 8, St Louis, 2013, Mosby/Elsevier.)

The dentin that is found between the tubules is **intertubular** (in-ter-**tube**-u-lar) **dentin**. Intertubular dentin is highly mineralized but less so than peritubular dentin.

Dentin can also be categorized by its relationship to the enamel and pulp (Figure 13-9). **Mantle dentin** is the first predentin that forms and matures within the tooth near the DEJ and underneath the enamel. Mantle dentin shows a difference in the direction of the mineralized collagen fibers compared with the rest of the dentin, having fibers that are perpendicular to the DEJ. Large diameter collagen fibers called *von Korff fibers* are associated with this type of dentin. Mantle dentin also has more peritubular dentin than the later formed inner dentin and thus has higher levels of mineralization.

Deep to the mantle dentin is the layer of dentin around the outer wall of pulp, the **circumpulpal** (serk-um-**pul**-pal) **dentin**, which makes up the bulk of the dentin in a tooth. This type forms and matures after mantle dentin. The collagen fibers of circumpulpal dentin are mainly parallel to the DEJ, compared with those of mantle dentin.

Dentin can also be categorized according to the time that it was formed within the tooth (Figure 13-10). **Primary dentin** is formed in a tooth before the completion of the apical foramen(s) of the root, which is the opening in the root's pulp canal. Most of the dentin in the tooth was formed during this time period. Primary dentin is characterized by its regular pattern of dentinal tubules.

Secondary dentin is formed after the completion of the apical foramen(s) and continues to form throughout the life of the tooth. Secondary dentin is formed more slowly than primary dentin; thus it makes up less of the dentin in the tooth. As it is being formed by the odontoblasts lined up along the dentin-pulp interface, the secondary dentin fills in the pulp chamber along its outer wall. This secondary time period of dentinogenesis is noted for its only slightly irregular pattern of tubules, but it has the same mineral content.

Microscopically, a dark line shows the junction between the primary and secondary dentin that results from an abrupt change in the course of the odontoblasts during appositional growth as the tooth's apex or apices are completed (see Figure 13-10). Most of the secondary dentin fills in on the roof and floor of the pulp chamber, causing recession of the pulp. This is especially noted in molar teeth and is important in determining the form of cavity preparation for certain restorative treatment.

One type of dentin, **tertiary dentin** (or reparative dentin or reactive dentin) is formed quickly in local regions in response to a localized injury to the exposed dentin (see Figure 13-10) (discussed next).

Clinical Considerations for Dentin Pathology

Apart from dentin that is resorbed during the shedding of primary teeth, the dentin formed is mostly stable during the life of the tooth. However, in a few cases dentin can become resorbed in permanent teeth, but the cause is unknown (idiopathic) and can involve either an internal or external resorption process. It can be noted radiographically, but it is hard to discern between the two processes. In contrast, when the process begins on the external surface of the root and then penetrates through the cementum into dentin (usually not into the pulp), it can lead to a pinkish crown color noted clinically from the granulation tissue seen beneath the translucent enamel.

Similar but much more serious than the resorption process in dentin is when the dentinal tubules serve as an entry mechanism for cariogenic microorganisms as the carious process begins to extend from the enamel to form **dentinal caries** (Figure 13-11). Microscopically, the microorganisms can be seen actually using the dentinal tubules as chutes that allow them to move toward the inner placed pulp due to their connection with the odontoblasts in the outer pulpal wall. When caries extends into the dentin from enamel (see enamel caries discussion in **Chapter 12**), the carious process moves more rapidly because of the increased organic composition of dentin as compared with enamel. In addition, because of the primary curvature of the dentinal tubules, the pulp may be affected at a more apical level than the level at which the external injury (such as caries) occurred. The cavity preparation process during restorative treatment considers this curvature of the tubules when carious dentin is removed. Light-induced devices

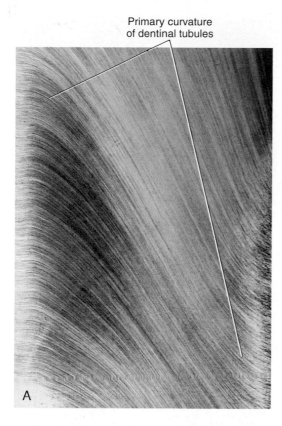

Primary curvature
of dentinal tubules

A

Secondary curvature
of dentinal tubules

Branching of
dentinal tubules

B

FIGURE 13-7 Curvature of the dentinal tubules in dentin. **A,** Primary curvature. **B,** Secondary curvature *(smaller circle)* with branching noted near the dentinoenamel junction *(larger circle)*. (From the Dr. Bernhard Gottlieb Collection, courtesy of James McIntosh, PhD, Assistant Professor Emeritus, Department of Biomedical Sciences, Baylor College of Dentistry, Dallas, TX.)

TABLE 13-1	Dentin Types	
TYPE	**LOCATION AND CHRONOLOGY**	**HISTOLOGIC FEATURES**
Peritubular dentin	Wall of tubules	Highly mineralized
Intertubular dentin	Between the tubules	Highly mineralized
Mantle dentin	Outermost layer near dentinoenamel junction underneath enamel	First dentin formed
Circumpulpal dentin	Layer around outer pulpal wall	Dentin formed after mantle dentin
Primary dentin	Formed before completion of apical foramen	Formed more rapidly; more mineralized than secondary
Secondary dentin	Formed after completion of apical foramen	Formed slower; less mineralized than primary
Tertiary dentin	Formed as a result of localized injury to exposed dentin	Irregular course of tubules

but neighboring undifferentiated mesenchymal cells of the pulp can move to the area and become odontoblasts (discussed further later in this chapter). This type of tertiary dentin is considered to be *reparative dentin.* If the tertiary dentin is formed by existing odontoblasts, it is considered to be *reactive dentin.* For both types, if there is a more rushed timetable for dentin formation, the tubules in tertiary dentin may assume a more irregular course than in secondary dentin as noted microscopically.

A certain type of tertiary dentin, *sclerotic dentin* (or transparent dentin), is often found in association with the chronic injury of caries and is noted in increased amounts as the tooth ages. In this type of dentin, the odontoblastic processes die and leave the dentinal tubules vacant. These hollow dentinal tubules then become retrofilled and, finally, occluded by a mineralized substance similar to peritubular dentin. This type of dentin may be involved, in fact, with prolonging pulp vitality because it reduces the permeability of dentin. Clinically, this is noted with presence of arrested caries in older dentitions; it appears as a dark, smooth, and shiny area.

Certain medications placed during cavity preparation with restorative treatment can promote secondary dentin formation and thus help protect the underlying pulp after outer dentin is lost due to caries or even from cavity preparation. During cavity preparation, the dental tubules are also usually sealed with certain preparations for less sensitivity post restoration.

When cutting dentin in cavity preparation, there is production of a smear layer, which is composed of adherent dental biofilm debris. It is about 1 micron thick and its composition reflects the underlying dentin, although different quantities and qualities of smear layer can be produced by the various instrumentation techniques. Its function is presumed to be protective, as it lowers dentin permeability. However, it masks the underlying sound dentin and interferes with attempts to bond dental restorative material to the dentin.

When dentin is exposed as a result of caries, cavity preparation, gingival recession, or attrition, the open dentinal tubules may be painful for the patient as discussed earlier, causing dentinal hypersensitivity (hi-per-sen-si-tiv-it-ee). However, many times it is the microscopic anatomy of the tooth that is the culprit; the enamel and cementum do not meet, leaving a gap with dentin exposed at the CEJ interface area a

that measure changes in laser fluorescence of hard tissue can now allow dental professionals to better diagnose early carious lesions.

Tertiary dentin forms quickly in local regions in response to a localized injury to the exposed dentin (see Figure 13-10). The dentinal injury could be due to caries, cavity preparation, attrition, or gingival recession. Tertiary dentin thus forms underneath the exposed dentinal tubules along the outer pulpal wall, trying to seal off the injured area. The dentinal injury could be due to caries, cavity preparation, attrition, or recession. Odontoblasts in the area of the affected tubules may perish because of the injury,

FIGURE 13-8 Cross sections of dentinal tubules composed of peritubular dentin *(arrows)* containing odontoblastic processes *(Odp)* and surrounded by intertubular dentin. **A,** Scanning electron microscope. **B,** Light microscope. **C,** Transmission electron micrograph showing close-up view starting at the mineralization front and extending to predentin. (From Nanci A: *Ten Cate's oral histology,* ed 8, St Louis, 2013, Mosby/Elsevier.)

third of the time (see Figure 14-7). In addition, the protective layers of both cementum and dentin can be inadvertently removed as a result of scaling with hand instruments, initiating sensitivity that may or may not be temporary. Branching of the dentinal tubules containing the live odontoblastic processes throughout dentin adds to the overall level of exposure.

Certain additional situations may additionally trigger the short, sharp pain of dentinal hypersensitivity. This includes stimuli such as thermal changes (cold water spray or ice); mechanical irritation (vibrations from instrumentation, dental handpieces, or ultrasonics); dehydration (stream of air or heat during cavity preparation); or chemical exposure (foods such as thick or hypertonic sweet, salty, or sour fluids;

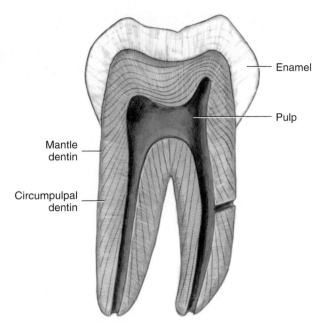

FIGURE 13-9 Main types of dentin and relationship to the enamel and pulp: mantle dentin and circumpulpal dentin.

FIGURE 13-10 Microscopic section of various types of dentin showing the relationship to the time of formation (from early to late): primary (P), secondary (S), and tertiary (T) with a dark line at the junction of the primary and secondary dentin (arrows) caused by an abrupt change in the course of the odontoblasts during appositional growth. Note also the more irregular course of dentinal tubules in tertiary dentin than in secondary dentin. (From the Dr. Bernhard Gottlieb Collection, courtesy of James McIntosh, PhD, Department of Biomedical Sciences, Baylor College of Dentistry, Dallas, TX.)

FIGURE 13-11 Photomicrograph of the dentinal caries showing the cariogenic microorganisms entering the deeper dentin (D) through the dentinal tubules (arrows). Note that cementum (C) has already been invaded by the cariogenic microorganisms from the dental biofilm or plaque (P) covering the root area. (From Perry DA, Beemsterboer PL, Essex G: *Periodontology for dental hygienists,* ed 4, St Louis, 2014, Saunders/Elsevier.)

tooth-colored restorative materials; or vital whitening agents). By contrast, the pain from other tooth-related situations (such as from caries and pulpal or gingival infections) is usually dull and chronic in nature.

However, dentinal hypersensitivity is often a type of diffuse pain, making localization to a specific tooth difficult for the dental professional, as well as for the patient. This pain may wrongly be interpreted as caries, pulpal or gingival infections, or soft tissue inflammation. Because of the chronic nature of attrition and gingival recession, the pain present may not be as painful as other forms of dentinal exposure because both of these are gradual processes, allowing time for subtle changes to occur in the dentinal tubules to close them off from the stimulation (discussed later). Dentinal hypersensitivity can occur within both of the dentitions and associated tooth types as well as all their surfaces but is especially evident in premolars and canines, usually on the facial and cervical regions.

The still controversial but widely accepted hydrodynamic theory of dentinal hypersensitivity suggests that it is due to changes in the dentinal fluid associated with the processes (Figure 13-12). This mechanism may be due to one or more of the following: evaporation and loss of dentinal fluid, movement of the fluid, and ionic changes in the fluid. These changes in the dentinal fluid are then transmitted to the afferent axon present in some dentinal tubules near the dentin-pulp interface, thus sending a painful message to the pulp and then on to the brain (see later discussion of pulp innervation). Possibly, that is the reason the previously mentioned painful stimuli are involved in dentinal hypersensitivity, because they are involved with dentinal fluid movement within the tubule, and because local anesthetics do not block sensation when they are placed on the surface of exposed dentin, as they would with a fully innervated tissue. However, in the

STIMULATION

Exposed dentin

Dentinal tubule

Change in dentinal fluid

Odontoblastic process

Possible nerve location

Odontoblast cell body in pulp tissue

Pain message sent to brain

FIGURE 13-12 Possible mechanisms involved in the hydrodynamic theory of dentinal hypersensitivity. Stimulation of the exposed dentinal tubules such as with cold water (*red arrow*) causes changes in the dentinal fluid, which is then transmitted to the nerves associated with the odontoblast cell bodies in the pulp.

future, more than one theory may be used to fully explain surface dentinal hypersensitivity.

Dentinal hypersensitivity can be treated somewhat successfully with solutions applied either by professionals or within over-the-counter products available to patients. These desensitizing agents either temporarily block the exposed open ends of the dentinal tubules (similar to the process of tooth staining) or interfere with nerve transmission. However, restorations sometimes are the only permanent method to reduce hypersensitivity of the exposed dentinal surface in severe cases. Methods that will fully seal the exposed dentinal tubules, and thus prevent any dentinal hypersensitivity, are being studied.

DENTIN HISTOLOGY

When mature dentin is examined microscopically, certain features (such as dentinal tubules and most types of dentin) are easily noted. However, the dentinal process within tubules is hard to discern microscopically. Other microscopic features are also noted and will be discussed further. These features can occur in both primary and secondary dentin.

The **imbrication** (im-bri-kay-shun) **lines of von Ebner** (eeb-ner) are incremental lines or bands in a microscopic section of dentin that can be likened to the growth rings of trees; they are also similar to the incremental lines of Retzius noted in enamel (Figure 13-13). These lines show the incremental nature of dentin during the apposition stage of tooth development and run at 90° to the dentinal tubules. With each daily 4-μm increment of dentin by the odontoblasts, the orientation of the deposited collagen fibers differs slightly. More severe changes occur every fifth day, giving rise at every 20 μm to an imbrication line as noted.

The **contour lines of Owen** are a number of adjoining parallel imbrication lines that are also present in a microscopic section of

FIGURE 13-13 Imbrication lines of von Ebner that transverse the dentinal tubules in dentin, with their direction noted (*arrow*). Note the regular pattern of dentin formation. (From the Dr. Bernhard Gottlieb Collection, courtesy of James McIntosh, PhD, Assistant Professor Emeritus, Department of Biomedical Sciences, Baylor College of Dentistry, Dallas, TX.)

FIGURE 13-14 Pronounced contour line of Owen, the neonatal line (*arrows*), as well as other parallel adjacent contour lines in dentin (*D*) underlying enamel (*E*). Note that they tend to appear together as a series of dark bands. (From the Dr. Bernhard Gottlieb Collection, courtesy of James McIntosh, PhD, Assistant Professor Emeritus, Department of Biomedical Sciences, Baylor College of Dentistry, Dallas, TX.)

dentin. These specific imbrication lines demonstrate a disturbance in body metabolism that affects the odontoblasts by altering their formation efforts, and they tend to appear together as a series of dark bands. The most pronounced contour line is the neonatal line that occurs during the trauma of birth (Figure 13-14). Other contour lines can occur in conjunction with the clinically visible tetracycline stain of the teeth, in which the antibiotic taken systemically during tooth development becomes chemically bound to the dentin in varying amounts

FIGURE 13-15 Tomes granular layer *(arrows)* in dentin *(D)* near the dentinocemental junction, beneath layers of cementum *(C)*. (From the Dr. Bernhard Gottlieb Collection, courtesy of James McIntosh, PhD, Assistant Professor Emeritus, Department of Biomedical Sciences, Baylor College of Dentistry, Dallas, TX.)

(see Figure 3-19). Most of this intrinsic stain can be lightened with vital whitening, evening out the tooth color, or dental restorations can be used.

Another feature of dentin is Tomes (tomes) **granular layer**, which is most often found in a microscopic section of dentin in the peripheral part beneath the root's cementum, adjacent to the DCJ (Figure 13-15). However, the area only looks granular because of its spotty microscopic appearance; the cause of the visible change in this region of dentin is unknown. It may be due to less mineralized areas of dentin having an increased level of interglobular dentin or the presence of branching of the terminal parts of dentinal tubules found near the DCJ, similar to that noted near the DEJ. It is unknown if it has any clinical significance. The DCJ itself is less distinct junction than the DEJ because these two types of tissue intermingle in the root of the tooth.

AGING DENTIN

With aging, the diameter of the dentinal tubule narrows because of deposition of peritubular dentin on the inner wall. This narrowing may be related to the decreased ability of pulp to react to various stimuli with age. In addition, the passageways of the tubules to the pulp are not as wide open as when younger; thus the stimuli are not transmitted as rapidly and in as large amounts as they were previously (discussed further in regard to pulp). Studies show the complete obliteration of older tubules with mineralization of the associated odontoblastic processes.

With age, odontoblasts also undergo cytoplasmic changes, including a reduction in organelle content. As discussed previously, dentin becomes more exposed as a result of both attrition and gingival recession, which may or may not lead to dentinal hypersensitivity (discussed earlier). Assessing age from the dentition constitutes an important step in constructing an identity profile of a decedent. Instead of microscopic features related to the aging process, dentinal translucency is one of the best morphohistologic parameters to use for dental age estimation, not only in terms of accuracy but also simplicity, along with use of related software and digital devices.

PULP PROPERTIES

The pulp is the innermost soft tissue of the tooth and appears radiolucent (dark) because it is less dense than the radiopaque (or lighter) hard tissue of the tooth (see Figure 2-5). The pulp of a tooth is a connective tissue with all the components of such tissue (discussed later in this chapter). During tooth development, the pulp forms from the central cells of the dental papilla (see Figure 6-7). During odontogenesis, when the predentin forms around the dental papilla, the innermost tissue is considered pulp (see Figures 6-10 and 6-11). Thus, pulp has a background similar to that of dentin because both are derived from the dental papilla of the tooth germ.

One important consideration that relates to the dentin-pulp complex is that the pulp is involved in the support, maintenance, and continued formation of dentin because the cell bodies of the odontoblasts remain along the outer pulpal wall (discussed later). Another function of the pulp is sensory because the cell bodies associated with the afferent axons in the dentinal tubules are located among this layer of odontoblasts. All sensations directed to the pulp are perceived by the brain as only the sensation of pain. Therefore, extreme temperature changes and response to touch such as vibrations that affect the pulp or dentin by way of the pulp's nerves are perceived only as painful stimuli. Thus the pulp being a sensory organ dictates that local anesthesia needs to be administered for pain control during many dental procedures.

Pulp also serves a nutritional function for itself as well as dentin because the dentin contains no blood supply of its own. Dentin depends on the pulp's vascular supply and associated tissue fluids for its nutrition. Nutrition is obtained through the dentinal tubules and their connection to the odontoblasts' cell bodies that line the outer pulpal wall.

Finally, the pulp has a protective function because it is involved in the formation of secondary dentin or tertiary dentin, which increases the coverage of the pulp. In addition, if the pulp suffers any injury that also involves the odontoblasts, its undifferentiated mesenchyme contains cells that can differentiate into fibroblasts, which then create fibers and intercellular substances, as well as odontoblasts, to create more dentin. The pulp also has white blood cells (WBCs) within its vascular system and surrounding tissue; these allow triggering of inflammatory and immune responses.

PULP ANATOMY

The large mass of pulp is contained within the **pulp chamber** of the tooth (Figure 13-16). The shape of each pulp chamber corresponds directly to the overall shape of the tooth and thus is individualized for every tooth (see **Chapters 16 and 17**). The pulpal tissue in the pulp chamber has two main divisions: coronal pulp and radicular pulp.

The **coronal pulp** is located in the crown of the tooth. Smaller extensions of coronal pulp into the cusps of posterior teeth form the **pulp horns**. These pulp horns are especially prominent in the permanent dentition under the buccal cusp of premolars and in the primary dentition under the mesiobuccal cusp of molars. In contrast, pulp horns are not found on anterior teeth and all pulp horns recede with age. To prevent exposure of the pulpal tissue, these regions must be taken into consideration during cavity preparation with restorative treatment, such as the use of radiographs to locate them.

The **radicular** (rah-**dik**-u-lar) **pulp**, or root pulp, is the part of the pulp located in the root of the tooth; it is also called the *pulp canal* by patients. The radicular pulp extends from the cervical part of the tooth to each apex of the tooth. This part of the pulp has openings from the pulp through the cementum into the surrounding periodontal ligament (PDL). These openings include each apical foramen and possibly accessory canals.

The **apical foramen** (ay-pi-kl for-ay-men) is the opening from the pulp into the surrounding PDL near each apex of the tooth. If more than one foramen is present on each root, the largest one is designated as the apical foramen, and the rest are considered accessory foramina.

This opening is surrounded by layers of cementum but still permits arteries, veins, lymphatics, and nerves to enter and exit the pulp from the PDL, allowing the tooth to remain vital (Tables 13-2 and 13-3). Thus, communication between the pulp and the PDL is possible because of the apical foramen. Each apical foramen is the last part of the tooth to form; it forms after the crown erupts into the oral cavity. In developing teeth, each foramen is large and centrally located. As the tooth matures, each foramen becomes smaller in diameter and is offset in position. Each foramen may be located at the anatomic apex of each of the roots but is usually located slightly more occlusal from each apex.

Accessory canals may also be associated with the pulp and are extra openings from the pulp to the PDL (Figure 13-17; see Figure 13-16). Accessory canals are also called *lateral canals* because they are usually located on the lateral surface of the roots of the teeth, but this is not always the case because they can be found anywhere along the root surface. Accessory canals form when Hertwig epithelial root sheath encounters a blood vessel during root formation. Root structure then forms around the blood vessel, forming the accessory canal. Not all teeth have these canals, and they are present in differing amounts in the various tooth types.

Thus teeth have a variable number of these canals, which sometimes poses problems during endodontic therapy or root canal treatment (discussed later). Radiographs do not always indicate the number or position of these canals, unless they are examined with instruments using radiopaque materials during this therapy. Gingival recession may expose the opening of an accessory canal, especially in the furcation area, possibly causing the spread of infection into the pulp from caries or periodontal disease.

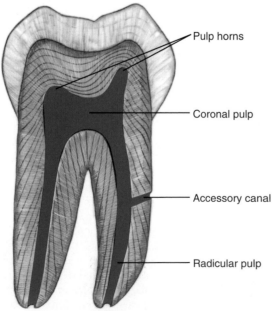

FIGURE 13-16 Anatomy of pulp.

PULP HISTOLOGY

Because pulp is a connective tissue, it has all the components of such tissue: intercellular substance, tissue fluid, certain cells, lymphatics, vascular system, nerves, and fibers (Figure 13-18). As in all forms of connective tissue, the fibroblasts are the largest group of cells in the pulp (see Figure 8-5). The odontoblasts are the second largest group of cells in the pulp, but only their cell bodies are located in the pulp. The odontoblasts are located only along the outer pulpal wall.

In addition to fibroblasts and odontoblasts, the pulp contains an undifferentiated mesenchyme type of stem cells, *dental pulp stem cells* (DPSCs). These cells are a rich resource for the dentin-pulp complex because they can transform into fibroblasts or odontoblasts if either cell population is reduced after injury.

The pulp also contains WBCs in its tissue and vascular supply, but levels are usually low, unless the cells are ready to be triggered by an inflammatory or immune reaction. The red blood cells are located in the extensive vascular supply. The fibers present in the pulp are mainly collagen fibers and some reticular fibers; the pulp contains no elastic

TABLE 13-2	Arterial Supply to Permanent Teeth and Periodontium
TEETH AND ASSOCIATED PERIODONTIUM	**MAJOR BRANCHES OF MAXILLARY ARTERY**
Posterior maxillary and periodontium	Posterior superior alveolar artery
Anterior maxillary and periodontium	Infraorbital artery
Mandibular and periodontium	Inferior alveolar artery

(From Fehrenbach MJ, Herring SW: *Illustrated anatomy of the head and neck*, ed 4, Philadelphia, 2012, Saunders/Elsevier.)

TABLE 13-3	Nerve Supply to the Permanent Teeth and Periodontium
TEETH AND ASSOCIATED PERIODONTIUM	**BRANCHES OF TRIGEMINAL NERVE OR FIFTH (V) CRANIAL NERVE**
Maxillary anterior teeth, maxillary anterior facial periodontium	Anterior superior alveolar nerve from maxillary nerve (V$_2$)
Maxillary anterior lingual periodontium	Nasopalatine nerve from maxillary nerve (V$_2$)
Maxillary posterior teeth, maxillary posterior buccal periodontium	Middle superior alveolar and posterior superior alveolar nerve from maxillary nerve (V$_2$)
Maxillary posterior lingual periodontium	Greater palatine nerve from maxillary nerve (V$_2$)
Mandibular teeth and facial periodontium of the mandibular anterior teeth and premolars	Inferior alveolar nerve from mandibular nerve (V$_3$)
Mandibular posterior buccal periodontium	Long buccal nerve from mandibular nerve (V$_2$)
Mandibular lingual periodontium	Lingual nerve from mandibular nerve (V$_2$)

(From Fehrenbach MJ, Herring SW: *Illustrated anatomy of the head and neck*, ed 4, Philadelphia, 2012, Saunders/Elsevier.)

The figure labels (for Figure 13-16): Pulp horns, Coronal pulp, Accessory canal, Radicular pulp fibers. Also present are an extensive vascular supply and rudimentary lymphatics.

Two types of nerves are associated with the pulp, including both myelinated nerves (20% to 30%) and unmyelinated nerves (70% to 80%) (see **Chapter 8**). They are mostly nociceptors that relay predominately the sensation of pain, such as can occur with injuries to the pulp. This can include mechanical or chemical injury and temperature extremes, all which can occur with cavity preparation (see

earlier discussion with dentin). The myelinated nerves are the axons of sensory or afferent neurons that are located in the dentinal tubules in dentin. The associated nerve cell bodies are located between the odontoblasts' cell bodies in the odontoblastic layer of the pulp. The unmyelinated nerves are associated with the blood vessels. The nerve fibers originate from the mandibular and maxillary branches of the trigeminal nerve and have their cell bodies in the trigeminal ganglion.

PULP ZONES

Four zones are evident when the pulp is viewed microscopically: odontoblastic layer, cell-free zone, cell-rich zone, and pulpal core (Table 13-4; see Figure 13-18). This chapter discusses these zones in order, from the outermost zone closest to the dentin to the center of the pulp.

The first zone of pulp closest to the dentin is the *odontoblastic layer*. This zone lines the outer pulpal wall. It consists of a layer of the cell bodies of odontoblasts, whose odontoblastic processes are located in the dentinal tubules in the adjacent dentin. The odontoblasts are capable of forming secondary or tertiary dentin along the outer pulpal wall. If this occurs, the odontoblasts realign on the pulpal side next to this newly-formed dentin. In addition, the cell bodies of the afferent axons from the dentinal tubules in dentin are located between the cell bodies of the odontoblasts.

The next zone, nearest to the odontoblastic layer and inward from the dentin, is considered the *cell-free zone*, but it is anything but empty. This zone was so named because it appears to be virtually free of cells, but this is only true when using lower-power magnification. In reality, this zone consists of fewer cells in contrast to the odontoblastic layer, but it is not entirely cell free. A nerve and capillary plexus is also located in this zone. No secondary or tertiary dentin is formed here initially, but newly formed dentin may encroach upon this zone.

The next zone after the cell-free zone is the *cell-rich zone*, inward from dentin. The cell-rich zone, as its name implies, has an increased density of cells compared with the cell-free zone but still does not contain as many cells as the odontoblastic layer. This zone also has a more extensive vascular supply than does the cell-free zone.

The final zone of pulp is the *pulpal core*, which is in the center of the pulp chamber. This zone consists of many cells and an extensive

FIGURE 13-17 Accessory canal *(arrow)* located in the root, which is composed of pulp *(P)* and dentin *(D)* covered by cementum. Note that the accessory canal is open to the periodontal ligament *(PDL)*. (From the Dr. Bernhard Gottlieb Collection, courtesy of James McIntosh, PhD, Assistant Professor Emeritus, Department of Biomedical Sciences, Baylor College of Dentistry, Dallas, TX.)

FIGURE 13-18 Zones of pulp deep to the dentin *(D)*, from the outer three zones to inner zone of the pulpal core, with the its location noted *(arrow)*. (From the Dr. Bernhard Gottlieb Collection, courtesy of James McIntosh, PhD, Assistant Professor Emeritus, Department of Biomedical Sciences, Baylor College of Dentistry, Dallas, TX.)

vascular supply. Except for its location, it is very similar to the cell-rich zone.

AGING PULP

The pulp horns recede with aging. Also with increased age, the pulp undergoes a decrease in intercellular substance, water, and cells as it fills with an increased amount of collagen fibers. This decrease in cells is especially evident in the reduced number of undifferentiated mesenchymal cells. Thus, the pulp becomes more fibrotic with increased age, leading to a reduction in the regenerative capacity of the pulp due its loss of these cells. Also, the overall pulp cavity may be smaller by the addition of secondary or tertiary dentin, thus causing pulp recession. The lack of sensitivity associated with older teeth is due to receded pulp horns, pulp fibrosis, addition of dentin, or possibly all these age-related changes; many times restorative treatment can proudly be performed without local anesthesia on older dentitions.

The pulp's apical foramen may also become obliterated with deposits of cementum over time, leading to blockage of blood vessels serving the tissue, especially the veins (see **Chapter 14**). This can result in vascular congestion and then pulpal necrosis, resulting slowly in painless tooth death without any evidence of caries, periodontal disease, or endodontic infection.

Clinical Considerations for Pulp Pathology and Repair

Pulp stones (or denticles) are sometimes present in the pulp (Figure 13-19). These can be mineralized masses of dentin complete with dentinal tubules and odontoblastic processes (also known as true); in other cases, they are amorphous in structure (also known as false). They can be free or unattached to the outer pulpal wall, or they can be attached to the dentin at the dentin-pulp interface. Pulp stones are formed during tooth development and also later as the pulp ages, and they may be due to microtrauma. They are quite common and may fill most of the pulp chamber. They are detected as radiopaque masses in radiographs and are only a problem possibly during endodontic therapy.

Knowing the exact anatomy of a tooth's pulp chamber using radiographs, especially the extension of the pulp horns into the overlying cusps, is important when practicing safe restorative dentistry. However,

TABLE 13-4	Microscopic Zones in Pulp
ZONES (FROM OUTER TO INNER ZONES)	**MICROSCOPIC FEATURES**
Odontoblastic layer	Lines outer pulpal wall and consists of cell bodies of odontoblasts, which may form secondary dentin, causing cell bodies to realign themselves; cell bodies of afferent axons from dentinal tubules located between cell bodies of odontoblasts
Cell-free zone	Contains fewer cells than odontoblastic layer; nerve and capillary plexus located here
Cell-rich zone	Contains increased density of cells compared with cell-free zone and more extensive vascular supply
Pulpal core	Located in center of pulp chamber; similar to cell-rich zone with many cells and extensive vascular supply

FIGURE 13-19 Pulp stones in multirooted teeth. **A,** Microscopic section. **B,** Radiograph *(arrows)*. (**A,** From the Dr. Bernhard Gottlieb Collection, courtesy of James McIntosh, PhD, Assistant Professor Emeritus, Department of Biomedical Sciences, Baylor College of Dentistry, Dallas, TX. **B,** Courtesy of Margaret J. Fehrenbach, RDH, MS.)

when the pulp is injured by cavity preparation through mechanical or chemical injury, and even by extensive caries or other types of injury, it may undergo inflammation with **pulpitis** (pul-**pie**-tis). This inflammation of pulpitis initially remains localized within the confines of the dentin. However, the pressure from this confined pulpitis can result in extreme pain as the inflammatory edema presses on the afferent nerves contained in the pulp (see earlier discussion).

Pulpitis can later cause a pulpal infection in the form of a periapical abscess or cyst in the surrounding periodontium, spreading through the apical foramen or, possibly, an accessory canal. This is an example of the communication between the pulp and the surrounding periodontium, where disease states can extend between the tissue types, ending up to involve both. However, rarely does infection or other diseases of the periodontium involve the pulp.

If the pulp dies from the infection, it must be surgically removed. An inert radiopaque rubbery material (gutta-percha) is then placed within the pulp chamber, including each radicular pulp (or root canal) during endodontic therapy (or root canal treatment). When the pulp is removed by this treatment, the tooth is no longer vital, because its nutritional source from the vascular pulpal tissue has been removed. Thus, the endodontically treated tooth may darken and become brittle and break during mastication. The darkening is due to leftover degradative products from pulpal necrosis with the death of the pulp tissue that were passed along the dentinal tubules.

A full-coverage restorative crown is placed on the treated natural crown to protect it from breaking and to prolong retention of the tooth, as well as to improve its appearance if tooth colored. Internal or external nonvital whitening may also be necessary to reduce darkening with certain esthetic restorations, or if coverage is deferred. If an abscess or cyst formation develops in the periodontium as a result of pulpitis, further surgery (apicoectomy) must be performed to remove the apical lesion.

Dental professionals must try to prevent injury to the pulp during preventive procedures and restorative treatment. Such iatrogenic injury to the pulp can result from the heat or vibrations emitted by an older dental handpiece during cavity preparation, as well as excessive coronal polishing, causing mechanical injury. The pulp can also undergo chemical injury by various restorative materials placed during cavity preparation (see earlier discussion). Newer water-cooled handpieces with rapid rotation, which minimize the heat and vibrations on the tooth, as well as selective polishing techniques, are now used successfully to reduce the incidence of pulpal damage.

Liners are also currently placed over dentin when using toxic chemical restorative materials to prevent future pulpal damage. Then cement bases are placed after the liner, to protect the pulp from restorations that can serve as thermal conductors, such as gold inlays/crowns or silver amalgams. Tertiary types of dentin will also fill in around the sensitive pulp after the restoration has been placed within 6 months to a year, thereby reducing pulpal pain.

The vitality of the dentin-pulp complex, during health and after injury, depends on pulpal tissue cell activity and the signaling processes that regulate the cell's behavior. This is especially true regarding the DPSCs present. Research has led to a better understanding of the molecular control of cellular behavior. Growth factors play a pivotal role in signaling the events of tissue formation and repair in the dentin-pulp complex. Harnessing these growth factors can provide exciting opportunities for biologic approaches to dental tissue repair and the blueprint for replacement tissue engineering of the tooth. These approaches offer significant potential for improved clinical management of dental disease and maintenance of tooth vitality.

In addition, work is continuing directly with the DPSCs, because this particular type of stem cell has the future potential to differentiate into a variety of other cell types that were originally derived from the embryonic mesenchyme, including muscle, bone, cartilage, and fat, as well as dental tissue, such as dentin, cementum, PDL, and lamina propria. The DPSCs are most viable in primary teeth; permanent molars (such as thirds) also have the cells, though fewer. Processing has to be quick after removal, and the freezing process is the same as used to store cord blood stem cells. Teeth that merely fall out may have damaged pulp and may not be a useful source, especially if viability standards are not set.

The potential for using DPSCs for dental repair, however, remains unclear. Research continues related to using cord blood stem cells to regrow tissue and possibly to help address diseases like Parkinson and Alzheimer diseases, spinal cord injury, cerebrovascular accident, thermal injury, cardiovascular disease, diabetes, osteoarthritis, and rheumatoid arthritis.

In addition, identification of the genes controlling odontoblast differentiation might lead to development of methods enabling induction of tertiary dentin formation under carious lesions. Identification of the genes active during dentinogenesis might lead to recognition of regulatory factors, which would cause secondary dentinogenesis to proceed at the rate of primary dentinogenesis, so that present-day restorations would become a thing of the past.

CHAPTER 14

Periodontium: Cementum, Alveolar Process, and Periodontal Ligament

ⓔ Additional resources and practice exercises are provided on the companion Evolve website for this book: http://evolve.elsevier.com/Fehrenbach/illustrated.

●●● LEARNING OBJECTIVES

1. Define and pronounce the key terms in this chapter.
2. Give an overview of periodontium properties, including its components.
3. Identify each individual component of the periodontium on a diagram.
4. Discuss cementum properties and the clinical considerations with cementum structure, integrating it into patient care.
5. Discuss cementum development, histology, types, and repair as well as the clinical considerations for cementum pathology, integrating it into patient care.

6. Discuss alveolar process properties, including jaw anatomy and histology.
7. Discuss the clinical considerations with the alveolar process, integrating it into patient care.
8. Describe periodontal ligament properties.
9. Identify the fiber groups of the periodontal ligament on a diagram and discuss the functions assigned to each of them.
10. Discuss the clinical considerations for periodontal ligament pathology and repair, integrating it into patient care.

PERIODONTIUM PROPERTIES

To understand the pathologic changes that occur during the disease states involving the **periodontium** (per-e-o-**don**-she-um), dental professionals must first appreciate the histology of the healthy periodontium. Thus, the underlying histologic features of these components provide a clue to the clinical appearances noted with the periodontium, whether in a healthy or diseased state.

The periodontium consists of both the supporting soft and hard dental tissue between the tooth and the alveolar process, as well as parts of the tooth and alveolar process (Figure 14-1). The periodontium serves to support the tooth in its on-going relationship to the alveolar process. Thus, the periodontium includes the cementum, alveolar process, and periodontal ligament (PDL), as well as each of the individual components of each type of tissue. Some clinicians may include various types of gingival tissue in the category of the periodontium, but it has only a minor role in the support of the tooth (see **Chapter 10**).

CEMENTUM PROPERTIES

The cementum is the part of the periodontium that attaches the teeth to the alveolar process by anchoring the PDL (Figure 14-2). However, in a healthy patient, the cementum is not clinically visible because it usually covers the entire root, overlying Tomes granular layer in

dentin, which is not usually exposed in a healthy oral cavity. Cementum helps provide a protective cover over the open dentinal tubules within the root dentin if exposure occurs.

Cementum is a hard tissue that is thickest at the tooth's apex or apices and in the interradicular areas of multirooted teeth (50 to 200 μm) and thinnest at the **cementoenamel** (see-**men**-to-ih-**nam**-l) **junction (CEJ)** at the cervix of the tooth (10 to 50 μm). Unlike bone, cementum has no nerve supply and is also avascular (without blood vessels), receiving its nutrition through its own imbedded cells from the surrounding vascular PDL. However, like the other dental hard tissue of both dentin and the alveolar process, cementum can form throughout the life of the tooth, including after eruption (see Table 6-2).

Mature cementum is by weight 65% inorganic or mineralized material, 23% organic material, and 12% water. This crystalline formation of mature cementum consists mainly of calcium hydroxyapatite with the chemical formula of $Ca_{10}(PO_4)_6(OH)_2$. The calcium hydroxyapatite found in cementum is similar to that found in higher percentages in both enamel and dentin, but more closely resembles the percentage found in bone tissue, such as the alveolar process. Other forms of calcium are also present. The organic components include collagen glycoproteins, and proteoglycans with mainly Type I collagen as wel as lesser amounts of other types.

Because of its mineral level, cementum appears more radiolucent (or darker) than either enamel or dentin, but it appears more radiopaque (or lighter) than pulp when viewed on radiographs; however, any cemental layer(s) near the CEJ may not be viewable on radiographs due to its thinness (see Figure 14-22).

Clinical Considerations with Cementum Structure

In certain situations, when cementum is initially exposed from gingival recession (such as occurring during chronic advanced periodontal disease), it is a dull pale yellow, lighter than dentin but darker than enamel's whitish shade (discussed later). When instruments are used against its surface, the exposed cementum feels grainy compared with the harder dentin and the even harder, smoother enamel surfaces. However, when cementum is exposed through gingival recession, it quickly undergoes abrasion by mechanical friction because of its low mineral content and thinness, exposing the underlying dentin (see Figure 13-1). The exposure of the deeper dentin can lead to extrinsic staining and dentinal hypersensitivity (see **Chapter 13**).

Studies are showing that such histologic features may result in an increased risk of cemental (see-men-tal) caries. The incidence of cemental caries increases in older adults as gingival recession occurs from either trauma or periodontal disease. It is a chronic condition that forms a large, shallow lesion and slowly invades first the root's cementum and then dentin to cause a chronic infection of the pulp (Figure 14-3). Because dental pain is a late finding, many lesions are not detected early, resulting in restorative challenges and increased tooth loss. Xerostomia (or dry mouth), poor manual dexterity for adequate homecare, and poor nutrition in older adults can complicate cemental caries, and all of these issues must be addressed during dental treatment of these patients.

Increased controversy surrounds treatment of periodontal disease that involves the removal of the outer layers of cementum during root scaling performed during nonsurgical periodontal therapy. Dental biofilm and the related hardened calculus are associated with the cemental surface of the root deep inside an active periodontal pocket (Figures 14-4 and 14-5; see also **Chapter 10**). In the past, it was believed that bacterial toxins (or endotoxins) could be absorbed into the outer part of cementum from the adjacent dental biofilm and that these outer layers of "toxic" cementum must be removed by manual scaling for the dentogingival junctional tissue to heal and form a more occlusal epithelial attachment. Now it is believed that these toxins are loosely adherent to the cementum and that the cementum does not need to be mechanically removed by scaling, but, instead, ultrasonic devices can flush these toxins from the cementum without removing any of the associated hard tissue. Root scaling performed during nonsurgical periodontal therapy is only to be used to remove hardened calculus. More ultrastructural studies in this area are necessary as more evidence-based therapies of periodontal disease are considered.

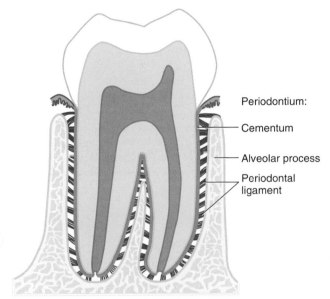

FIGURE 14-1 Periodontium with its components.

Periodontium:

— Cementum

— Alveolar process

— Periodontal ligament

Junctional epithelium

Epithelial attachment

Lamina propria of marginal gingiva

Gingival fiber group

Sharpey fibers

Alveolar crest of alveolar bone proper

Periodontal ligament

Enamel

Mantle dentin

Cementoenamel junction

Dentinocemental junction

Tomes granular layer in dentin

Cementoblasts

Cementocytes in cementum

FIGURE 14-2 Cementum and its relationship to both the tooth and the alveolar bone proper with Sharpey fibers from the periodontal ligament inserting into both tissue types. Note the Tomes granular layer in the adjacent underlying dentin.

CEMENTUM DEVELOPMENT

The development of cementum has been subdivided into a prefunctional stage, which occurs throughout root formation, and a functional stage, which starts when the tooth is in occlusion and continues throughout life.

Cementum, which develops from the dental sac, forms on the root dentin after the disintegration of Hertwig epithelial root sheath (see Figure 6-20). This disintegration allows the undifferentiated cells of the dental sac to come into contact with the newly formed surface of root dentin, inducing these cells to become cementoblasts. The cementoblasts then disperse to cover the root dentin area and undergo cementogenesis, laying down cementoid. Unlike ameloblasts and odontoblasts, which leave no cellular bodies in their secreted products during the later steps within the apposition stage, many of the cementoblasts become entrapped by the cementum they produce, becoming cementocytes (Figure 14-6). Again, cementum is more similar to the alveolar process with its osteoblasts becoming entrapped osteocytes.

When the cementoid reaches the full thickness needed, the cementoid surrounding the cementocytes becomes mineralized, or matured, and is then considered cementum. As a result of the appositional growth of cementum over the dentin, the dentinocemental junction (DCJ) is formed. This interface is not as defined, either clinically or microscopically as that of the dentinoenamel junction (DEJ)—given that cementum and dentin are of common developmental background, unlike enamel and dentin.

CEMENTUM HISTOLOGY

Cementum is composed of a mineralized fibrous matrix and cells. The fibrous matrix consists of both Sharpey fibers and intrinsic nonperiodontal fibers (see Figure 14-2). **Sharpey (shar**-pee) **fibers** are collagen fibers from the PDL that are partially inserted into the outer surface of the cementum at 90° or perpendicular. They are inserted on the other end, into the alveolar process, at the same angulation. These fibers are organized to function as a ligament between the tooth and alveolar process. The intrinsic non-PDL fibers of the cementum are collagen fibers made by the cementoblasts and laid down in a nonorganized pattern, yet all these fibers still run parallel to the DCJ.

The cells of cementum are the entrapped cementoblasts, the cementocytes (see Figure 14-6). Each cementocyte lies in its lacuna (plural, lacunae), similar to the pattern noted in bone. These lacunae also have **canaliculi** (kan-ah-**lik**-u-lie) or canals. Unlike those in bone, however, these canals in cementum do not contain nerves, nor do they radiate outward. Instead, the canals are oriented toward the PDL and

FIGURE 14-3 Cemental caries with invasion into the adjacent dentin. Pulpal involvement is a late finding due to the initial shallowness of the lesions. (Courtesy of Margaret J. Fehrenbach, RDH, MS.)

FIGURE 14-4 Scanning electron micrograph of subgingival dental biofilm on the cemental root surface in a deep periodontal pocket. (Courtesy of Jan Cope, RDH, MS, Associate Professor, Oregon Institute of Technology, Klamath Falls, OR.)

FIGURE 14-5 Calculus (arrow) embedded within the cementum (C) that overlies the dentin (D). Note that dental biofilm or plaque (P) then overlies the rough calculus. Many times the calculus on the root is more mineralized than the underlying cementum or even dentin. (From Newman MG, Takei HH, Klokkevold PR: Carranza's Clinical periodontology, ed 12, St Louis, 2015, Saunders/Elsevier.)

contain cementocytic processes that exist to diffuse nutrients from the vascularized periodontal ligament; however, cementocytes in deeper layers may no longer be vital.

After the appositional growth of cementum in layers, the cementoblasts that do not become entrapped in cementum line up along the cemental surface for the entire length of the outer covering of the PDL. These cementoblasts can form subsequent layers of cementum if the tooth is injured (discussed later).

Three possible types of transitional interfaces may be present at the CEJ. The traditional view was that certain interfaces dominated in certain oral cavities. Studies with the scanning electron microscope indicate that the CEJ may exhibit all of these interfaces in an individual's oral cavity, and there is even considerable variation when one tooth is traced circumferentially (Figures 14-7 and 14-8) In some cases, the cementum may overlap the enamel at the CEJ (but less frequently than previously

FIGURE 14-6 Microscopic section of cellular cementum with its cementocytes within their lacunae and the canaliculi oriented toward the periodontal ligament for nutrition *(arrow)*. (From the Dr. Bernhard Gottlieb Collection, courtesy of James McIntosh, PhD, Assistant Professor Emeritus, Department of Biomedical Sciences, Baylor College of Dentistry, Dallas, TX.)

thought, at less than 15% of the cases). Thus novice clinicians may have difficulty discerning the CEJ from calculus deposits around the cervix with this situation. However, compared with the usually spotty placement and roughness of calculus, cementum exhibits a more uniform placement and as well as continual roughness when using an explorer.

Another possible interface that can occur with the CEJ is that the cementum and enamel may meet end-to-end, presenting no problems for either the clinician or patient, and it is the most common finding at about 52% of cases. Finally, another possible interface at the CEJ is that a gap may exist between the cementum and enamel, exposing dentin in about 33% of cases. Thus, patients may experience dentinal hypersensitivity (see Figure 13-12).

CEMENTUM TYPES

Two basic types of cementum are formed by cementoblasts: acellular and cellular (Figure 14-9, *A*, and Table 14-1). Acellular cementum (see-*men*-tum) consists of the first layers of cementum deposited at the DCJ and thus is also considered *primary cementum*. It is formed at a slower rate than other types and contains no embedded cementocytes. At least one layer of acellular cementum covers the entire outer surface of each root with many more layers covering the cervical one-third near the CEJ (see Figure 14-3). The width of acellular cementum never changes.

The other type of cementum is cellular cementum, sometimes called *secondary cementum* because it is deposited later than the primary type (see Figures 14-6 and 14-9, *B*). Cellular cementum consists of the last layers of cementum deposited over the acellular cementum, mainly in the apical one-third of each root. It is formed at a faster rate than acellular type, catching the cementoblasts during production, and thus many embedded cementocytes are found within it. Lining up at its periphery are cementoblasts located in the PDL, which allow the future production of more cellular cementum in response to tooth wear and movement and is also associated with repair of periodontal tissue.

Thus, the width of cellular cementum can change during the life of the tooth, especially at the apex or apices of the tooth (discussed next). This type of cementum is also common in interradicular areas. It is important to note that Sharpey fibers in acellular cementum are fully mineralized; those in cellular cementum are generally mineralized only partially at their periphery.

CEMENTUM REPAIR

Similar to bone tissue such as the alveolar process, cementum can undergo removal within the tissue as a result of trauma (Figure 14-10). This removal involves resorption of cementum by the odontoclast,

FIGURE 14-7 Phase-contrast image of the cementoenamel junction interface where cementum and enamel do not meet, leaving a gap where dentin is exposed *(arrow)*, which may lead to dentinal hypersensitivity. (Courtesy of P. Tambasco de Oliveira. From Nanci A: *Ten Cate's oral histology*, ed 8, St Louis, 2013, Mosby/Elsevier.)

FIGURE 14-8 Three interfaces (overlap, meet, and gap) present at the cementoenamel junction *(CEJ)* throughout a dentition, as well as points along the way *(arrows)*. **A,** Cementum may overlap enamel *(Overlap)*; may meet end-to-end *(Meet)*; may be a gap between enamel and cementum, leaving dentin exposed *(Gap)*. **B,** Ground sections of the same three interfaces with gap exposing dentin highlighted in last section *(arrows)*. (From Nanci A: *Ten Cate's oral histology,* ed 8, St Louis, 2013, Mosby/Elsevier.)

resulting in reversal lines. When viewed in a microscopic section of cementum, these reversal lines appear as scalloped lines, just as in bone. However, cementum is less readily resorbed than bone, an important consideration during orthodontic tooth movement (discussed later).

At the same time, there can be repair of traumatic resorption area by involving the appositional growth of cementum by cementoblasts in the adjacent PDL. Appositional growth of this recently formed protective cementum is noted by the arrest lines. These arrest lines when viewed in a microscopic section, look like smooth growth rings in a cross section of a tree. This is similar to what occurs in bone tissue, such as the alveolar process. Both reversal and arrest lines are prominent in cementum subjected to occlusal trauma or to orthodontic tooth movement, as well as during the shedding of primary teeth and eruption of the permanent tooth. However, unlike bone, cementum does not continually undergo

FIGURE 14-9 Two types of cementum on the root surface. **A,** Acellular cementum *(AC)* without cementocytes makes up the first layers deposited at the dentinocemental junction over the dentin *(D)*. **B,** Cellular cementum *(CC)* that contains embedded cementocytes *(arrows)* is the last of the layers deposited over the thin layer of acellular cementum *(AC)* adjacent to the dentin *(D)*. Cells adjacent to the periodontal ligament *(PDL)* are cementoblasts. (From the Dr. Bernhard Gottlieb Collection, courtesy of James McIntosh, PhD, Assistant Professor Emeritus, Department of Biomedical Sciences, Baylor College of Dentistry, Dallas, TX.)

TABLE 14-1	Cementum Types
ACELLULAR	**CELLULAR**
First layer(s) deposited	Formed after acellular layer(s)
At least one layer over entire root with many layers near cervical one-third	Layered over acellular, mainly in apical one-third, especially in interradicular region
Formed at slower rate	Formed at faster rate
No embedded cementocytes	Embedded cementocytes
Width constant over time	Can widen over time; layers can be added

FIGURE 14-10 Reversal lines and arrest lines in cementum with embedded cementocytes *(white arrows)* that has undergone repair due to severe trauma. On the surface of the cementum are the cementoblasts *(dark arrows)* within the surrounding periodontal ligament *(PDL)*. Note that the alveolar bone proper *(ABP)* has similar lines noted as a result of bone remodeling. (From the Dr. Bernhard Gottlieb Collection, courtesy of James McIntosh, PhD, Assistant Professor Emeritus, Department of Biomedical Sciences, Baylor College of Dentistry, Dallas, TX.)

remodeling or repair as part of its history, but only when severely traumatized. Additionally, aging does not result in a change in mineral content of cementum like bone, but its permeability may lessen.

Clinical Considerations for Cementum Pathology

Cementicles (see-men-ti-kuls) are mineralized spherical bodies of cementum found either attached to the cemental root surface or lying free in the PDL (Figure 14-11). They form from the appositional growth of cementum around cellular debris in the PDL, possibly as a result of microtrauma to Sharpey fibers. They become attached or fused from the continued appositional growth of cementum and may be noted on radiographs.

FIGURE 14-11 Cementicle attached to the cemental surface within the periodontal ligament (*arrow*). (From the Dr. Bernhard Gottlieb Collection, courtesy of James McIntosh, PhD, Assistant Professor Emeritus, Department of Biomedical Sciences, Baylor College of Dentistry, Dallas, TX.)

Cemental spurs can be found at or near the CEJ. These are symmetrical spheres of cementum attached to the cemental root surface, similar to enamel pearls. Cemental spurs result from irregular deposition of cementum on the root and may be noted on radiographs. Both cementicles and cemental spurs can present some clinical problems in differentiating them from calculus; however, because they are hard, they are not easily removed. Thus, they may also interfere with periodontal therapy and homecare and may need to be removed through periodontal surgery.

Hypercementosis (hi-per-see-men-**toe**-sis) is the excessive production of cellular cementum, which mainly occurs at the apex or apices of the tooth (Figure 14-12). It may be present on radiographs as a radiopaque (or lighter) mass at each root apex. This condition can result from occlusal trauma caused by excessive occlusal forces and during certain pathologic conditions (such as chronic periapical inflammation), as well as systemic conditions (generalized level with Paget disease). It may also be a compensatory mechanism in response to attrition to increase occlusal tooth height, keeping the dentition in functional occlusion. However, such overgrowth of deposits form bulbous enlargements on the roots and may interfere with extractions, especially if adjacent teeth become fused, such as with concrescence (see Box 6-1, Q). It may also result in pulpal necrosis if at a severe level by blocking blood supply via the apical foramen (see **Chapter 13**).

In contrast, an unwanted side effect of rapid orthodontic therapy can be root apex resorption, reducing the overall length of the tooth, which is especially noted with permanent maxillary incisors (discussed later). The risk of tooth mobility is also increased. However, with new bioefficient orthodontic therapy being utilized, this effect has been minimized. In addition, thankfully cementum is resistant to resorption in a younger dentition during orthodontic therapy, unlike the alveolar process.

FIGURE 14-12 Hypercementosis at the root apices due to traumatic occlusal forces on permanent mandibular molar teeth. **A,** Microscopic section with tooth components identified: dentin (*D*), cementum (*C*), and radicular pulp (*P*). **B,** Radiograph. (**A,** From the Dr. Bernhard Gottlieb Collection, courtesy of James McIntosh, PhD, Assistant Professor Emeritus, Department of Biomedical Sciences, Baylor College of Dentistry, Dallas, TX; **B,** courtesy of Margaret J. Fehrenbach, RDH, MS.)

FIGURE 14-13 Alveolar process with its microscopic components is identified, including osteocytes in lacunae, as well as arrest and reversal lines, deep to the gingiva and adjacent to the periodontal ligament (*PDL*) and deeper cementum. Note that there has been a slight resorption of the alveolar crest showing the beginning of periodontitis. (From the Dr. Bernhard Gottlieb Collection, courtesy of James McIntosh, PhD, Assistant Professor Emeritus, Department of Biomedical Sciences, Baylor College of Dentistry, Dallas, TX.)

ALVEOLAR PROCESS PROPERTIES

The **alveolar** (al-vee-o-lar) **process** is that part of either the maxilla or mandible that supports and protects the teeth. The alveolar process is also that part of the periodontium to which the cementum of the tooth is attached through the PDL (Figure 14-13). The term alveolar process will be used mainly in this textbook since it has a clinical connotation; whereas, the other term used, *alveolar bone*, has mainly a histologic background.

The alveolar process is a hard, mineralized tissue with all the components of other bone tissue (see Figure 8-9). It is important to note that alveolar process is more easily remodeled than cementum, thus allowing orthodontic tooth movement (discussed later). When viewing a microscopic section, the remodeled alveolar process shows arrest lines and reversal lines, as does all bone tissue.

Like all bone, mature alveolar process is by weight 60% inorganic material or mineralized, 25% organic material, and 15% water. This crystalline formation consists mainly of calcium hydroxyapatite with the chemical formula of $Ca_{10}(PO_4)_6(OH)_2$. The calcium hydroxyapatite in the alveolar process is similar to that found in higher percentages in both enamel and dentin but is most similar to the levels in cementum (see Table 6-2). The minerals of potassium, manganese, magnesium, silica, iron, zinc, selenium, boron, phosphorus, sulfur, chromium, and others are also present but in smaller amounts.

JAW DEVELOPMENT

Both the maxilla and mandible develop from tissue of the first branchial arch, or mandibular arch. The maxilla forms within the fused maxillary processes of the mandibular arch, and the mandible forms within the fused mandibular processes of the mandibular arch. Both jaws also start as small centers of intramembranous ossification located around the stomodeum. These centers then increase in diameter, growing into the mature jaws (see **Chapter 8**). In addition, both jaws also have several skeletal units during development, and these are related to the overall morphology, or form, of the bones. Each of these units is influenced in its growth pattern by some adjacent structure that acts on the developing bone.

The maxilla's primary center of intramembranous ossification for each half of the maxilla appears around the seventh week of prenatal development. It is located at the termination of the infraorbital nerve, just superior to the dental lamina of the primary maxillary canine tooth in each maxillary process. Secondary ossification centers, the zygomatic, orbitonasal, nasopalatine, and intermaxillary, then appear and fuse rapidly with the primary centers. The two intermaxillary centers generate the alveolar process and primary palate region.

The subsequent growth of the maxilla can be subdivided into several skeletal units: the basal body unit, which develops beneath the infraorbital nerve, surrounding it to form the infraorbital canal; the orbital unit, which responds to the growth of the eyeball; the nasal unit, which depends on nasal septal cartilage for its growth; the alveolar unit, which forms in response to the maxillary teeth; and the pneumatic unit, which reflects maxillary sinus expansion. The primary bone initially formed in the maxilla is soon replaced by secondary bone as the face and oral cavity develop.

During the sixth week of prenatal development, on each side of the embryo's mandibular arch, a primary ossification center appears in the angle formed by the division of the inferior alveolar nerve and its incisive and mental branches, on the lateral aspect of Meckel cartilage, a rod derived from the first branchial arch or mandibular arch (see Figures 4-11 and 5-3).

In the seventh week, the first bone tissue in the body of the mandible forms. Bone development spreads rapidly from the angle anterior to the midline. The anterior bone forms around Meckel cartilage to produce a trough with medial and lateral plates that unite inferiorly around the incisive nerve. This trough extends to the midline on the embryo, where it comes into close approximation with a similar trough from the other side.

These two separate bilateral centers of ossification of the mandibular arch remain separated at the mandibular symphysis until shortly after birth. The trough turns into the mandibular canal as bone is formed over the incisive nerve joining the lateral and medial plates of initial bone.

Bone development in the mandibular arch also spreads posteriorly toward the point where the mandibular nerve is divided into its lingual and inferior alveolar branches. This ossification initially forms a gutter, which later evolves into a canal that contains the inferior alveolar nerve.

The mandible subsequently develops as several skeletal units: a condylar unit that forms the articulation with the temporal bone; the body of the mandible, which is the center of all growth of the mandible; the angular unit, which forms in response to the lateral pterygoid and masseter muscles; the coronoid unit, which forms in response to the temporalis muscle development; and the alveolar unit, which forms in response to the mandibular teeth.

Because it acts as a temporary supporting structure in the embryonic mandible, almost all of Meckel cartilage disappears as the mandible develops. The primary bone formed along Meckel cartilage is soon replaced by secondary bone. Secondary cartilage appears between the tenth and fourteenth weeks of prenatal development to form the head of the condyle, part of the coronoid process, and the mental protuberance. Separate from Meckel cartilage, the coronoid cartilage becomes incorporated into the expanding intramembranous bone of the ramus and disappears before birth. In the mental region, a similar situation occurs as the cartilage there disappears when the mandibular processes fuse at the mandibular symphysis (see Figure 1-9).

The condylar cartilage appears initially as a cone-shaped structure and is the primordium of the condyle. Chondrocytes differentiate in the center and increase by interstitial and appositional growth. By the middle of fetal life, most of the condylar cartilage is replaced with bone as a result of endochondral ossification, but its superior end persists into puberty. Thus, the condylar cartilage acts as a growth center for the temporomandibular joint (see **Chapter 8** and Figures 8-13 and 19-4).

Clinical Considerations during Jaw Development

The developmental dental anomaly of anodontia, in which tooth germ(s) are congenitally absent, may affect the development of the alveolar processes of the associated jaw (see Box 6-1, *A-B*). This occurrence can prevent the alveolar processes of either the maxilla or the mandible from developing locally. Proper development is impossible because the alveolar unit of each dental arch only forms in response to the tooth germs in the area. Instead only basal bone will be present in each one of the involved areas of the jaws (discussed next).

JAW ANATOMY AND HISTOLOGY

Each mature jaw, either the maxilla or mandible, is composed of two types of bone tissue with differing physiologic functioning (Figure 14-14). The part that contains the roots of the teeth is the alveolar process, which is also called the alveolar bone or alveolar ridge. The part apical to the roots of the teeth is the basal (bay-sal) bone, which then forms the body of the maxilla or body of the mandible, and thus is not part of the periodontium. Both the alveolar process and basal bone are covered by periosteum.

The alveolar process or alveolar bone is divided into the alveolar bone proper and the supporting alveolar bone. Microscopically, both the alveolar bone proper and the supporting alveolar bone have the same components: fibers, cells, intercellular substances, nerves, blood vessels, and lymphatics (see **Chapter 8**; see Figure 14-13).

The alveolar bone proper (ABP) makes up the lining of the tooth socket or alveolus (plural, alveoli) (see Figure 14-14). Although the ABP is composed of compact bone, it may be called the *cribriform plate* because it contains numerous holes where Volkmann canals with its nerves and blood vessels pass from the ABP into the PDL. The ABP is also called *bundle bone* because Sharpey fibers, a part of the fibers of the PDL, are inserted here (Figure 14-15). Similar to those of the cemental surface, Sharpey fibers in ABP are each inserted at 90° or perpendicular to the alveolar process to mediate the anchorage of the tooth, but are fewer in number, although thicker in diameter than those present in cementum. As in cellular cementum, Sharpey fibers in bone are generally mineralized only partially at their periphery. The attached gingiva along with the periosteum of the ABP serves as a mucoperiosteum (see **Chapter 9**).

The ABP consists of plates of compact bone that surround the tooth and assume the shape of the tooth. The ABP varies in thickness from 0.1 to 0.5 mm. The part of the ABP that is present on radiographs is considered the lamina dura (lam-i-nah dur-ah), which is uniformly radiopaque (or lighter) (Figure 14-16). The integrity of the lamina dura is important when studying radiographs for pathologic lesions.

The alveolar crest is the most cervical rim of the ABP (Figure 14-17). In a healthy situation, the alveolar crest is slightly apical to the CEJ by approximately 1 to 2 mm. The alveolar crests of neighboring teeth are also uniform in height along the jaw in a healthy jaw.

A part of the alveolar crest that is between neighboring teeth is present on periapical and bite-wing radiographs as a radiopaque (or lighter) triangle at the most coronal part of the interdental septum or bone (see Figure 14-16, *A*). This anatomic representation can be used for educating patients about bone loss levels occurring with periodontal disease; however, it shows only the levels of ABP interproximally, limited to two dimensions. In reality, bone loss occurs in three dimensions and at any surface adjacent to the tooth root and in varying amounts around it.

The supporting alveolar bone (SAB) consists of both cortical bone and trabecular bone. The cortical (kor-ti-kal) bone consists of a plate of compact bone on both the facial and lingual surfaces of the alveolar process; thus the term *cortical plate* is also used to describe this part of the alveolar process (see Figure 14-15). These cortical plates are usually about 1.5 to 3 mm thick over posterior teeth, but the thickness is highly variable around anterior teeth. The cortical bone is not visible on periapical or bitewing radiographs but only on occlusal radiographs as a uniformly radiopaque (or lighter) bony sheet, facial and lingual to the teeth (see Figure 14-16, *B*).

The trabecular (trah-bek-u-lar) bone consists of cancellous bone (or spongy bone) that is located between the ABP and the plates of cortical bone (see Figure 14-15). Only the parts of trabecular bone between the teeth and between the roots are ever present on any type of radiographs, and this trabecular bone appears less uniformly radiopaque and more porous than the uniformly radiopaque lamina dura of the ABP.

The alveolar process that separates two neighboring teeth is the interdental (in-ter-den-tal) septum (or interdental bone) (Figure 14-18). It is present on both periapical and bitewing radiographs (see Figure 14-17). The interdental septum consists of both the compact bone of the ABP and cancellous bone of the trabecular bone. The alveolar process that separates the roots of the same tooth is the interradicular (in-ter-rah-dik-u-lar) septum (or interradicular bone) (Figure 14-19). The interradicular septum consists of both ABP and trabecular bone; however, only a part of the interradicular

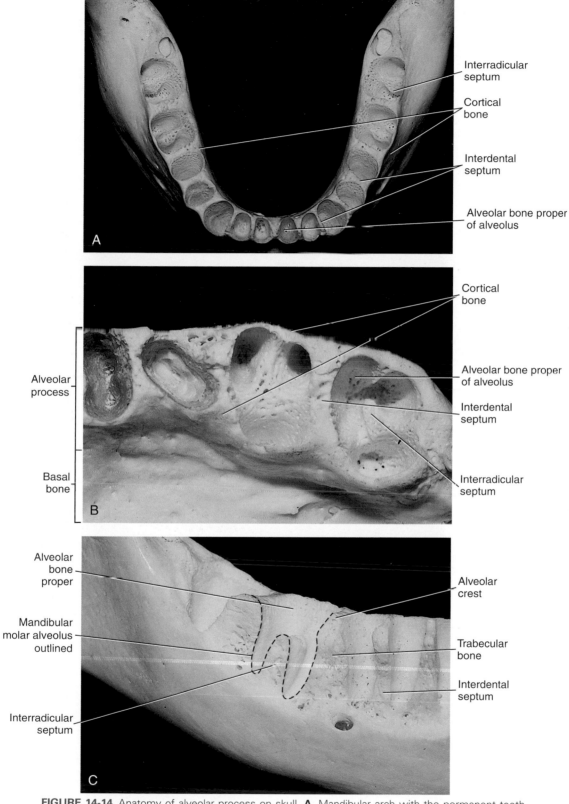

FIGURE 14-14 Anatomy of alveolar process on skull. **A,** Mandibular arch with the permanent teeth removed. **B,** Part of the maxilla with the teeth removed demonstrating the surrounding cribriform plate of the alveolar bone proper of the alveolus. **C,** Cross section of the mandible with the teeth removed and a mandibular molar alveolus highlighted *(dashed lines)*. (Courtesy of Margaret J. Fehrenbach, RDH, MS.)

septum is ever present on periapical or bitewing radiographs (see Figure 14-17).

Clinical Considerations with Dental Procedures and Pathology Involving Alveolar Process

Bone remodeling can be forced with orthodontic therapy to produce tooth movement for repositioning (Figure 14-20). The bands, wires, or appliances put pressure on one side of the tooth and adjacent alveolar process, creating a *compression zone* in the PDL. This compression in the PDL leads to bone resorption. On the opposite side of the tooth and bone, a *tension zone* develops in the PDL and causes the deposition of new bone. Thus, the tooth or teeth are slowly moved along the jaw to achieve a dentition that works in harmony (see **Chapter 20**). In this way, the width of the space between the alveoli and the root is kept about the same.

Mesial (me-ze-il) drift (or physiologic drift) is the natural movement phenomenon in which all the teeth move slightly toward the midline of the oral cavity over time (see Figure 20-21). This can cause crowding late in life of a once-perfect dentition. It occurs quite slowly, depending mostly on the degree of wear of the contact points between adjacent teeth and on the number of missing teeth. Overall,

FIGURE 14-15 Microscopic section of the insertion of Sharpey fibers from the periodontal ligament into the alveolar bone proper in the root area. Note the Haversian system within the cortical bone as well as the alveolar bone proper. (From Nanci A: *Ten Cate's oral histology,* ed 8, St Louis, 2013, Mosby/Elsevier.)

FIGURE 14-16 Radiographic landmarks of the alveolar process of the mandible. **A,** Periapical radiograph. **B,** Occlusal radiograph. Tooth components are also identified: enamel *(E)*, dentin *(D)*, and pulp *(P)*. (Courtesy of Margaret J. Fehrenbach, RDH, MS.)

the amount of movement may total no more than 1 cm over a lifetime. However, this crowding may lead to poor homecare in the region as well as less than optimal esthetics.

After extraction of a tooth, the clot in the alveolus fills in with immature bone, which later is remodeled into mature secondary bone. However, with the loss of teeth, a patient becomes edentulous

(e-den-tu-lus), either partially or completely, and the surrounding alveolar process progressively undergoes resorption (Figure 14-21). The bony trabeculae supporting the alveoli also decrease in number and in thickness as the alveolar process itself becomes thinner. In contrast, the underlying basal bone of the body of the maxilla or mandible remains less affected, however, because it does not need the presence of teeth to remain viable. Thus, the alveolar process depends on the functional stimulation from teeth during mastication and speech for preservation of its structure.

Resorption of the alveolar process can occur in higher levels in postmenopausal women who experience a shortage of estrogen, which usually helps maintain bone density; however, severe bone loss levels may occur with the onset of osteoporosis. The placement of a denture, either partial or full, or a bridge can somewhat mimic the stimulation of the teeth in the alveolar process. Over time, however, some amounts of the alveolar process are lost even with these types of tooth replacements, especially if the prosthesis produces excessive compression of the underlying bone. Loss of the alveolar process also accompanies the aging process but is increased in clinical conditions where blood supply is compromised and hypoxia (reduced oxygen) occurs, such as following severe inflammation, radiation trauma, or bone fracture.

Occlusal drift or supereruption within the alveolar process can also occur with loss of teeth, especially if involved with the permanent posterior teeth (see Figures 17-43 and 17-56). The exact mechanism that causes drifting of the dentition is still controversial; it may be an adjustment process to retain balance among the various components of the masticatory apparatus, or may just be related to the wear of the proximal and occlusal tooth surfaces.

The loss of the alveolar process due to aging, coupled with attrition of the teeth, causes also a progressive loss of height of the lower third of the vertical dimension of the face when the teeth are in maximum intercuspation (Figure 14-22; see Figures 1-3 and 1-10 for comparison and **Chapter 20**). The extent of this loss is determined based on clinical judgment using the Golden Proportions. This part of the vertical dimension is important in determining the way in which the teeth and jaws function. In addition, a proper amount of height in the lower third of the face reduces the amount of facial wrinkles and lines around the mouth as the skin ages, sags, and loses its resilience (see **Chapter 8**). With the loss of vertical dimension in the lower third, older patients can take on a cartoon "Popeye" facial appearance that is esthetically displeasing and results in poor functioning of the teeth and jaws.

FIGURE 14-17 Photomicrograph of the alveolar crest of the alveolar bone proper *(ABP)* and its relationship to the root covered by cementum *(C)* with the alveolar crest fibers of the periodontal ligament *(PDL)* inserting Sharpey fibers into both tissue types. Note that there is slight resorption of the alveolar crest showing the beginning of periodontitis. (From the Dr. Bernhard Gottlieb Collection, courtesy of James McIntosh, PhD, Assistant Professor Emeritus, Department of Biomedical Sciences, Baylor College of Dentistry, Dallas, TX.)

FIGURE 14-18 Microscopic section of interdental septum or bone *(B)* found between the roots of two neighboring teeth *(T)* and surrounded on each side by the horizontal group of the periodontal ligament *(PDL)*. (From the Dr. Bernhard Gottlieb Collection, courtesy of James McIntosh, PhD, Assistant Professor Emeritus, Department of Biomedical Sciences, Baylor College of Dentistry, Dallas, TX.)

FIGURE 14-19 Microscopic section of interradicular septum or bone between two roots *(B)* of a mandibular molar and surrounded on each side by the interradicular group of the periodontal ligament *(PDL)*. The molar's roots are composed of dentin *(D)* and cementum *(C)*. (From the Dr. Bernhard Gottlieb Collection, courtesy of James McIntosh, PhD, Assistant Professor Emeritus, Department of Biomedical Sciences, Baylor College of Dentistry, Dallas, TX.)

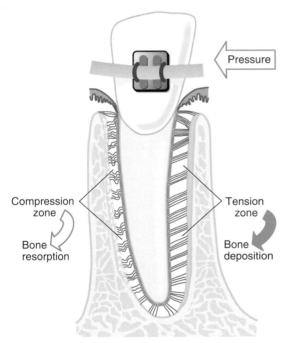

FIGURE 14-20 Process of tooth movement during orthodontic therapy. Appliances put pressure on one side, creating a zone of compression in the periodontal ligament on the opposite side, which leads to bone resorption. On the same side, a zone of tension develops causing deposition of new bone. Thus, the tooth or teeth are slowly moved along the jaw.

Ideally, a dental implant is placed in an edentulous area, which preserves the integrity of the bone, provides adequate stimulation, and serves as a permanent replacement for a lost tooth or teeth, preventing further loss of vertical dimension (Figure 14-23). An implant has a core part made of titanium that is surgically implanted in the alveolar process of either jaw with an attached prosthetic superstructure of a tooth or denture; the high success rate of these current implants has now been demonstrated.

The deeper core of the implant has an open structure, allowing bone to bond to it over a short time, so as to undergo osseointegration of the implant to the surrounding alveolar process. However, unlike natural teeth having an insertion of the principal fiber groups of the PDL into the alveolar process via Sharpey fibers that allows supported

tooth movement, an implant has no movement. Instead, the implant makes direct contact with the alveolar process, as well as with the surrounding connective tissue and superficial epithelium, the *periimplant tissue*. Research has shown that a sulcular epithelium that consists of the circular fibers of the gingival tissue surrounds and also attaches to the superior part of the implant by hemidesmosomes in tissue that structurally resembles a junctional epithelium. After osseointegration and healing of the tissue, a prosthetic superstructure of a tooth or denture is then attached to the surgical part of the implant.

Studies have shown that failure to obtain and maintain this cellular junction may lead to apical migration of the epithelium on the bone-implant interface, possible soft tissue encapsulation of the implant, and eventual implant failure resulting from mobility. Thus, special devices are needed for professional care and homecare of an implant's prosthetic superstructure to remove any deposits and prevent periimplant disease. Sadly, most patients with implants have a history of inadequate homecare that led to the initial tooth loss.

In addition, the placement of an immediate load implant upon extraction of a noninfected tooth or teeth is now available. For this placement to be considered successful adequate bone must exist and a sufficiently large implant must be placed; once placed, the implant must be able to resist occlusal forces. The temporary prosthetic superstructure must be adjusted so that no forces are placed on it during function; meeting these criteria allows osseointegration. After a period of 9 weeks, a permanent prosthetic superstructure can be placed, shortening treatment time by 4 to 6 months.

During the chronic advanced periodontal disease of periodontitis, the localized alveolar process is also lost (Figure 14-24; see Figure 10-12 and discussion in **Chapter 10**). This bone loss may be due to an overresponse of the immune system and the activation of certain osteoclast populations; among the bioactive agents implicated are cytokines and prostaglandins. Cytokines are small proteins that function as signaling compounds for the white blood cells, which are necessary to the inflammatory response (see **Chapter 8**). Examples of cytokines include the various interleukins (ILs), such as IL-1, IL-6, and IL-1β, and tumor necrosis factor-alpha (TNF-α).

When periodontitis initially develops or as it progresses, hard and soft tissue destruction is by both collagen and extracellular matrix (ECM) degradation. This degradation is primarily by proteinases, protein-degrading enzymes. There are many types of proteinases, including a group called *matrix metalloproteinase (MMP)*; more than 25 MMPs have currently been identified, and broadly categorized into six groups.

FIGURE 14-21 Edentulous states with resultant changes in the alveolar process. **A,** A partially edentulous case from the extraction of the posterior teeth with loss of the alveolar process of the mandibular posterior sextant with only the basal bone remaining. **B,** A complete edentulous skull from a past full mouth extraction of the teeth with the bone loss of both the alveolar processes with only basal bone remaining. (Courtesy of Margaret J. Fehrenbach, RDH, MS.)

FIGURE 14-22 Loss of vertical dimension in the inferior third of the face in 20-year increments (age 20, age 40, and age 60) as the bone from alveolar process is lost from the jaws. The permanent teeth themselves have also undergone a reduction in height by slight attrition, the mechanical wear of the masticatory surface. Note the increase in facial wrinkles and lines around the mouth caused by these orofacial changes. This amount due to aging can be dramatically increased with tooth loss, severe periodontal disease, or increased levels of attrition.

FIGURE 14-23 Single-tooth implant placed in the mandible. **A,** Clinical photograph after prosthetic replacement. **B,** Previous radiograph. Note that the implant had successfully undergone osseointegration of the titanium core and the prosthetic suprastructure could then be placed to replace a missing permanent mandibular second premolar due to partial anodontia. (**A** and **B,** From Newman MG, Takei HH, Klokkevold PR: *Carranza's Clinical periodontology,* ed 12, Philadelphia, 2015, Saunders/Elsevier.)

FIGURE 14-24 Bone loss caused by the chronic advanced periodontal disease of periodontitis. **A,** Microscopic section of periodontitis occurring between a lateral incisor *(L)* and a canine *(C)* demonstrating calculus *(Ca)* and a periodontal pocket with suppuration *(S).* **B,** Close-up view showing bone resorption *(R)* from the alveolar bone proper *(ABP)* due to osteoclast activity beneath the inflammation in the periodontal ligament *(PDL);* areas of fibrosis *(F)* are also noted in reaction. **C,** Radiograph showing severe bone loss from previously healthy levels *(outline)* on permanent mandibular incisors. This bone loss initially involved the alveolar crest and moved apically as the periodontitis progressed. (**A** and **B,** From Newman MG, Takei HH, Klokkevold PR: *Carranza's Clinical periodontology,* ed 12, Philadelphia, 2015, Saunders/Elsevier. **C,** Courtesy of Margaret J. Fehrenbach, RDH, MS.)

Several of these degrade collagen, including MMP-1, MMP-8, and MMP-13, thereby being classified as collagenases. Assessment of MMP in either the tissue of periodontium, gingival cervical fluid, or saliva may serve as an important future biomarker in diagnosis of periodontal diseases and also for prognostic follow-up. Targeted therapy aimed at reducing effects of MMP may serve as a useful adjunct for treatment of periodontitis. At this time, a subantimicrobial dose (SD) of doxycycline is used during periodontal therapy to inactivate collagenase.

The bone loss is first evident in the most coronal part of the ABP, the alveolar crest, which looks moth-eaten both microscopically and radiographically (see Figures 14-13 and 14-24). As the loss of the alveolar process slowly progresses apically, the tooth becomes increasingly mobile, also increasing the risk of future tooth loss. Prevention of further loss of the alveolar process, and thus management of the periodontal disease, is important in the dental treatment plan for these patients and may include the homecare removal of oral deposits, surgical procedures to increase self-cleansing, and even the use of SD of antibiotics.

Bone grafting may be included during surgical periodontal therapy especially during implant placement. The bone graft is sourced from either the alveolar process or other bone (such as the chin) and even from other sources (such as cadavers), possibly with the use of guided tissue regeneration (GTR) membrane. GTRs are surgical procedures that utilize barrier membranes to direct the growth of new bone and soft tissue at sites having insufficient volumes or dimensions for proper function, esthetics, or prosthetic restoration. The use of GTR is based on the long-recognized concept that fibroblasts from the PDL as well as undifferentiated mesenchyme have the potential to re-create the original periodontal attachment.

Using GTR to treat narrow intrabony defects and class II mandibular furcations has been very successful, as has its use to support bone growth on an alveolar process and to allow stable placement of the implant. However, GFR offers limited benefits in the treatment of other types of periodontal defects. Bone repair is also being enhanced by the use of platelet-rich plasma (PRP) in the alveolus with both bone defect treatment and with implant placement (see **Chapter 8**). Treatments for the management of osteoporosis involving the jaws may be used in the future in more localized bone loss within the alveolar process.

The density of the alveolar process in a given area also determines the route that dental infection takes with abscess formation, as well as the efficacy of local infiltration of the agent during the administration of local anesthesia. In addition, the differences in alveolar process density determine the easiest and most convenient areas of bony fracture to be used if needed during tooth extraction of impacted teeth (see Figure 17-62).

Finally, with occlusal trauma, the part of the ABP present on radiographs as the lamina dura may become thickened in response, along with the widening of the PDL space (discussed later and see **Chapter 20**). Thus the ABP becomes thicker with the individual bony trabeculae supporting the alveoli also increasing in number and in thickness as well.

There can also be loss of integrity of the lamina dura when studying radiographs for pathologic lesions such as with bone cancer, giving various aggressive radiolucent presentations that appear "moth-eaten", with an ill-defined zone of multiple small radiolucencies that may coalesce or be permeative with numerous tiny radiolucencies in between the residual bone trabeculae.

PERIODONTAL LIGAMENT PROPERTIES

The PDL is that part of the periodontium that provides for the attachment of the teeth to the surrounding ABP by way of the root cementum (see Figure 14-1). The width of the PDL ranges from 0.15 to 0.38 mm, with its thinnest part around the middle third of the root. The PDL appears on radiographs as the **periodontal** (pare-ee-o-don-tal) **ligament space** which is a radiolucent (or darker) area located between the denser radiopaque (or lighter) lamina dura of the ABP and the similar radiopaque (or lighter) cementum (see Figure 14-16).

The PDL is an organized fibrous connective tissue that also maintains the gingival tissue in proper relationship to the teeth. In addition, the PDL transmits occlusal forces from the teeth to the bone, allowing for a small amount of movement and acting as a shock absorber for the soft tissue structures around the teeth, such as the nerves and blood vessels (see **Chapter 20**). Other functions of the PDL are discussed in detail later in this chapter. In general, these other functions include serving as the periosteum for both the cementum and the alveolar process. Cells in the PDL also participate in the development and resorption of the hard tissue of the periodontium. Additionally, it has blood vessels that provide nutrition for the cells of the ligament and surrounding cells of the cementum and the alveolar process.

Finally, the PDL and its nerve supply provide a most efficient proprioceptive mechanism, allowing us to feel even the most delicate forces applied to the teeth and any displacement of the teeth resulting from these forces (such as metal foil in candy wrappers). Unlike the soft connective tissue of the pulp, the PDL not only transmits pain, but also touch, pressure, and temperature sensations.

Even after patients have endodontic therapy (root canal treatment) and the tooth becomes nonvital, they may feel some level of discomfort when biting down or when the clinician taps the teeth when measuring tooth percussion sensitivity. This discomfort is not due to sensations from the removed pulp tissue but from sensations garnered within the still present PDL. This is as it receives pressure from even the slightest intrusive movements of the tooth during mastication.

Similar to the alveolar process, the PDL develops from the dental sac of the tooth germ (see Figure 6-20). Unlike other connective tissue of

FIGURE 14-25 Microscopic section of the periodontal ligament *(PDL)*, which is located between the alveolar bone proper *(ABP)* and cementum *(C)*, inserting Sharpey fibers into both tissue types. (From the Dr. Bernhard Gottlieb Collection, courtesy of James McIntosh, PhD, Assistant Professor Emeritus, Department of Biomedical Sciences, Baylor College of Dentistry, Dallas, TX.)

the periodontium, however, the PDL does not show any overwhelming changes related to aging but its width does decrease with age.

Because the PDL is a connective tissue, it has all the components of a connective tissue, such as intercellular substance, cells, and fibers (Figure 14-25; see **Chapter 8**). It has mainly Type I collagen as well as lesser amounts of other types.

The PDL also has a vascular supply, lymphatics, and nerve supply, which enter the apical foramen of the tooth to supply the pulp (see **Chapter 13**). Two types of nerves are found within the PDL. One type is afferent (or sensory), which is a myelinated nerve and transmits sensations that occur within the PDL (as discussed earlier); the other type is an autonomic sympathetic nerve, which regulates the blood vessels (see **Chapter 8**).

PERIODONTAL LIGAMENT CELLS

The PDL has all the cells that are found in most connective tissue, such as the cells of blood and endothelium (Figure 14-26). And like all connective tissue, the fibroblast is the most common cell in the PDL, producing fibers and intercellular substance (see Figure 8-5). Studies have demonstrated that these fibroblasts further appear to function as mechanosensing entities that regulate collagen-secretory and collagen-remodeling activities according to the level of strain in the ligament. Mechanical challenge also plays an important role during the activation of periodontal fibroblasts in response to injury.

The PDL also has cells that are not present in other connective tissue, such as a line of cementoblasts along the cemental surface of the root. Osteoblasts are also present in the PDL at the periphery of the adjacent ABP. In addition, the PDL has osteoclasts as well as odontoclasts. Each of these specific cell types can form either cementum or bone, or even resorb the respective tissue, depending on the need of the periodontium or the demands of the adjacent environment. Also present are undifferentiated mesenchymal cells, which can differentiate into any of these cells if any of these cell populations are injured. Thus, the PDL serves as a protective periosteum for both the root cementum and adjacent ABP.

In addition, the epithelial rests of Malassez (ERM) are present within the PDL (see Figure 14-26). These groups of epithelial cells are stranded in mature PDL after the disintegration of Hertwig epithelial root sheath during the formation of the root (see Figures 6-19 and 6-20). Studies are now demonstrating that these cell rests play an active role and can be activated to participate in PDL repair and regeneration.

The ERM can also become cystic, usually forming nondiagnostic, radiolucent apical lesions that can be present on radiographs. This occurs as a result of chronic periapical inflammation after pulpitis occurs. These cysts must be surgically removed and then observed for recurrence on follow-up visits.

FIGURE 14-26 Microscopic section of the periodontal ligament *(PDL)* that includes a layer of osteoblasts *(O)* on the periphery of the alveolar bone proper *(ABP)* with a line of cementoblasts *(C)* on the cemental surface of the tooth *(T)*. Note the epithelial rests of Malassez in the periodontal ligament *(white arrows)*. (From the Dr. Bernhard Gottlieb Collection, courtesy of James McIntosh, PhD, Assistant Professor Emeritus, Department of Biomedical Sciences, Baylor College of Dentistry, Dallas, TX.)

PERIODONTAL LIGAMENT FIBER GROUPS

The PDL is wider near the apex and cervix of the tooth and narrower between these two end points of cementum and bone. All the fibers in the PDL are collagen in structure. Most of the fibers are considered **principal fibers**. The principal fibers are not found as individual fibers but are organized into groups or bundles according to their orientation to the mature tooth and related function; these bundles resemble spliced ropes. Each is approximately 5 µm in diameter. Histologists refer to these groups by various names, but this textbook uses the most commonly used names by the dental community. Whether nonorganized collagen fibers or secondary fibers of the PDL form an indifferent or intermediate plexus alongside the principal fibers remains controversial.

During mastication and speech, certain forces are exerted on a tooth, such as rotational, tilting, extrusive, or intrusive. The principal fibers of the PDL distribute these forces, protecting its soft tissue and allowing some give when they occur—similar to a rubber band attached at both ends to two hard objects. The fibers can accomplish this task because the ends of each fiber are anchored within both cementum and the ABP, or in cementum alone from adjacent roots or teeth. The ends of the principal fibers that are within either cementum or ABP are considered Sharpey fibers (see Figure 14-17). Sharpey fibers are each partially inserted into the hard tissue of the periodontium at 90° or perpendicular to either cemental or bony surface as discussed earlier. Studies show that the fiber bundles go the length of the PDL space and then branch along the two end points of cementum and bone, increasing the strength of the ligament.

ALVEOLODENTAL LIGAMENT

The main principal fiber group is the **alveolodental** (al-vee-o-lo-dent-al) **ligament**, which consists of five fiber subgroups: alveolar crest, horizontal, oblique, apical, and interradicular on multirooted teeth (Figure 14-27; Table 14-2). If viewed on sagittal section or from a facial or lingual view of the PDL, the fiber subgroups have different orientations from the cervix to the apex or apices. If the alveolodental ligament is viewed on cross section, the fiber subgroups appear as spokes of a wheel around the tooth (Figure 14-28). Thus, the overall function of the alveolodental ligament is to resist

FIGURE 14-27 Diagram of a sagittal section of a multirooted tooth and periodontal ligament. Fiber subgroups of the alveolodental ligament are identified: alveolar crest group, horizontal group, oblique group, apical group, and interradicular group. Note Sharpey fibers within both the alveolar bone proper and cementum.

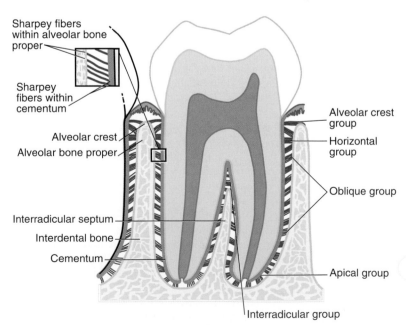

Sharpey fibers within alveolar bone proper

Sharpey fibers within cementum

Alveolar crest

Alveolar bone proper

Interradicular septum

Interdental bone

Cementum

Alveolar crest group

Horizontal group

Oblique group

Apical group

Interradicular group

rotational forces or twisting of the tooth in its alveolus. Each of the five fiber subgroups also has its own specific function related to its differing orientation to the tooth.

The alveolar crest group of the alveolodental ligament is attached to the cementum just below the CEJ and runs in an inferior and outward direction to insert into the alveolar crest of the ABP. Its function is to resist tilting, intrusive, extrusive, and rotational forces.

The horizontal group of the alveolodental ligament is just apical to the alveolar crest subgroup and runs at 90° to the long axis of the tooth from cementum to the ABP, just inferior to its alveolar crest. Its function is to resist tilting forces, which work to force the tooth to tip mesially, distally, lingually, or facially, and to resist rotational forces.

The oblique (o-bleek) group of the alveolodental ligament is the most numerous of the fiber subgroups and covers the apical two-thirds of the root (Figure 14-29). This subgroup runs from the cementum in an oblique direction to insert into the ABP more coronally. Its function is to resist intrusive forces, which try to push the tooth inward, as well as rotational forces.

The apical group of the alveolodental ligament radiates from cementum around the apex of the root to the surrounding ABP, forming the base of the alveolus. Its function is to resist extrusive forces, which try to pull the tooth in an outward manner, and rotational forces.

The interradicular group of the alveolodental ligament is found only between the roots of multirooted teeth. This subgroup runs from the cementum of one root to the cementum of the other root(s) superficial to the interradicular septum and thus has no bony attachment. This subgroup works together with the alveolar crest and apical subgroups to resist intrusive, extrusive, tilting, and rotational forces.

FIGURE 14-28 Cross section of the tooth composed of cementum *(C)* and dentin *(D),* highlighting the spokelike arrangement of the fibers subgroups of alveolodental ligament *(arrows),* in most cases running between the cementum and alveolar bone proper *(ABP)* of the surrounding alveolus. (From the Dr. Bernhard Gottlieb Collection, courtesy of James McIntosh, PhD, Assistant Professor Emeritus, Department of Biomedical Sciences, Baylor College of Dentistry, Dallas, TX.)

TABLE 14-2	Alveolodental Ligament Fiber Subgroups	
FIBER SUBGROUPS	**LOCATION**	**FUNCTION**
Alveolar crest group	Attached to cementum just below cementoenamel junction and runs in inferior and outward direction to insert into alveolar crest of alveolar bone proper	To resist tilting, intrusive, extrusive, and rotational forces
Horizontal group	Just apical to alveolar crest group and runs 90° to the long axis of tooth from cementum to alveolar bone proper, just inferior to alveolar crest	To resist tilting forces and rotational forces
Oblique group	Runs from cementum in oblique direction to insert into alveolar bone proper more coronally	To resist intrusive forces and rotational forces
Apical group	Radiates from cementum around root apex to surrounding alveolar bone proper, forming base of alveolus	To resist extrusive forces and rotational forces
Interradicular group (on multirooted teeth)	Runs from the cementum of one root to cementum of other root(s) superficial to interradicular septum and thus has no bony attachment superficial to interradicular septum	To resist intrusive, extrusive, tilting, and rotational forces

FIGURE 14-29 Photomicrograph of a tooth at the location of the oblique group of the periodontal ligament *(PDL)* that runs from the cementum *(C)* in an oblique direction *(arrow)* to insert more coronally into alveolar bone proper *(ABP);* makes up the bulk of the alveolodental ligament. Having both cemental and bony attachments, its function is to resist intrusive forces, which try to push the tooth inward, as well as rotational forces. (From the Dr. Bernhard Gottlieb Collection, courtesy of James McIntosh, PhD, Assistant Professor Emeritus, Department of Biomedical Sciences, Baylor College of Dentistry, Dallas, TX.)

INTERDENTAL LIGAMENT

Another principal fiber other than the alveolodental ligament is the **interdental ligament** (or transseptal ligament) (Figures 14-30 and 14-31). This principal fiber inserts mesiodistally or interdentally into the cervical cementum of neighboring teeth, at a height coronal to the alveolar crest of the ABP and apical to the base of the junctional epithelium. Thus, the fibers traverse from cementum to cementum without any bony attachment, connecting all the teeth of the arch. Its function is to resist rotational forces and thus to hold the teeth in interproximal contact.

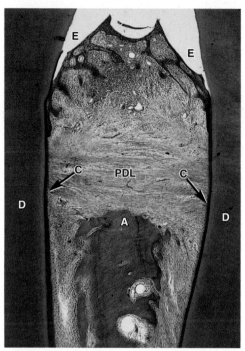

FIGURE 14-30 Microscopic section of interdental ligament of the periodontal ligament *(PDL)*, which is located between the cementum *(C with arrow)* of two neighboring teeth with their dentin *(D)* and enamel (space, *E*) and coronal to the alveolar crest of the alveolar bone proper *(ABP)*. (From the Dr. Bernhard Gottlieb Collection, courtesy of James McIntosh, PhD, Assistant Professor Emeritus, Department of Biomedical Sciences, Baylor College of Dentistry, Dallas, TX.)

FIGURE 14-31 Interdental ligament, which inserts mesiodistally or interdentally into the cervical cementum of neighboring teeth coronal to the alveolar crest of the alveolar bone proper; thus it does not have any bony attachment. Its function is to resist rotational forces and thus hold the teeth in interproximal contact.

GINGIVAL FIBER GROUP

Some histologists also consider the **gingival** (jin-ji-val) **fiber group** to be part of the principal fibers of the PDL, and so it will be discussed here for completeness (Figure 14-32). These are a separate but adjacent group that is found within the lamina propria of the marginal gingiva (see Figure 10-1). These include the fiber subgroups of the circular and dentogingival ligament, as well as the alveologingival and dentoperiosteal ligaments, but other terms may also be used for these fiber groups. They do not support the tooth in relationship to the jaws such as the principle fibers of the PDL, which resist any forces of mastication or speech; rather, the gingival fiber group supports only the marginal gingiva in an effort to maintain its relationship to the tooth.

The circular ligament encircles the tooth, as shown on a cross section of a tooth, interlacing with the other gingival fiber subgroups. Like "pulling the purse strings" of the gingiva, it helps to only maintain gingival integrity.

The dentogingival ligament is the most extensive of the gingival fiber group. It inserts in the cementum on the root, apical to the epithelial attachment, and extends into the lamina propria of the marginal and attached gingiva. Thus, the dentogingival ligament has only one mineralized attachment to the cementum. The dentogingival ligament works with the circular ligament to maintain gingival integrity, mainly of the marginal gingiva.

The alveologingival ligament radiates from the alveolar crest of the ABP and extend coronally into the overlying lamina propria of the marginal gingiva. It helps to attach the gingiva to the ABP because of its one mineralized attachment to bone. The dentoperiosteal ligament courses from the cementum, near the CEJ, across the alveolar crest. The dentoperiosteal ligament anchors the tooth to the bone and protects the deeper PDL.

> ### Clinical Considerations for Periodontal Ligament Pathology and Repair
>
> To a lesser extent, orthodontic therapy also affects the PDL similar to the alveolar process (discussed earlier, see Figure 14-20). On the side under tension, the PDL space will become wider; with the side under pressure, it will become narrower. The interdental ligament is also responsible for the memory of tooth positioning within each dental arch. Therefore, a sufficiently prolonged retention period must be allowed to reattach the interdental ligament fully to its new position and thereby ensure the maintenance of the clinical stability of tooth

Interdental ligament

Facial surface of tooth

Cross-sectioned tooth

Cementoenamel junction

Interdental papilla

Alveolar crest
Alveolar bone proper
Alveolodental fibers

Cementum

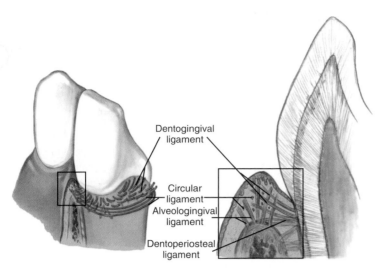

FIGURE 14-32 Fiber subgroups of the gingival fiber group: circular ligament, dentogingival ligament, alveologingival ligament, and dentoperiosteal ligament. These are located in the lamina propria of the marginal gingiva and support only the gingival tissue in order to maintain its relationship to the tooth.

position established during orthodontic therapy. This is because the turnover time for the interdental ligament is not as rapid as the alveolodental ligament. Retainers, removable and permanent, are used to maintain this desirable alignment.

Many times the inflammation associated with the pulp or pulpitis travels through the apical foramen to involve the periodontium, thus causing apical inflammation and destruction (see **Chapter 13**). Surgery may have to be performed to remove the apical lesion (apicoectomy).

It is important to note that occlusal trauma does not cause periodontal disease but can accelerate the progression of existing disease with certain changes noted in the PDL. When traumatic forces of occlusion are placed on a tooth, the PDL widens to take the extra forces (see **Chapter 20**). The width of the ligament can even double in size, as the individual principal fiber bundles become thicker. Thus, early occlusal trauma can be viewed on radiographs as a widening of the radiolucent (or darker) PDL space between the radiopaque (or lighter) lamina dura of the ABP and the similar radiopaque (or lighter) cementum (Figure 14-33). Thickening of the lamina dura, which represents the ABP, is also possible with occlusal trauma in response to the overall loss of the alveolar process (see earlier discussion).

Advanced occlusal trauma is additionally noted by the late manifestation of increased mobility of the tooth and possibly the presence of pathologic tooth migration (Figure 14-34). This mobility and migration is due to the further weakened periodontium when even the occlusal forces need not be at abnormal levels if the periodontal support is reduced; the width is compensated for by the deposition of cementum.

Changes can also be noted microscopically in the PDL as a result of advanced occlusal trauma: thrombosis, dilation, and edema of the blood supply; hyalinization of the collagen fibers; the presence of an inflammatory infiltrate; and nuclear changes in the osteoblasts, cementoblasts, and fibroblasts. No microscopic changes are noted in the gingival collagen fibers or in the adjacent junctional epithelium with occlusal trauma. However, studies show that microscopic changes distinct from existing early periodontal disease are reversible if the causes of trauma are eliminated. Conversely, a reduction in function leads to narrowing of the ligament and a decrease in number and thickness of the fiber bundles compounding the initial trauma.

The PDL also undergoes drastic changes with the chronic advanced periodontal disease of periodontitis that involves the deeper structures of the periodontium. The fibers of the PDL become

FIGURE 14-33 Early occlusal trauma noted radiographically with a widening of the radiolucent periodontal ligament space *(arrow)* between the radiopaque lamina dura of the alveolar bone proper and the similarly radiopaque cementum; thickening of the lamina dura in response is also possible. (Courtesy of Margaret J. Fehrenbach, RDH, MS.)

FIGURE 14-34 Pathologic tooth migration caused by the weakened periodontium in which the occlusal forces need not be at an abnormal level if the periodontal support is already reduced by periodontal disease. (Courtesy of Margaret J. Fehrenbach, RDH, MS.)

FIGURE 14-35 Microscopic section of two adjacent suprabony periodontal pockets in an interdental space. Note the horizontal arrangement of the interdental ligament even with the presence of active periodontitis *(arrow)*. (From Newman MG, Takei HH, Klokkevold PR, Carranza FA: *Clinical periodontology*, ed 12, St Louis, 2015, Saunders/Elsevier.)

disorganized, and their attachments to either the ABP or cementum through Sharpey fibers are lost because of the resorption of these two hard dental tissue types (see Figures 10-12 and 14-24). The first fibers involved with periodontitis are the alveolar crest group of the alveolodental ligament, which is located at the most coronal level to the adjacent alveolar process.

The destruction of the PDL with periodontitis then progresses further in an apical manner similarly to the destruction of the alveolar process, affecting (in order) the horizontal, then oblique, then apical, and then the interradicular subgroups, if present. The teeth involved in advancement of periodontal disease become increasingly mobile, moving in directions that indicate the amount and type of fiber group lost, such as buccal to lingual or with downward pressure, as the periodontitis progresses inward to the apices of the teeth.

Thus, the principal fiber group that remains the longest in the presence of active periodontitis, despite the previous destruction of the entire adjacent alveolodental ligament, is the interdental ligament (Figure 14-35). The interdental ligament keeps reattaching itself in a more apical manner as the periodontitis proceeds apically so that the teeth are at least held in interproximal contact. Thus, when teeth become severely mobile interproximally (from mesial to distal) after mobility in other directions is already present, the prognosis is poor because now there is the further destruction of the interdental ligament. Mobility and its amount and direction per tooth should be charted in the patient record to achieve an overall prognosis for a dentition with periodontitis.

The use of GTR is not only involved in the treatment of the loss of the alveolar process (as discussed earlier) but also will assist with the repair of the resultant disorganization of the PDL caused by periodontitis. Using this method to both increase alveolar process levels and strengthen the PDL, a membrane of various materials allows only osteoblasts and fibroblasts to produce either bone or PDL fibers at the diseased site. GTR is becoming even more successful because the membrane type now being used results in less inflammation at the site.

CHAPTER **15**

Overview of Dentitions

Additional resources and practice exercises are provided on the companion Evolve website for this book: ⓔ
http://evolve.elsevier.com/Fehrenbach/illustrated.

●●●LEARNING OBJECTIVES

1. Define and pronounce the key terms in this chapter.
2. Describe the two dentitions and the relationship to each other.
3. Recognize tooth types and outline the tooth numbering systems.
4. Assign the correct universal or international number for a tooth and its correct dentition period on a diagram or a skull and for a tooth model or a patient.
5. Define each dentition period and discuss the clinical considerations concerning each dentition period, integrating it into patient care.
6. Use the correct dental anatomy terminology and discuss the clinical considerations concerning tooth anatomy, integrating it into patient care.
7. Use the correct orientational tooth terms and discuss the clinical considerations concerning tooth surfaces, integrating it into patient care.
8. Identify tooth forms and discuss the clinical considerations concerning them, integrating it into patient care.

DENTITIONS

The term *dentition* is used to describe the natural teeth in the jaws. As described in **Chapter 6** in relationship to tooth development, a person has two dentitions during a lifetime: a primary dentition and a permanent dentition.

The first dentition present is the primary dentition (Figure 15-1). Child patients and their supervising adults consider the primary teeth to be the *baby teeth*. An older term for the primary dentition is the *deciduous dentition*. This term is derived from the concept that the primary dentition is shed (just as deciduous trees shed leaves) and replaced entirely by the permanent dentition. Thus, the permanent dentition is the second dentition to develop (Figure 15-2). The permanent dentition is also sometimes considered the *secondary dentition,* and the permanent teeth are called the *adult teeth.* By recent convention (or convenience), clinicians seem to prefer to mix and match terms when referring to the two dentitions, as in *primary dentition* and *permanent dentition.*

The permanent dentition is also sometimes mistakenly considered the *succedaneous dentition* because most of these permanent teeth succeed primary predecessors. However, dental professionals must remember that the molars of the permanent dentition are nonsuccedaneous because they are without any primary predecessors; only the anteriors and premolars of the permanent dentition are succedaneous.

Development of the primary dentition, eruption and shedding of the primary teeth, and development of the permanent dentition were discussed further in **Chapter 6,** which can be reviewed before the discussion of specific tooth anatomy.

TOOTH TYPES

Teeth comprise around 20% of the surface area of the oral cavity—maxillary more so than mandibular teeth. Tooth types of both arches within the primary dentition include 8 incisors, 4 canines, and 8 molars, for a total of 20 teeth (see Figure 15-1). The anatomy of the primary dentition is discussed further in **Chapter 18.**

Tooth types of both arches within the permanent dentition include 8 incisors, 4 canines, 8 premolars, and 12 molars, for a total of 32 teeth (see Figures 2-4 and 15-2). Note that only the permanent dentition has premolars; in contrast, the primary dentition does not have premolars. The detailed anatomy of the permanent dentition is discussed further in **Chapter 16** (anterior teeth) and **Chapter 17** (posterior teeth).

TOOTH DESIGNATION

The primary teeth and the permanent teeth are both designated by the Universal Numbering System (UNS) (Figure 15-3). This system is the most widely used in the United States for the designation of

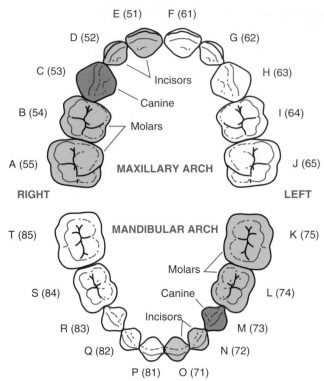

FIGURE 15-1 Primary dentition during the primary dentition period with tooth types and Universal numbering identified (with International numbering in parentheses).

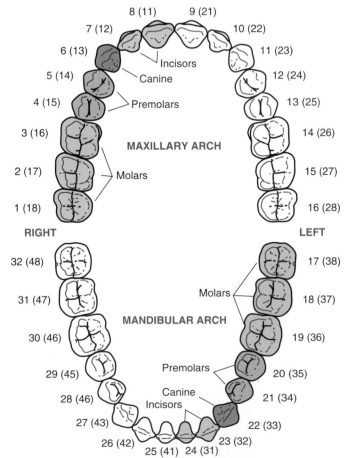

FIGURE 15-2 Permanent dentition during the permanent period with tooth types and Universal numbering identified (with International numbering in parentheses).

both dentitions, because it is adaptable to electronic data. With the UNS, the primary teeth are designated from each other in a consecutive arrangement by using capital letters, *A* through *T*, starting with the maxillary right second molar, moving clockwise, and ending with the mandibular right second molar (see Figure 15-1).

The permanent teeth are designated from each other in the UNS in consecutive arrangement as the patient is observed from in front by using the digits *1* through *32*, starting with the maxillary right third molar, moving clockwise, and ending with the mandibular right third molar (see Figure 15-2). The clockwise convention also is also used when charting restorations or periodontal conditions in the oral cavity for a patient. When speaking about a certain tooth such as the permanent maxillary right central incisor, the clinician calls it "number eight."

However, the need for a system that can be used internationally, as well as by electronic data transfer, is recognized; thus the acceptance of the International Numbering System (INS) (or International Designation System) by the International Standards Organization (ISO) and the World Health Organization (WHO) (see Figure 15-3). With this system, the teeth are designated from each other by using a two-digit code. The first digit of the code indicates the quadrant (see later discussion under general dental terms), and the second indicates the tooth's position in this quadrant. This is based on the system of the Fédération Dentaire Internationale (FDI).

Thus with the INS, the digits *1* through *4* are used for quadrants in a clockwise manner in the permanent dentition, and digits *5* through *8* are used in a clockwise manner for those quadrants of the primary dentition. For the second digit, which indicates the tooth, the digits *1* through *8* are used for the permanent teeth, starting at the midline and numbering in a distal direction. The digits *1* through *5* are then used for the primary dentition, again starting at the midline and numbering in a distal direction. When speaking about a certain tooth such as the permanent maxillary right central incisor, the clinician calls it "number one–one."

Another system that is commonly used in orthodontic therapy is the Palmer Notation Method also known as the *Military Numbering System* (see Figure 15-3). It is helpful with this dental specialty because it allows immediate discussion of the teeth that require prompt treatment, and it can produce an easy to view graphic mapping of the dentitions. In this system, the teeth are designated from each other with a right-angle symbol indicating the quadrants and arch, with the tooth number placed inside, similar in numbering to INS that superseded it.

DENTITION PERIODS

Although there are only two dentitions, there are three dentition (den-**tish**-in) periods throughout a person's lifetime because the two dentitions overlap in time: primary, mixed, and permanent (Table 15-1). Each patient should be assigned a dentition period to allow the most effective dental treatment for that period. This specificity is especially important with the consideration of orthodontic therapy, because growth during certain dentition periods can be maximized to allow expansion of the jaws and movement of the teeth.

PRIMARY DENTITION PERIOD

The first dentition period is the primary dentition period (see Figure 15-1). This period begins with the eruption of the primary mandibular central incisors. Thus, this period occurs between approximately 6 months and 6 years of age (see Figure 6-22, *A,* for chronologic order, Table 18-1 for approximate ages, and Figure 20-5 for sequence). Only the primary teeth are present during this time, with their full eruption

Maxillary Arch

Molars		Canine	Incisors				Canine	Molars	
A	B	C	D	E	F	G	H	I	J
55	54	53	52	51	61	62	63	64	65
E⌋	D⌋	C⌋	B⌋	A⌋	⌊A	⌊B	⌊C	⌊D	⌊E

E⌉	D⌉	C⌉	B⌉	A⌉	⌈A	⌈B	⌈C	⌈D	⌈E
85	84	83	82	81	71	72	73	74	75
T	S	R	Q	P	O	N	M	L	K

Mandibular Arch

Right	Left

I   Universal Numbering System

II   International Numbering System

III   Palmer Notation Method

A

FIGURE 15-3 Tooth designation systems including Universal Numbering System, International Numbering System, and Palmer Notation Method. **A,** For the primary teeth.

Continued

completed at 30 months, usually when the primary second molars are in occlusion. The jaws are beginning to also grow further during this period to accommodate the coming larger and more numerous permanent teeth. This period usually ends when the first permanent tooth erupts—the permanent mandibular first molar.

MIXED DENTITION PERIOD

The mixed dentition period follows the primary dentition period (Figure 15-4; see **Chapter 6**). This period occurs between approximately 6 and 12 years of age. Both primary and permanent teeth are present during this transitional stage. During this time, both shedding of primary teeth and eruption of permanent teeth begin after their crowns are completed. Thus, this period begins with eruption of the first permanent tooth, a permanent mandibular first molar, which is guided by the distal surface of the primary second molar. This period usually ends with shedding of the last primary tooth, which generally occurs from age 11 to 12.

The color differences between the primary and permanent teeth become apparent during this middle phase, as any supervising adult

has noticed in the child and routinely and enviously points it out to the dental professionals. The primary crowns are lighter in color than the darker permanent crowns owing to the fact that the permanent teeth having less opaque enamel, and thus the underlying yellow dentin is more visible (see Figure 18-4). Also more evident is the difference in the crown size and root length between the smaller and shorter primary teeth and the larger and longer permanent teeth.

The jaws undergo the fastest and most noticeable growth during this period, consistent with the onset of puberty, to accommodate the larger size and number of permanent teeth. Women shed their primary teeth and receive their permanent teeth slightly earlier than men, possibly reflecting their earlier overall physical maturation achieved.

PERMANENT DENTITION PERIOD

The final dentition period is the permanent dentition period (see Figure 15-2). This period begins with shedding of the last primary tooth. Thus, this dentition period begins approximately after 12 years of age. Included is the eruption of all the permanent teeth, except for teeth that are congenitally missing or impacted and cannot erupt,

	Molars			Premolars		Canine	Incisors				Canine	Premolars		Molars		
Maxillary Arch																
I	1	2	3	4	5	6	7	8	9	10	11	12	13	14	15	16
II	18	17	16	15	14	13	12	11	21	22	23	24	25	26	27	28
III	8⌋	7⌋	6⌋	5⌋	4⌋	3⌋	2⌋	1⌋	⌊1	⌊2	⌊3	⌊4	⌊5	⌊6	⌊7	⌊8

III	8⌉	7⌉	6⌉	5⌉	4⌉	3⌉	2⌉	1⌉	⌈1	⌈2	⌈3	⌈4	⌈5	⌈6	⌈7	⌈8
II	48	47	46	45	44	43	42	41	31	32	33	34	35	36	37	38
I	32	31	30	29	28	27	26	25	24	23	22	21	20	19	18	17
Mandibular Arch																
	Right							Left								

I   Universal Numbering System

II   International Numbering System

III   Palmer Notation Method

B

FIGURE 15-3, cont'd Tooth designation systems including Universal Numbering System, International Numbering System, and Palmer Notation Method. **B,** For the permanent teeth.

TABLE 15-1	Dentition Periods with Clinical Considerations		
	PRIMARY DENTITION PERIOD	**MIXED DENTITION PERIOD**	**PERMANENT DENTITION PERIOD**
Approximate time span	~6 months to ~6 years	~6 years to 12 years	After ~12 years
Teeth marking start of period	Eruption of primary mandibular central incisor	Eruption of permanent mandibular first molar	Shedding of the last primary tooth
Dentition present	Primary	Primary and permanent	Usually permanent
Growth of jaws	Beginning	Fastest and most noticeable	Slowest and least noticeable

(All data from Nelson S: *Wheeler's dental anatomy, physiology and occlusions,* ed 10, Philadelphia, 2015, Saunders/Elsevier.)

usually involving the third molars (see Figure 6-22, *B,* for chronologic order; Table 15-2 and **Appendix D** for approximate ages; and Figure 20-6 for sequence).

The permanent teeth are usually the only teeth present during this period. Growth of the jaws is not as noticeable because it slows and then eventually stops. Thus, little growth of the jaws occurs overall during this period, given that puberty has passed. Tooth types tend to erupt in pairs so that, if any asymmetry exists in a patient, a radiograph of the area may be required. When a child patient is unusually early or

late regarding the usual sequential eruption of teeth, the biologic family dental history should be reviewed for developmental anomalies.

Clinical Considerations for Dentition Periods

The clinical considerations associated with both the primary and the permanent dentition periods are discussed later in each appropriate chapter. However, the mixed dentition period also has characteristic physiologic and psychological effects. This dentition period is sometimes

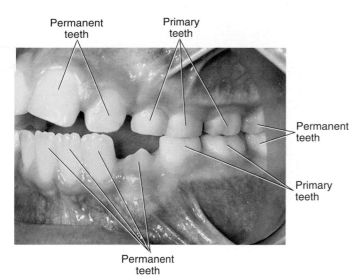

Permanent teeth

Primary teeth

Permanent teeth

Primary teeth

Permanent teeth

FIGURE 15-4 Mixed dentition period with its primary and permanent teeth identified. (Courtesy of Margaret J. Fehrenbach, RDH, MS.)

TABLE 15-2	Approximate Eruption and Root Completion Ages for Permanent Teeth (in Years)	
TOOTH TYPE	**ERUPTION**	**ROOT COMPLETION**
Maxillary Teeth		
Central incisor	7 to 8	10
Lateral incisor	8 to 9	11
Canine	11 to 12	13 to 15
First premolar	10 to 11	12 to 13
Second premolar	10 to 12	12 to 14
First molar	6 to 7	9 to 10
Second molar	12 to 13	14 to 16
Third molar	17 to 21	18 to 25
Mandibular Teeth		
Central incisor	6 to 7	9
Lateral incisor	7 to 8	10
Canine	9 to 10	12 to 14
First premolar	10 to 12	12 to 13
Second premolar	11 to 12	13 to 14
First molar	6 to 7	9 to 10
Second molar	11 to 13	14 to 15
Third molar	17 to 21	18 to 25

(All data from Nelson S: *Wheeler's dental anatomy, physiology and occlusions*, ed 10, Philadelphia, 2015, Saunders/Elsevier.)

considered an *ugly duckling stage* because of the differing tooth colors, disproportionately sized teeth, and various clinical crown heights. The patient's smile shows temporary edentulous areas and crowding. Additionally, in many cases, the surrounding gingiva responds to all these changes, as well as hormonal fluctuations, by becoming inflamed.

Homecare may be difficult for patients during the mixed dentition period because these changes, such as crowding, may promote dental biofilm retention. Child patients and supervising adults must

be reminded to be especially diligent about homecare and be reassured that this stage is only temporary. Early interceptive orthodontic therapy may also be initiated during this dentition period; a series of panoramic radiographs is important for monitoring tooth development (see Figure 6-27, *A*, and **Chapter 20**).

If in the primary and/or mixed dentition gingival inflammation is only slight with little dental biofilm formation but bone loss around the newly erupted permanent first molars and mandibular anteriors is severe, early aggressive periodontitis (previously referred to as *juvenile periodontitis*) may be suspected. Early intervention in this serious periodontal disease can prevent further bone loss.

DENTAL ANATOMY TERMINOLOGY

Dental professionals must be able to understand and correctly use dental anatomy terminology. **Dental anatomy** is the area of the dental sciences dealing with the morphology or form of the teeth, both the crown and root. Restorative dentistry uses many specific dental anatomy terms when discussing treatment and pathology. Periodontal therapy of the teeth also necessitates using many of these detailed terms, such as *line angles,* when performing procedures such as probe readings of the gingival sulcus that surrounds each tooth.

GENERAL DENTAL TERMS

As noted earlier, each tooth is surrounded and supported by the bone of the tooth socket, or alveolus (plural, alveoli) (Figure 15-5). Each alveolus is located in the alveolar process, or tooth-bearing part of each jaw. Each alveolar process of the jaws is also considered a dental arch—either the maxillary arch or the mandibular arch.

The teeth in the maxilla are the maxillary teeth; the teeth in the mandible are the mandibular teeth (see Figure 15-5). Occlusion is the method by which the teeth of the mandibular arch come into contact with those of the maxillary arch. The term *occlusion* is also used to describe the anatomic alignment of the teeth and the relationship to the rest of the masticatory system (see **Chapter 20**).

Teeth can also be described according to the position in each dental arch and in relationship to the midline (Figure 15-6). The incisors and canines are considered anterior teeth because they are closer to the midline. In contrast, the molars (and premolars, if present) are considered posterior teeth because they are farther from the midline.

Each dental arch has a midline, an imaginary vertical plane that divides the arch into two approximately equal halves—a right and a left (see Figure 15-6). The midline is similar to the median, or midsagittal, plane of the body. The midline is an important consideration in the evaluation of a patient's smile. Thus, each dental arch can be further divided into two **quadrants** (**kwod**-rints), with four quadrants in the entire oral cavity. Thus, teeth are described as being located in one of the four quadrants: maxillary right quadrant, maxillary left quadrant, mandibular right quadrant, and mandibular left quadrant. This designation is useful when planning a course of dental treatment for a patient, because it allows the treatment of one or more oral regions at a time.

The correct sequence of words when describing an individual tooth using a **D-A-Q-T System** is based on the tooth within its quadrant: *D* for dentition, *A* for arch, *Q* for quadrant, and *T* for tooth type. An example of this would be the written description of the permanent *(D)* mandibular *(A)* left *(Q)* first premolar *(T)*.

Some dental treatment plans also include the use of **sextants** (**sextants**), which further divide each dental arch into three parts according to the relationship to the midline: right posterior sextant, anterior sextant, and left posterior sextant (see Figure 15-6). An example is

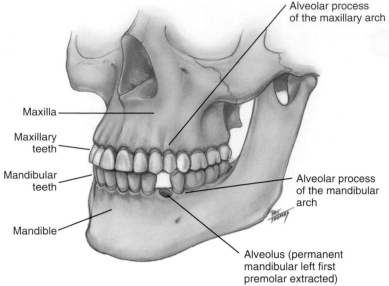

FIGURE 15-5 Permanent dentition with the maxillary arch and mandibular arch as well as associated structures identified.

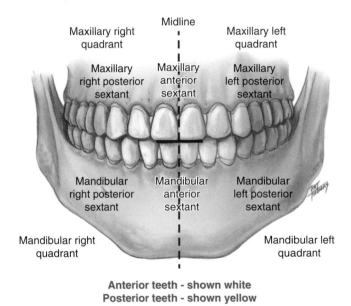

Anterior teeth - shown white
Posterior teeth - shown yellow

FIGURE 15-6 Permanent dentition with the anterior and posterior teeth, midline, quadrants, and sextants identified.

TABLE 15-3	International Standards Organization Designation of Areas of Oral Cavity
AREA	**NUMBER**
Oral cavity	00
Maxillary arch	01
Mandibular arch	02
Maxillary right quadrant	10
Maxillary left quadrant	20
Mandibular left quadrant	30
Mandibular right quadrant	40
Maxillary right sextant	03
Maxillary anterior sextant	04
Maxillary left sextant	05
Mandibular left sextant	06
Mandibular anterior sextant	07
Mandibular right sextant	08

that the permanent maxillary right central incisor is in the maxillary anterior sextant of the permanent dentition. This division follows the mapping of oral nerve pathways, especially in the maxillary arch. Thus, the use of sextants can be useful in dental treatment plans for regions, such as those that use local anesthesia for patient pain control like periodontal therapy.

To prevent miscommunication globally, the ISO also includes the designation of areas in the oral cavity (used also in the tooth designation system). A two-digit number designates these areas, and at least one of the two digits is zero (Table 15-3). An example of this system is that *00* designates the entire the oral cavity, and *01* designates the maxillary arch only.

TOOTH ANATOMY TERMS

Each tooth consists of a crown and one or more roots (Figure 15-7; see Figure 2-5). The crown has dentin covered by enamel, and each root

has dentin covered by cementum. The inner part of the dentin of both crown and root also covers the pulp cavity of the tooth. The pulp cavity has a pulp chamber, pulp canal (or canals) with an apical foramen (or foramina), and possibly pulp horn (or horns).

In this textbook, the illustrations of the head and neck, as well as any structures related to them, are oriented according to the patient's head being in anatomic position unless otherwise noted (see **Appendix A**). This is the same as if the patient were being viewed straight on while sitting upright in the dental chair. Thus, maxillary teeth show the root superior to the crown; mandibular teeth show the root inferior to the crown (see Figure 15-3).

Orientation of the dental chart is traditionally from the dental professional's view (i.e., the patient's right corresponds to the notation chart's left). The designations "left" and "right" on the chart, however, nonetheless correspond to the patient's left and right, respectively. Other dental charts may show each of the teeth "unfolded" so that

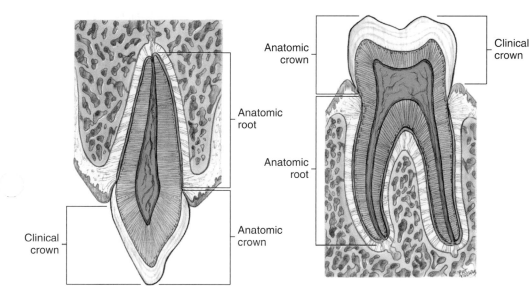

FIGURE 15-7 Anterior and posterior tooth showing the involved dental tissue.

FIGURE 15-8 Anterior and posterior tooth showing the anatomic crown and root, as well as the clinical crown. The clinical root is not shown because this is a healthy periodontal situation without gingival recession, which would have an exposed clinical root.

the facial, occlusal or incisal, and lingual surfaces of the teeth can be noted.

The enamel of the crown and cementum of the root usually meet close to the cementoenamel junction (CEJ), an external line at the neck or cervix of the tooth (see Figure 14-8). There are three possible interfaces at the CEJ, and multiple situations are possible on one tooth or even one surface of the tooth. At the CEJ, the cementum over the neck of each tooth may overlap the enamel, the enamel may meet the cementum edge to edge, or a small area of underlying dentin may be exposed because there is a gap between the enamel and cementum. The CEJ usually feels smooth or evenly grainy or has a slight groove when explored.

Parts of the crown and root of a tooth can also be designated using more specific terms in order to assist the clinician during patient dental charting (Figure 15-8). The anatomic crown is the part covered by enamel. It remains mostly constant throughout the life of the tooth, except for attrition and other physical wear. The clinical crown is that part of the anatomic crown that is visible and not covered by the gingiva. Its height is determined by the location of the marginal gingiva. The clinical crown of a tooth can change over time, especially with gingival recession as the marginal gingiva recedes toward the root (see Figure 13-1). This textbook, when discussing the crown of a

tooth, refers to the anatomic crown of a healthy tooth unless designated otherwise.

Similarly, the anatomic root is that part of the root covered by cementum. The clinical root of a tooth is that part of the anatomic root that is visible, subject to variability over time, again related to gingival recession (see Figure 10-10). This textbook, when discussing the root of a tooth, refers to the anatomic root of a healthy tooth unless designated otherwise.

Some clinicians describe features of a tooth related to the root axis line (RAL), which is an imaginary line representing the long axis of a tooth, drawn in a way to bisect the root (and thus the crown) into two halves (see Figure 20-9). When viewing the root axis lines of the teeth overall, it is important to note that the tooth's crown and root are never strictly vertically placed within the alveolar process but have some degree of angulation as discussed in **Chapter 20.**

Teeth may have one or more roots, but all the roots of both dentitions have common traits. All roots are widest at the CEJ and taper toward the apex of the tooth. Roots have more bulk on the facial surface than on the lingual surface. The root tapers more dramatically on the lingual surface. Many surfaces of the roots have depressions, or root concavities. These indentations in the root surface commonly occur on the proximal root surfaces of anteriors and posteriors and the buccal and lingual surfaces of molars. An area between two or more of these roots is a furcation; see further discussion in **Chapter 17** and see Table 17-1.

Clinical Considerations with Tooth Anatomy

Certain restorations may cover the entire anatomic crown area; these are full artificial crowns (or what patients call *caps*). Post and core may be placed within the crown and root to help with the buildup of restorative materials to support an individual restoration.

A full artificial crown should ideally cover the entire prepared anatomic crown, but enlarged gingival tissue or loss of anatomic crown structure may require a surgical periodontal procedure called *crown lengthening* to increase the amount of the clinical crown and reduce the surrounding gingival tissue by removal. However, many clinicians feel that a restored artificial crown should be partial if possible, avoiding the CEJ region that is in contact with the gingival tissue in order to preserve tissue health. In a dentition case with poorer prognosis, a root (or roots) may be retained without the crown(s) if there is enough structure and periodontal attachment to support a removable prosthesis, such as an overdenture.

Historically in dental education, the importance of clinical crown anatomy was emphasized with limited emphasis on clinical root anatomy. Subsequently, dental professionals have seen an increased educational emphasis placed on detailed knowledge of root anatomy. This change in emphasis is due to a new recognition of the importance of precise periodontal root instrumentation to achieve oral health in cases of disease, as well as preserving of the crown of the teeth by restorations. Initially, pocket analysis using periodontal probes yields the situational root morphology and deposit level in a patient with periodontal disease. Once root morphology is understood and the patient's periodontal needs ascertained, the dental professional can also choose the most effective treatment plan, including instrumentation. In addition, the awareness of root morphology will prevent the destruction of the root by overinstrumentation by hand.

Root concavities should be carefully explored during instrumentation appointments and charted in the patient's record. These concavities can become exposed to the oral environment due to periodontal disease but still be hidden to the clinician under a periodontal pocket, presenting complications during periodontal or even endodontic instrumentation and homecare. Treatment failures have been linked to deposits remaining either after therapy or with continued poor homecare, because these deposits contribute to the continuation of the disease process. However, a significantly greater attachment loss occurs for root surfaces with proximal root grooves as compared with those that lack proximal root grooves.

Whereas these concavities can act as predisposing factors in the periodontal disease process, the depressions also increase the attachment area, producing a root shape more resistant to damaging occlusal forces. Thus, root contours present both harmful and protective effects that must be considered individually in the patient's periodontal prognosis.

Performing periodontal debridement of roots and associated furcations involves a set instrumentation treatment plan; the best approach is to treat each root as a separate tooth when access permits, with a combination of strokes using instruments, air polisher, or ultrasonic.

Until recently, clinicians were not able to visualize the root surface unless access was gained by periodontal flap surgery to fold back the overlying oral mucosa. Instead they had to rely only on tactile sense and resultant mental picture to understand the subgingival topography. However, with the recent development of endoscopic technology, with its small camera that can fit within a deepened sulcus, clinicians

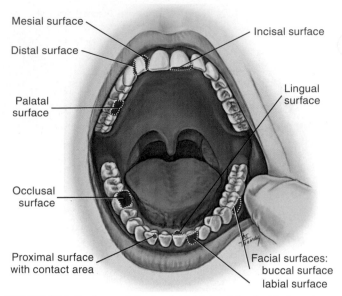

FIGURE 15-9 Surfaces of the teeth highlighted *(red)* with the orientational relationship to other oral cavity structures noted as related to the midline and to other teeth.

today are able to see the root surface in real time. When incorporated into more clinical practice settings in the future, such devices may change the way many dental procedures are performed.

ORIENTATIONAL TOOTH TERMS

Each tooth has five surfaces: facial, lingual, masticatory, mesial, and distal surfaces. Thus, each tooth is like a box with sides. Some of the surfaces of the tooth are identified by the orientational relationship to other orofacial structures, similar to the designation of the soft tissue of the oral cavity (Figure 15-9; see Figure 2-1). The tooth surface closest to the surface of the face is termed facial. The facial tooth surface closest to the lips is termed labial. Those facial tooth surfaces closest to the inner cheek are termed buccal. Therefore, the anterior teeth have a labial surface, and posterior teeth have a buccal surface.

The tooth surface closest to the tongue is termed lingual. Those lingual surfaces closest to the palate on the maxillary arch are sometimes also termed palatal. The **masticatory (mass**-ti-ka-tor-ee) **surface** is the chewing surface on the most superior surface of the crown. This is the **incisal (in**-sigh-zl) **surface** for anterior teeth and the **occlusal (ah-kloo**-zl) **surface** for posterior teeth.

The masticatory surfaces of both anterior and posterior teeth have linear elevations, or **ridges**, which are named according to location. The masticatory surfaces of both canines and posterior teeth also have at least one major elevation, the **cusp (kusp)**; cusps contribute to a significant part of the tooth's surface. Maxillary and mandibular canines both have one cusp, and the maxillary premolars and the mandibular first premolars usually have two cusps. Mandibular second premolars frequently have three cusps: one buccal and two lingual. Maxillary molars have two buccal cusps and two lingual cusps; a minor fifth cusp may form on these teeth (cusp of Carabelli). In contrast, mandibular molars may have five or four cusps.

Surfaces of both the crown and the root are also defined by the relationship to the midline (see Figure 15-9). The surface closest to the midline is termed the **mesial (me**-ze-il); the surface farthest away from the midline is termed the **distal (dis**-tl).

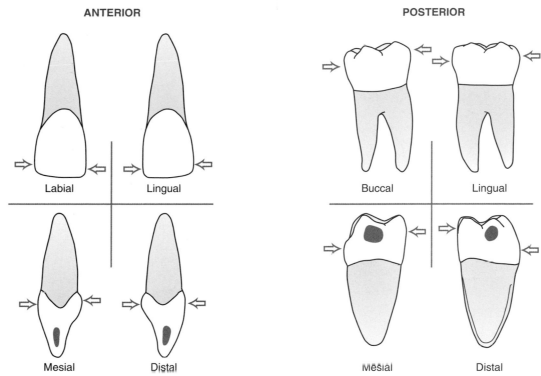

ANTERIOR

Labial   Lingual

Mesial   Distal

POSTERIOR

Buccal   Lingual

Mesial   Distal

FIGURE 15-10 Anterior and posterior teeth with the height of contour for each surface noted *(open arrows)* and contact areas highlighted *(red).*

Together, both the mesial and the distal surfaces between adjacent teeth are termed the **proximal** (prok-si-mal). In other words, either surface of a tooth that is next to an adjacent tooth is referred to as a proximal surface, which may therefore be either the mesial or the distal surface. The area between adjacent tooth surfaces is the **interproximal** (in-ter-prok-si-mal) **space**.

It is noted when viewing teeth overall that the proximal CEJ curvature is greatest on the anterior and the least on the posterior teeth. However, this curvature is approximately similar on mesial and distal surfaces of the two teeth that face each other. In addition, on any given tooth, the height of the CEJ curvature is greater on the mesial aspect of that tooth than it is on the distal aspect.

The area where the crowns of adjacent teeth in the same arch physically touch each adjacent proximal surface is the **contact area** or, as referred to by clinicians, the *contact* (see Figure 15-9). Its presence is checked when dental floss is passed between two teeth and some resistance is felt.

The contact areas on the mesial and distal surfaces are usually also considered the location of the height of contour on the proximal surfaces when in an ideal alignment (Figure 15-10). Thus the **height of contour** (or crest of curvature) is the greatest elevation of the tooth either incisocervically or occlusocervically on a specific surface of the crown when viewing its profile from the labial or buccal and the lingual. The crown also has a facial or lingual height of contour that is easily seen when viewing the crown's profile from the mesial and the distal. The facial and lingual surfaces of a tooth also have a height of contour that is easily seen when viewing the tooth's profile from the proximal aspect.

When two teeth in the same arch come into contact, the curvatures next to the contact areas form spaces considered **embrasures** (em-**bray**-zhers) (Figure 15-11). These consist of triangular-shaped spaces between two teeth, created by the sloping away of the mesial and distal surfaces, and may diverge facially, lingually, occlusally, or

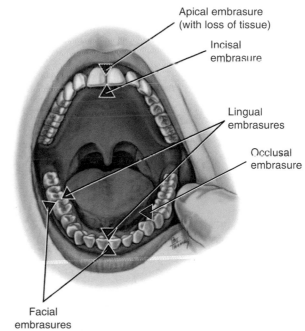

FIGURE 15-11 Embrasures highlighted *(red triangles)* that form between two teeth created by the sloping away of the mesial and distal surfaces, which may diverge facially, lingually, incisally/occlusally, or apically with loss of tissue.

apically with loss of tissue. The embrasures are continuous with the interproximal spaces between the teeth, and there is an increasing angle of the occlusal embrasures anterioposteriorly. They form spillways between teeth to direct food away from the gingiva. Also, they provide a mechanism for teeth to be more self-cleansing. Finally, the

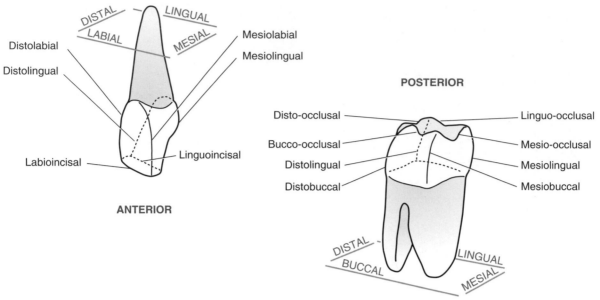

FIGURE 15-12 Anterior and posterior tooth with the designation of line angles of the crown.

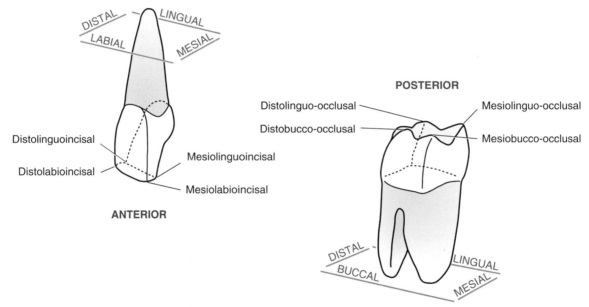

FIGURE 15-13 Anterior and posterior tooth with the designation of point angles of the crown.

embrasures protect the gingiva from undue frictional trauma but still provide the proper degree of stimulation to the tissue.

All these tooth contours (such as contact areas, heights of contour, and embrasures) are important in the function and health of the masticatory system (see **Chapter 20**). These specific forms and alignments of the teeth serve to shelter the vulnerable gingivosulcular area from damage and help to stabilize the position of the teeth within each dental arch.

Each tooth can also be divided by imaginary lines to designate specific crown areas of the tooth. A **line angle** is formed by the lines that are created at the junction of two crown surfaces, and the name is derived by combining the names of those two surfaces (Figure 15-12). When combining terms such as *mesial* and *labial*, the *al* from the end of the first surface is dropped and an *o* is added and combined with the second surface, thus creating *mesiolabial*. If the first letter of the second word results in doubling a vowel, a hyphen is placed between

the words, such as *mesio-occlusal*. An example of line angle designation would be the mesiolabial line angle, which is the junction of the mesial and labial surfaces.

Posterior teeth have eight line angles per tooth: mesiobuccal, distobuccal, mesiolingual, distolingual, mesio-occlusal, disto-occlusal, buccoocclusal, and linguo-occlusal. Anterior teeth have only six line angles per tooth: mesiolabial, distolabial, mesiolingual, distolingual, labioincisal, and linguoincisal. Anteriors have fewer line angles than posteriors because the mesial and distal incisal line angles are rounded; thus, the mesioincisal and distoincisal line angles are practically nonexistent.

A **point angle** is another way to determine a specific area of the crown (Figure 15-13). The junction of three surfaces of the crown, the point angle, takes its name from those three surfaces. Each tooth has four point angles. Examples of point angle designations are mesiolabioincisal for an anterior tooth or mesiobucco-occlusal for a posterior tooth.

ANTERIOR

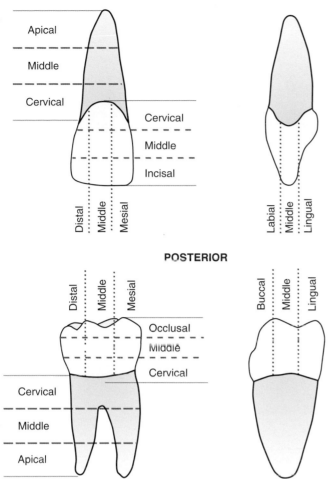

POSTERIOR

FIGURE 15-14 Anterior and posterior tooth with the designation of crown and root thirds. Note that the root can only be divided into thirds horizontally.

Finally, a crown surface can be divided both horizontally and vertically into three parts, or *thirds*, to designate specific tooth areas (Figure 15-14). An example is the middle third of the labial surface of an anterior tooth's crown. However, the root can be divided into thirds only horizontally. An example of designating a third area on a tooth root is the cervical third of the buccal surface of a posterior tooth's root. In comparison, the root is can only be divided vertically into halves by the RAL as discussed earlier, such that the halves when viewing the tooth from the mesial or distal are designated as labial or buccal and lingual; the halves when viewing the tooth from the labial or buccal are designated as mesial and distal.

Note that in reference to line angles, point angles, thirds, or even a direction, there is an accepted sequencing of combined names of the involved surfaces. The accepted sequence allows that the one term *mesial* precedes the term *distal* and also that both *mesial* and *distal* precede all other terms. The terms *labial, buccal,* and *lingual* follow *mesial* or *distal* but precede *incisal* or *occlusal* in any combination.

Clinical Considerations for Tooth Surfaces

The tooth's angles, height of contour, and spaces define the front or face of a tooth when the design of a patient's smile is considered, because these features are noted first when contemplating someone's smile.

Altering placement and shape of these features changes the face of a tooth and its perceived size and the appearance of the smile. Note that ideally the mesial part of the face and silhouette of a tooth is more angled vertically than the distal part of the face of a tooth.

After studying the surfaces of a tooth, dental professionals must be careful to note that access to the proximal surfaces and the interproximal space is more difficult than access to facial and lingual surfaces, although line angles can also present difficulties. These access challenges occurs for the patient during homecare, as well as for the clinician during instrumentation and restorative treatment.

TOOTH FORM

Each tooth type as already discussed has a specific form, no matter which dentition it is in (Table 15-4). This tooth form is related to the function during mastication for the tooth type, as well as to its role in speech and esthetics. The form and function of each tooth type are similar for both the primary and permanent dentitions.

The incisors function as instruments for biting and cutting food during mastication, because of the triangular proximal form of their crowns. The canines, because of the tapered shape and the prominent cusp of their crowns, function to pierce or tear food during mastication.

The premolars, which are found only in the permanent dentition, assist the canines in piercing and tearing food because of prominent cusps of their crowns during mastication. The premolars also assist the molars in grinding food during mastication because of the crown's wide masticatory surface, the occlusal surface. Finally, as the teeth with the largest and strongest crowns, the molars function in grinding food during mastication, assisted by the premolars. The wide masticatory surface, the occlusal surface of the molars, with the prominent cusps, function during mastication.

Tooth types also have tooth forms of the crown that roughly follow specific geometric shapes. Certain general shapes of the crown outline can be seen for each tooth type when viewing from each of the four perspectives; these specific shapes will be discussed in more detail in **Chapters 16 and 17** with each individual tooth type. As already discussed, the crowns of the incisors are triangular from mesial or distal views with the apex of the triangle at the masticatory surface of the tooth, the incisal surface, and its base at the cervix. From labial and lingual views, the crown outline of incisors is trapezoidal, or four-sided with only two parallel sides; the longer of the two parallel sides is toward the incisal surface.

Morphologically, canines can be considered a transitional tooth between incisors and premolars in the permanent dentition. Similar to the incisors, the crowns of canines are triangular from mesial and distal views as are all anteriors but are pentagonal or five-sided from labial or lingual views.

Only found in the permanent dentition, premolars are considered also morphologically to be a transitional tooth between canines and molars. From buccal and lingual views, the premolars' crowns are pentagonal, or five-sided, similar to canines.

For maxillary premolars, the crown outline from mesial or distal views is trapezoidal, or four-sided with only two parallel sides; the longer of the two parallel sides is toward the occlusal surface. In contrast, the mandibular premolars' crowns are rhomboidal from mesial or distal views, or four-sided having the opposite sides parallel. The rhomboidal outline is inclined lingually, thus allowing correct intercuspal contact of the mandibular tooth with the maxillary antagonists.

Similar to the maxillary premolars, the maxillary molars' crowns are trapezoidal in shape when viewed from the mesial or distal, as are all maxillary posteriors while the mandibular molars are rhomboidal

TABLE 15-4	Tooth Forms

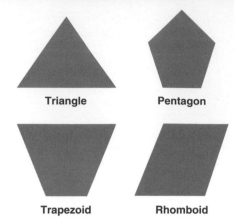

Triangle   Pentagon

Trapezoid   Rhomboid

TOOTH TYPE	TOOTH FORMS OF CROWNS WITH GEOMETRIC SHAPES	FUNCTION DURING MASTICATION
Incisors	 Labial Mesial Labial Mesial **PERMANENT MAXILLARY AND MANDIBULAR RIGHT INCISORS**	Biting and cutting because of triangular proximal form
Canines	 Labial Mesial Labial Mesial **PERMANENT MAXILLARY AND MANDIBULAR RIGHT CANINES**	Pierce or tear food because of tapered shape and prominent cusp

Continued

TABLE 15-4	Tooth Forms—cont'd	
TOOTH TYPE	**TOOTH FORMS OF CROWNS WITH GEOMETRIC SHAPES**	**FUNCTION DURING MASTICATION**
Premolars*	 Buccal Mesial Buccal Mesial **PERMANENT MAXILLARY AND MANDIBULAR RIGHT FIRST PREMOLARS**	Assist canines because of prominent cusps and assist molars because of broad masticatory surface
Molars	 Buccal Mesial Buccal Mesial **PERMANENT MAXILLARY AND MANDIBULAR RIGHT FIRST MOLARS**	Grinding food because of largest and strongest crowns, with wide masticatory surface and prominent cusps

*Premolars are only found in the permanent dentition.

from the same views as are all mandibular posteriors. In contrast, when viewed from the buccal or lingual, the molars' crown outline for both arches is trapezoidal.

Clinical Considerations for Tooth Form

Variation of teeth within a particular tooth type is a given and is always of interest to clinicians. The individual tooth form and its related function can be lost as a result of attrition, caries, and trauma or even extraction and shedding with complete loss of the tooth. Functional tooth form that has been lost can be approximated by restorative treatment, in many cases, using artificial crowns as discussed earlier or replacement bridges, partial or complete and fixed or removable dentures, as well as implants (see Figure 14-23). If not restored or replaced, this change in form over time can affect mastication, especially in older patients, who may change to a softer diet that may be poor nutritionally.

Because the specific shape of a tooth varies in each person and possibly within a dentition, a mold of the restored crown is made when integrating artificial crowns within an individual dentition. The goal is to match as closely as possible the shape of the patient's teeth on the opposite side so that the arch appears symmetrical and the crowns fit the space provided. This mold is selected by comparing it with a mold guide of white plastic model crowns provided by various manufacturers. The shade of the tooth is also a consideration (see **Chapter 12**).

CONSIDERATIONS FOR DENTAL ANATOMY STUDY

It is important to note that **Appendix C** in this textbook includes charts of the measurements of the permanent dentition. Student dental professionals should note that the values are mean values of ideal teeth; real teeth vary in size among patients and do not always directly reflect proportionate jaw size. Student dental professionals should also note that most of the descriptions in this textbook are also of ideal teeth. For consistency, the professionally drawn figures are larger than life-size; however, size relationships among teeth are retained, similar to those to be drawn and also illustrated in the flashcards from the *Workbook for Illustrated Dental Embryology, Histology, and Anatomy.* Also included are directions on how to draw each of the teeth which allows the student dental professional to further study each of the features of each individual tooth.

These drawn ideal teeth within the figures also have no wear or pathology, similar to plastic or plaster teeth. Extracted tooth specimens may be real but have detractions too. The detailed features on most extracted tooth specimens are sometimes harder to see because of signs of wear on both the crown and even the root apex, and the teeth may also show the trauma related to caries and restorative treatment. Examining a healthy dentition in a dental setting does present the teeth to best advantage.

However, many of the specific distinguishing features of a tooth can be seen only when holding an extracted tooth specimen. Thus extraction allows both the anatomic crown and the anatomic root to be viewed at once. In contrast, fewer features can be seen clinically when parts of the CEJ and root are covered by gingival tissue and only the clinical crown is visible. However, clinical views of the teeth are still important for observation of overall tooth arrangements and relationships.

Thus, extracted teeth provide a more realistic form of dental anatomy than plastic or plaster teeth, because they have more clearly formed cusps, ridges, fossae, and pits; variations of the ideal tooth form can thus be seen. Extracted teeth can also provide an opportunity to view relatively rare, as well as more common dental anomalies. However, infection control procedures must be followed when handling extracted teeth; see the *Workbook for Illustrated Dental Embryology, Histology, and Anatomy* for detailed procedures. When studying dental anatomy, all opportunities for observation must be considered for the most effective level of expertise to be achieved: extracted tooth specimens, plastic or plaster teeth, and dentitions in a clinical setting.

CHAPTER 16

Permanent Anterior Teeth

Additional resources and practice exercises are provided on the companion Evolve website for this book:
http://evolve.elsevier.com/Fehrenbach/illustrated.

●●●●LEARNING OBJECTIVES

1. Define and pronounce the key terms in this chapter.
2. Identify the permanent anterior teeth and discuss their properties and the clinical considerations concerning them, integrating it into patient care.
3. Identify the permanent incisors and their general features and discuss their clinical considerations, integrating it into patient care.
4. Describe the general and specific features of the permanent maxillary incisors and discuss the clinical considerations concerning them, integrating it into patient care.
5. Describe the general and specific features of the permanent mandibular incisors and discuss the clinical considerations concerning them, integrating it into patient care.
6. Identify the permanent canines and their general features and discuss their clinical considerations, integrating it into patient care.
7. Describe the general and specific features of the permanent maxillary canines and discuss the clinical considerations concerning them, integrating it into patient care.
8. Describe the general and specific features of the permanent mandibular canines and discuss the clinical considerations concerning them, integrating it into patient care.
9. Assign the correct names and universal or international tooth number for each permanent anterior tooth on a diagram or a skull and for a tooth model or a patient.
10. Demonstrate the correct location of each permanent anterior tooth on a diagram, a skull, and a patient.

PERMANENT ANTERIOR TEETH PROPERTIES

Permanent anterior teeth include the incisors and canines (Figure 16-1; see Figures 2-4 and 15-2). All anterior teeth are thought to be composed of four developmental lobes, three labial lobes (mesiolabial, middle labial, and distolabial), and one lingual lobe (Figure 16-2). Two vertical labial developmental depressions outline the separations between the labial developmental lobes: the mesiolabial and distolabial developmental depressions. Lobe discussion, as was noted in **Chapter 6**, is controversial but is included for completeness when discussing in detail the various tooth types.

All permanent anterior teeth are succedaneous, which means that each one replaces the primary tooth of the same type. The development and shedding of the primary dentition as well as the development of the permanent dentition can be reviewed in **Chapter 6**.

The long crown of an anterior tooth has an incisal surface, which is considered the incisal (in-sigh-zl) ridge, which is its masticatory surface (Figure 16-3). The crown outline of anteriors is triangular when viewed from the proximal with the apex at the incisal ridge and the base of the triangle at the cervix (Figure 16-4; see Table 15-4). These teeth are wider mesiodistally than labiolingually when compared with posteriors. For anteriors, the height of contour for both the crown's labial and lingual surfaces is in the cervical third. Each contact area of anteriors is usually centered labiolingually on their proximal surfaces and has a smaller area than the contacts of posterior teeth (see Figure 15-10). On each proximal surface, the cementoenamel junction (CEJ) curvature of all anteriors is greater than that of the posteriors.

The lingual surfaces of all anteriors have a cingulum (sin-gu-lum), which is a raised, rounded area on the cervical third of the lingual surface in varying degrees of prominence or development (Figure 16-5). The cingulum corresponds to the lingual developmental lobe. Ridges may also be present on the lingual surface. The lingual surface on anteriors is bordered mesially and distally on each side by a rounded raised border, the marginal ridge.

FIGURE 16-1 Permanent anterior teeth identified, which include the incisors and canines. (Courtesy of Margaret J. Fehrenbach, RDH, MS.)

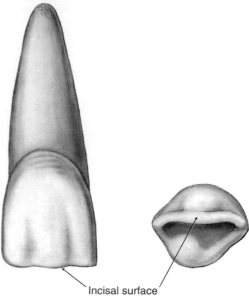

FIGURE 16-3 Example of an incisal surface on a permanent anterior tooth.

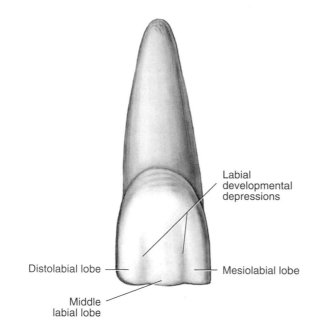

Labial View

FIGURE 16-2 Example of lobe development in a permanent anterior tooth.

Some anteriors have a more complex lingual surface with a fossa (fos-ah) (plural, fossae [fos-ay]), which is a shallow, wide depression (Figure 16-6). Some may also have developmental pits, which are located in the deepest part of each fossa. Other anteriors may have on their lingual surface a developmental groove (or primary groove), a sharp, deep, V-shaped linear depression that marks the junction between the developmental lobes.

In addition, a supplemental groove (or secondary groove) may also be present on the lingual surface of anteriors, which is a shallower, more irregular linear depression than the developmental groove (see Figure 16-6). Supplemental grooves branch from the developmental grooves but are not always present in the same pattern on each different tooth type. In general, the more anterior the tooth is located in the arch, the fewer supplemental grooves are present and the less pronounced the lingual surface.

Anteriors usually have a single root, with some exceptions. Each root of the maxillary anterior teeth has great lingual and slight distal inclination (see Figure 20-9). Each root of the mandibular anterior

teeth varies in angulation from nearly vertical to great lingual inclination, with the canines possibly having a slight distal root inclination.

Clinical Considerations with Permanent Anterior Teeth

Patients may have difficulty in maintaining homecare of anteriors because their dental arch position naturally may allow the lips to overhang the teeth. Thus, patients may provide care only to the incisal two-thirds of the labial surface of the crowns of anteriors, especially missing the associated cervical area and labial gingival tissue; this may also make instrumentation or restoration difficult. Mouth breathing may also dry the maxillary labial gingival tissue, causing inflammation.

Instrumentation and restorative treatment may also be compromised in the area where the greater curvature of the CEJ is present interproximally on anteriors, and where accessibility is limited as well as having the teeth in close proximity. The grooves on the lingual surface of anteriors may present areas for dental biofilm retention if they extend to the root and are near the adjacent gingival tissue; for this reason, the grooves may need to be reduced with minor odontoplasty.

When the anterior teeth are restored or undergo orthodontic therapy, the Golden Proportions can be useful guidelines to balance the size of the teeth with one another (see Figure 1-10). These guidelines designate the ideal width of the maxillary lateral incisor as a factor of 1.0×, the width of the central incisors as 1.618×, and the width of the canines as 0.168×, all when observed in two dimensions from the labial aspect. Other formulas state that the maxillary central should be 60% wider than the lateral, and the lateral should be 60% wider than the canine, as measured from the midline to the mesial aspect. In addition, each incisor should also ideally have an 8:10 width-to-length ratio.

Consideration of smile design may involve the drawing of a line following the ideal outline formed by the incisal ridges of the maxillary anterior teeth; the ideal line should be 1 to 3 mm parallel or equidistant to the lower lip line. Straight smiles are perceived as more masculine, and more curved smiles are perceived as more feminine. In addition, if the upper lip line appears to be convex instead of concave compared with the lower lip line, the smile will be perceived as more youthful (see Figure 14-22). Some variation of one's smile will occur with aging due to a noticeable loss of elasticity in the lips, which results in sagging, prominence of the mandibular anterior teeth, and diminution of the maxillary anterior teeth.

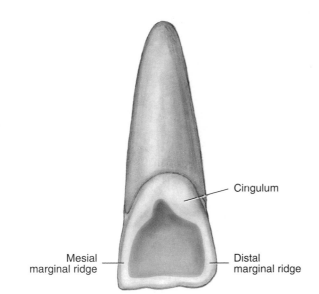

Height of contour ⇒
Height of contour ⇒
⇐ **Height of contour**
⇐ **Height of contour**

Cementoenamel junction curvature

Height of contour

Contact area

Labial View   **Proximal View**

FIGURE 16-4 Example of a permanent anterior tooth with the various heights of contour and contact area identified.

Cingulum

Mesial marginal ridge   Distal marginal ridge

FIGURE 16-5 Example of lingual surface features on a permanent anterior tooth.

PERMANENT INCISORS

GENERAL FEATURES OF PERMANENT INCISORS

Permanent incisors are the eight most anterior teeth of the permanent dentition with four in each dental arch (Table 16-1). The two types are the central incisors and the lateral incisors. The centrals are closest to the midline, and the laterals are the second teeth from the midline. One of each type is present in each quadrant of each dental arch. Both types are mesial to the permanent canines when the permanent dentition is fully erupted. The permanent incisors are succedaneous and replace the primary incisors of the same type. On occasion, the permanent incisors seem to spread out across the arch as a result of open spacing during initial eruption, especially in the maxillary arch, but with the eruption of the permanent canines, these spaces often close (see Figure 15-4).

Incisors function as instruments for biting and cutting food during mastication because of their incisal ridge, triangular proximal form, and arch position (see Table 15-4). They also support the lips and facial muscles as well as maintain vertical dimension of the face. Additionally, they contribute to overall arch appearance. Finally, they are involved during the articulation of speech and assist in guiding jaw closure as the teeth come together.

From both the labial and lingual, the crown outline of incisors is trapezoidal, or four-sided, with only two parallel sides. The longer of the two parallel sides is toward the incisal surface (see Table 15-4).

When newly erupted, each incisor also has three mamelons (mam-ah-lons), which are rounded enamel extensions on the incisal ridge from the labial or lingual views (Figures 16-7). The mamelons are considered by some histologists to be extensions from the three labial developmental lobes (see **Chapter 6**).

The incisors are also the only permanent teeth with two incisal angles formed from the incisal ridge and each proximal surface (see Figure 16-7). Incisors of both types are the only permanent teeth with a nearly straight incisal ridge, which is a linear elevation on the masticatory or incisal surface of these anteriors when newly erupted—thus the name *incisors*.

The lingual surface has a cingulum that corresponds to the lingual developmental lobe, although its prominence or development differs for each type of incisor (see Figure 16-7). These teeth also have a lingual fossa and marginal ridges on the lingual surface, again in differing developmental levels for each type of incisor. The height of contour for both labial and lingual surfaces of all incisors is at the cervical third, as is the case for all anteriors.

Clinical Considerations with Permanent Incisors

Because of the anterior position of the incisors, esthetic concerns are important during restorative procedures. However, restorative replacement of any part of the incisal surfaces of these teeth after traumatic fracture may also be difficult to maintain owing to their function in biting and cutting food during mastication.

The mamelons on the incisal ridges of incisors usually undergo slight attrition, the wearing away of a tooth surface caused by tooth-to-tooth contact, shortly after eruption as the teeth move into occlusion. Thus, mamelons are usually most noticeable immediately after

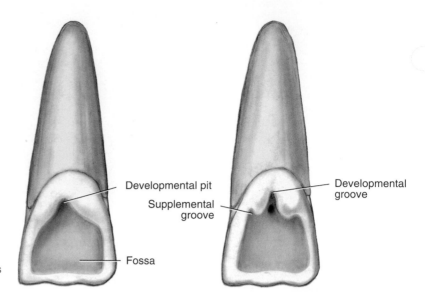

Developmental pit

Supplemental groove

Developmental groove

Fossa

FIGURE 16-6 Additional examples of lingual surface features on a permanent anterior tooth.

TABLE 16-1	Permanent Incisors			
	MAXILLARY CENTRAL INCISOR	**MAXILLARY LATERAL INCISOR**	**MANDIBULAR CENTRAL INCISOR**	**MANDIBULAR LATERAL INCISOR**
Universal number	#8 and #9	#7 and #10	#24 and #25	#23 and #26
International number	#11 and #21	#12 and #22	#31 and #41	#32 and #42
General crown features	Incisal ridge, incisal angles, cingulum, marginal ridges, lingual fossa			
Specific crown features	Widest crown mesiodistally. Greatest CEJ curve and height of contour. Pronounced distal offset cingulum and marginal ridges, with wide and deep lingual fossa	Greatest crown variation. Like a smaller central. Pronounced lingual surface, with centered cingulum and prominent marginal ridges	Smallest and simplest tooth. Symmetric. Small centered cingulum, with less pronounced marginal ridges and lingual fossa	Like a larger mandibular central. Not symmetric. Appears twisted distally. Small, distally placed cingulum, with mesial marginal ridge longer than distal marginal ridge
Height of contour	Cervical third			
Mesial contact	Incisal third			
Distal contact	Junction of incisal and middle thirds	Middle third	Incisal third	Incisal third
Distinguish right from left	Sharper mesioincisal angle and rounder distoincisal angle. More pronounced mesial CEJ curvature			
General root features	Single root			
Specific root features	Triangular in cross section. Overall conical shape. No proximal root concavities. Rounded apex	Oval in cross section. Same or longer than central but thinner. Overall conical shape. No proximal root concavities. Root curves distally, with sharp apex	Elliptic on cross section. Root is longer than the crown. Pronounced proximal root concavities can give a double-rooted appearance.	

CEJ, Cementoenamel junction.

eruption, becoming less detectable as the teeth undergo some level of attrition over time.

If mamelons are still present on the incisal ridges long after eruption, it is because these teeth are not in occlusion where they usually undergo some level of attrition, such as with an anterior open bite relationship (Figure 16-8, *A*). Many young adults do not like the appearance of mamelons and sometimes request to have them removed by minor odontoplasty; some patients even request restorative treatment to achieve straighter-appearing incisal ridges.

Part of the reason that the mamelons are so noticeable if present long after eruption is that these extensions are made of enamel with no dentin layer underneath. This factor and their thinness contribute overall to the striking translucent appearance, as opposed to the rest of the clinical crown, which is usually more opaque than the mamelons. With the addition of vital tooth whitening (or bleaching), incisal translucencies from mamelons or incisal ridges may become even more noticeable.

In addition, after eruption the incisal ridges can now appear even more flattened from the labial, lingual, or incisal views due

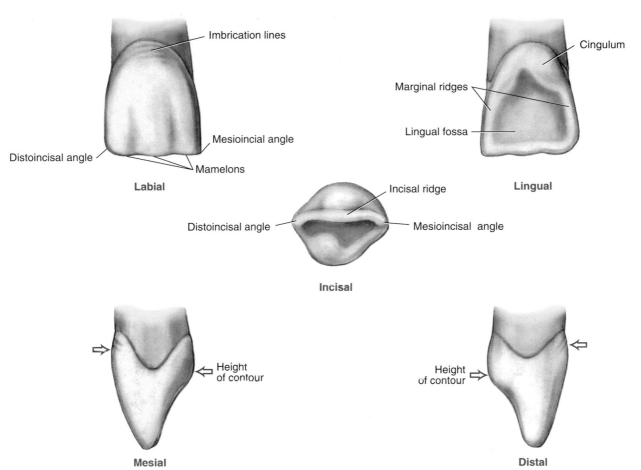

Imbrication lines

Cingulum

Marginal ridges

Lingual fossa

Distoincisal angle

Mesioincial angle

Mamelons

Labial

Lingual

Incisal ridge

Distoincisal angle

Mesioincisal angle

Incisal

Height
of contour

Height
of contour

Mesial

Distal

FIGURE 16-7 Views of a newly erupted permanent incisor with the features noted.

FIGURE 16-8 Incisal surface on permanent incisors. **A,** Mamelons present on the incisal ridges of newly erupted permanent mandibular incisors in a mixed dentition, which have been kept from attrition due to an anterior open bite. In contrast, through attrition the mamelons have been lost on the already erupted same tooth type on the maxillary arch. **B,** Lateral view of both permanent maxillary and mandibular incisors altered by higher levels of attrition on the incisal surfaces, which have transitioned from incisal ridges to incisal edges *(dark outlines)*. (Courtesy of Margaret J. Fehrenbach, RDH, MS.)

to attrition and each becomes an incisal edge (see Figure 16-8, *B*). Thus with this arrangement, the incisal edges of the maxillary and mandibular incisors are now usually parallel to one another and occlude correctly during mastication. However, with increased attrition the maxillary incisors' incisal edges can show lingual inclination, and the mandibular incisors can have a labial inclination to their incisal edges, as well as translucency (see Figure 16-9, *C*).

The crown of a permanent maxillary incisor can be affected with dens in dente (see Box 6-1, *G, H*). This disturbance may leave the tooth with a deep lingual pit resulting from invagination of the enamel organ into the dental papilla. This pit may lead to pulpal exposure and pathology. Dens in dente may be hereditary and is more common with a maxillary lateral incisor.

The crowns of permanent incisors, similar to molars, can be affected in children with congenital syphilis. A pregnant woman infected with syphilis transmits the spirochete *Treponema pallidum,* a sexually transmitted microorganism, to her fetus via the placenta. This microorganism may cause localized enamel hypoplasia, which can result in Hutchinson incisors (hutch-in-sun) occurring during tooth development (see Figure 3-17, *A*). A Hutchinson incisor has a crown with a screwdriver shape from the labial view and is wider cervically and narrow incisally with a notched incisal ridge. Restorative treatment of these teeth may improve their oral appearance. Children may also have other developmental anomalies, such as blindness, deafness, and paralysis from congenital syphilis.

A sharp, small extra cusp, or *talon cusp* (means like a claw), occasionally appears as a projection from the cingulum of incisor teeth and can happen within both dentitions. These types of cusps can interfere with occlusion, and even minor odontoplasty may be a hazardous procedure. They often contain a prominent pulp horn, which is at an increased risk of pulpal exposure during restorative procedures.

PERMANENT MAXILLARY INCISORS
GENERAL FEATURES

Permanent maxillary incisors are the four most anteriorly placed teeth of the maxillary arch. Each has a crown that is larger in all dimensions, especially mesiodistally, compared with a mandibular incisor. In addition, the labial surfaces are rounder from the incisal aspect with the tooth tapering toward the lingual.

The central and lateral incisors of the maxillary arch both resemble each other more than they resemble the similar type of incisors of the opposing arch. Generally, a maxillary central incisor is larger than a maxillary lateral incisor, but overall they have a similar form. Both types of maxillary incisors are wider mesiodistally than labiolingually.

All lingual surface features, including the marginal ridges, lingual fossa, and cingulum, are more prominent on the maxillary incisors than on the mandibular incisors. Finally, the incisal ridge is just labial to the long axis of the root from either proximal view.

Each root is short compared with those of other maxillary teeth and usually is without root concavities. However, the presence of bulbous and pronounced crowns may create deep mesial and distal concavities at the CEJ.

If a maxillary incisor has increased prominence of the lingual marginal ridges and a deeper lingual fossa, it may be considered to have a shovel-shaped form (Figure 16-9, *A*). It can also have an accentuated cingulum with deepened grooves, or have an incisal edge with severe attrition, giving it a lingual inclination (see Figure 16-9, *B* and *C*, respectively). In addition, supragingival tooth deposits, such as dental biofilm and stain, can collect in the prominent lingual surface concavities of maxillary incisors (see Figure 16-9, *D*).

The lingual pit is another lingual feature that if present on the maxillary incisors can be at increased risk of caries development due to both increased dental biofilm retention and the weakness of the enamel forming the walls of the pit (Figure 16-10, *A-C*; see Figure 12-4, *A*). If the lingual pit is deep, a developmental disturbance of dens in dente must be considered, and needed changes must be made in the patient's treatment plan (discussed earlier). Also present may be a vertically-placed linguogingival groove that originates in the lingual pit and extends cervically and slightly distally onto the cingulum (see Figure 16-10, *D*). It is more common on maxillary laterals, possibly resulting in caries.

Clinicians need to be aware of these lingual pit and groove patterns on maxillary incisors when they examine a dentition in order to determine the patient's caries risk level. All pits and grooves must be checked for decay with an explorer and mirror. Light-induced devices that measure changes in laser fluorescence of hard tissue allow dental professionals to better diagnose early lesions in pits and grooves. Maxillary incisors with deep pit and groove patterns but without incipient decay should have enamel sealants placed as soon as they erupt. If dental caries occur or an enamel sealant does not remain on the lingual surface, tooth-colored restorative materials can be used to achieve a more esthetic appearance, and thus the past history of the lingual pit may not now be easy to discern clinically.

During instrumentation or restoration, the proximal surfaces of these teeth are more accessible from the lingual than the labial approach because of the increased tapering of the tooth to the lingual. Dental professionals

FIGURE 16-9 Lingual views of extracted permanent maxillary incisors. **A,** Shovel shape to lingual surface. **B,** Accentuated cingulum with deepened grooves. **C,** Attrition on incisal surface with formation of an incisal edge from the incisal ridge with lingual inclination. **D,** Stain in the deepened lingual fossa. (Courtesy of Margaret J. Fehrenbach, RDH, MS.)

FIGURE 16-10 Lingual views of extracted permanent maxillary incisors. **A,** Lingual pit. **B,** Lingual pit with caries. **C,** Lingual pit caries repaired. **D,** Linguogingival groove with caries. (Courtesy of Margaret J. Fehrenbach, RDH, MS.)

must be careful to check for deposits in any mesial and distal root concavities at the CEJ if this area is exposed as a result of gingival recession.

Finally, the competency of the lips to maintain a lip seal, when at a resting posture, can affect the overall position of the maxillary incisors (see Figure 20-31). Competent lips allow these tooth ridges to be inferior to the lower lip border, helping to maintain the level of inclination. Incompetent lips that fail to provide a lip seal do not control this inclination and may even allow the maxillary incisors to be anterior to the lower lip, exaggerating already buccally-inclined teeth and possibly becoming lingually-inclined. A tongue thrust is a complicating factor that may be associated with this occlusal challenge (see Figure 20-28).

PERMANENT MAXILLARY CENTRAL INCISORS #8 AND #9 (#11 AND #21)

Specific Overall Features Permanent maxillary central incisors erupt between 7 to 8 years of age with root completion at age 10

(Figure 16-11). Thus, these teeth usually erupt after the mandibular central incisors. Many child patients want these two teeth to come in fast to fill their wide open anterior arch space when they shed their two primary maxillary central incisors, as in the old song, "All I Want for Christmas Is My Two Front Teeth."

The maxillary central incisors are the most prominent teeth in the permanent dentition because of both their large size and their anterior arch position. In addition, they are the largest of all the incisors, and the two usually share a mesial contact area. They have the widest crown mesiodistally of any permanent anterior tooth.

The maxillary central incisor has a single conical root, smooth and slightly straight, usually with a rounded apex. Thus, the root is thick in the cervical third and narrows through the middle to the blunt apex, and it is one and one-half times the length of the crown. The root is also about the same length, or shorter, but wider than the lateral of the same arch. Bulbous crowns may create deep mesial and distal concavities at CEJ. The root is oval or egg-shaped in cervical cross section, being slightly wider on the labial surface and narrower at the lingual.

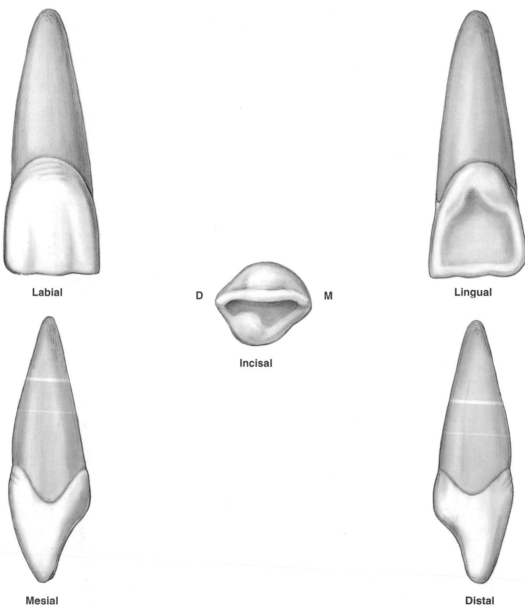

Labial   **D** **M**   **Lingual**

Incisal

Mesial   **Distal**

FIGURE 16-11 Views of a permanent maxillary right central incisor.

The pulp cavity mirrors the shape of the tooth; there is only one root canal that is considerably large (Figure 16-12). The pulp chamber of the maxillary central incisor has three sharp elongations: the mesial, distal, and central pulp horns. These pulp horns correspond to the three labial developmental lobes of the tooth. The central pulp horn is usually shorter than the other two and more rounded.

Labial View Features The crown of a maxillary central incisor is narrowest at the cervical third and becomes wider toward the incisal ridge on the labial surface (see Figure 16-11). The incisal ridge is nearly straight. Two labial developmental depressions may extend the length of the crown from the cervical to the incisal, showing the division of the surface into three labial developmental lobes. The crown usually has imbrication lines, or slight ridges, that run mesiodistally in the cervical third, and between them are the grooved perikymata (see **Chapter 12**). The CEJ on the labial surface has more curvature to the distal.

From the labial view, both incisal angles can be seen on the maxillary central incisor. The overall mesial outline is slightly rounded with a sharp mesioincisal angle. The overall distal outline is even rounder with a definite rounded distoincisal angle. The difference in sharpness of the central's mesioincisal and distoincisal angle *helps to distinguish the maxillary right central incisor from the left.*

The mesial contact with the other maxillary central is in the incisal third (see Figure 16-7). The distal contact with the maxillary lateral is at the junction of the incisal and the middle third, located farther cervically than the mesial contact.

Lingual View Features The lingual surface of the crown of a maxillary central incisor is narrower overall than the labial surface (see Figure 16-11). The CEJ usually has more curvature to the distal. The single cingulum is wide and well-developed in size, as well as being located slightly off center toward the distal.

From the lingual view, the mesial marginal ridge is longer than the distal marginal ridge. The single lingual fossa is wide yet shallow and is located immediately incisal to the cingulum. The lingual fossa varies in depth and diameter. Outlining the incisal border of the lingual fossa, the raised linguoincisal ridge is on the same level as the bordering marginal ridges.

Variations can occur on the lingual surface of the tooth (Figure 16-13). A horizontally placed lingual groove may be present (although it is more common on maxillary laterals), separating the cingulum from the lingual fossa. The lingual groove may make the cingulum appear scalloped along its borders. A lingual pit may also be present at the incisal border of the cingulum in the lingual groove. Also present may be a vertically placed linguogingival groove, which originates in the lingual pit and extends cervically and slightly distally onto the cingulum.

Proximal View Features The CEJ curvature on the mesial surface is deep incisally and has the greatest depth of curvature of any tooth surface in the permanent dentition, which *helps to distinguish the maxillary right central incisor from the left* (see Figure 16-11). The height of contour for both the labial and lingual surfaces is also greater on this tooth than on any tooth in the permanent dentition and is located at the cervical third, as in all incisors.

The incisal ridge is located slightly labial to the long axis of the tooth. The incisal outline is also sloped toward the lingual from its longest and, also, most labial part. The distal view is similar to the mesial, although the curvature of the CEJ is less on the distal than on the mesial surface.

Incisal View Features Overall, the shape of the crown of a maxillary central incisor from the incisal view is triangular with the labial outline broadly rounded (see Figure 16-11). This is a useful view for

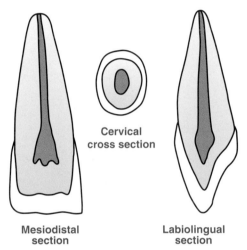

Cervical cross section

Mesiodistal section

Labiolingual section

FIGURE 16-12 Pulp cavity of a permanent maxillary right central incisor.

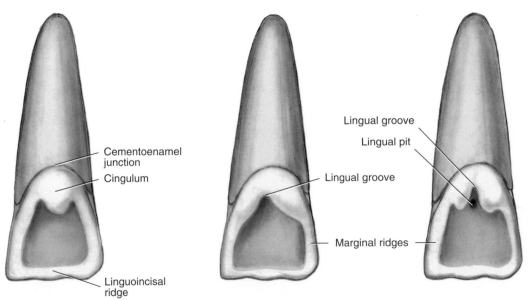

Cementoenamel junction

Cingulum

Linguoincisal ridge

Lingual groove

Lingual groove

Lingual pit

Marginal ridges

FIGURE 16-13 Lingual surface variations of the permanent maxillary right central incisor with the lingual fossae highlighted.

observing the slight distal placement of the cingulum. On the lingual surface of the incisal view, the mesial marginal ridge again appears longer than the distal marginal ridge. Note that the incisal ridge lies just labial to the long axis of the root.

Clinical Considerations with Permanent Maxillary Central Incisors

The incisal ridge, or even the entire maxillary central incisor, is especially at risk for traumatic fracture or tooth displacement because of the tooth's more anterior and labial position as well as its early eruption into the oral cavity. Because of these two factors and without full root completion, the entire tooth in a child may undergo avulsion (ah-**vul**-shin), which is complete displacement of the tooth from the tooth socket or alveolus, resulting from extensive trauma to the area. Even if the tooth only undergoes fracture, pulpal pathology may occur in the tooth and result in the need for endodontic therapy or loss of tooth vitality as the pulp dies.

An open contact, or diastema (di-ah-**ste**-mah), can also exist between the maxillary central incisors. It can be a wide, and to some patients, unattractive space. Both the cause and treatment of this type of diastema are controversial. Treatment may involve surgical release to reduce the impact of a tight maxillary labial frenum, with or without additional orthodontic therapy. Incisors may appear *winged* when looking at the patient's smile. This is not a disturbance of development, but rather a case of tooth rotation, usually bilateral rotation to the mesial. This can be corrected with orthodontic therapy. Finally, in consideration of a patient's smile design, the central incisors should dominate the perspective in such a way that each adjacent tooth appears to get smaller as one moves distally down the dental arch.

One common location for a supernumerary tooth is between the two maxillary central incisors, which is considered a mesiodens (me-ze-oh-denz) (see Box 6-1, *C, D*). This developmental anomaly is due to the presence of an extra tooth germ resulting from an abnormal initiation process during tooth development, forming a supernumerary tooth. The presence of this extra tooth may affect spacing in the maxillary arch, whether it is erupted or not. The involved tooth may also have a dwarfed root, which results in a lack of periodontal support for the tooth and thus may negatively affect the prognosis of the tooth if it is involved in periodontal disease.

PERMANENT MAXILLARY LATERAL INCISORS #7 AND #10 (#12 AND #22)

Specific Overall Features Permanent maxillary lateral incisors erupt between 8 and 9 years of age with root completion at age 11 (Figure 16-14). Thus, these teeth usually erupt after the maxillary central incisors.

The crown of a maxillary lateral incisor has the greatest degree of variation in form of any permanent tooth, except for the third molars. This tooth resembles a maxillary central incisor in all views of the tooth but is smaller and has a slightly rounder crown. This tooth when examined as an extracted tooth is frequently confused with a small permanent mandibular canine, but the root usually has no depressions on the proximal surface, which is common on a mandibular canine.

A maxillary lateral incisor has a single conical root that is relatively smooth and straight but may curve slightly to the distal. Its crown is one to one and one-half times shorter than the length of the root. The root is also about the same length as or longer than the central, but it is thinner, particularly mesiodistally, as well as being wider labiolingually. The shape of the root on cross section is oval. A linguogingival groove may be present on the root and possibly continue on the crown. The apex of the root is not rounded like the central but is sharp.

The pulp cavity of the maxillary lateral incisor is simple in form with a single pulp canal and a pulp chamber (Figure 16-15). The pulp chamber does not have three sharp pulp horns as it does in a maxillary central incisor; instead, it usually has one rounded form or two less-sharp pulp horns: a mesial and distal pulp horn.

Labial View Features Labial developmental depressions and imbrication lines on the labial surface are less common on a maxillary lateral than on a central incisor (see Figure 16-14). The crown is smaller than that of a central incisor and less symmetrical.

However, it generally resembles a central in its mesial outline, with the mesial contact with the maxillary central at the incisal third. The distal outline is always rounder than the central and has a more cervical distal contact area with the maxillary canine at the middle third or at the junction of the incisal and the middle third.

From the labial view, both incisal angles are rounder on a maxillary lateral than on a central incisor. Although similar to a central incisor, a maxillary lateral has different incisal angles from the labial. The lateral's mesioincisal angle is sharper than the distoincisal angle, which *helps to distinguish the maxillary right lateral incisor from the left.*

Lingual View Features The lingual surface of the crown of a maxillary lateral incisor is narrower than the labial surface, as is the case with a central (see Figure 16-14). It has a prominent, yet centered and narrower cingulum than does a central incisor, with a deeper lingual fossa. The marginal ridges are pronounced: The longer mesial marginal ridge is nearly straight, and the shorter distal marginal ridge is quite straight. The linguoincisal ridge is also noticeably well developed in size.

Variations can occur on the lingual surface of the tooth (Figure 16-16). On the lingual surface, a horizontal lingual groove that separates the cingulum from the lingual fossa is more common on a maxillary lateral and better developed than on a central. A lingual pit is more common on a lateral than on a central and is located on the incisal surface of the cingulum, along the lingual groove.

Additionally present on the lingual surface may be a vertical linguogingival groove that originates in the lingual pit and extends cervically and slightly distally onto the cingulum. The linguogingival groove may extend onto the root surface. The linguogingival groove is also more common on this tooth than on a maxillary central. Rarely, the root has a deep distolingual marginal groove, a developmental groove that begins on the distal marginal ridge on the lingual surface and extends onto the root.

Proximal View Features The crown of a maxillary lateral incisor is triangular on a mesial view, as are all anterior teeth (see Figure 16-14 and Table 15-4). The CEJ curvature is similar to that of a central, although it is not as deeply curved on a lateral. Also similar to a central, a lateral's CEJ is more curved on the mesial surface than the distal of this tooth, *which helps to distinguish the maxillary right lateral incisor from the left.* The incisal ridge is usually labial to the long axis of the tooth. The distal view is similar to that of the mesial, although the CEJ is not as deeply curved.

Incisal View Features The outline of the crown of a maxillary lateral incisor is round or oval from the incisal view, not triangular, as is a central (see Figure 16-14). The crown's mesiodistal measurement is somewhat wider than the labiolingual measurement. Thus, the labial surface of the lateral is rounder than that of a central.

Clinical Considerations with Permanent Maxillary Lateral Incisors

Open contacts that seem unattractive to some patients may be easily visible in this region of the dental arch due to variations in form, as well as asymmetry in both tooth size and position across the

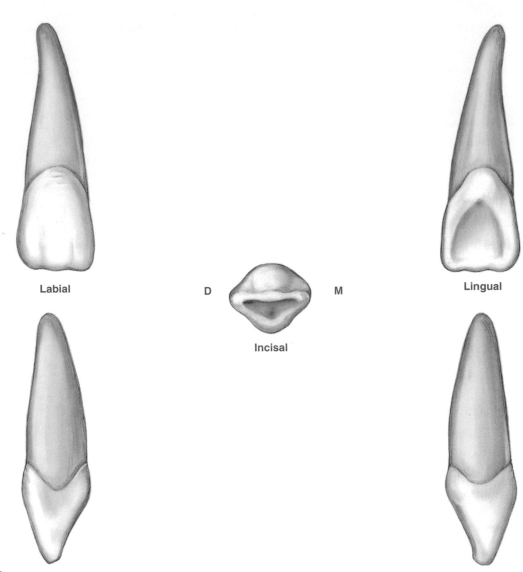

FIGURE 16-14 Views of a permanent maxillary right lateral incisor.

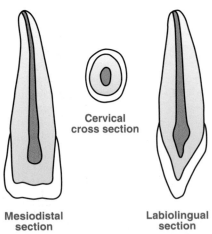

FIGURE 16-15 Pulp cavity of a permanent maxillary right lateral incisor.

maxillary arch (see Figure 20-24). Because of the variations in form as well as the possibility of developmental disturbances, maxillary lateral incisors present challenges during preventive, restorative, and orthodontic procedures.

The linguogingival groove on the tooth can be considered an adverse factor because tooth deposits can accumulate in the niche-like groove. This feature then can track periodontal destruction apically following the pathway of the groove, resulting in the formation of a localized periodontal lesion, such as an abscess. A deeper mean probing pocket depth and a greater degree of severe gingivitis are usually present with this situation. Careful and repeated pocket depth probing with associated root exploration is essential to monitor these high-risk areas for periodontal complications in a patient with such a feature.

A maxillary lateral incisor is one of the most common teeth of the permanent dentition to exhibit partial microdontia (see Box 6-1, *E*). This disturbance leads to a smaller lateral incisor crown, or peg lateral, present either unilaterally or bilaterally. This disturbance occurs in the process of proliferation during tooth development. It may be hereditary or may result from other factors. To improve appearance, prosthetic treatment may be performed to increase the crown size of the tooth.

The maxillary laterals are also more commonly involved in partial anodontia and thus may be congenitally missing (see Box 6-1, *A*). This disturbance results from an absence of the appropriate individual tooth germ(s) in the area, unilaterally or bilaterally. This occurs at around 1-2% of the time, resulting from a failure in the initiation

Lingual groove

Cingulum

Lingual pit

Mesial marginal ridge

Distal marginal ridge

Linguoincisal ridge

Linguogingival groove

Lingual pit

Distolingual marginal groove

FIGURE 16-16 Variations of the lingual surface of the permanent maxillary right lateral incisor with the lingual fossae highlighted.

process during tooth development. Partial anodontia may present esthetic challenges for patients and can also result in complications with occlusion; thus, these missing teeth may require a prosthetic replacement such as an implant, bridge, or partial denture.

Finally, a maxillary lateral may have one or more tubercles, or accessory cusps, on the cingulum. The dilaceration of the crown or root, showing angular distortion may occur, making extraction and endodontic treatment difficult.

PERMANENT MANDIBULAR INCISORS
GENERAL FEATURES

Permanent mandibular incisors are the smallest teeth of the permanent dentition and the most symmetrical when first erupted. More uniformity in form is seen with these teeth than with any other of the permanent dentition. The lateral and central incisors of the mandibular arch resemble each other more than do the similar types of incisors of the maxillary arch.

Generally, a mandibular lateral is slightly larger than a central, exactly the opposite of the situation in the maxillary arch. The incisal ridge is just lingual to the long axis of the root. Each mandibular incisor has a crown that is wider labiolingually than mesiodistally, which is also unlike the maxillary incisors. Both mandibular incisors also have less pronounced lingual surface features than the maxillary incisors, including those of the cingulum, lingual fossa, and marginal ridges.

The root is longer than the crown for both incisors (see Figures 16-18 and 16-20). The root of a mandibular incisor is elliptic, an elongated oval on cervical cross section. Thus, the root is extremely narrow on the labial and lingual surfaces and wide on both proximal surfaces. Proximal root concavities are also present on both types of mandibular incisors and, if deep enough, give the teeth a double-rooted appearance.

Clinical Considerations with Permanent Mandibular Incisors

With attrition, the wearing away of a tooth surface caused by tooth-to-tooth contact, the incisal ridge can drastically change on the mandibular incisors as it becomes an incisal edge (see **Chapter 20**). Excessive attrition can even sometimes create a bow-shaped wear pattern on

FIGURE 16-17 Clinical view of severe attrition noted on the incisal surface of the permanent mandibular incisors as well as canines. (Courtesy of Margaret J. Fehrenbach, RDH, MS.)

the incisal edge from the incisal view, exposing the underlying dentin (Figure 16-17). The exposed dentin is more porous and can become unattractively intrinsically stained, or it can be affected by dentinal hypersensitivity (see Figure 13-12).

Although the concavities of the lingual surfaces of all mandibular incisors are less pronounced than that of maxillary incisors, supragingival tooth deposits (such as dental biofilm, calculus, and stain) tend to collect in the concavities. This buildup of deposits is aided by the mandibular incisors' position in the oral cavity near the duct openings of both the submandibular and sublingual salivary glands in the floor of the mouth. Saliva, with its mineral content, is released from these glands, causing the dental biofilm to mineralize quickly into supragingival calculus, along with the addition of stain. The addition of mesial drift over time can also add to increased deposit levels on these teeth from crowding (see Figure 20-21).

Instrumentation or restoration may be more difficult in this area because many patients have overlapping mandibular incisors owing to inadequate mandibular arch size and other occlusal factors. This crowding increases with age because of the physiologic process of mesial drift, even after orthodontic therapy, which can also complicate homecare. And if the incisors tip incisally back toward the tongue, instrumentation or restoration becomes extremely difficult, and use of a mouth mirror for indirect vision is essential.

Labial

Mesial

M D

Incisal

Lingual

Distal

FIGURE 16-18 Views of a permanent mandibular right central incisor.

Prolonged hand instrumentation can narrow even further the already narrow labial and lingual root surfaces of the mandibular incisors. The crowns of the teeth can thus be placed in jeopardy during mastication because of unsupported cervical enamel. Finally, the proximal surface of the roots can be difficult to explore with instruments or treat restoratively because of the limited interproximal space and the ovoid root shape, and the presence of proximal root concavities may also increase this difficulty.

PERMANENT MANDIBULAR CENTRAL INCISORS #24 AND #25 (#31 AND #41)

Specific Overall Features Permanent mandibular central incisors erupt between 6 and 7 years of age with root completion at age 9 (Figure 16-18). Thus, these teeth usually erupt before the maxillary central incisors. They are the smallest and simplest teeth of the permanent dentition; thus they are smaller than the lateral incisors of the same arch. Due to its smallness, the tooth has only one antagonist in the maxillary arch. This tooth and the maxillary third molar are the only teeth that have one antagonist; all others have two. Equally different is that the two mandibular centrals usually share a mesial contact area.

This tooth has a simple root, which is widest labiolingually and then mesiodistally. The root is a narrow oval in cross section. The root has pronounced proximal root concavities, which vary in both length and depth, and a shallow depression extends longitudinally along the midportion of root. The pulp cavity of the mandibular central is quite simple because it has a single pulp canal and three pulp horns (Figure 16-19).

Labial View Features The crown of a mandibular central incisor is quite symmetrical from the labial view, having a fan shape (see Figure 16-18). The imbrication lines and developmental depressions usually are not present or are extremely faint. The mesial contact with the other mandibular central is at the incisal third. The distal contact with the lateral incisor is also at the incisal third.

From the labial view, both the incisal angles, mesioincisal angle and distoincisal angle, are sharp or only slightly rounded; the mesioincisal angle is slightly sharper than the distoincisal angle, which *helps to distinguish the mandibular right central incisor from the left*. Nevertheless, differentiating between the right and left central incisors is often difficult. The mesial and distal outlines are nearly straight from the CEJ to the relatively straight incisal ridge.

Lingual View Features The crown outline of a mandibular central incisor is narrower on the lingual surface than the labial, which is

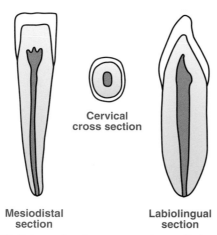

**Cervical
cross section**

**Mesiodistal
section**

**Labiolingual
section**

FIGURE 16-19 Pulp cavity of a permanent mandibular right central incisor.

the reverse of the labial view (see Figure 16-18). However, its outline of the crown is the most symmetrical of all incisors, either maxillary or mandibular. Overall, the lingual surface is less pronounced and has a small, centered cingulum.

On the lingual surface, the single lingual fossa is barely noticeable; therefore, the mesial marginal ridge and distal marginal ridge are barely noticeable as well. And because the cingulum is centered, the faint mesial and distal marginal ridges both have the same length.

Proximal View Features The CEJ curvature is higher incisally on the mesial than on the distal surface, which *helps to distinguish the mandibular right central incisor from the left* (see Figure 16-18). The incisal ridge is usually straight but can be rounded and is lingual to the long axis of the root. The distal view is similar to the mesial view of the tooth, except that the CEJ curves less incisally on the distal than on the mesial surface.

Incisal View Features The mandibular central incisor has a nearly symmetrical crown outline (see Figure 16-18). The incisal ridge is usually at 90°, or perpendicular, to the labiolingual axis of the crown of the tooth and overall it is just lingual to the long axis of the root. The labiolingual measurement is also wider than the mesiodistal measurement on incisal view. Again, on the lingual surface, the faint mesial marginal ridge and distal marginal ridge are both the same length.

Clinical Considerations with Permanent Mandibular Central Incisors

Root proximation with the contralateral mandibular central incisor may cause access difficulty for homecare and instrumentation. Developmental disturbances are rarely noted in the mandibular central incisors. One rare exception is that the teeth may have an accessory root or bifurcated root with the two branches having labial and lingual orientations.

PERMANENT MANDIBULAR LATERAL INCISORS #23 AND #26 (#32 AND #42)

Specific Overall Features Permanent mandibular lateral incisors erupt between 7 and 8 years of age with root completion at age 10 (Figure 16-20). Thus, these teeth usually erupt after the mandibular central incisors. The tooth is slightly larger overall than a central; there is also more variation overall in form too. The crown

is also slightly larger than that of a central, but it resembles a central in most other ways. From both the labial and lingual views, the crown appears tilted or twisted distally in regard to the long axis of the tooth; this gives the impression that the tooth has been bent at the CEJ.

The single root of a mandibular lateral is usually straight, slightly longer, and wider than that of a central. The root, like that of a mandibular central, has pronounced proximal root concavities, especially on the distal surface. These vary in both length and depth. The pulp cavity for this tooth is quite simple because it has a single pulp canal and three pulp horns (Figure 16-21).

Labial View Features The crown of a mandibular lateral incisor is not as symmetrical as that of a central and appears tilted or twisted distally on the root from the labial view (see Figure 16-20). The tooth is not symmetrical because the distal outline is slightly rounder and shorter compared with the slightly flatter and longer mesial outline. The incisal angles are different: The mesioincisal angle of the incisal ridge is sharper than the distoincisal angle, which *helps to distinguish the mandibular right lateral incisor from the left.* The labial developmental depressions are deeper than on the central incisors of the same arch.

From the labial view, the mesial contact with a mandibular central incisor is in the incisal third. The distal contact with a mandibular canine is in the incisal third but is located more cervically than the mesial contact.

Lingual View Features The crown of a mandibular lateral incisor lacks bilateral symmetry and again appears tilted or twisted distally on the root from the lingual view with its outline the reverse of the labial view (see Figure 16-20). Overall, the lingual surface has more prominent features as compared to the lingual surface of a central incisor. The small single cingulum lies just distal to the long axis of the root.

Thus on the lingual surface, both the mesial marginal ridge and the distal marginal ridge are more developed than on a central, and the mesial marginal ridge is longer than the distal marginal ridge. A single lingual fossa is also present, but a lingual pit is rarely present on a lateral, although this happens more often than on a central.

Proximal View Features The greater height of the CEJ curvature on the mesial than on the distal surface *helps to distinguish the mandibular right lateral incisor from the left* (see Figure 16-20). Also, from the mesial view, more of the lingual surface is visible because of the distal tilt or twist of the incisal ridge. The distal view is similar to the mesial view of the tooth, but the CEJ is curved less on the distal than the mesial surface.

Incisal View Features A rounder appearance is noted both labially and lingually from the incisal view of a mandibular lateral incisor as compared with that of a central (see Figure 16-20). The entire incisal ridge is not straight mesiodistally as it is in a central; instead, the incisal ridge curves toward the lingual in its distal part. Additionally the incisal angles are noticeably different: The distoincisal angle is visibly at a distinctly lingual location compared to the mesioincisal angle, and the cingulum appears displaced toward the distal. Again, on the lingual surface, the mesial marginal ridge is longer than the distal marginal ridge.

Clinical Considerations with Permanent Mandibular Lateral Incisors

Developmental disturbances are rare in a mandibular lateral incisor, as is the case with the central of the same arch. One rare exception is that the tooth may have an accessory root or bifurcated root with the two root branches having labial and lingual orientation.

Labial

Lingual

M   D

Incisal

Mesial

Distal

FIGURE 16-20 Views of a permanent mandibular right lateral incisor.

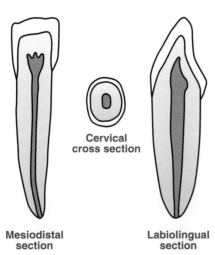

Mesiodistal
section

Cervical
cross section

Labiolingual
section

FIGURE 16-21 Pulp cavity of a permanent mandibular right lateral incisor.

PERMANENT CANINES

GENERAL FEATURES OF PERMANENT CANINES

Permanent canines are the four anterior teeth located at the corners of each quadrant for each dental arch (Table 16-2). Thus, it is the third tooth from the midline in each quadrant, distal to the incisors and mesial to the posteriors. The permanent canines are succedaneous and replace the primary canines of the same type.

Patients commonly call them the *eyeteeth;* an older term that was also used was *cuspids* because they were the only teeth in the permanent dentition with one cusp. The more commonly used term of *canines* comes from the Latin word for dog because they resemble dogs' teeth. Patients often complain of the slightly deeper yellow color of their permanent canines compared with their incisors, which is due to increased thickness and thus opaqueness. This property is placed in prosthetic teeth to mimic a more natural look.

TABLE 16-2	Permanent Canines		
	MAXILLARY CANINE		**MANDIBULAR CANINE**
Universal number	#6 and #11		#22 and #27
International number	#13 and #23		#33 and #43
General crown features	Single cusp with tip and slopes, labial ridge, cingulum, lingual ridge, marginal ridges, and lingual fossae		
Specific crown features	Longest tooth in arch		
	Prominent lingual surface. Sharp cusp tip		Less pronounced lingual surface. Less sharp cusp tip
Height of contour	Labial: Cervical third Lingual: Middle third		
Mesial contact	Junction of incisal third and middle thirds		Incisal third
Distal contact	Middle third		Junction of incisal and middle thirds
Distinguish right from left	Shorter mesial cusp slope, with more pronounced mesial CEJ curvature. More cervical contact on distal		
	More cervical contact on distal, with shorter distal outline on labial view with depression between the distal contact and CEJ		Shorter and rounder distal outline on labial view, with a shorter mesial slope than distal
General root features	Long, thick single root		
Specific root features	Oval on cross section. Proximal root concavities. Blunt root apex		Oval on cross section. Proximal root concavities, with developmental depressions on mesial and distal, giving tooth double-rooted appearance. Pointed apex

CEJ, Cementoenamel junction.

Because of their tapered shape and prominent cusp, the canines function to pierce or tear food during mastication (see Table 15-4). And because of their arch position, they serve as a major support of facial muscles and keep the overall vertical dimension of the face intact. Without their presence intact, facial contours cannot be maintained, and a loss of height occurs in the lower third of vertical dimension. Anatomists consider the canines the cornerstones of the dental arch because of their arch position, tooth form, and function.

The canines also support the incisors and premolars in their functions during mastication and speech. During occlusal movement, these teeth act as guideposts (see Figure 20-13). In this respect, they serve as a protective functional device for a type of mandibular movement that is termed *lateral deviation* (see **Chapter 20**). Finally, they can help relieve any excessive horizontal forces imposed on posteriors.

The canines are the most stable teeth in the dentition, one reason being their long root length, which offers an increased amount of periodontal tissue support. In addition, the proximal root concavities help to provide an increased periodontal anchorage for these teeth. Thus, these teeth have a significantly reduced risk of loss as a result of periodontal disease or traumatic injury, usually making them the last teeth present in an overall failing dentition. The canines (or many times only the roots) often serve as the stabilizing anchors for replacements of lost teeth in prosthetic procedures, such as the placement of partial fixed or removal dentures and permanent bridges. These teeth are also important esthetically because each one holds the skin of the labial commissure in its position, reducing the appearance of any deep lip lines or wrinkles present as the skin has a tendency to cave in here with increasing age.

Dental caries usually do not usually occur with canines, which is another factor that makes them an extremely stable tooth in the dentition. This is because the crown generally has a less pronounced form that promotes self-cleansing and does not easily retain dental biofilm or other deposits.

Both the maxillary and mandibular canines resemble one another (Figure 16-22). The crown of each is about the same size and, when viewed from the proximal, appears triangular like all anterior teeth (see Table 15-4). When viewed from the labial or lingual, however, its crown outline appears pentagonal with five sides. Canines are also wider labiolingually than the incisors, even wider than maxillary central incisors.

Similar to the other anteriors, each of the canines has an incisal ridge on its masticatory surface (see Figure 16-22). Different from the incisors is the cusp (kusp) tip, which is in line with the long axis of the root for both maxillary and mandibular canines when first erupted. Because of the presence of the cusp tip, the incisal ridge is divided into two cusp (kusp) slopes or ridges, rather than being nearly straight across like the incisors.

The mesial cusp slope is usually shorter than the distal cusp slope for both the maxillary and mandibular canines when they first erupt. The mesial cusp slope of a maxillary canine occludes with the distal cusp slope of a mandibular canine. The length of these cusp slopes and position of the cusp tip can change with attrition (discussed later).

The canines are the only teeth in the permanent dentition with a centrally placed vertical labial (lay-be-al) ridge (see Figure 16-22). This labial ridge is a result of greater development of the middle labial developmental lobe in comparison with the mesial and distal labial developmental lobes. Mamelons are usually not present on the incisal ridge as they are on incisors, but a small notch may be seen on either cusp slope. The height of contour on labial and lingual surfaces is in the cervical third for the canines, similar to all anteriors.

Each canine also has a cingulum and marginal ridges on its lingual surface, similar to the incisors (Figure 16-23). The cingulum corresponds to the lingual developmental lobe, as in the incisors, but is larger than on any incisor. As with the incisors, however, its crown is narrower on the lingual surface than on the labial surface with the crown tapering lingually.

In addition, canines have a centrally placed vertical lingual ridge that extends from the cusp tip to the cingulum. The lingual ridge creates two separate and shallow lingual fossae between it and the

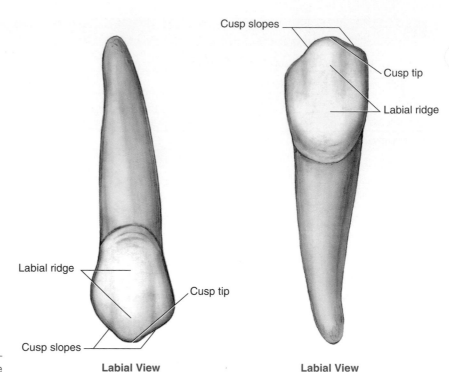

FIGURE 16-22 Labial views of newly erupted permanent canines with features noted; both teeth resemble each other.

Labial View
Permanent Maxillary Right Canine

Labial View
Permanent Mandibular Right Canine

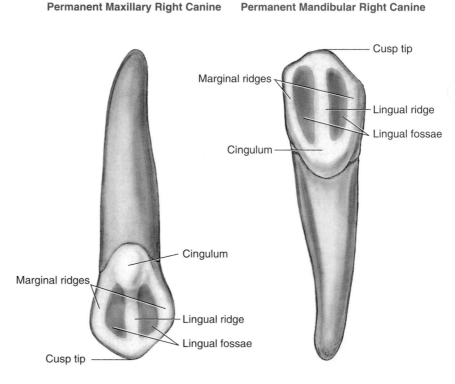

FIGURE 16-23 Lingual views of permanent canines and their features with lingual fossae highlighted; both teeth resemble each other.

Lingual View
Permanent Maxillary Right Canine

Lingual View
Permanent Mandibular Right Canine

bordering marginal ridges; these lingual fossae are more pronounced on the maxillary canines than on the mandibular.

The permanent canines are the longest teeth in the dentition. Each has a particularly long, thick root, and the root is usually one and one-half times the length of the crown. The long and large root is externally manifested in the jaws by the vertically oriented and labially placed bony ridge of the alveolar process called the *canine eminence,* which is especially noted on the maxillary arch. The root is oval or egg-shaped on cervical cross section (see Figures 16-26 and 16-29). Proximal root concavities are located on both proximal root surfaces.

Clinical Considerations with Permanent Canines

Changes can occur in the length of each canine cusp slope and in the position of the usually centered cusp tip. With attrition, the lengths of the cusp slopes are often altered due to this wearing away of a tooth

FIGURE 16-24 Lateral view of permanent canines altered on the incisal surfaces by attrition. The cusp tip of maxillary canines is now placed more to the distal of center with mesial displacement of the cusp tip for the mandibular canine. This also lengthens the mesial cusp slope, as well as shortening the distal one for the maxillary canines, while it shortens the mesial cusp slope and lengthens the distal one for the mandibular canines. (Courtesy of Margaret J. Fehrenbach, RDH, MS.)

surface caused by tooth-to-tooth contact and the overall narrower incisal ridges become wider incisal edges similar to worn incisors (Figure 16-24). With wear, each cusp tip of the maxillary canines is placed more to the distal of center with mesial displacement of the cusp tip for the mandibular canine. This wear also lengthens the mesial cusp slope and shortens the distal slope for the maxillary canines, while it shortens the mesial cusp slope and lengthens the distal slope for the mandibular canines. The related wear pattern on a canine from the incisal view can appear either diamond-shaped or triangular.

It is also noted that proximal surfaces of the canines are more accessible from the lingual than the labial approach during instrumentation or restoration. This is because of the convergence of the proximal surfaces toward the lingual.

PERMANENT MAXILLARY CANINES #6 AND #11 (#13 AND #23)
SPECIFIC OVERALL FEATURES

Permanent maxillary canines erupt between 11 and 12 years of age with root completion between ages 13 and 15 (Figure 16-25). Thus, these teeth usually erupt after the mandibular canines, after the maxillary incisors, and possibly after the maxillary premolars.

The crown of a maxillary canine is similar in length, or even shorter, than that of a maxillary central incisor. Labiolingually, the crown is considerably wider than that of a central incisor, but a canine crown is noticeably narrower mesiodistally. The cingulum on the lingual surface is more developed and larger than that of a central incisor of the same arch, making the tooth stronger during mastication.

A maxillary canine does somewhat resemble a mandibular canine. However, the cusp is more developed and larger, and the cusp tip is sharper as on all maxillary teeth. In addition, the entire lingual surface features of the maxillary canine are more prominent, including the lingual ridge and marginal ridges.

Finally, an entire maxillary canine is as long as a mandibular canine, but the crown is as long as, or slightly shorter, than that of a

mandibular canine. The long root is single and has a blunt apex; it is the longest root in the maxillary arch. Developmental depressions are evident on both proximal surfaces of the root but are especially pronounced on the distal surface owing to the distal prominence of crown at CEJ. Moderate to deep proximal concavities are also possible. The pulp cavity consists of a single pulp canal and a large pulp chamber (Figure 16-26). The pulp chamber usually has only one pulp horn.

LABIAL VIEW FEATURES

The mesial half of the crown of a maxillary canine resembles the nearby incisor, and the distal half resembles the nearby premolar, showing the transition in form from the incisors to the premolars in the maxillary arch (see Figure 16-25). Usually, both imbrication lines and perikymata are present in the cervical third of the surface, especially in newly erupted teeth (see Figure 12-9).

Two faint and vertical mesial and distal labial developmental depressions extend from the cervical to the incisal and separate the three labial developmental lobes. These depressions are located on either side of the centrally placed vertical labial ridge, and this ridge is most noticeable in the incisal part of the labial surface.

The mesial outline of the labial surface of the maxillary canine is usually rounded from the mesial contact area to the CEJ, but overall it is straighter than the distal outline. The distal outline is shorter than the mesial outline and usually has a depression between the distal contact area and the CEJ, which *helps to distinguish the maxillary right canine from the left*. From the labial view, the mesial and distal contacts are on two different levels of the tooth, which also *helps to distinguish the maxillary right canine from the left*. The mesial contact with the lateral incisor is at the junction of the incisal and the middle third. The distal contact with the first premolar is more cervical because it is at the middle third.

As previously discussed, the single cusp is round, and the mesial cusp slope of a maxillary canine is shorter than the distal cusp slope when first erupted, which again *helps to distinguish the maxillary right canine from the left*. The CEJ on the labial surface is evenly curved toward the root.

LINGUAL VIEW FEATURES

The mesial, distal, and incisal lingual outlines of a maxillary canine are similar to those on the labial view of the tooth (Figure 16-27). The overall dimension of the lingual surface is less than that of the labial surface, however, because the both mesial and distal surfaces converge slightly toward the lingual. The cingulum is large and usually less pronounced and is centered mesiodistally on the lingual surface.

The lingual surface also has a prominent mesial marginal ridge and distal marginal ridge. A centrally placed vertical lingual ridge is also present from the cingulum to the cusp tip, separating two lingual fossae—the shallow but visible mesiolingual fossa and distolingual fossa. Each of the major features of this tooth are "variations on a theme": The cingulum and incisal half of the lingual surface are sometimes separated by a shallow lingual groove, and this groove may contain a lingual pit near its center, or the pit may also be present without the lingual groove.

PROXIMAL VIEW FEATURES

The mesial and distal aspects present a triangular outline (see Figure 16-25 and Table 15-4). They resemble the maxillary incisors but are stronger looking, especially in the cingulum region. The CEJ curves

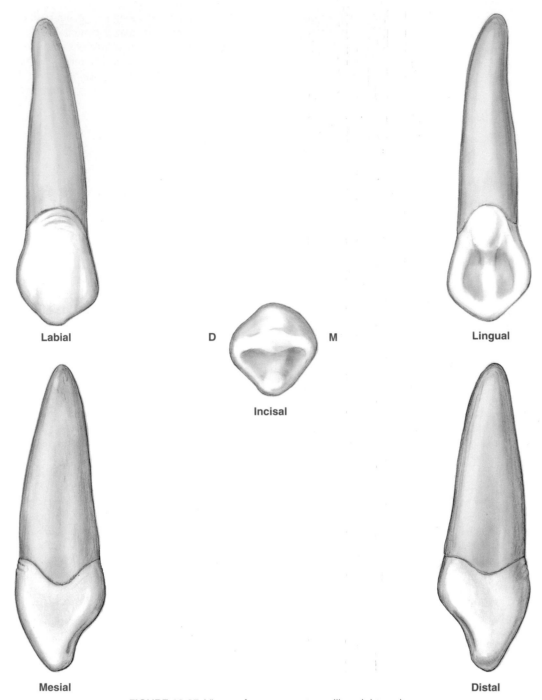

Labial

D   M

Incisal

Lingual

Mesial

Distal

FIGURE 16-25 Views of a permanent maxillary right canine.

higher incisally on the mesial than on the distal surface, *which helps to distinguish the maxillary right canine from the left*. The cusp tip is toward the labial. The distal view of the tooth is similar to the mesial view, but the CEJ curvature is less on the distal than on the mesial surface.

INCISAL VIEW FEATURES

Again, the labiolingual width of a maxillary canine is large in comparison with that of any other anterior tooth, making it an extremely strong tooth during mastication (see Figure 16-25). Additionally,

the crown outline is asymmetrical; the mesial part of the crown has greater labiolingual bulk. The distal part of the crown appears thinner than the mesial and gives the impression of being stretched to make contact with the first premolar.

More specifically, the mesial half of the labial outline is quite rounded, and the distal half is frequently concave. The distal half of the lingual outline is also frequently concave because the distal fossa is deeper and thus more pronounced. The mesial marginal ridge is longer than the distal marginal ridge. The cusp slopes seem to form a nearly straight line; the tip of the cusp is displaced labially and mesial to the central long axis.

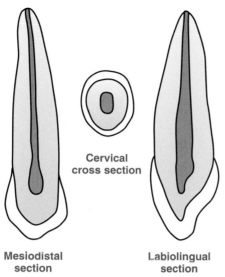

FIGURE 16-26 Pulp cavity of a permanent maxillary right canine.

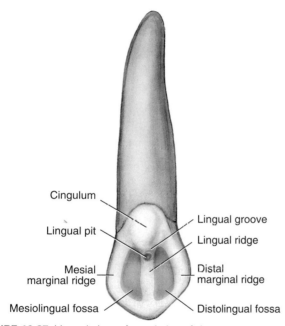

FIGURE 16-27 Lingual view of a variation of the permanent maxillary right canine and features with lingual fossae highlighted.

Clinical Considerations with Permanent Maxillary Canines

Because the maxillary canines erupt after the maxillary incisors and possibly the maxillary premolars, their expected dental arch space often is partially closed. Because of this they may erupt labially or lingually to the surrounding teeth. The maxillary canines may also fail to erupt fully, remaining impacted (im-pak-ted) within the alveolar process. An impacted tooth is an unerupted or partially erupted tooth that is positioned against another tooth, bone, or even soft tissue in a way that makes complete eruption unlikely. As a result, surgical exposure and maintenance orthodontic therapy may be needed, which may in some cases be prevented by careful evaluation of mixed dentition, and institution of any needed interceptive orthodontic therapy. Finally, developmental cyst formation may occur within the dental tissue of an impacted crown of a maxillary canine, resulting in a dentigerous cyst.

The cingula on the maxillary canines may exhibit tubercles or extra cusps that are located near the most incisal level of the cingulum. A lingual pit is often associated with the presence of tubercles. In addition, the distal prominence of the crown is at the CEJ, which may cause instrumentation and restoration difficulties on the distal root surface. The root of maxillary canines may also undergo distorted angulations or dilaceration, and there may be several curvatures along its length. With root curvature in the apical third, the root is usually curved distally.

PERMANENT MANDIBULAR CANINES #22 AND #27 (#33 AND #43)
SPECIFIC OVERALL FEATURES

Permanent mandibular canines erupt between 9 and 10 years of age with root completion between ages 12 and 14 (Figure 16-28). Thus, these teeth usually erupt before the maxillary canines and after most of the incisors have erupted.

A mandibular canine closely resembles a maxillary canine. Although the entire tooth is usually as long, a mandibular canine is narrower labiolingually and mesiodistally than a maxillary canine. The crown of this tooth can be equal to in length, or even longer than that of a maxillary canine.

The single cusp is not as well developed in size, and the two cusp ridges are thinner labiolingually than those of a maxillary canine. The single cusp tip usually is not as sharp. In addition, the cusp tip is lined up with the long axis of the root, but it is sometimes positioned lingually, similar to the mandibular incisors.

The lingual surface of the crown of a mandibular canine is less pronounced than that of a maxillary canine, having a less developed cingulum and two marginal ridges. Thus, the lingual surface of this crown more closely resembles the form of the lingual surface of the adjacent mandibular lateral incisors, despite the added feature of a lingual ridge.

The single root of a mandibular canine may be as long as that of a maxillary canine but is usually somewhat shorter, although it still has the longest mandibular root. The root has a slight mesial inclination. The mesial developmental depression on the root is more pronounced and often deeper compared with that of a maxillary canine. A distal developmental depression similar to the mesial one is also apparent. These proximal concavities may extend the full length of the root. These depressions may be extremely pronounced, to the point of creating a labial and lingual component in the apical third and giving the tooth a double-rooted appearance. The root apex is also more pointed on this tooth than on a maxillary canine.

The pulp cavity of a mandibular canine resembles that of a maxillary canine in that they both usually have a single pulp canal and a large pulp chamber (Figure 16-29). There is also only one pulp horn. The major difference is that a mandibular canine may have two separate pulp canals. If the tooth has two canals, one is placed labially and the other lingually; the canals may join at the apex or have separate apical foramina.

LABIAL VIEW FEATURES

The labial surface on a mandibular canine is not as rounded as that on a maxillary canine, especially in the incisal two-thirds of the tooth (see Figure 16-28). In contrast, however, a mandibular canine is generally rounder than a mandibular incisor.

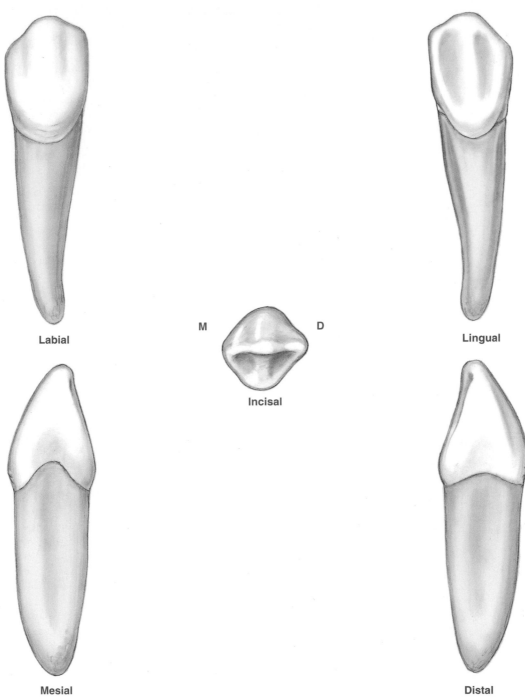

Labial

Lingual

M   D

Incisal

Mesial

Distal

FIGURE 16-28 Views of a permanent mandibular right canine.

Imbrication lines are not usually present on the labial surface, unlike a maxillary canine. Two faint and vertically placed mesial and distal labial developmental depressions separate the three labial lobes, similar to the maxillary canine and incisors. These depressions are located on either side of the centrally placed vertical labial ridge, which is not as prominent as that of a maxillary canine.

From the labial view, the mesial outline is almost a straight line from the mesial contact to the CEJ, straighter than on a maxillary canine. The distal outline is shorter and rounder than the mesial outline, similar to that of a maxillary canine, which *helps to distinguish the mandibular right canine from the left.*

From the labial view, similar to a maxillary canine, the mesial and distal contacts are on different levels of the tooth, which also *helps to distinguish the mandibular right canine from the left.* The mesial contact with the lateral incisor is in the incisal third. The distal contact with the first premolar is at the junction of the incisal and middle thirds, at a more cervically placed location than that on the mesial side.

As discussed earlier, the cusp slopes are different: The mesial cusp slope of a mandibular canine is shorter than the distal cusp slope when first erupted from the labial view, which again *helps to distinguish the mandibular right canine from the left.* With attrition, the central cusp tip moves to the mesial, shortening the already short mesial

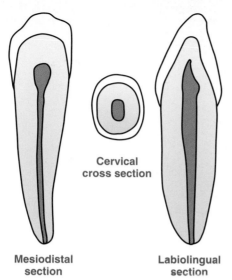

FIGURE 16-29 Pulp cavity of a permanent mandibular right canine.

Mesiodistal section

Cervical cross section

Labiolingual section

cusp slope and further lengthening the distal cusp slope. The CEJ is evenly curved toward the root.

LINGUAL VIEW FEATURES

The lingual surface is less pronounced, except for the faintly demarcated features of a lingual ridge, mesial marginal ridge, distal marginal ridge, and two lingual fossae, the distolingual fossa and mesiolingual fossa (see Figure 16-28). The less developed cingulum on a mandibular canine is not centered as on a maxillary canine but lies distal to the long axis of the root. In addition, the cingulum also does not extend as far incisally as it does in the maxillary canines. Rarely are there any lingual pits or lingual grooves on this surface.

PROXIMAL VIEW FEATURES

A mandibular canine is, again, similar to a maxillary canine from a mesial view with a similar triangular shape and pointed cusp on the crown (see Figure 16-28 and Table 15-4). However, a less developed cingulum and thinner marginal ridges are seen. The cusp tip is more lingually inclined without incisal wear, unlike the labially placed cusp tip on a maxillary canine.

The CEJ curvature on the mesial surface is more toward the incisal when compared to the same surface of a maxillary canine. Additionally, the CEJ curve is more toward the incisal on the mesial surface than the distal on this same tooth, which *helps to distinguish the mandibular right canine from the left*. The distal view is similar to the mesial aspect. The one exception is that the CEJ is curved less on the distal than on the mesial surface.

INCISAL VIEW FEATURES

A mandibular canine from this view is similar to a maxillary canine, but it is slightly more symmetrical compared with the maxillary tooth (see Figure 16-28). Additionally, the crown is wider labiolingually than mesiodistally and is offset toward the mesial. The less developed cingulum is offset toward the distal. This placement still gives the tooth only a slight asymmetrical appearance from this view, less than a maxillary canine.

The mesial marginal ridge is longer than the distal marginal ridge. The labial outline is also rounder mesiodistally than that of the mandibular incisors because of the slightly more pronounced labial ridge.

Clinical Considerations with Permanent Mandibular Canines

The dilaceration of the root can also occur with a mandibular canine, similar to a maxillary canine (see **Chapter 6**). Another developmental disturbance that may occur is an accessory root or bifurcated root in the apical third with labial and lingual root branches. This tooth is the anterior tooth most likely to have a bifurcated root, although this still is rare.

CHAPTER 17

Permanent Posterior Teeth

ⓔ Additional resources and practice exercises are provided on the companion Evolve website for this book:
http://evolve.elsevier.com/Fehrenbach/illustrated

●●●LEARNING OBJECTIVES

1. Define and pronounce the key terms in this chapter.
2. Identify the permanent posterior teeth and discuss their properties and the clinical considerations concerning them, integrating it into patient care.
3. Identify the permanent premolars and their general features and discuss their clinical considerations, integrating it into patient care.
4. Describe the general and specific features of the permanent maxillary premolars and discuss the clinical considerations concerning them, integrating it into patient care.
5. Describe the general and specific features of the permanent mandibular premolars and discuss the clinical considerations concerning them, integrating it into patient care.
6. Identify the permanent molars and their general features and discuss their clinical considerations, integrating it into patient care.
7. Describe the general and specific features of the permanent maxillary molars and discuss the clinical considerations concerning them, integrating it into patient care.
8. Describe the general and specific features of the permanent mandibular molars and discuss the clinical considerations concerning them, integrating it into patient care.
9. Assign the correct names and universal or international tooth number for each permanent posterior tooth on a diagram or a skull and for a tooth model or a patient.
10. Demonstrate the correct location of each permanent posterior tooth on a diagram, a skull, and a patient.

PERMANENT POSTERIOR TEETH PROPERTIES

The permanent posterior teeth include the premolars and molars (Figure 17-1; see Figures 2-4 and 15-2). The crown of each has an occlusal surface as its masticatory surface, bordered by the raised marginal ridges that are located on both the distal surface and mesial surface (Figure 17-2). The occlusal surface also has two or more cusps. Some anatomists liken a cusp to a *gothic pyramid* with four **cusp** (kusp) **ridges** descending from each cusp tip. Between these cusp ridges are sloping areas, or four **inclined cuspal** (kusp-al) **planes**. These planes are named by combining the names of the two cusp ridges that are between them. Some inclined planes are functional and thus involved in the occlusion of the teeth (see **Chapter 20**).

The occlusal surface of permanent posteriors creates an inner **occlusal** (ah-kloo-zl) **table** bordered by the marginal ridges (Figure 17-3). It is important to note that the discussion of the maxillary first premolar has extensive coverage of its occlusal table since it is the first posterior tooth discussed in this chapter; this information can then be related to the occlusal tables of other posterior teeth.

There are also **triangular ridges**, which are cusp ridges that descend from the cusp tips toward the central part of the occlusal table (Figure 17-4). They are so named because the slopes of each side of the ridge are inclined in a way that resembles two sides of a triangle. Thus, the triangular ridges are specifically named for the cusps to which they belong. Additionally present on many posteriors is a **transverse** (trans-**vers**) **ridge**, a collective term given to the joining of two triangular ridges crossing the occlusal table transversely, or from the labial to the lingual outline.

Each shallow and wide depression on the occlusal table is a **fossa** (fos-ah) (plural, **fossae** [**fos**-ay]). One type of fossa on posteriors, the **central fossa**, is located at the convergence of the cusp ridges in a central point, where the grooves meet. Another type of fossa is the **triangular fossa**, which forms a triangular shape at the convergence of the cusp ridges, and is associated with the termination of the triangular grooves (discussed next). Located in the deepest parts of some of the

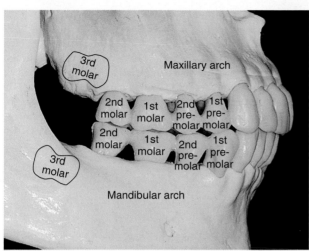

FIGURE 17-1 Permanent posterior teeth identified on a skull, which include the premolars and molars. Note that the third molars have not erupted yet. (Courtesy of Margaret J. Fehrenbach, RDH, MS.)

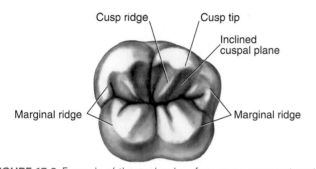

FIGURE 17-2 Example of the occlusal surface on a permanent posterior tooth with its features noted.

A

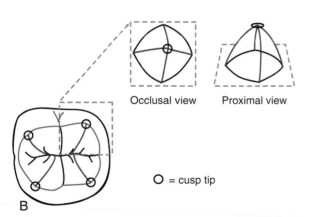

B

FIGURE 17-3 Occlusal views of a permanent posterior tooth. **A,** Occlusal table highlighted. **B,** Triangular ridges highlighted with a close-up of the *gothic pyramid* shape of the cusp that many anatomists refer to when discussing these features.

fossae are occlusal pits; each developmental pit is a sharp pinpoint depression where two or more grooves meet.

Developmental grooves (or primary grooves) are also found on the occlusal table. The developmental grooves on each different posterior tooth type are located in the same place and are thought to mark the junction between the developmental lobes. The grooves are sharp, deep, V-shaped linear depressions. The most prominent developmental groove on posteriors is the central groove, which generally travels mesiodistally and separates the occlusal table buccolingually. Lobe discussion, as was noted in **Chapter 6,** is controversial but is included for completeness when discussing in detail the various tooth types.

Other developmental grooves are marginal grooves, which cross the marginal ridges and serve as spillways, allowing food to escape during mastication. Finally, there are triangular grooves that separate a marginal ridge from the triangular ridge of a cusp and at their terminations form the triangular fossae.

In contrast, supplemental grooves (or secondary grooves) appear as shallower, more irregular linear depressions on the occlusal table (Figure 17-5). Supplemental grooves branch from the developmental grooves, but these grooves are not always present in the same pattern on the occlusal table of each different tooth type. In general, the more posterior a tooth is located in the dental arch, the more supplemental

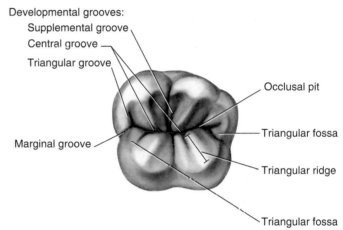

FIGURE 17-4 Example of the other features of the occlusal table on a permanent posterior tooth, including the central groove with the triangular fossae highlighted.

FIGURE 17-5 Example of supplemental grooves on the occlusal surface of an extracted permanent posterior tooth, the maxillary third molar. The more posterior a tooth is located in the dental arch, the more supplemental grooves are present. (Courtesy of Margaret J. Fehrenbach, RDH, MS.)

grooves are present, such that the occlusal table appears more wrinkled. Grooves are sometimes called *fissures*.

For posteriors, the height of contour for the crown's buccal surface is in the cervical third, and for the lingual surface it is in the middle third (Figure 17-6). When compared with anteriors, most of the posteriors are wider labiolingually than mesiodistally, except for the mandibular molars.

In another comparison with anteriors, the contact areas of posteriors are wider, usually located at the buccal of center, and nearer to the same level on each proximal surface (see Figure 15-10). In addition, on each proximal surface is a cementoenamel junction (CEJ) curvature that is less pronounced on the posteriors than on the anteriors. In fact, the CEJ is often quite straight for posteriors.

Like anterior teeth, **multirooted** premolars and molars originate as a single root on the base of the crown (Figure 17-7). This part on these posterior teeth is considered the **root trunk**. The cervical cross section of the root trunk initially follows the form of the crown. Unlike anteriors, the root of a posterior tooth divides from the root trunk into the correct number of root branches for its tooth type (see Figure 6-21). This can be with either two roots, which means it is **bifurcated** (bi-fer-kay-ted), or with three roots, which means it is **trifurcated** (try-fer-kay-ted). In some cases, a bifurcated tooth may additionally have **root fusion** with little of the remaining root trunk being truly bifurcated.

An area between two or more of these root branches, before they divide from the root trunk, is a **furcation** (fer-kay-shin) (Table 17-1; see Figure 17-7). The spaces between the roots at the furcation are the **furcation crotches**. Bifurcated teeth with two roots, such as the maxillary first premolar and mandibular molars, have two furcation crotches; trifurcated teeth with three roots, such as maxillary molars, have three furcation crotches. Such crotches can be located on various surfaces, depending on tooth type—each with a slightly different individual configuration. With periodontal health, these features of the root(s) are covered by the alveolar process as well as overlying gingival tissue.

Clinical Considerations for Permanent Posterior Teeth

The complex pit and groove patterns on the occlusal surface of posteriors can put them at an increased risk of caries (Figure 17-8). This susceptibility is due to increased dental biofilm retention and the weakness of enamel forming the walls of the pits and grooves (see Figure 12-4, *A*). Clinicians need to be aware of these pit and groove patterns on the posteriors when they examine dentitions to assess the patient's caries risk level. Thus the pits and grooves (or fissures) must be checked for decay with an explorer and mirror. In addition, using light-induced devices that measure changes in laser fluorescence of hard tissue allows dental professionals to better diagnose early lesions in pits and grooves. Posteriors with deep pit and groove patterns, but without incipient decay, should have enamel sealants applied as soon as possible.

PERMANENT PREMOLARS

GENERAL FEATURES OF PERMANENT PREMOLARS

Permanent premolars are the most anteriorly placed posteriors in the permanent dentition (Figure 17-9; Table 17-2). Each dental arch has four premolars, two to each quadrant.

There are two types of premolars: first premolar and second premolar. One of each type is present in each quadrant of each dental arch. The first is closer to the midline at the fourth position from it. The second is next to the first premolar and is in the fifth position from the midline. Both types are distal to the permanent canine and mesial to the permanent first molar when full eruption of the permanent dentition has occurred. Permanent premolars are succedaneous because the first and second premolars replace the primary first and second molars, respectively.

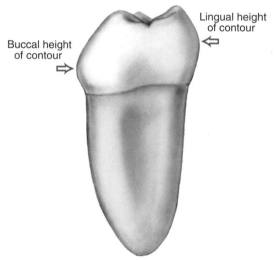

FIGURE 17-6 Height of contour on a permanent posterior tooth.

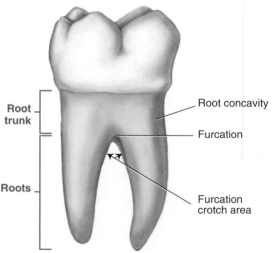

FIGURE 17-7 Buccal root features of both a permanent maxillary and a mandibular molar.

TABLE 17-1	Permanent Posterior Tooth Furcations and Furcation Crotches

FURCATIONS AND FURCATION CROTCHES

Maxillary Right First Premolar

B L
14 mm
1/2 7 mm

Mesial Aspect

L B
14 mm
1/2 7 mm

Distal Aspect

Maxillary Right First Molar*

DB L MB
12 mm   13 mm   12 mm
1/2 4 mm

Buccal Aspect

MB L
12 mm   13 mm
2/3 3 mm

Mesial Aspect

MB
L DB
13 mm   12 mm
1/2 5 mm

Distal Aspect

Mandibular Right First Molar*

3 mm
1/2
D M
14 mm

Buccal Aspect

4 mm
1/2
M D
14 mm

Lingual Aspect

*Second and third molars for each arch are similar to first, but have longer root trunks so that furcations of more posterior molars are located more apically and with roots closer together, creating tighter furcation entrances.

(All data from Nelson S: *Wheeler's dental anatomy, physiology, and occlusion,* ed 10, Philadelphia, 2015, Saunders/Elsevier.)

Premolars function to assist the molars in grinding food during mastication because of the broad occlusal surface and the prominent cusps. Premolars also assist the canines in piercing and tearing food with those cusps. The crown outline from the buccal and lingual is pentagonal, or five-sided, similar to the canines (see Table 15-4). These teeth, along with the canines, also help maintain the height of the lower third of the vertical dimension of the face, supporting the facial muscles, especially those muscles at the labial commissures. Thus, the premolars are involved in both esthetics and speech, less so than the anteriors, but more so than the molars.

An older term for a premolar was *bicuspid* because of the usual presence of two cusps on the occlusal surface, which is one more cusp than in the canines. However, the mandibular second premolar frequently has three cusps. Thus, the term *premolar* is more widely used because these teeth are located anterior to the molars.

FIGURE 17-8 Example of a complex pit and groove pattern on the occlusal surface of an extracted permanent posterior tooth. (Courtesy of Margaret J. Fehrenbach, RDH, MS.)

Finally, along with the cusps, the occlusal surface of a premolar, similar to all posteriors, has marginal ridges, triangular ridges, developmental grooves, and occlusal pits. The boundaries of the occlusal surface, created by these marginal ridges and cusp ridges, form the inner occlusal table.

As posterior teeth, premolars have a shorter crown than anterior teeth. The buccal surface is rounded and has a prominent centrally located vertical **buccal (buk-al) ridge** (Figure 17-10). The buccal ridge of premolars is similar to the labial ridge of the canines and may be related to the increased development of the middle buccal lobe. Two buccal developmental depressions are noted on each side of the buccal ridge. The height of contour for premolars is in the cervical third on the buccal surface, similar to all anteriors. And the height of contour on the lingual is in the middle third like all posteriors.

Most premolars usually have one root, except for the permanent maxillary first premolar, which has two roots. Whether one or two roots are present, all have proximal root concavities present.

Clinical Considerations for Permanent Premolars

In some cases, a permanent premolar can be extracted in each quadrant during orthodontic therapy to improve dental arch spacing. If a premolar has been extracted, the distinctive pit and groove patterns on the occlusal surface will help in identifying the remaining premolar when the arch space from the extraction is lost, unless the tooth has been restored. However, orthodontic therapy tends instead to now include expansion of the jaw, if needed, instead of removing premolars so as to retain a more natural rounded curved shape to the arches. If extraction is unavoidable, first premolars are usually extracted more often than second premolars. Additionally, premolars present difficulties in instrumentation of the root because they have proximal root concavities, especially on the mesial of the maxillary first premolar.

TABLE 17-2	**Permanent Premolars**			
	MAXILLARY FIRST PREMOLAR	**MAXILLARY SECOND PREMOLAR**	**MANDIBULAR FIRST PREMOLAR**	**MANDIBULAR SECOND PREMOLAR**
Universal number	#5 and #12	#4 and #13	#21 and #28	#20 and #29
International number	#14 and #24	#15 and #25	#34 and #44	#35 and #45
General crown features	Occlusal table with marginal ridges and cusps with tips, ridges, inclined planes, grooves, fossae, and pits			
	Buccal ridge			
Specific crown features	Larger than second. Buccal cusp longer of two cusps. Long central groove. Mesial surface features unlike second	Smaller than first. Two cusps same length. Short central groove, with increased supplemental grooves. No mesial surface features like first	Smaller than second. Smaller lingual cusp of two cusps. Mesial surface features	Larger than first. Usually three cusps with: Y-shaped groove pattern or two cusps with H- or U–shaped groove pattern. Increased supplemental grooves
Mesial and distal contact*	Just cervical to junction of occlusal and middle thirds			
Distinguish right from left	Longer mesial cusp slope than distal cusp slope, with mesial features: deeper CEJ curvature, marginal groove, developmental depression	Lingual cusp offset to the mesial	Shorter mesial cusp slope than distal cusp slope, with mesial surface features: deeper mesial CEJ curvature and mesiolingual groove	Distal marginal ridge more cervically located, thus more occlusal surface visible from distal view
General root features	Two roots with root trunk		Single root	
Specific root features	Elliptic on cross section. Proximal root concavities		Oval or elliptic on cross section. Proximal root concavities	

CEJ, Cementoenamel junction.
*Height of contour of posteriors for the buccal is in cervical third and lingual in middle third.

PERMANENT MAXILLARY PREMOLARS
GENERAL FEATURES

Both types of maxillary premolars resemble each other more than the mandibular premolars resemble each other (see Figures 17-11 and 17-17). However, a maxillary first premolar is larger than a maxillary second premolar. In contrast, a mandibular first premolar is smaller than a mandibular second premolar. In keeping though, both maxillary premolars erupt earlier than the mandibular premolars.

The crown of a maxillary premolar is shorter occlusocervically than that of the nearby maxillary canine, but is slightly longer than that of the adjacent molars. The crown outline from each proximal aspect is trapezoidal, or four-sided with only two parallel sides, similar to all maxillary posteriors (see Table 15-4). The maxillary premolars are composed of four developmental lobes: three buccal and one lingual.

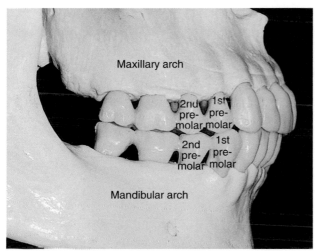

FIGURE 17-9 Permanent premolars identified on a skull. (Courtesy of Margaret J. Fehrenbach, RDH, MS.)

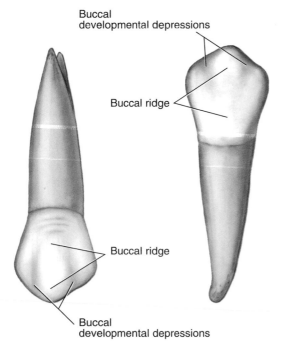

FIGURE 17-10 Buccal features of permanent premolars and their similar features.

The crown is also centered over the root and shows no lingual inclination, unlike the mandibular premolars, which are like other mandibular posteriors. They also have a greater buccolingual width than mesiodistal width compared with the mandibular premolars or other mandibular posterior teeth when viewed from the occlusal. The crown outline for both maxillary premolars is somewhat hexagonal from this view, or six-sided, and it is almost oval compared with the rounder mandibular premolars.

Both maxillary premolars have two cusps of almost equal size. In contrast, the mandibular premolars can have more than two cusps, but any lingual cusps are always smaller. Like all premolars, these cusps are centered over the long axis of the tooth from either proximal view.

The roots of the maxillary premolars are shorter than the maxillary canine's roots, but the root length is the same as that of the molars. The roots show slight lingual and distal inclination. The roots on cervical cross section are elliptic, or an elongated oval, but which may be slightly altered by proximal root concavities.

Clinical Considerations for Permanent Maxillary Premolars

The roots of maxillary premolars may penetrate the anterior part of the maxillary sinus as a result of accidental trauma or during tooth extraction because of the close relation of these roots to the sinus walls, which can occur with other maxillary posterior teeth (see Figure 11-22). To complicate matters, the discomfort of sinusitis can be mistakenly interpreted as tooth-related from the maxillary premolar, and vice versa. Thus, radiographs of the questionable tooth and maxillary sinus, as well as other diagnostic tests are necessary to determine the cause of the discomfort.

PERMANENT MAXILLARY FIRST PREMOLARS #5 AND #12 (#14 AND #24)

Specific Overall Features Permanent maxillary first premolars erupt between 10 and 11 years of age with root completion between ages 12 to 13 (Figure 17-11). These teeth erupt distal to the primary maxillary canines or the open arch space, and thus are the succedaneous replacements for the primary maxillary first molars.

The crown of a maxillary first premolar has an angular shape with a sharply defined outline compared with a maxillary second premolar's more rounded shape. The tooth's two cusps are also sharply defined with the buccal cusp usually about 1 mm higher than the lingual cusp. The central groove on the occlusal surface is also longer on the maxillary first premolar than on the second. The tooth appears bent mesially when viewed from the occlusal compared with the second premolar of the same arch.

Most maxillary first premolars are bifurcated, having two root branches in the apical third: a buccal root and lingual (or palatal) root. This is unlike the other premolars, which are single-rooted. However, maxillary first premolars originate as a single root on the base of the crown, as do other premolars as well as anteriors; this part is considered the root trunk.

A cervical cross section of the root trunk of the bifurcated tooth follows the crown form. The root trunk usually makes up half the length of the entire root, and the root branches make up the other half. The roots are rounded overall and taper to sharp apices. The buccal root is larger but not longer than the lingual root. However, root anatomy can get even more complex with this tooth. The root trunk can also have undergone root fusion with little of the remaining root trunk being truly bifurcated.

Because the maxillary first molar has both a buccal and lingual root, it also has two furcations, which are located on both the mesial and distal surfaces (see Table 17-1). Both of these furcations are located midway on the root surface, with both 7 mm from the CEJ.

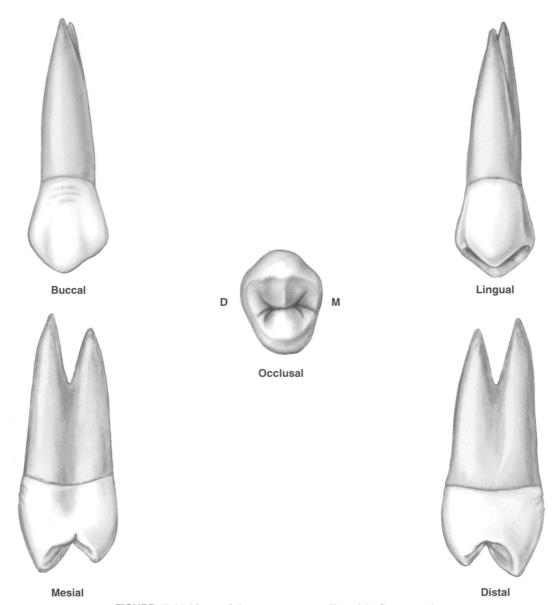

Buccal

D   M

Occlusal

Lingual

Mesial

Distal

FIGURE 17-11 Views of the permanent maxillary right first premolar.

In addition, a distinct mesial root concavity is present on the root trunk of the maxillary first premolar, extending from the contact area to the bifurcation. An additional mesial surface groove on the root puts this tooth possibly at an increased risk for periodontal disease because it allows an increased deposit level (see earlier discussion). The distal surface has a groove but it is reduced in depth, creating a more less-risky convex or flat surface.

If a single root is present, as is the case in about 20% of the cases, it is wider buccolingually than mesiodistally, both the buccal and lingual surfaces are rounded, and the root is tapered to a blunt apex. In cross section, the root becomes kidney shaped. A single root also has a deep and wide mesial surface root concavity, which ranges from relatively shallow to deep enough to almost bifurcate the root. Trifurcated teeth have been occasionally found with this tooth with two buccal roots and a single lingual root.

The pulp cavity for a bifurcated tooth usually shows two pulp horns (one for each cusp) and two pulp canals (one for each root) (Figure 17-12). Even if there is only one undivided root like the maxillary second premolar, two pulp canals are usually found, although they often combine apically to form one apical foramen.

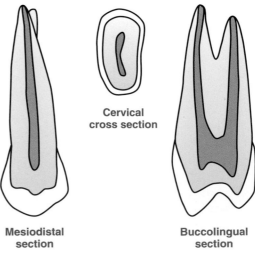

Cervical cross section

Mesiodistal section

Buccolingual section

FIGURE 17-12 Pulp cavity of the permanent maxillary right first premolar.

Buccal View Features The crown of a maxillary first premolar is the widest mesiodistally of all the premolars (Figure 17-13). This tooth's crown is wide at the level of the contact areas, becoming narrower at the CEJ, which is similar to the adjacent maxillary canine. The mesial contact with the maxillary canine is just cervical to the junction of the occlusal and middle thirds. The distal contact with the maxillary second premolar is the same, just cervical to the junction of the occlusal and middle thirds.

The mesial and distal outlines of the crown of the maxillary first premolar are both almost straight from the contact areas to the CEJ, but the mesial outline is more rounded. Both of these outlines converge more toward the cervical than they do on the maxillary second premolars. Imbrication lines and perikymata are found on the buccal surface, and these extend mesiodistally in the cervical third. The CEJ curvature of the tooth is evenly rounded toward the apex of the tooth and has less depth than on anterior teeth.

The buccal cusp of a maxillary first premolar is high and sharp, located slightly distal to the long axis of the tooth because the two cusp slopes of the buccal cusp are not equal in height. This tooth is the only tooth in the permanent dentition that has a buccal cusp with the mesial cusp slope longer than the distal cusp slope, which *helps to distinguish the maxillary right first premolar from the left.* This relationship of the cusp slopes usually exists upon eruption but any attrition may change it. A bulge may be found occasionally on the buccal cusp of this tooth.

Lingual View Features The lingual surface of the maxillary first premolar is rounded in all directions but is smaller than the buccal surface (see Figure 17-11). The shorter lingual cusp is sharp but not as sharp as the buccal cusp and is offset toward the mesial. Thus, the cusp slopes of the lingual cusp are again not equal in length. From the lingual aspect, however, the mesial cusp slope is shorter than the distal cusp slope.

Proximal View Features On the mesial surface of the crown of a maxillary first premolar, the mesial marginal ridge is present on the concave occlusal margin. A mesial marginal groove is also sometimes present (Figure 17-14). This developmental groove crosses the mesial marginal ridge and extends from the occlusal to the middle third of the crown, lingual to the contact area.

Also the mesial surface usually has a mesial developmental depression located cervical to the contact area, crossing the CEJ, and extending onto the root. On the root, the depression joins a deep developmental root concavity between the roots. The CEJ curvature is more occlusally located on the mesial than on the distal surface. All of these prominent mesial features from the proximal view *help to distinguish the maxillary right first premolar from the left.*

The distal surface is similar to the mesial, except that it does not have a depression, and more of the occlusal surface shows because the distal marginal ridge is more cervically located than is the mesial marginal ridge (see Figure 17-11). A distal marginal groove is sometimes located across the distal marginal ridge, but this distal groove is shallower than the similar groove on the mesial surface. Additionally, the CEJ curvature on the distal surface is not as deep cervically as the mesial.

Occlusal View Features The outline of the occlusal surface of a maxillary first premolar is somewhat hexagonal, or six-sided, but is wider buccolingually than mesiodistally (Figure 17-15). The buccal ridge (or buccal cusp ridge of the buccal cusp, as discussed later) is prominent on the buccal margin, and the lingual margin of the

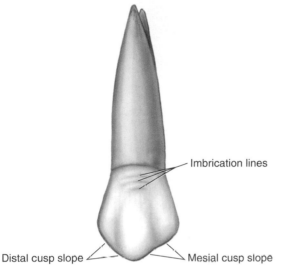

FIGURE 17-13 Buccal features of the permanent maxillary right first premolar.

Imbrication lines

Distal cusp slope   Mesial cusp slope

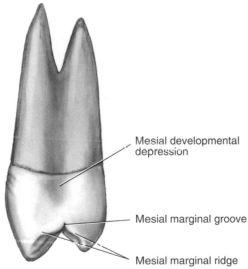

FIGURE 17-14 Mesial features of the permanent maxillary right first premolar.

Mesial developmental depression

Mesial marginal groove

Mesial marginal ridge

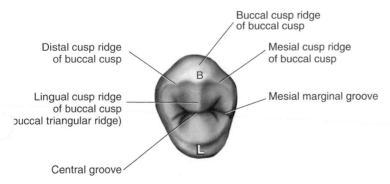

Buccal cusp ridge of buccal cusp

Distal cusp ridge of buccal cusp

Mesial cusp ridge of buccal cusp

Lingual cusp ridge of buccal cusp (buccal triangular ridge)

Mesial marginal groove

Central groove

FIGURE 17-15 Occlusal features of the permanent maxillary right first premolar with the occlusal table highlighted.

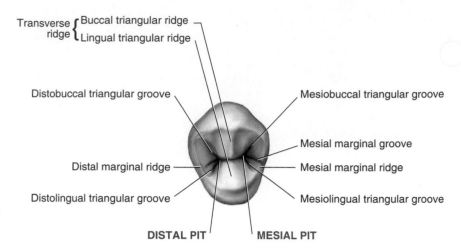

FIGURE 17-16 Additional occlusal features of the permanent maxillary right first premolar with the fossae highlighted.

occlusal outline is almost a semicircle. However, both the mesial and distal margins are straight as they converge toward the lingual. Thus, the lingual part of the tooth is narrower mesiodistally than the buccal part. When the mesial marginal groove is prominent, it may create a dip in the mesial margin.

Occlusal Table Components The buccal cusp of a maxillary first premolar is sharper and higher than the lingual cusp. The occlusal function of the buccal cusp involves only its lingual surface. Four buccal cusp ridges descend from the buccal cusp tip, each named for its location: buccal, lingual, mesial, and distal. Because this is the first occlusal table of a posterior tooth under discussion in this chapter, this text provides specific details on each of the occlusal table features; this information can then be related to the occlusal tables of other posterior teeth.

The buccal cusp ridge of the buccal cusp extends cervically from the cusp tip on the buccal surface and corresponds to the buccal ridge. The lingual cusp ridge extends lingually from the buccal cusp tip to the central groove (or buccal triangular ridge or buccal part of the transverse ridge, as discussed later). The mesial cusp ridge of the buccal cusp extends mesially from the cusp tip to the mesiobucco-occlusal point angle. The distal cusp ridge extends distally from the buccal cusp tip to the distobucco-occlusal point angle.

Between the cusp ridges are four buccal-inclined cuspal planes, named for the two cusp ridges they are between: mesiobuccal, mesiolingual, distobuccal, and distolingual. However, only the mesiolingual- and distolingual-inclined cuspal planes function during occlusion.

The lingual cusp of the maxillary first premolar is rounder, less sharp, and shorter than the buccal cusp. This cusp is also located well to the lingual and offset to the mesial. Again, there are four lingual cusp ridges and four lingual-inclined cuspal planes similar to those associated with the buccal cusp, but all the lingual-inclined cuspal planes are functional in occlusion. This is because the entire lingual cusp functions during occlusion, unlike the buccal cusp.

Extending mesiodistally, across the occlusal table of the maxillary first premolar, is a long central groove, evenly dividing the tooth buccolingually. The central groove is a developmental groove that is sharply defined; it is deep and V-shaped. A few supplemental grooves appear irregular in shape and shallower because they branch from the central groove. Thus, the occlusal surface is relatively less pronounced compared with the adjacent maxillary second premolar.

The lingual cusp ridge, which runs from the buccal cusp tip to the central groove, is also termed the *buccal triangular ridge* (Figure 17-16). The buccal cusp ridge of the lingual cusp is also termed the *lingual triangular ridge* because it runs from the lingual cusp tip to the central groove. Perpendicular to the central groove is a *transverse*

ridge, which is the collective term given to the joining of the buccal triangular ridge and the lingual triangular ridge.

The central groove of the maxillary first premolar also crosses to the mesial marginal ridge, which is shorter than the distal marginal ridge. Extending from the central groove, another developmental groove, the mesial marginal groove, crosses the mesial marginal ridge and travels onto the mesial surface of the tooth.

Descending down the slope of the buccal cusp and just inside the distal and mesial marginal ridges are two developmental grooves: the mesiobuccal triangular groove and the distobuccal triangular groove. Across the occlusal table, the lingual cusp also has two developmental grooves: the mesiolingual triangular groove and the distolingual triangular groove.

Each of these triangular grooves ends in a triangular-shaped depression, the triangular fossa. These fossae include: the deeper mesial triangular fossa that surrounds the mesiobuccal triangular groove and the shallower distal triangular fossa that surrounds the distobuccal triangular groove. The boundaries of the mesial triangular fossa are the mesial marginal ridge, the transverse ridge, and the mesial cusp ridges of the two cusps. The distal triangular fossa has boundaries similar to those of the mesial fossa in a mirror-image fashion. Within the deepest parts of these fossae are the occlusal pits, the mesial pit, and distal pit, respectively. These developmental pits are connected by the central groove on the occlusal table.

PERMANENT MAXILLARY SECOND PREMOLARS #4 AND #13 (#15 AND #25)

Specific Overall Features Permanent maxillary second premolars erupt between 10 and 12 years of age with root completion between ages 12 and 14 (Figure 17-17). These teeth erupt distal to the permanent maxillary first premolars and thus are the succedaneous replacements for the primary maxillary second molars.

A maxillary second premolar resembles a first premolar, except that its crown is less angular and more rounded. Additionally, more crown variations, especially in its occlusal surface anatomy, are noted in this tooth as compared with maxillary first premolars.

Unlike a maxillary first premolar, a maxillary second premolar usually has only a single root, but it may occasionally have two roots. The dimensions between the maxillary second and the first premolars are usually about the same overall, except for greater root length of the second. The mesial root concavity is not as pronounced as in a first premolar. The pulp cavity of this tooth has two pulp horns and one single pulp canal (Figure 17-18).

Buccal View Features The buccal cusp of a maxillary second premolar is neither as long nor as sharp as that of a maxillary first

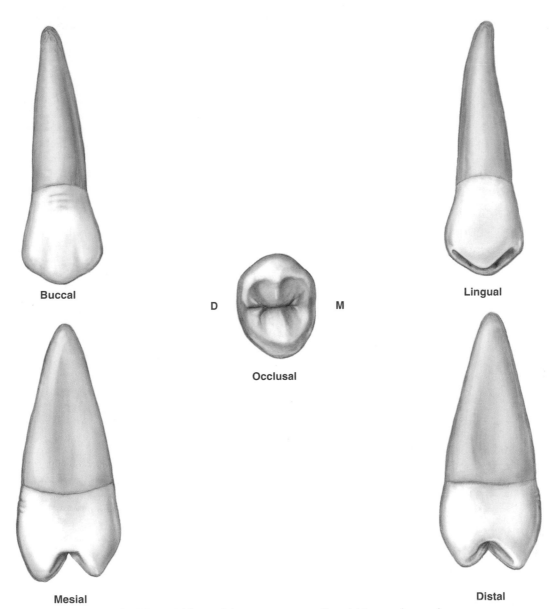

Buccal

Lingual

D   M

Occlusal

Mesial

Distal

FIGURE 17-17 Views of the permanent maxillary right second premolar.

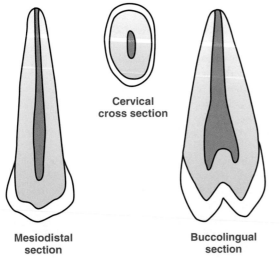

Cervical
cross section

Mesiodistal
section

Buccolingual
section

FIGURE 17-18 Pulp cavity of the permanent maxillary right second premolar.

premolar (see Figure 17-17). All other features of the buccal surface of a maxillary second are similar to those of the first. Again, the mesial contact with a maxillary first premolar is just cervical to the junction of the occlusal and middle thirds on the buccal surface. The distal contact with a maxillary first molar is the same, just cervical to the junction of the occlusal and middle thirds.

Lingual View Features All lingual surface features of a maxillary second premolar are similar to those of a maxillary first premolar (see Figure 17-17). One exception is that the lingual cusp is larger, almost the same height as the buccal cusp on a maxillary second premolar. In addition, the lingual cusp is slightly displaced to the mesial, which *helps to distinguish the maxillary right second premolar from the left*. In addition, less of the occlusal surface is seen from this view because the crown is longer on the lingual.

Proximal View Features The mesial surface of a maxillary second premolar is similar to that of a maxillary first premolar, except that the cusps are closer to being the same size, and no mesial developmental depression is present on either the crown or root. Instead, this area cervical to the contact area is rounder (see Figure 17-17). In addition, this tooth has no mesial marginal groove. Both the contact areas and

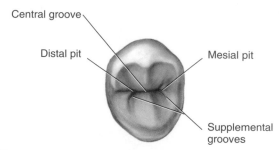

FIGURE 17-19 Occlusal features of the permanent maxillary right second premolar with the occlusal table highlighted.

mesial marginal ridge are more cervically located than those on a maxillary first premolar. The distal surface is the same as the mesial surface without any distal marginal groove, but the contact area is larger.

Occlusal View Features The outline of the occlusal surface of a maxillary second premolar is more rounded and larger overall than that of a maxillary first premolar from the occlusal view (see Figure 17-17). Thus, the overall hexagonal outline of the crown from the occlusal is more difficult to see.

Occlusal Table Components The central groove is shorter on a maxillary second premolar than on a maxillary first premolar (Figure 17-19). Thus when this groove ends in a mesial pit and distal pit at each of its ends, the pits are closer together and more to the middle on the occlusal table.

Other features and the overall anatomy of this tooth's occlusal surface are similar to those of a maxillary first premolar. An exception is that the maxillary second premolar has numerous supplemental grooves radiating from the central groove. This gives the tooth a more wrinkled appearance compared with a maxillary first premolar.

> **Clinical Considerations for Permanent Maxillary Second Premolars**

With premature loss of a primary maxillary second molar, the developing permanent maxillary first molar inclines and drifts mesially. The developing permanent maxillary second premolar is prevented from eruption because its arch leeway space is nearly closed (see **Chapter 20**). This situation can allow the maxillary second premolar to become impacted against the first molar. An impacted tooth is an unerupted or partially erupted tooth, which is positioned against another tooth, bone, or even soft tissue, making complete eruption unlikely. Additionally, the leeway space can be compromised if the permanent maxillary second molar erupts before the maxillary second premolars, the arch perimeter significantly shortened, and occlusal disharmony is likely to occur, as with a malocclusion. These related complications may be prevented by careful evaluation of patients with a mixed dentition present and use of interceptive orthodontic therapy, such as space maintainers (see Figure 20-4), as well as tooth replacement.

PERMANENT MANDIBULAR PREMOLARS
GENERAL FEATURES

Mandibular premolars do not resemble each other as much as do the maxillary premolars (see Figures 17-20 and 17-26). Although a maxillary first premolar is larger overall than the second premolar, a mandibular first premolar is smaller than a mandibular second premolar. Both mandibular premolars generally erupt into the oral cavity later than do the maxillary premolars.

Quite distinct from maxillary premolars, the buccal outline of the crown of all mandibular premolars shows a strong lingual inclination when viewed from the proximal, which is similar to all mandibular posterior teeth. The permanent mandibular premolars also have an equal buccolingual and mesiodistal width when viewed from the occlusal, making the outline almost round. In addition, both types of premolars have a similar buccal outline of both the crown and root.

The mesial and distal contact areas of mandibular premolars are on nearly the same level. Similar CEJ curvatures are also found on both premolars. From each proximal view, both the crown outlines of mandibular premolars are rhomboidal, or four-sided, having the opposite sides parallel, which is like all mandibular posteriors (see Table 15-4). The crowns thus incline lingually on their root bases, bringing the cusps of these mandibular teeth into proper occlusion with their maxillary antagonists and the distribution of forces along their long axes.

Unlike the maxillary premolars, both of which have two cusps of almost equal size, the mandibular premolars can have more than two cusps; however, any lingual cusp is always smaller than the buccal cusp.

These mandibular premolars usually have a single root; the angulation of the roots of mandibular premolars may show slight distal inclination. The root on cervical cross section is either oval or egg-shaped or elliptic, which is an elongated oval; these shapes may be slightly altered by the presence of proximal root concavities. These proximal root concavities are most frequently found on the mesial surface of the root.

> **Clinical Considerations for Permanent Mandibular Premolars**

Both types of mandibular premolars can present difficulties during instrumentation or restoration due to narrow lingual surfaces combined with the lingual inclination of the crown, especially with subgingival placement. In addition, patients may have difficulty performing adequate homecare because of the lingual inclination of the crown, which causes some patients to miss the cervical interface with the associated lingual gingival tissue and take care of only the occlusal surface with a toothbrush. Proximity of the nearby tongue also can make homecare procedures and instrumentation or restoration more difficult on the lingual surface.

PERMANENT MANDIBULAR FIRST PREMOLARS #21 AND #28 (#34 AND #44)

Specific Overall Features Permanent mandibular first premolars erupt between 10 and 12 years of age with root completion between ages 12 and 13 (Figure 17-20). These teeth erupt distal to the permanent mandibular canines and thus are the succedaneous replacements for the primary mandibular first molars.

A mandibular first premolar resembles a mandibular canine in many more ways than it does a mandibular second premolar. This is true despite the fact that any premolar is smaller overall than a canine. However, the buccolingual width of this tooth is similar to that of a mandibular canine. Thus, a mandibular first premolar shows the transition in form in the dental arch from the narrower canine to the wider molar-like second premolar.

A mandibular first premolar has a buccal cusp that is long and sharp and is the only functional cusp during occlusion, which is similar to a mandibular canine. The lingual cusp of a mandibular first premolar is usually small and nonfunctioning. The lingual cusp, then, is similar in appearance to the cingulum found on some maxillary canines, but it can vary considerably. Finally, the occlusal surface of the mandibular first premolar has a similar outline and slopes sharply to the lingual, and the mesiobuccal cusp ridge is shorter than the distobuccal cusp ridge; all features are similar to the mandibular canine.

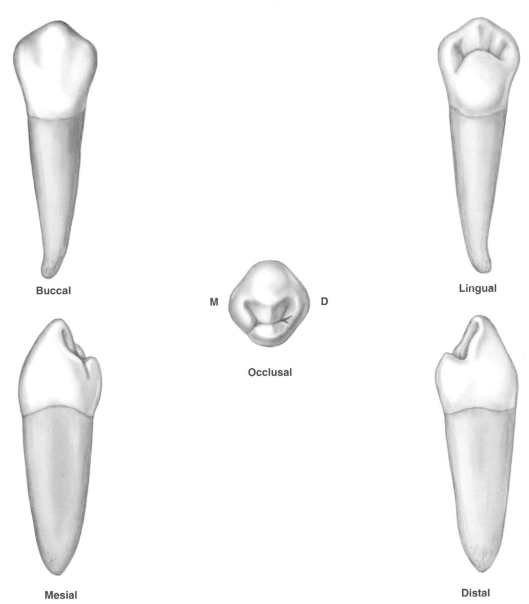

Buccal

Lingual

M   D

Occlusal

Mesial

Distal

FIGURE 17-20 Views of the permanent mandibular right first premolar.

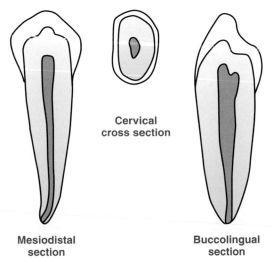

Cervical cross section

Mesiodistal section

Buccolingual section

FIGURE 17-21 Pulp cavity of the permanent mandibular right first premolar.

A mandibular first premolar has a smaller and shorter root than a mandibular second premolar, although it is closer to the length of a second premolar than to that of a mandibular canine. The buccal aspect of the root is more conical, but the lingual aspect is tapered. A deep groove may be found on the distal root surface. The tooth occasionally has a bifurcated root with the root divided into buccal and lingual root branches.

The pulp cavity of this tooth consists of two pulp horns and a single pulp canal (Figure 17-21). Each pulp horn is located within a cusp. The buccal pulp horn is more pronounced, and the lingual pulp horn is smaller and less significant.

Buccal View Features The outline of the crown of a mandibular first premolar from the buccal is nearly symmetrical (see Figure 17-20). The middle developmental lobe is visibly well developed, resulting in a prominent buccal ridge and a large, pointed buccal cusp. In contrast, the buccal ridge is not as prominent as on a maxillary first premolar. Two buccal developmental depressions are often seen separating the three buccal lobes. Imbrication lines are not usually present on the buccal surface.

The buccal cusp is also located slightly to the mesial of the center of the crown, again similar to a mandibular canine. Thus, the two cusp slopes of the premolar are not equal in length. The mesial cusp slope of the buccal cusp is shorter than the distal cusp slope, which *helps to distinguish the mandibular right first premolar from the left*.

The mesial outline of the mandibular first premolar is slightly concave from the mesial contact to the CEJ. The distal outline is rounder and shorter. Again, the mesial contact with the maxillary first premolar is just cervical to the junction of the occlusal and middle thirds. The distal contact with the maxillary first molar is the same, just cervical to the junction of the occlusal and the middle third.

Lingual View Features The lingual surface is much narrower than the buccal on a mandibular first premolar, with the crown tapering to the lingual (Figure 17-22). Most of both the mesial and distal surfaces, therefore, can be seen from the lingual. The lingual cusp is small and nonfunctional during occlusion, and the lingual cusp tip is often pointed.

Because the lingual cusp is small, most of the occlusal surface can also be seen from this view. The lingual cusp tip lines up with the buccal triangular ridge. The mesial fossa and distal fossa are on each side of this ridge. A developmental groove, the mesiolingual groove, usually separates the mesial marginal ridge from the mesial cusp slope of the small lingual cusp.

Proximal View Features From the mesial, the crown of a mandibular first premolar tilts noticeably toward the lingual at the cervix, as do all mandibular posteriors (see Figure 17-20). Thus, the buccal outline is longer than the lingual outline. This lingual inclination of the crown also places the buccal cusp tip almost over the root axis line. Thus, the lingual cusp tip is usually in line vertically with the lingual surface of the cervical part of the root. The transverse ridge slopes at a 45° angle from the buccal cusp tip to the occlusal surface and then nearly flattens out to the lingual cusp tip.

The mesial marginal ridge is nearly parallel to the angulation of the transverse ridge at a more cervical level; the slope of the mesial marginal ridge is similar to that of anteriors. The mesiolingual groove, again, can be seen near the lingual margin. The CEJ curvature is also more occlusal on the mesial surface. Both these mesial surface features *help to distinguish the mandibular right first premolar from the left*.

The distal view of the mandibular first premolar is somewhat similar to the mesial, except for the absence of a groove near the lingual margin. And the distal marginal ridge is much more developed than that of the mesial, and its continuity is unbroken by any deep developmental grooves. Additionally, the distal marginal ridge does not show quite as steep a slope toward the lingual, as is present on the mesial.

Occlusal View Features The crown outline of the mandibular first premolar is diamond shaped from the occlusal with a notch in the mesial outline at the mesiolingual groove (Figure 17-23). The prominent buccal ridge is located on the buccal margin. The lingual margin is much shorter than the buccal margin. The mesial margin is slightly rounded to nearly straight, except in the area near the mesiolingual groove. The distal margin is even more rounded than the mesial margin.

Occlusal Table Components Both the cusps and transverse ridge of the mandibular first premolar are offset to the mesial, leaving the distal part of the tooth larger than the mesial part (see Figure 17-23). The larger and functioning buccal cusp has four buccal cusp ridges and four functioning buccal-inclined cuspal planes, all of which are named for their location. The lingual cusp ridge of the buccal cusp is also considered the buccal triangular ridge.

The lingual cusp is quite small, usually no more than half the height of the buccal cusp. It also has four lingual cusp ridges and four lingual-inclined cuspal planes. The buccal cusp ridge of the buccal cusp is also considered the lingual triangular ridge.

The transverse ridge is composed of the joining of the buccal triangular ridge of the lingual cusp and the lingual triangular ridge of

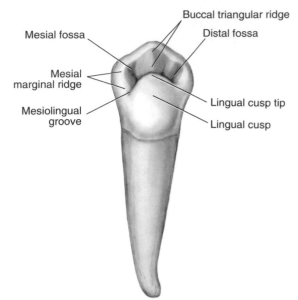

FIGURE 17-22 Lingual features of the permanent mandibular right first premolar with the occlusal table highlighted.

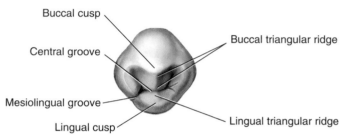

FIGURE 17-23 Occlusal features of the permanent mandibular right first premolar with the occlusal table highlighted.

the buccal cusp. The buccal triangular ridge is longer than the lingual, thus making up a greater part of the transverse ridge. The transverse ridge is perpendicular to the central groove. This groove, which slightly separates the two triangular ridges, is sometimes rather indistinct, and thus the two triangular ridges appear to be continuous.

The mesial marginal ridge closely resembles the angulation of the marginal ridges of anterior teeth, especially the canine. This is because it slopes from the buccal to the lingual at a 45° angle (Figure 17-24). The mesial marginal ridge is less prominent and shorter than the distal marginal ridge. The distal marginal ridge also does not have quite as steep a slope toward the lingual.

The mesial fossa and distal fossa, and associated deeper mesial pit and distal pit, are also found on the occlusal table. The mesial fossa is shallower than the distal, and although both are circular, the mesial fossa is slightly more linear. The mesial pit is the junction of the central groove, mesiolingual groove (previously described on the lingual and mesial aspects), and mesiobuccal triangular groove (similar in location to that of the maxillary premolars). The distal pit is the junction of the central groove, distal marginal groove, distolingual triangular groove, and distobuccal triangular groove.

Clinical Considerations for Permanent Mandibular First Premolars

When mandibular first premolars have Class I metallic (amalgam or gold) restorations that fill the both mesial and distal occlusal pits, these restorations are sometimes nicknamed *snake eyes* because of the eye-like roundness presented (Figure 17-25). This type of restoration

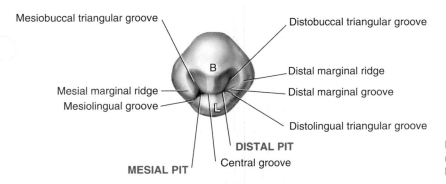

FIGURE 17-24 Additional occlusal features of the permanent mandibular right first premolar with the fossae highlighted.

FIGURE 17-25 Metallic restorations on the permanent mandibular first premolar in the oral cavity, which are considered to be like snake eyes *(arrow)*. (Courtesy of Margaret J. Fehrenbach, RDH, MS.)

can also be noted on the occlusal surface of mandibular second premolars. Tooth-colored restorative materials are now more commonly placed on the occlusal surface of these smaller posterior teeth to achieve a more esthetic appearance.

PERMANENT MANDIBULAR SECOND PREMOLARS #20 AND #29 (#35 AND #45)

Specific Overall Features The permanent mandibular second premolars erupt between 11 and 12 years of age with root completion between ages 13 and 14 (Figure 17-26). These teeth erupt distal to the mandibular first premolars and thus are the succedaneous replacements for the primary mandibular second molars.

There are two forms of the mandibular second premolars: three-cusp type (the tricuspidate form) and two-cusp type (the bicuspidate form; Figure 17-27). Unlike mandibular first premolars, the more common (55% frequency) three-cusp type has three cusps: the one large buccal cusp composed of the three buccal lobes and the two smaller lingual cusps composed of the two lingual lobes (see Figure 17-26). Thus, the three-cusp type is composed of total five developmental lobes: three buccal and two lingual.

Similar to mandibular first premolars, the less common (45% frequency) two-cusp type has a larger buccal cusp and a single smaller lingual cusp (Figure 17-28). The two-cusp type is thus composed of a total of four developmental lobes: three buccal and one lingual.

The two types of this tooth differ mainly in their occlusal features, but other surface features are similar. Both types of mandibular second premolars have more supplemental grooves than the first premolar of the same arch. The three-cusp type also appears more angular from the occlusal view, and the two-cusp type appears more rounded.

Although a mandibular first premolar resembles a mandibular canine, the more common three-cusp type of mandibular second premolar resembles a small molar because its lingual cusps are well developed, which places both marginal ridges horizontal and superior on the occlusal table. A more efficient occlusion thus results with the premolars in the opposite arch, which is similar to the molars. A mandibular second premolar thus represents the transition in form from a narrow canine-like first premolar to the wider molars.

The single root of a mandibular second premolar is larger and longer than that of a first premolar but shorter than both types of maxillary premolars. Proximal root concavities are pronounced. In addition, the apex of this tooth is blunter than that of a first molar or of the maxillary premolars.

The pulp cavity of the three-cusp type shows three pointed pulp horns (see Figure 17-28). Two pulp horns are present with the two-cusp type. No matter the number of pulp horns, all pulp horns are more pointed in the mandibular second premolar than the first.

Buccal View Features A mandibular second premolar has a shorter buccal cusp than does a mandibular first premolar (see Figure 17-26). The cusp slopes of the buccal cusp are also more rounded. The mesial contact and distal contact are both wide and at the same location, just cervical to the junction of the occlusal and middle thirds.

Lingual View Features From the lingual, a mandibular second premolar shows considerable differences from a first premolar (Figure 17-29). The lingual cusp or cusps, depending on the type, are longer. Thus, less of the occlusal surface can be seen from this view. Because the lingual cusp is still smaller than the buccal cusp, however, a small part of the buccal margin of the occlusal surface may be seen.

And the differences between its two types can also be noted. In the three-cusp type, the mesiolingual cusp is wider and longer than the distolingual cusp. A developmental groove, the lingual groove, is located between the cusps, extending a short distance on the lingual surface and usually distal to the center of the crown because the mesiolingual cusp is wider.

With the two-cusp type of the mandibular second premolar, the single lingual cusp development is at an equal height with the mesiolingual cusp of the three-cusp type but is higher than that of a first premolar of the same arch. The two-cusp type has no groove noted lingually but does show a distolingual developmental depression where the lingual cusp ridge joins the distal marginal ridge.

Proximal View Features From the mesial, a mandibular second premolar has a shorter buccal cusp and is located more to the buccal than a first premolar (see Figure 17-26). Therefore, the distance between the cusp tips of this tooth is shorter than for the first. In addition, the crown is wider buccolingually, and the lingual cusp or cusps are larger. The mesial marginal ridge is perpendicular or 90° to the long axis of the tooth. There is no mesiolingual groove.

The distal view is similar, although more of the occlusal surface can be seen from this view because the distal marginal ridge is more

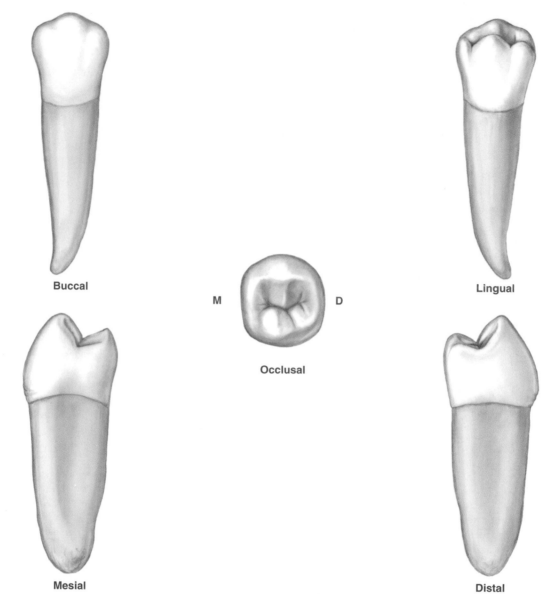

Buccal

M D

Occlusal

Lingual

Mesial

Distal

FIGURE 17-26 Views of the permanent mandibular right second premolar of the three-cusp type.

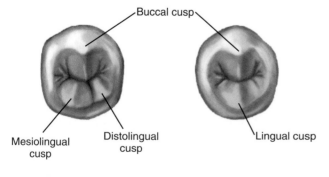

Buccal cusp

Mesiolingual cusp

Distolingual cusp

Lingual cusp

Three-cusp type

Two-cusp type

FIGURE 17-27 Occlusal views of the two types of permanent mandibular right second premolars: three-cusp type and two-cusp type with the occlusal table highlighted.

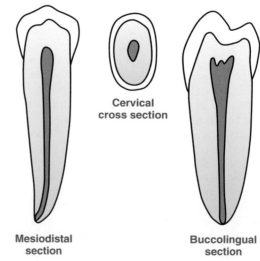

Cervical cross section

Mesiodistal section

Buccolingual section

FIGURE 17-28 Pulp cavity of the permanent mandibular right second premolar of the three-cusp type.

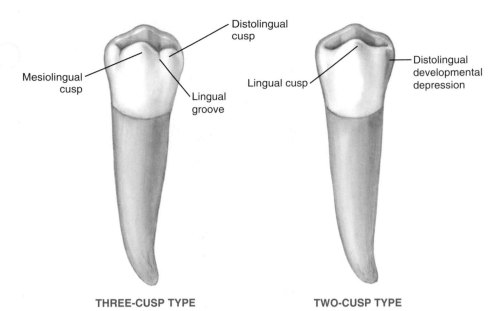

THREE-CUSP TYPE

Distolingual
cusp

Mesiolingual
cusp

Lingual
groove

TWO-CUSP TYPE

Lingual cusp

Distolingual
developmental
depression

FIGURE 17-29 Lingual views of both types of permanent mandibular right second premolars with the occlusal table highlighted.

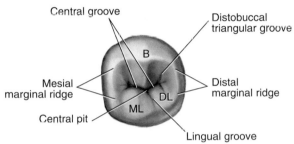

Central groove

Distobuccal
triangular groove

B

Mesial
marginal ridge

Distal
marginal ridge

DL

Central pit

ML

Lingual groove

FIGURE 17-30 Occlusal view of the three-cusp type of permanent mandibular right second premolar showing the Y-shaped groove pattern with the occlusal table highlighted.

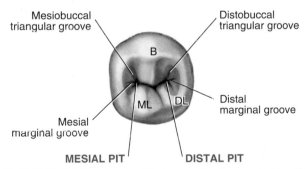

Mesiobuccal
triangular groove

Distobuccal
triangular groove

B

Mesial
marginal groove

ML

DL

Distal
marginal groove

MESIAL PIT   **DISTAL PIT**

FIGURE 17-31 Additional occlusal features of the three-cusp type of permanent mandibular right second premolar with the fossae highlighted.

cervically located than the mesial marginal ridge, which *helps to distinguish the mandibular right second premolar from the left.*

Occlusal View Features The general shape of the crown outline of a mandibular second premolar is more nearly square, especially in the three-cusp type, than a mandibular first premolar (see Figure 17-26). The convergence of the mesial and distal margins toward the lingual is equally severe.

Occlusal Table Components In both the three-cusp and two-cusp types of mandibular second premolar, the buccal cusp is similar. Thus, the two types are the same in that part of the occlusal table, which is buccal to the mesiobuccal and distobuccal cusp ridges.

Each of the cusps has buccal ridges, triangular ridges, and cuspal inclined planes, which are each named for their location and orientation.

On the three-cusp type, the cusps are separated by two developmental grooves, a V-shaped central groove, and a linear lingual groove (Figure 17-30). The lingual groove extends lingually between the two lingual cusps and ends on the lingual surface of the crown just below the meeting of the lingual cusp ridges. These two grooves together form a distinctive Y-shaped groove pattern on the occlusal table.

On the three-cusp type, a deep central pit is located at the junction of the central groove and the lingual groove, toward the lingual. The central pit is also more to the distal between the mesial marginal ridge and distal marginal ridge because the mesiolingual cusp is wider than the distolingual cusp. Some anatomists prefer to separate the central groove on this tooth into two grooves: a mesial groove and a distal groove.

On the three-cusp type of a second mandibular premolar, the mesial part of the central groove travels in a mesiobuccal direction and ends in a mesial pit surrounded by a mesial triangular fossa just distal to the mesial marginal ridge, which is often crossed by a mesial marginal groove (Figure 17-31). The distal part of the central groove travels in a distobuccal direction, is slightly shorter than the mesial groove, and ends in a distal pit surrounded by a distal triangular fossa mesial to the distal marginal ridge.

These triangular fossae are shallow, irregularly shaped, but overall more linear in form than the triangular fossae of the maxillary premolars. In addition, a mesiobuccal triangular groove, which extends into the mesial pit, is on the occlusal table. The distobuccal triangular groove, distolingual triangular groove, and possibly a distal marginal groove also extend into the distal pit.

In contrast, the two-cusp type is rounder lingual to the buccal cusp ridges (Figure 17-32). The mesial and distal margins converge slightly, making the lingual part narrower than the buccal, but never to the degree of a mandibular first premolar. The larger and longer buccal cusp is seen directly opposite the smaller and shorter lingual cusp. On the two-cusp type, a central groove on the occlusal table travels in a mesiodistal direction.

The central groove is most often crescent shaped, forming a U-shaped groove pattern on the occlusal table. Less often, the central groove may be straight, forming an H-shaped groove pattern on the occlusal table. The lingual cusp of the type with the H-shaped groove pattern is larger and sharper than the one with the U-shaped

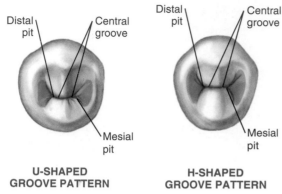

U-SHAPED GROOVE PATTERN

H-SHAPED GROOVE PATTERN

FIGURE 17-32 Occlusal views of the two-cusp type of permanent mandibular right second premolar showing the U-shaped and H-shaped groove patterns with the fossae highlighted.

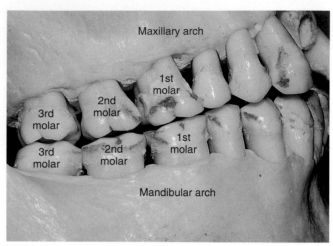

FIGURE 17-33 Permanent molars identified per arch on a skull. (Courtesy of Margaret J. Fehrenbach, RDH, MS.)

groove pattern and is often offset to the mesial. The buccal cusp for both occlusal groove patterns of the two-cusp type has four functional inclined planes during occlusion, and the lingual cusp has two.

The central groove of the two-cusp type with either groove pattern has its terminal ends centered in the mesial fossa and distal fossa, which are circular depressions having supplemental grooves radiating from them. Some two-cusp types have a mesial pit and a distal pit centered in mesial and distal fossae instead of an unbroken central groove; most have a distolingual developmental depression crossing the distolingual cusp ridge. None of the two-cusp types have a lingual groove or central pit.

Clinical Considerations for Permanent Mandibular Second Premolars

With any premature loss of a primary mandibular second molar, the developing permanent mandibular first molar inclines and drifts mesially in a mixed dentition. The developing permanent mandibular second premolar is prevented from eruption because its arch leeway space is nearly closed (see Figure 20-3). This situation can allow the mandibular second premolar to become impacted against the first molar. An impacted tooth is an unerupted or partially erupted tooth that is positioned against another tooth, bone, or even soft tissue, making complete eruption unlikely. Additionally, the leeway space can be compromised if the permanent mandibular second molars erupt before the mandibular second premolars, the arch perimeter is significantly shortened, and occlusal disharmony is likely to occur as with a malocclusion. These complications may be prevented by careful evaluation of patients with mixed dentition and use of interceptive orthodontic therapy, such as with space maintainers, as well as tooth replacement.

Permanent mandibular second premolars are also commonly involved in partial anodontia and thus may be congenitally missing (see Box 6-1, *B*). With this disturbance, the appropriate individual tooth germ(s) in the area is absent because of failure of the initiation process during tooth development; this condition can be bilateral or unilateral. A careful patient evaluation needs to be performed when primary mandibular second molars are retained either in a mixed or permanent dentition, including radiographs. Missing permanent teeth may require prosthetic replacement (such as an implant) because they can result in complications with spacing and occlusion.

However, these retained primary molars, without the presence of the underlying succedaneous permanent teeth may not be shed for many years. Thus, these primary teeth can serve as functioning stand-ins for the permanent premolar teeth and should not be extracted unless they are involved in caries or root pathology, or are uncomfortably mobile.

PERMANENT MOLARS

GENERAL FEATURES OF PERMANENT MOLARS

Permanent molars are the most posteriorly placed posterior teeth of the permanent dentition, distal to the premolars (Figure 17-33). Molars are also the largest teeth in the dentition. Each dental arch usually has six molars with three in each quadrant, if all have erupted. The name *molar* comes from the Latin word for *grinder*, which is one of the functions of the molar teeth.

There are three types of molars: first molars, second molars, and third molars. The first molars and second molars are called the *6-year molars* and *12-year molars*, respectively, because of their eruption times.

The third molars, also known as the *wisdom teeth*, are extremely variable in their eruption time, as well as in their anatomic size and form. They were given this unusual nickname in ancient times when it was thought that only educated men had this important type of molar. Many dental professionals jokingly argue against the wisdom sometimes shown in newly minted young adults, given that these teeth erupt between 17 and 21 years of age. Eruption of the third molars usually marks the end of the growth of the jaws.

Only the permanent dentition has three types of molars; the primary dentition only has two types. One of each type of molar is present in each quadrant of each dental arch. The first molars are closer to the midline, at the sixth position from it, and at the same time, they are distal to the permanent second premolars when full eruption of the permanent dentition has occurred. The second molars are distal to the first molars and are in the seventh position from the midline. Finally, the third molars are distal to the second molars and are in the eighth position from the midline.

All three types of molars erupt in order distal to the primary second molars, long after all the primary teeth have erupted and are functioning. Thus, all the permanent molars are nonsuccedaneous because they do not replace any primary teeth. These teeth usually have enough space as they progressively erupt because of the continued elongation of the facial bones during development (except in some cases for third molars, as discussed later).

Having the largest and strongest crowns of the permanent dentition, the molars, assisted by the premolars, function in grinding food during mastication (see Table 15-4). This grinding function is possible because molars have wide occlusal surfaces with prominent cusps.

Developmental groove

Cusp

Cusp ridge

Occlusal developmental pit

Supplemental groove

Marginal ridge

FIGURE 17-34 Occlusal view of a permanent molar with the occlusal table highlighted.

FIGURE 17-35 Exposed root surface on the permanent mandibular first molar of a skull due to advanced periodontal disease, which also exposed the buccal furcation and buccal furcation crotch *(circled)*. (Courtesy of Margaret J. Fehrenbach, RDH, MS.)

These teeth also support the soft tissue of the cheek, especially the facial muscles, because they maintain the height of the lower third of the vertical dimension of the face and alveolar process. Thus, the molars are involved in both esthetics and speech, but less so than the premolars, due to their more posterior position. When viewed from the buccal or lingual, the molars' crown outline for both arches is trapezoidal, or four-sided, with only two parallel sides; the longer of the two parallel sides is toward the occlusal surface (see Table 15-4).

The first molar is overall the largest, and the second and third are each progressively smaller. Each molar has an extremely large crown compared with the rest of the permanent dentition, but the crown is shorter occlusocervically in contrast to the teeth anterior to it. Each buccal surface of a molar has a prominent **cervical (ser-vi-kal) ridge** in the cervical one-third, running mesiodistally.

Like all posterior teeth, molars have an occlusal surface with usually three or more cusps, of which at least two are buccal cusps (Figure 17-34). Unlike anterior teeth and premolars, molars do not exhibit buccal developmental depressions. Evidence of developmental lobe separation is in the developmental grooves on the occlusal table.

In addition to having cusps, the occlusal table of the molar is bordered by its cusp ridges and marginal ridges. The occlusal table of molars is even more complex than that of premolars because it has more developmental grooves, supplemental grooves, and occlusal pits.

Grooves and pits are located not only on the occlusal surface of both maxillary and mandibular molars but also on the lingual surfaces of maxillary molars and buccal surfaces of mandibular molars, in some cases.

In addition, molars usually are multirooted. Maxillary molars usually have three root branches (trifurcated), and mandibular molars have two (bifurcated) (see Figure 17-7). Molars, like other teeth, originate as a single root on the base of the crown, which is considered the root trunk. The cervical cross section of root trunk follows the form of the crown, but the root then divides from the root trunk into the number of root branches for its type (see Figure 6-21). Multiple roots give molars increased periodontal support.

As discussed earlier in this chapter, an area between two or more of these root branches, before they divide from the root trunk, is a furcation (see Figure 17-7 and Table 17-1). The spaces between the roots at the furcation are the furcation crotches. Teeth with two roots (such as mandibular molars) have two furcation crotches; teeth with three roots (such as maxillary molars) have three furcation crotches. Such crotches can be located on either the buccal surfaces and the lingual surfaces, or on the buccal, mesial, and distal surfaces, depending on tooth type, each with a slightly different individual configuration. The furcation crotches may be close to the CEJ or far from it. Root concavities are also found on many of the root branches of molar teeth, as well as on the associated furcal surfaces. In a molar, the root canals join the deeper pulp chamber apical to the CEJ. With periodontal health, these features of the root(s) are covered by the alveolar process as well as overlying gingival tissue.

Clinical Considerations for Permanent Molars

Even though it is a common procedure during adolescence, third molar removal remains a controversial procedure. Still it is felt that around 25% of patients need to have their third molars removed before age 25. Often, patients are not aware of any difficulties associated with their third molars. More than 40% of adult patients who never had their third molars removed during adolescence may develop infection, caries, cyst formation, or associated periodontal disease by age 45, thus requiring extraction. In addition, the risk of surgical complications in adults with removal is increased by approximately 30% compared with adolescents. However, automatically removing functioning third molars is not the norm if they are not causing any overriding complications. Thus, an evaluation of the third molars by age 25 is generally recommended.

With the loss of periodontal support caused by periodontitis, the furcations, furcation crotches, and root concavities of the molars can lose their periodontal support in varying degrees resulting in furcation involvement (Figure 17-35; see Table 17-1). The horizontal component of a furcation invasion can be measured and classified by using a Nabors probe within a periodontal pocket, because if gingival recession has occurred, they can become clinically exposed. Dental biofilm and other deposits can be retained in the exposed furcation crotches and root concavities, leading to further periodontal disease. Molars are lost to advanced periodontal disease more than single rooted teeth partially due to the presence of furcations.

Performing periodontal debridement of roots and associated furcations involves a set instrumentation treatment plan; the best approach is to treat each root as a separate tooth when access permits, with a combination of strokes using instruments, air polisher, or ultrasonic. The distal surface is instrumented first, followed by the buccal, lingual, and mesial surfaces. Lastly, the concavity is debrided. Furcation involvement should be suspected in the presence of a 4-mm periodontal probe reading on a multirooted tooth adjacent to a buccal or lingual furcation. In some cases, especially in mandibular molars where the bifurcation is located only 3 mm from the cervical line, invasion can occur in the early stages of periodontitis with attachment loss of only 2 to 4 mm.

Therefore, furcation crotches and root concavities on these molars present a challenge during both instrumentation and performance of homecare in the area due to lack of access. Approximately half of molar furcations are too narrow for access even by instruments or devices, decreasing the prognosis of therapy if periodontally involved.

FIGURE 17-36 Dilaceration of an extracted permanent mandibular first molar and permanent mandibular second molar on a radiograph, respectively. (From Ibsen OAC, Phelan JA: *Oral pathology for dental hygienists,* ed 6, St Louis, 2014, Saunders/Elsevier.)

To allow better access, the furcations of a tooth may be reduced by minor odontoplasty, and any occluding gingival tissue is removed during surgical intervention. In addition, when roots are extremely close to each other, access to interproximals may be even more difficult. The cervical ridge on molars also presents challenges during instrumentation or restoration around the cervical area.

Finally, awareness of root trunk dimensions and their relationship to the furcations is critical to the periodontal prognosis of a molar. There is also a strong correlation between length of the root trunk and furcation invasion by advanced periodontal disease. Short root trunks are most commonly found buccally on both maxillary and mandibular molars, whereas long root trunks are more commonly found mesially in both maxillary molars. Additionally, short root length is associated with longer root trunks, and these long root trunks are more commonly found on the second molars than on the first molars.

Permanent molar teeth may have one or more tubercles (or accessory cusps) on the occlusal surface. In addition, similar to incisors, the molars may be affected in children with congenital syphilis. The spirochete *Treponema pallidum,* a sexually transmitted microorganism, is passed from an infected pregnant woman to her fetus via the placenta. This microorganism may cause localized enamel hypoplasia and result in mulberry molars (mull-bare-ee), a disturbance that occurs during tooth development (see Figure 3-17, *B*). This tooth has a crown with an abnormally shaped occlusal surface characterized by berry-like nodules or tubercles of enamel instead of cusps. Children with this condition may also have other developmental anomalies, such as blindness, deafness, and paralysis caused by congenital syphilis. Treatment using full-coverage crowns may be performed to improve the appearance of these teeth.

Another developmental disturbance associated mainly with molars is the enamel pearl (see Box 6-1, *R, S*). Mainly found on the buccal surfaces of second molars, these deposits of enamel apical to the level on the CEJ have a tapered form and extend into root furcation areas. They are present on over 28% of maxillary and 17% of mandibular molars and on most mandibular molars with isolated furcation involvement. These teeth were also found to have deeper root concavities compared with teeth that lacked cervical enamel projections. Unlike calculus, which it somewhat resembles radiographically, the

enamel pearl cannot be removed by instrumentation. Instead, it must undergo minor odontoplasty to restore the contour of the tooth.

Finally, dilaceration of the root(s) can also occur, making extraction and endodontic treatment challenging (Figure 17-36; see **Chapter 6**). Another developmental disturbance that can be present is root fusion, which creates deep developmental grooves when the molar roots fuse. These can function as hidden niches to accumulate deposits that are not easily accessible to either periodontal therapy or homecare procedures. The highest prevalence of permanent molars with root fusion occurs in maxillary second molars, followed by mandibular second molars, maxillary first molars, and finally, mandibular first molars; women present an overall higher incidence of root fusion than men.

PERMANENT MAXILLARY MOLARS
GENERAL FEATURES

Permanent maxillary molars erupt between 6 months and 1 year after the corresponding permanent mandibular molars (Table 17-3; see Figures 17-39, 17-44, and 17-47). They are usually the first permanent teeth to erupt into the maxillary arch. In addition, maxillary molars are overall the largest and strongest teeth of the maxillary arch. They are usually shorter occlusocervically than are the crowns of teeth anterior to them, but they are larger still in all other measurements compared to other maxillary teeth.

All maxillary molars are wider buccolingually than mesiodistally; in contrast, the mandibular molars are wider mesiodistally. From the occlusal, the outline of the crown of maxillary molars is rhomboidal, or four-sided, with opposite sides parallel (see Table 15-4). Like all maxillary posteriors, the crown outline is trapezoidal from each proximal view—again four-sided but with only two parallel sides. In addition, the crown is also centered over the root and shows no lingual inclination, similar to maxillary premolars, but unlike mandibular molars.

Each maxillary molar usually has four major cusps with two cusps on the buccal part of the occlusal table and two on the lingual (Figure 17-37). An **oblique** (obleek) **ridge** is a unique feature present on the occlusal table of most maxillary molars except the third molar. This type of transverse ridge crosses the occlusal table obliquely, forming by the union of the triangular ridge of the distobuccal cusp and distal

TABLE 17-3	Permanent Maxillary Molars		
	MAXILLARY FIRST MOLAR	**MAXILLARY SECOND MOLAR**	**MAXILLARY THIRD MOLAR**
Universal number	#3 and #14	#2 and #15	#1 and #16
International number	#16 and #26	#17 and #27	#18 and #28
General crown features	Occlusal table with marginal ridges and cusps with tips, inclined planes, ridges, grooves, fossae, and pits		
	Buccal cervical ridge		
Specific crown features	Largest tooth in arch and largest crown in dentition. Prominent oblique ridge. Four major cusps, with buccal cusps almost equal in height. Fifth minor cusp of Carabelli associated with mesiolingual cusp	Smaller crown than first. Heart-shaped or rhomboidal crown outline, with three or four cusps. Less prominent oblique ridge. Mesiobuccal cusp longer than distobuccal cusp. Distolingual cusp smaller than on first or absent. No fifth cusp	Smaller crown than second and variable in form. Heart-shaped or rhomboidal crown outline, with three or four cusps
Mesial contact*	Junction of occlusal and middle thirds	Middle third	Middle third
Distal contact*	Middle third	Middle third	None
Distinguish right from left	Mesiolingual cusp outline longer and larger but not as sharp as distolingual cusp outline		Distobuccal cusp shorter than mesiobuccal cusp. Roots curve distally
General root features	Three roots		
Specific root features	Furcations well removed from CEJ. Root trunks and root concavities.		Usually fused roots, curving distally
	Divergent roots		Less divergent roots

CEJ, Cementoenamel junction.
*Height of contour of posteriors for the buccal is in cervical third and lingual in middle third.

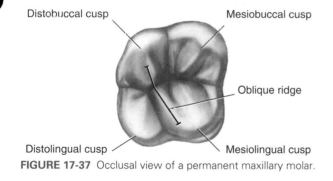

Distobuccal cusp
Mesiobuccal cusp
Oblique ridge
Distolingual cusp
Mesiolingual cusp

FIGURE 17-37 Occlusal view of a permanent maxillary molar.

cusp ridge of the mesiolingual cusp. In contrast, an oblique ridge is never present on mandibular molars.

Maxillary molars usually have three root branches, or are trifurcated, unlike mandibular molars, which usually have only two root branches because they are bifurcated (see Figure 17-7). These roots of the maxillary molar roots include: the mesiobuccal, distobuccal, and lingual (or palatal). The lingual root is usually the largest and longest for all these molars.

The farther distal a molar is in the maxillary arch, the shorter and more varied in size, shape, and curvature are the roots. The roots also become less divergent (or divided) on the teeth located farther distally, being less parallel with each other. Thus, a first molar has longer, more divergent roots than a third molar and has more consistency in the root's size, shape, and curvature. Roots of maxillary molars show increased lingual inclination but only moderate distal inclination.

Because maxillary molars are trifurcated, there are usually three furcations, which are located on the buccal, mesial, and distal surfaces (see Figure 17-7 and Table 17-1). All furcations on maxillary teeth usually begin near the junction of the cervical and middle thirds of the root. The buccal furcation is located midway between the mesial and

FIGURE 17-38 Lingual pit on an extracted permanent maxillary first molar. (Courtesy of Margaret J. Fehrenbach, RDH, MS.)

distal surfaces. The mesial and distal furcations are both located more to the lingual than the buccal surface. Root concavities are found on the mesial surface of the mesiobuccal root, the lingual surface of the lingual root, and all three furcal surfaces.

Clinical Considerations for Permanent Maxillary Molars

A possible lingual pit on the lingual surface of maxillary molars is at an increased risk of caries (Figure 17-38). This is due to both increased

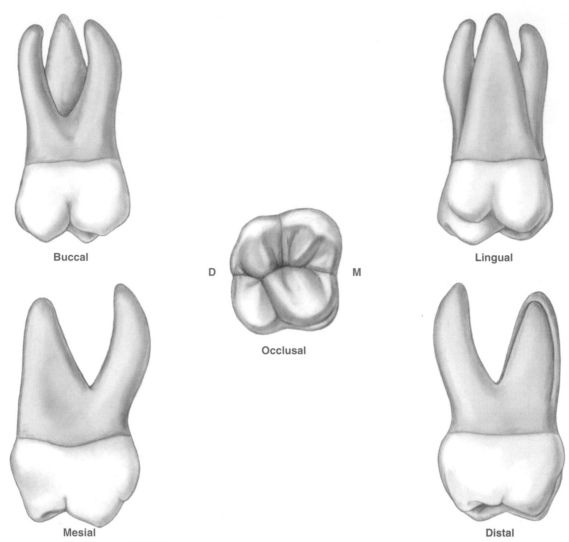

Buccal

Lingual

D   M

Occlusal

Mesial

Distal

FIGURE 17-39 Views of the permanent maxillary right first molar.

dental biofilm retention and the thinness of enamel forming the walls of the pit (see **Chapter 12**). An enamel sealant could be placed on the lingual pit of the erupting teeth. However, because of the histology of enamel in the area, enamel sealants do not bond as easily on any lingual surface as on the occlusal surface, so a full restoration procedure may be needed. A tooth-colored restorative material can be used to achieve a more esthetic appearance and provide protection or even to repair caries; thus the past presence of the lingual pit may not now be easy to discern clinically.

The roots of maxillary molars may penetrate the middle and posterior parts of the maxillary sinus as a result of accidental trauma, or during tooth extraction because of the close relation of these roots to the sinus walls, as can occur with other maxillary posteriors (see Figure 11-22). To complicate matters, the discomfort of sinusitis can be mistakenly interpreted as tooth-related from the maxillary molars, and vice versa. Thus, radiographs of the questionable tooth and maxillary sinus, as well as other diagnostic tests become necessary to determine the cause of the discomfort in this area.

Also due to the arch position of maxillary molars and with the natural overhang of the cheek, instrumentation, restoration, and homecare of the buccal surface may be difficult. In addition, furcation entrances of the maxillary molars can be very narrow, making access limited when desired.

Maxillary molars are some of the most common teeth of the permanent dentition to be involved in concrescence (see Box 6-1, *Q*). Concrescence is the union of the root structure of two or more teeth through the cementum only. The teeth involved are initially separate but join because of excessive cementum deposition surrounding one or more teeth following eruption. It occurs as a result of traumatic injury or crowding of the teeth in the area during the stages of apposition and maturation of tooth development. This disturbance may present complications during extraction and endodontic treatment; thus, preoperative radiographs are important.

PERMANENT MAXILLARY FIRST MOLARS #3 AND #14 (#16 AND #26)

Specific Overall Features Permanent maxillary first molars erupt between 6 and 7 years of age with root completion between ages 9 and 10 (Figure 17-39). Thus, these teeth are the first permanent teeth to erupt into the maxillary arch. They erupt distal to the primary maxillary second molars and thus are nonsuccedaneous, having no primary predecessors.

The maxillary first molar is the largest tooth in the maxillary arch, as well as having the largest crown in the permanent dentition. It has a much more complex crown form than the nearby maxillary premolars. However, of all the maxillary molars, the first is the least variable in form.

This tooth is composed of five developmental lobes: two buccal and three lingual. These are named in the same manner as their associated cusps: mesiobuccal, distobuccal, mesiolingual, distolingual, and an additional minor cusp may be located on the lingual surface (discussed later). Evidence of lobe separation can be found in the developmental grooves on the occlusal surface.

The roots of maxillary first molars are larger and more divergent than those of the second molars, and they are more complex in form than those of the maxillary premolars. The roots are also twice as long as the crown. The lingual (or palatal) root is the largest and longest, inclining lingually to extend beyond the crown outline. It has a banana-like curvature toward the buccal. A vertical depression may be present on the direct palatal surface of the root that is more pronounced at the cervical third.

The mesiobuccal root is the second largest and longest and is inclined both mesially and buccally, having its apical third curve distally. The distobuccal root is the smallest, shortest, and thus the weakest of the three. This root inclines both distally and buccally, having its apical one-third curve mesially. Both the mesiobuccal and distobuccal roots have an extreme curvature that when viewed together makes them look like the handles on a set of pliers.

The furcations of the maxillary first molar are well removed from the CEJ of the tooth (see Table 17-1). But the concavity depths are only 0.1 mm to 0.75 mm, limiting homecare procedures and instrumentation (see earlier discussion). The midway-placed buccal furcation on the buccal surface is about 4 mm apical to the CEJ.

The mesial furcation is located two-thirds of the way across the mesial surface from the buccal aspect, or one-third of the way from the lingual aspect due to the large mesiobuccal root. Thus the mesial furcation is not centered and it is wider buccolingually than mesiodistally; its entrance is dictated by the size of mesiobuccal root. The mesial furcation is 3 mm from the CEJ; a better approach for homecare procedures and instrumentation is from the lingual aspect.

The distal furcation is 5 mm from the CEJ; it is located halfway between the buccal and lingual on the distal surface. Approach for homecare procedures and instrumentation is first from the buccal aspect and then from the lingual aspect. The distal furcation is predisposed to develop periodontal disease due to the proximity of the divergent distobuccal root to the adjacent second molar, limiting access to its already narrow furcation entrance.

The pulp cavity of a maxillary first molar usually has one pulp horn for each major cusp (Figure 17-40). Thus, the four pulp horns include: the mesiobuccal, distobuccal, mesiolingual, and distolingual. Three main pulp canals are usually present, one for each of the three roots. The lingual pulp canal is the largest, the distobuccal is the smallest, and the mesiobuccal is between these two in size. The tooth sometimes has four pulp canals with two pulp canals in the mesiobuccal root.

Buccal View Features   The general shape of a maxillary first molar from this view is trapezoidal, with the longer parallel side toward the occlusal (see Figure 17-39 and Table 15-4). The entire buccal surface is larger than that of the adjacent premolar. Despite this fact, the occlusocervical measurement is slightly smaller.

Parts of all four major and functioning cusps seen from this view include: the mesiobuccal cusp, distobuccal cusp, mesiolingual cusp, and distolingual cusp. This is because the two lingual cusps are slightly offset to the distal relative to the buccal cusps. The occlusal outline of the mesiobuccal cusp is wider, but the distobuccal cusp tip is sharper. However, the two buccal cusps are nearly the same height, and the mesiolingual cusp tip is seen between them.

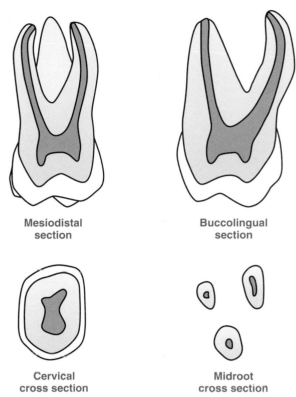

Mesiodistal section

Buccolingual section

Cervical cross section

Midroot cross section

FIGURE 17-40   Pulp cavity of the permanent maxillary right first molar.

The occlusal outline of a maxillary first molar is divided symmetrically by the buccal groove. This developmental groove extends between the two buccal cusps, and overall is parallel to the long axis of the tooth. It then runs apically about halfway to the CEJ, where it can fade out or end in a buccal pit or even end in two short, slanting grooves, with or without a buccal pit.

The mesial outline is flat from the CEJ occlusally to the mesial contact. The mesial contact is at the junction of the occlusal and middle thirds. This mesial contact is initially with a primary maxillary second molar until that tooth is shed; later the tooth's contact is with the permanent second premolar after it erupts. As noted occlusally from the mesial contact, the mesial outline is rounded.

Instead of being flat like the mesial, the distal outline of the maxillary first molar is rounded or convex from the CEJ to the occlusal surface. The distal contact is in the middle third. However, no distal contact with a tooth occurs until the permanent maxillary second molars erupt. The CEJ is slightly but irregularly curved apically but with less curvature than that on teeth anterior to it. A sharp dip or point may be observed just occlusal to the furcation area.

Lingual View Features   The lingual surface of the maxillary first molar is almost as wide mesiodistally as the buccal surface, as well as trapezoidal (see Figure 17-39). However, the lingual surface is more rounded or convex than the buccal. Both the mesial and distal outline and CEJ curvature are about the same, except that the distal outline is shorter because the distolingual cusp is smaller than the distobuccal cusp. Being the largest cusp on the occlusal surface, the mesiolingual cusp outline is much longer and larger, but the cusp is not as sharp as the distolingual cusp, which *helps to distinguish the maxillary right first molar from the left.*

Commonly arising from the lingual surface of the mesiolingual cusp of the maxillary first molar is a fifth nonfunctioning cusp, the cusp of Carabelli (kare-ah-bell-ee), named for its discoverer (see Figure 17-38). This minor cusp is set apart from the rest of the mesiolingual

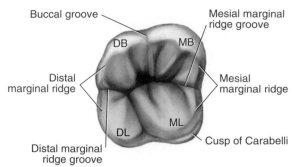

FIGURE 17-41 Occlusal features of the permanent maxillary right first molar with the occlusal table highlighted.

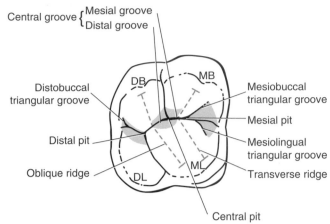

FIGURE 17-42 Additional occlusal features of the permanent maxillary right first molar with the fossae highlighted.

cusp by its associated **cusp of Carabelli groove**. Its presence can be variable; it is not present in all dentitions. If present, this small cusp, and its equally small groove, varies in prominence from tooth to tooth.

Similar to the buccal surface, the lingual surface has a distolingual groove that divides the occlusal outline into two unequal parts. And dissimilar to the buccal surface, only the two lingual cusps can be seen from this view. The distolingual groove usually ends in a lingual pit in the middle of the lingual surface, but it also may fade out.

Proximal View Features The only two cusps of the maxillary first molar that are seen from the mesial are the mesiobuccal cusp and mesiolingual cusp (see Figure 17-39). A mesial marginal groove usually notches the mesial marginal ridge about midway along its length. The contact area on the mesial is situated slightly to the buccal.

The distal view is the same as the mesial, the exception being that the mesial cusp tips are seen projecting beyond the outline of the distobuccal cusp and distolingual cusp from proximal. The distal marginal ridge is less prominent and dips farther cervically than on the mesial with a distal marginal groove halfway along its length. On both proximal views, the CEJ usually curves slightly toward the occlusal and may even be a straight line on some teeth on the distal.

Occlusal View Features The overall rhomboidal outline of the occlusal surface of a maxillary first molar is seen from the occlusal view, because it is four-sided, with opposite sides parallel (Figure 17-41). The buccal outline is divided unequally into two parts by the buccal groove with the mesial part longer than the distal part. The lingual outline is also divided unequally into two parts by the distolingual groove with the mesial part longer and less rounded than the distal part.

The mesial marginal ridge is longer and more prominent than the distal marginal ridge. Both marginal ridges are crossed by a mesial marginal ridge groove and distal marginal ridge groove, respectively. Because this is the first molar discussed, an extensive coverage of the occlusal table follows, and this information can be applied to the other molars, especially the maxillary molars.

Occlusal Table Components On the maxillary first molar, the two marginal ridges and two cusp ridges of the four major cusps are found bordering the occlusal table on the buccal and lingual margins (Figure 17-42). Each major cusp has a triangular ridge and three other cusp ridges. Also present with each major cusp are four inclined cuspal planes.

The mesiobuccal cusp has a sharp cusp tip and is the second largest cusp. It has a mesial cusp ridge that extends from the cusp tip to the mesiobuccal occlusal point angle. The mesiobuccal cusp on the first maxillary first molar is important in classifying the permanent dentition using Angle classification of malocclusion in relation to the mandibular arch (see Table 20-1).

The distal cusp ridge of the mesiobuccal cusp runs from the cusp tip to the buccal groove. The buccal cusp ridge passes from the cusp

tip to the CEJ on the buccal surface. Finally, the lingual cusp ridge runs from the cusp tip to the central groove and is also considered the triangular ridge of the mesiobuccal cusp. The mesiobuccal cusp has four inclined planes with all the lingual parts functional in occlusion.

The distobuccal cusp has the sharpest cusp tip and is the third largest cusp. Its triangular ridge, cusp ridges, and inclined planes are named similarly to those of the mesiobuccal cusp.

The mesiolingual cusp is the largest cusp with a rounded cusp tip. Its cusp ridges are similar to those of the other cusps, except that the distal triangular ridge extends from the mesiolingual cusp tip in an oblique distobuccal direction. There the distal triangular ridge meets the lingual triangular ridge of the distobuccal cusp to form the defining prominent oblique ridge. The mesiolingual cusp also has four inclined planes, all of which are functional in occlusion. A typical transverse ridge is also present and is formed by the buccal triangular ridge of the mesiolingual cusp and the lingual triangular ridge of the mesiobuccal cusp.

The distolingual cusp is the smallest of the major cusps and is the most variable of this group. The triangular ridge, cusp ridges, and inclined planes are similar to those of other cusps, except that all of the inclined planes are functional in occlusion.

The smallest cusp, when present on the maxillary first molar, is the minor and nonfunctional cusp, the cusp of Carabelli, with its associated cusp of Carabelli groove.

Four fossae are also present, along with associated developmental grooves and occlusal pits: central, mesial triangular, distal triangular, and distal. The central fossa is mesial to the oblique ridge and has a central pit in its most central, deepest part. The central pit divides the central groove into two parts: a mesial groove and a distal groove. Thus, the central pit is at the junction of three developmental grooves: buccal, mesial, and distal.

Three triangular grooves are present: mesiobuccal triangular groove, mesiolingual triangular groove, and distobuccal triangular groove. The buccal groove extends onto the buccal surface. The mesial groove, as part of the central groove, extends from the central pit to the mesial pit. The mesial pit is in the mesial triangular fossa, distal to the mesial marginal ridge. Thus, the mesial pit is at the junction of four developmental grooves: mesial, mesiobuccal triangular, mesiolingual triangular, and mesial marginal.

As part of the central groove, the distal groove usually extends from the central pit across the oblique ridge to the distal pit; it can also be considered the transverse groove of the oblique ridge. The distal pit is in the distal triangular fossa, mesial to the distal marginal ridge,

FIGURE 17-43 Changes that can occur in the permanent dentition when the maxillary first molar is lost. Arch undergoes mesial inclination and drift of the maxillary second molar into the adjacent open space with supereruption of the mandibular first molar into opposing space.

making the distal pit located at the junction of five developmental grooves: distal, distolingual, distobuccal triangular, distal marginal, and distal lingual triangular. The last fossa noted is the distal fossa, a linear rather than circular depression that is distal and parallel to the oblique ridge and thus is within the distolingual groove. Along with the central groove and other developmental grooves, a few supplemental grooves can be present.

Clinical Considerations for Permanent Maxillary First Molars

Because of their arch position and because the permanent maxillary first molars are the first permanent teeth to erupt in the maxillary arch, they are considered important in the development of functional occlusion (see Table 20-1). The importance of their role in occlusion is demonstrated if this tooth is lost (Figure 17-43). Loss of this tooth now commonly results from periodontal disease, whereas, in the past, it resulted mainly from caries.

Loss of the tooth is followed by mesial inclination and mesial drift of the maxillary second molar into the open arch space, and the mandibular first molar, if present, also supererupts. Occlusion and then mastication are disabled, causing an increased risk of caries and possibly periodontal disease around the irregularly spaced teeth. Prosthetic replacement may prevent these situations.

The distobuccal surfaces of the permanent maxillary first molars may have increased supragingival tooth deposits. This is mainly due to the maxillary first molars' position in the oral cavity, opposite the duct openings of the parotid salivary glands on the inner cheek at the parotid papilla. Saliva, with its mineral content, is released from these glands, causing the dental biofilm to mineralize quickly into supragingival calculus.

PERMANENT MAXILLARY SECOND MOLARS #2 AND #15 (#17 AND #27)

Specific Overall Features Permanent maxillary second molars erupt between 12 and 13 years of age with root completion between ages 14 and 16 (Figure 17-44). These teeth erupt distal to the permanent maxillary first molars and thus are nonsuccedaneous, having no primary predecessors.

Much variation in the form of the maxillary second molars is observed, especially in the size of the distolingual cusp. The crown usually has four cusps similar to the four major cusps of the first molar

of the same arch, but it can also have three cusps. This tooth is composed of four developmental lobes, all named in the same manner as their associated cusps. Evidence of lobe separation can be found in the developmental grooves on the occlusal surface.

The three roots on maxillary second molars are smaller than the first molars. They are also less divergent, as well as placed at a more parallel position than on the first molars. The lingual root is still the largest and longest, extending beyond the crown outline, but it is usually straighter and not as curved toward the buccal as the same root of the first molars.

The layout for the furcations of the maxillary second molar is similar to the first, and the approach for homecare procedures and instrumentation is also the same (see Table 17-1 for general placement). Thus this tooth has three furcations: buccal, mesial, and distal. However, the furcation notches tend to be narrower in the second than those in the first molars with shallower depressions. Thus, the chance of fusion, especially of the buccal roots or even of all three roots, is greater for the second than for the first molars.

The pulp cavity of a maxillary second molar consists of a pulp chamber and three main pulp canals, one for each of the three roots (Figure 17-45). Each major cusp usually has one pulp horn, giving it four pulp horns: mesiobuccal, distobuccal, mesiolingual, and distolingual.

Buccal View Features A maxillary second molar is shorter occlusocervically and narrower mesiodistally than a first molar (see Figure 17-44). The buccal groove is located farther distally on the buccal surface of the second than the first. The mesiobuccal cusp is also longer and has a less sharp cusp tip than the distobuccal cusp. Both the mesial contact and distal contact are in the middle third.

Lingual View Features The distolingual cusp of the maxillary second molar is smaller and shorter than on the first molar and is sometimes not even present (see Figure 17-44). Thus, the outline of the largest cusp of the occlusal surface, the mesiolingual cusp, is much longer and larger, but the cusp is not as sharp as the distolingual cusp, which *helps to distinguish the maxillary right second molar from the left*. In addition, a fifth cusp (or cusp of Carabelli) usually does not exist as it does in the first. From this view, the cusp tips of both the distobuccal cusp and the mesiobuccal cusp can be seen.

A lingual pit is usually present at the end of the distolingual groove, which does not extend as far mesially or cervically as the groove on the first molar. Thus, the distolingual groove ends at a point that is occlusal and distal to the center of the lingual surface.

Proximal View Features From the mesial, the mesial contact area of a maxillary second molar is larger, and the cervical flattening or concavity is never as pronounced as in a first molar (see Figure 17-44). From the distal, both the distobuccal cusp and distolingual cusp are smaller on a second than a first molar, thus showing more of the occlusal surface. Note that no distal contact area is present until the third molar possibly erupts and moves into occlusion.

Occlusal View Features The general outline of the crown of a maxillary second molar is narrower mesiodistally than that of a maxillary first molar but is about the same width buccolingually (see Figure 17-44). Two types of more specific crown outlines are possible on this tooth when viewed from the occlusal: rhomboidal or heart-shaped (Figure 17-46). The more common rhomboidal type has four sides with opposite sides parallel; this type is similar to that of the first molar but with an even more accentuated outline. The heart-shaped type is the less common and is similar to the typical maxillary third molar.

Occlusal Table Components With the rhomboidal type on a maxillary second molar, the cusps present are similar to the major cusps of a maxillary first molar (see Figure 17-46). With the heart-shaped type, the distolingual cusp is quite small with the other three cusps completely overshadowing by their larger size. The distolingual

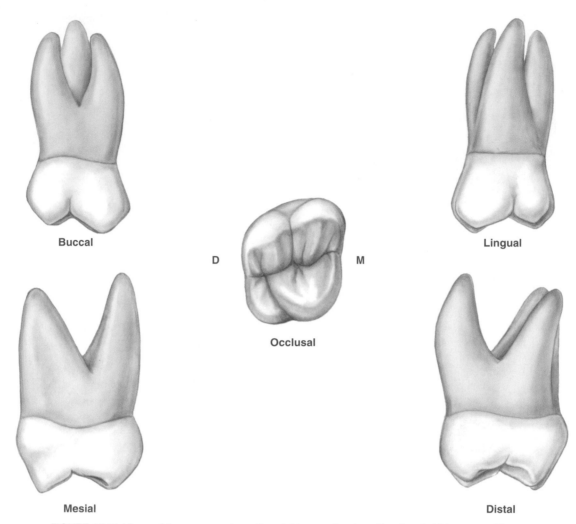

Buccal

D M

Occlusal

Lingual

Mesial

Distal

FIGURE 17-44 Views of the permanent maxillary right second molar with a rhomboidal crown outline.

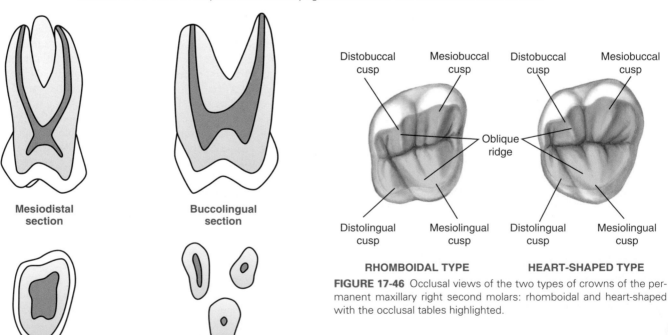

Mesiodistal section

Buccolingual section

Cervical cross section

Midroot cross section

FIGURE 17-45 Pulp cavity of the permanent maxillary right second molar with a rhomboidal crown.

Distobuccal cusp

Mesiobuccal cusp

Distobuccal cusp

Mesiobuccal cusp

Oblique ridge

Distolingual cusp

Mesiolingual cusp

Distolingual cusp

Mesiolingual cusp

RHOMBOIDAL TYPE

HEART-SHAPED TYPE

FIGURE 17-46 Occlusal views of the two types of crowns of the permanent maxillary right second molars: rhomboidal and heart-shaped with the occlusal tables highlighted.

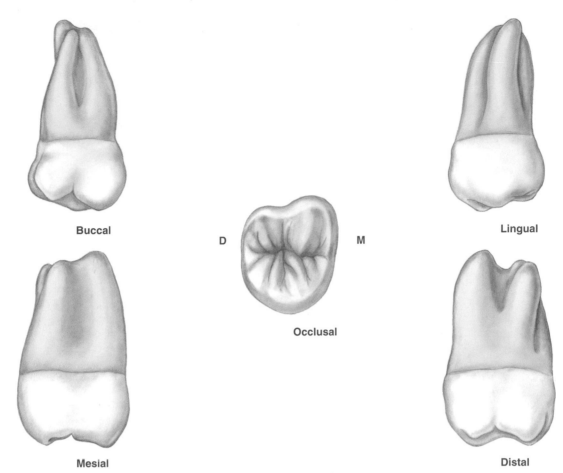

FIGURE 17-47 Views of the permanent maxillary right third molars with a heart-shaped occlusal outline.

cusp can sometimes even be absent in the heart-shaped type with the distolingual groove confined to the occlusal table.

The cusp ridges, triangular ridges, transverse ridge, oblique ridge, developmental grooves, fossae, and occlusal pits for both types of a second molar are similar to those of the first molar of the same arch. However, the defining oblique ridge is less prominent on the second than on the first molar. Instead, an increased number of supplemental grooves are usually present on the occlusal table of the second.

PERMANENT MAXILLARY THIRD MOLARS #1 AND #16 (#18 AND #28)

Specific Overall Features Permanent maxillary third molars may erupt between 17 and 21 years of age with root completion between ages 18 and 25 (Figure 17-47). If erupted, they are located distal to the permanent maxillary second molars and thus are nonsuccedaneous, having no primary predecessors.

The tooth's mesial contact is in the middle third, but it does not have a distal tooth contact because it may be the last tooth in each maxillary quadrant. In addition, because of its very distal arch position, the tooth has only one antagonist in the mandibular arch. This tooth and the very small mandibular central incisor are the only teeth that have one antagonist in the permanent dentition; all others have two.

In addition, this tooth is the smallest molar and most variable tooth in shape in the permanent dentition. Without any standard form observed for this tooth, describing a typical maxillary third molar is therefore difficult. It is smaller generally in all dimensions than a

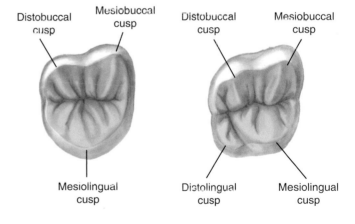

HEART-SHAPED TYPE   **RHOMBOIDAL TYPE**

FIGURE 17-48 Occlusal views of the two types of crown outlines of the permanent maxillary right third molars: heart-shaped and rhomboidal types with the occlusal table highlighted.

second maxillary molar, and its crown is poorly developed when compared with the other maxillary molars. The tooth is composed of four developmental lobes.

Two types of crown outlines are possible for a maxillary third molar when viewed from the occlusal (Figure 17-48). The most common type is heart-shaped, similar to a maxillary second molar but with more supplemental grooves present on the occlusal table. With the

FIGURE 17-49 Pulp cavity of the permanent maxillary right third molar.

FIGURE 17-50 Peg third molar of the permanent maxillary arch *(arrow)* in the oral cavity. (Courtesy of Margaret J. Fehrenbach, RDH, MS.)

heart-shaped type, the tooth usually has only three cusps: mesiobuccal, distobuccal, and mesiolingual; a distolingual cusp is not present.

If a fourth cusp is present, it is the rhomboidal type, having a small and nonfunctioning distolingual cusp, but without any oblique ridge present. For both types of occlusal surfaces, the distobuccal cusp is much shorter than the mesiobuccal cusp, which *helps to distinguish the maxillary right third molar from the left.*

All roots of the third are also poorly developed, like the crown, and shorter than that of a second molar. And similar to other maxillary molars, the maxillary third molars are trifurcated. However, the roots are sometimes so close together that they are fused, either partially or fully, and thus may give the appearance of a single root. The distobuccal root usually is the smallest and often is found tucked under the crown. The roots are curved distally, which also *helps to distinguish the maxillary right third molar from the left.*

The pulp cavity of a maxillary third molar may have a pulp chamber and three pulp canals (Figure 17-49). The tooth may sometimes have one large pulp canal with a fused root to as many as four pulp canals with four roots. The number of pulp horns varies and depends on the number of cusps; if there are three cusps, there are three pulp horns.

> **Clinical Considerations for Permanent Maxillary Third Molars**

Any homecare procedures, instrumentation or restoration may be difficult when these teeth are erupted because of their extreme posterior arch position. Many times, the tooth in each quadrant has heavy deposits and an increased risk of disease, either periodontally or with caries on not only the occlusal surface but also on the cervix of the buccal surface. Having the patient open less wide, actually helps accommodate any procedures on these teeth.

However, permanent maxillary third molars may also fail to erupt and remain impacted within the alveolar process. An impacted tooth is an unerupted or partially erupted tooth that is positioned against another tooth, bone, or even soft tissue in such a way that only partial eruption is likely, if at all. This impaction usually occurs because

the maxilla is underdeveloped, and space or arch length is insufficient to accommodate these teeth because they are the last to erupt in the maxillary arch; thus, surgical removal may be necessary (see earlier discussion). Finally, developmental cyst formation may occur within the dental tissue of an impacted crown, resulting in a dentigerous cyst.

Permanent maxillary third molars, along with the mandibular third molars, commonly exhibit partial anodontia and thus are congenitally missing (see **Chapter 6**). With this disturbance, the appropriate individual tooth germ(s) in the area is missing owing to failure of the initiation process during tooth development. However, the situation in this case usually has no harmful consequences.

This tooth also commonly exhibits partial microdontia, which leads to a smaller molar crown with one cusp, or **peg molar**, either unilaterally or bilaterally, owing to failure in the proliferation process during tooth development (Figure 17-50; see Box 6-1, *F*). This tooth may also have accessory roots, which can complicate extraction procedures.

PERMANENT MANDIBULAR MOLARS
GENERAL FEATURES

Permanent mandibular molars erupt between 6 months and 1 year before the corresponding permanent maxillary molars (Table 17-4; see Figures 17-51, 17-57, and 17-60). The crown has four or five major cusps, of which there are always two lingual cusps of about the same width. All mandibular molars are wider mesiodistally than buccolingually, which is similar to anterior teeth. In contrast, maxillary molars are wider buccolingually, as are all posterior teeth. Thus, from an occlusal view, the outline of the crown is also rectangular, four-sided, or pentagonal, five-sided.

Quite distinct from maxillary molars, the buccal crown outline of all mandibular molars also shows a strong lingual inclination when viewed from the proximal, like the nearby premolars. Thus, from each proximal view, the crown outline is rhomboidal, or four-sided, with opposite sides parallel, which is like all mandibular posterior teeth (see Table 15-4). The crown is thus inclined lingually on the root base, bringing the cusps of these mandibular teeth into proper occlusion with their maxillary antagonists and distributing the forces along the long axis.

Mandibular molars are usually bifurcated, having two roots, a mesial root and distal root (see Figure 17-7). Both of these roots show great to moderate distal root inclination. Because these teeth are bifurcated, there are two furcations located on the buccal and lingual surfaces midway between the proximal surfaces (see Table 17-1). These furcations are also at a level of one-fourth the root length from the CEJ. Root concavities are also found on the mesial surface of the mesial root and on furcal surfaces of both the mesial and distal roots.

TABLE 17-4 Permanent Mandibular Molars

	MANDIBULAR FIRST MOLAR	MANDIBULAR SECOND MOLAR	MANDIBULAR THIRD MOLAR
Universal number	#19 and #30	#18 and #31	#17 and #32
International number	#36 and #46	#37 and #47	#38 and #48
General crown features	Occlusal table with marginal ridges and cusps with tips, inclined planes, ridges, grooves, fossae, and pits		
	Buccal cervical ridge		
Specific crown features	First permanent tooth to erupt. Widest crown mesiodistally of dentition. Five cusps, with Y-shaped groove pattern. Buccal groove possibly ending in buccal pit	Smaller crown than first. Four cusps with cross-shaped groove pattern	Smaller crown than second
Mesial and distal contact*	Junction of occlusal and middle thirds	Middle third	Mesial: cervical third; Distal: none
Distinguish right from left	Distal cusp smallest with a sharp cusp	Difference in height of contour for buccal and lingual from each proximal surface and wider on the mesial than distal	Wider buccolingually on mesial than on distal
General root features	Two roots		
Specific root features	Furcations well removed from the CEJ. Root trunks and root concavities. Divergent roots	Furcations closer to CEJ. Root trunks and root concavities. Less divergent roots	Fused roots, irregularly curved, with sharp apices

CEJ, Cementoenamel junction.

*Height of contour of posteriors for the buccal is in cervical third and lingual in middle third.

Buccal

Mesial

M   D

Occlusal

Lingual

Distal

FIGURE 17-51 Views of the permanent mandibular right first molar.

The root concavities on the mesial root are especially deep if this root also has two root canals.

All three types of mandibular molars can present difficulties in instrumentation or restoration because of their narrow lingual surfaces combined with the lingual inclination of the crown; therefore, instrument placement subgingivally can be even more difficult.

In addition, patients may have difficulty in performing homecare procedures because of the lingual inclination of the crown. They may miss the cervical interface with the associated lingual gingival tissue and remove deposits from only the occlusal surface with a toothbrush. And the proximity of the tongue also makes homecare procedures, instrumentation or restoration more difficult on the lingual surface.

PERMANENT MANDIBULAR FIRST MOLARS #19 AND #30 (#36 AND #46)

Specific Overall Features The permanent mandibular first molars erupt between 6 and 7 years of age with root completion between ages 9 and 10 (Figure 17-51). These teeth are usually the first permanent teeth to erupt in the oral cavity. They erupt distal to the primary mandibular second molars and thus are nonsuccedaneous, having no primary predecessors.

The crown of a mandibular first molar usually has five cusps: three buccal and two lingual. Thus, these teeth are usually composed of five developmental lobes, like the maxillary first molars but unlike the other mandibular molars, which have four. The lobes are named for their associated cusps. Evidence of lobe separation is found in the developmental grooves on the occlusal surface. Occasionally, the distal cusp is missing and, even more rarely, the distal cusp can have an adjacent sixth cusp on larger sized ones.

The two roots, mesial and distal, of a mandibular first molar are both larger and more divergent than the second, leaving these roots widely separated buccally and no longer parallel to each other. The root trunk of the first is also shorter than that of the second. Both roots are usually the same length on the tooth, but if one is longer, it is the mesial root. The mesial root is also the wider and stronger of the two. If this molar has three roots, it is because the mesial root has developed both buccal and lingual root branches. **Fluting**, an elongated developmental depression, is present on many surfaces of the root branches. This is especially noted on the mesial surface of the mesial root; they are not observed on the distal surface of the distal root.

The midway-placed furcations on both the buccal and lingual surfaces are well removed from the CEJ at 3 mm for the buccal furcation and 4 mm for the lingual furcation (see Table 17-1). But the entrance diameters for both are small at only around 1 mm or less, making access to homecare procedures and instrumentation limited. And the buccal furcation entrance tends to be smaller than that of the lingual furcation.

The pulp cavity of a mandibular first molar is more likely to have three root canals: distal, mesiobuccal, and mesiolingual and five pulp horns (Figure 17-52). The distal pulp canal is much larger than the other two canals and is usually the only canal in the distal root. The mesial root usually has two pulp canals: mesiobuccal and mesiolingual. Rarely, these two mesial canals are joined with one single apical foramen, or only one pulp canal is found in the mesial root. Again, rarely, two canals are present in the distal root, just as in the case of the mesial root.

Buccal View Features The crown of a mandibular first molar is larger mesiodistally than occlusocervically (see Figure 17-51). It is also the widest tooth mesiodistally of any permanent tooth because

Mesiodistal section

Buccolingual section

Cervical cross section

Midroot cross section

FIGURE 17-52 Pulp cavity of the permanent mandibular right first molar.

it has a fifth major cusp. From this view, at least some part of all five cusps is visible.

The mesiobuccal cusp is the largest, widest, and highest cusp on the buccal side. The distobuccal cusp is slightly smaller, shorter, and sharper than the mesiobuccal cusp. The distal cusp, despite its name, is also considered a buccal cusp due to its position on that side; it is the lowest cusp and slightly sharper than the other two. The occlusal outline is divided into three sections by the two grooves, as they pass into the buccal surface: the mesiobuccal and distobuccal grooves. These sections of the crown's buccal surface decrease in size from the distal to the mesial.

The mesiobuccal groove on a first mandibular molar is important in classifying the permanent dentition using Angle classification of malocclusion in relation to the maxillary arch (see Table 20-1). The mesiobuccal groove extends straight cervically to a point about midway occlusocervically, but slightly mesial to the center mesiodistally, and usually ends in the buccal pit. However, it may also end in two short, slanting grooves or even fade out after a short distance. The distobuccal groove extends cervically, similarly to the mesiobuccal groove, but is slightly distal to the center mesiodistally, and usually ends in a distobuccal pit but sometimes just fades out.

A buccal cervical ridge, which has a mesiodistally oriented roundness in the cervical third of the buccal surface, is apparent. It is usually more prominent in its mesial part. In addition, a shallow concavity may extend mesiodistally in the middle third.

The mesial outline on a mandibular first molar is slightly concave from the contact area cervically and is rounded occlusal to the contact. The distal outline is more rounded than the mesial. Both the mesial contact and distal contact are at the junction of the occlusal and middle thirds.

Lingual View Features The lingual surface of a mandibular first molar is smaller than the buccal surface but the mesial and distal outlines of the lingual surface are similar to the buccal surface (see Figure 17-51). The occlusal outline is divided in this view by a lingual groove between the mesiolingual cusp and the distolingual cusp.

Proximal View Features The crown is smaller buccolingually than mesiodistally and cervico-occlusally (see Figure 17-51). The crown is also inclined toward the lingual, as are the other mandibular posterior teeth. Additionally, the crown outline from this view is rhomboidal, four-sided, with opposite sides parallel, because the surface is wider at the cervical than the occlusal (see Table 15-4).

The buccal outline on the mesial surface is usually rounded, especially at the buccal cervical ridge. The buccal cervical ridge is in the cervical third, where the height of contour is also located. The lingual outline on the mesial is either straight or slightly rounded from the CEJ to the height of contour in the middle third. It is then rounded from the height of contour to the occlusal. The CEJ is either straight or slightly curved occlusally, but it is always located at a more occlusal level on the lingual part of the mesial surface.

The mesial marginal groove notches the mesial marginal ridge on a mandibular first molar. It has a flattened or slightly concave area centrally located in the gingival third, which is comparable to the mesial root concavity of a maxillary first premolar.

The distal surface is similar to the mesial but smaller, especially in the buccolingual dimension. The distal marginal ridge is notched by the distal marginal groove and is located more cervically than the mesial marginal ridge.

Occlusal View Features The crown outline of the mandibular first molar is roughly pentagonal, or five-sided, with the fifth side created by the distal cusp from an occlusal view (see Figure 17-51). The distal part of the buccal outline converges toward the distal to create the fifth side of the outline. The buccal outline has rounded line angles, which is divided into three parts by the two buccal grooves, the mesiobuccal groove and the distobuccal groove. The length of each of the buccal cusps decreases distally, as noted from the buccal view.

The lingual outline is divided into two parts by the lingual groove. The mesial outline is divided into two parts by the mesial marginal groove. The distal outline, the shortest of the five sides, is divided by the distal marginal groove.

Occlusal Table Components The mandibular first molar usually has five functional cusps; listed from largest to smallest: mesiobuccal, mesiolingual, distolingual, distobuccal, and distal (Figure 17-53). The cusps listed from highest to lowest: mesiolingual, distolingual, mesiobuccal, distobuccal, and distal cusp. Each cusp has four cusp ridges, a triangular ridge, and four inclined cuspal planes.

The mesiobuccal cusp is the bulkiest cusp, although it has a blunt tip. Except for the distal cusp, the distobuccal cusp is the smallest of the larger cusps and has a rounded tip. The mesiolingual cusp is second in size to the mesiobuccal cusp and has the sharpest tip. The distolingual cusp is also quite sharp but is slightly smaller than the mesiolingual cusp. The distal cusp is the smallest of all the cusps and has a sharp cusp, which *helps to distinguish the mandibular right first molar from the left.*

The mandibular first molar has the most complex developmental groove pattern of all the permanent mandibular molars (Figure 17-54). A Y-shaped groove pattern is formed on the occlusal table around the cusps by the mesiobuccal groove, distobuccal groove, and lingual groove. Two marginal ridges border the occlusal table, the mesial marginal ridge and the distal marginal ridge. No transverse ridges are found on the occlusal table, unlike a maxillary first molar and a mandibular second molar.

The occlusal table also has three fossae: large central fossa, smaller mesial triangular fossa, and distal triangular fossa. Three pits are associated with the fossae: mesial pit, central pit, and distal pit. The central it is the also the deepest pit, dividing the central groove into two grooves, the mesial groove and distal groove.

The central pit is the junction of three grooves: mesiobuccal, distobuccal, and lingual. The mesial pit is the junction of four grooves:

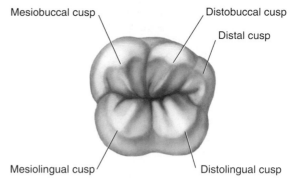

FIGURE 17-53 Occlusal features of the permanent mandibular right first molar.

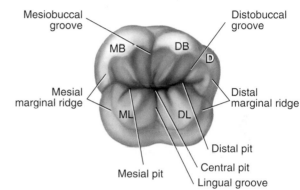

FIGURE 17-54 Additional occlusal features of the permanent mandibular right first molar with the occlusal table highlighted.

FIGURE 17-55 Buccal pit *(arrow)* on the permanent mandibular first molar of a skull. (Courtesy of Margaret J. Fehrenbach, RDH, MS.)

mesial, mesiobuccal triangular, mesiolingual triangular, and mesial marginal. The distal pit is the junction of three grooves: the distal, the distolingual, and distal marginal.

Clinical Considerations for Permanent Mandibular First Molars

Buccal pits that may occur on the buccal surface of mandibular first molars are at an increased risk of caries because of both increased dental biofilm retention and the thinness of enamel forming the walls of the pit (Figure 17-55; see **Chapter 12**). An enamel sealant could be placed on each buccal surface as the tooth begins to erupt.

Sealants on the buccal surface do not bond as easily as on the occlusal surface, however, because of the histology of the area. If caries occur, tooth-colored restorative materials can be used to achieve a more esthetic appearance, and thus the past presence of the buccal pit or associated restoration may not be easy to discern clinically.

FIGURE 17-56 Changes that can occur in the permanent dentition with the loss of the mandibular first molar. Teeth become inclined, and there is mesial drift of the mandibular second molar and possibly third molar with supereruption of the maxillary first molar into the opposing open space.

Because of their arch position, and because the permanent mandibular first molars are the first permanent teeth to erupt in the mandibular arch, they are considered important in regard to the development of occlusion (see Table 20-1). The importance of the role of this tooth in occlusion is shown when the tooth is lost (Figure 17-56). This loss might more easily occur because this tooth is the first permanent tooth to erupt into the oral cavity. It has a greater chance of being affected by caries because child patients are just beginning to master homecare procedures and dietary restrictions. In addition, early dental restorative intervention of the caries may be neglected with a newly present mixed dentition.

With the loss of the tooth, the mandibular second molar, and possibly the third molar, start to undergo mesial incline and mesial drift into the newly opened arch space, allowing the maxillary first molar to supererupt into the space. Occlusion and then mastication are disabled, and the risk of caries and possibly periodontal disease around the irregularly spaced teeth is greatly increased. Interceptive orthodontic therapy as well as tooth replacement is important to prevent these situations after tooth loss.

PERMANENT MANDIBULAR SECOND MOLARS #18 AND #31 (#37 AND #47)

Specific Overall Features The permanent mandibular second molars erupt between 11 to 13 years of age with root completion be-

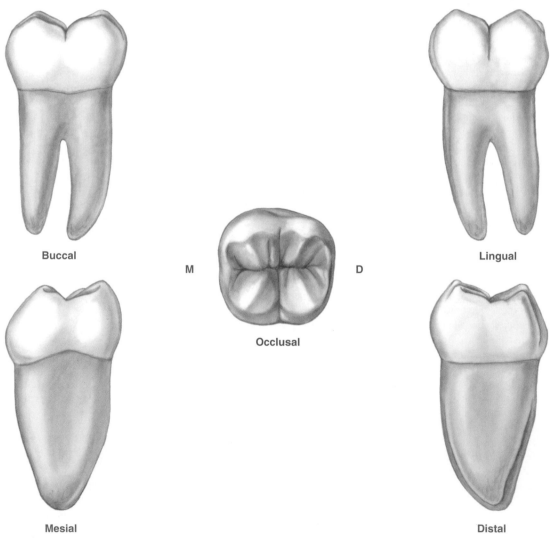

Buccal

Lingual

M   D

Occlusal

Mesial

Distal

FIGURE 17-57 Views of the permanent mandibular right second molar.

tween ages 14 to 15 (Figure 17-57). These teeth erupt distal to the permanent mandibular first molars and thus are nonsuccedaneous, having no primary predecessors.

The crown measurements of a mandibular second molar are generally smaller when compared to a first molar. The four cusps of a second are nearly equal in size compared with the five cusps of differing sizes of a first molar. Like the mandibular third molars, the mandibular second molars are usually composed of four developmental lobes, unlike the mandibular first molars, which are from five lobes. The lobes are named for the associated cusps, and the developmental grooves on the occlusal surface show lobe division.

The two roots of a mandibular second molar are smaller, shorter, and less divergent than those of a first molar, being more parallel to each other. However, the lack of root separation makes detection and deposit removal more difficult if exposed. The root trunk of a second is also longer than that of a first. The mesial root of the second is not as broad as that of a first, but the furcation is farther from the CEJ. The rest of the general layout of the furcations for the second is similar to the first (see Table 17-1 for general placement). However, all of the root depressions are shallower. And overall, root variability is greater in the second than in the first molar.

The pulp cavity of a mandibular second molar can have two pulp canals, with one for each root. However, it is more likely to have three pulp canals, similar to a mandibular first molar: distal, mesiobuccal, and mesiolingual canals; the latter two being together in the mesial root (Figure 17-58). The tooth usually has only four pulp horns, which correspond to the four cusps.

Buccal View Features   The buccal groove divides the same-size mesiobuccal cusp and distobuccal cusp of a mandibular second molar (see Figure 17-57). The mesial contact is at the junction of the occlusal and middle third. The distal contact is slightly cervical, but still at the junction of the occlusal and middle third.

Lingual View Features   The mesiolingual cusp and distolingual cusp have the same size and shape as the buccal cusps, although they have sharper cusp tips (see Figure 17-57). Because the crown converges lingually, a part of both the mesial and distal surfaces can be seen from this view.

Proximal View Features   The buccal height of contour is in the cervical third, and the lingual height of contour is in the middle third for the mandibular second molar (see Figure 17-57). The crown also tapers distally when viewed from the mesial aspect. That is because the molar is also wider buccolingually on the mesial surface than on the distal. Both these mesial surface features *help to distinguish the mandibular right second molar from the left*. The buccal cervical ridge is less pronounced on the second molar than on the first from the proximal.

The CEJ curvature on both proximal surfaces of a second is also less pronounced than that of a first. Neither the mesial nor distal marginal ridge is divided by a marginal groove.

Occlusal View Features   The outline of the crown of a mandibular second molar is rectangular, or four-sided (Figure 17-59). The tooth has four cusps, two buccal and two lingual cusps: mesiobuccal, distobuccal, mesiolingual, and distolingual. With this view, the occlusal surface of a second molar is considerably different from that of a first because there is no distal cusp, and all cusps are of equal size.

Occlusal Table Components   Unlike a mandibular first molar, this tooth has two transverse ridges (see Figure 17-59). The triangular ridges of the mesiobuccal and mesiolingual cusps meet to form a transverse ridge, as do the distobuccal and distolingual cusps. A cross-shaped groove pattern is formed where the well-defined central groove is crossed by the buccal groove and lingual groove, dividing the occlusal table into four parts that are nearly equal, like pastry buns in a pan. Cusp slopes on a second are less smooth than on a first because second molars have an increased number of supplemental grooves. There are three occlusal pits present: central, mesial, and distal.

PERMANENT MANDIBULAR THIRD MOLARS #17 AND #32 (#38 AND #48)

Specific Overall Features   The mandibular third molars may erupt between 17 to 21 years of age with root completion between ages 18 to 25 (Figure 17-60). If erupted, they are located distal to the permanent mandibular second molars and thus are nonsuccedaneous, having no primary predecessors. The tooth's rounded mesial contact when fully erupted is more cervical than any other mandibular molar, meeting at the cervical third, but it does not have a distal tooth contact because it may be the last tooth present in each mandibular quadrant.

Similar to maxillary thirds, the mandibular thirds are variable in shape, having no standard form. Thus, a typical mandibular third

Mesiodistal section   **Buccolingual section**

Cervical cross section   **Midroot cross section**

FIGURE 17-58 Pulp cavity of the permanent mandibular right second molar.

Central pit   Buccal groove
MB   DB
Mesial pit   Distal pit
Transverse ridge   Transverse ridge
ML   DL
Lingual groove

FIGURE 17-59 Occlusal features of the permanent mandibular right second molar with the occlusal table highlighted.

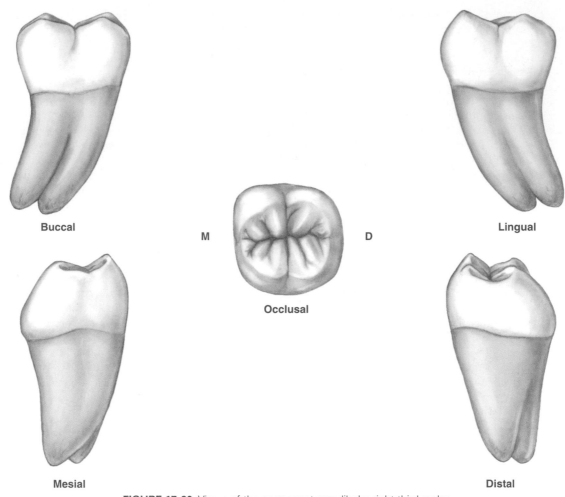

Buccal

M

D

Lingual

Occlusal

Mesial

Distal

FIGURE 17-60 Views of the permanent mandibular right third molar.

molar is difficult to describe. This molar usually is smaller in all dimensions than the second molar, and it sometimes is the same size as the first molar.

Like the mandibular second molars, the mandibular third molars are usually composed of four developmental lobes, unlike the mandibular first molars, which have five lobes. The lobes are named for the associated cusps, and the developmental grooves on the occlusal surface show lobe division.

The crown of a mandibular third molar tapers distally when viewed from the mesial aspect. That is because the molar is also wider buccolingually on the mesial surface than on the distal surface, which *helps to distinguish the mandibular right third molar from the left,* like all mandibular molars. The crown is usually smaller in all dimensions than that of a second molar.

The occlusal outline of the crown is more oval than rectangular, although the crown usually resembles that of a second molar. The two mesial cusps are larger than the two distal cusps. The occlusal surface appears quite wrinkled with an irregular groove pattern, numerous supplemental grooves, and deepened occlusal pits; if an excess of these features exists, the occlusal surface is described as *crenulated.*

A mandibular third molar usually has two roots that are fused, irregularly curved, and shorter than a mandibular second molar. Additionally, the roots are usually smaller in proportion to the crown and have sharp apices. The pulp cavity is usually similar to that of the second molars with four pulp horns and two or three pulp canals (Figure 17-61).

Mesiodistal section

Buccolingual section

Cervical cross section

Midroot cross section

FIGURE 17-61 Pulp cavity of the permanent mandibular right third molar.

Clinical Considerations for Permanent Mandibular Third Molars

Permanent mandibular third molars may also fail to erupt and remain impacted within the surrounding alveolar process (Figure 17-62), which occurs more frequently than with the maxillary counterparts. An impacted tooth is an unerupted or partially erupted tooth that is positioned against another tooth, bone, or even soft tissue, making complete eruption unlikely, and surgical removal may be necessary (see earlier discussion). This impaction usually occurs because the mandible is underdeveloped, and space or arch length is insufficient to accommodate these teeth, which are the last to erupt in the mandibular arch. They may also be partially erupted, causing the surrounding gingival tissue, which may even cover the occlusal surface (operculum), to have an increased risk of periodontal infections (pericoronitis) from poor homecare. Due to its arch position, this infection can become serious (with resultant Ludwig angina) and impact breathing.

Permanent mandibular third molars, as was the case with the maxillary third molars, are permanent teeth commonly involved in partial anodontia, being congenitally missing either unilaterally or bilaterally (see **Chapter 6**). With this disturbance, the appropriate individual tooth germ(s) in the area is missing because of a failure in the initiation process during tooth development. However, this situation usually has no harmful consequences.

FIGURE 17-62 Radiograph of an impacted permanent mandibular third molar. (Courtesy of Margaret J. Fehrenbach, RDH, MS.)

These teeth may also have accessory roots, which can complicate extraction procedures. Finally, developmental cyst formation may occur within the dental tissue of an impacted crown, resulting in a dentigerous cyst (see Figure 6-30).

CHAPTER 18

Primary Dentition

ⓔ Additional resources and practice exercises are provided on the companion Evolve website for this book:
http://evolve.elsevier.com/Fehrenbach/illustrated.

●●● LEARNING OBJECTIVES

1. Define and pronounce the key terms in this chapter.
2. Discuss primary teeth properties and the clinical considerations for primary dentition, integrating it into patient care.
3. Describe the general features of primary teeth and each primary tooth type as well as the specific features of each primary tooth.

4. Discuss the clinical considerations concerning primary molars, integrating it into patient care.
5. Assign the correct name and universal number for each primary tooth on a diagram and a patient.
6. Demonstrate the correct location of each primary tooth on a diagram and a patient.

PRIMARY TEETH PROPERTIES

The first set of teeth is the primary dentition (Figure 18-1). The primary dentition is shed and replaced by the permanent dentition, which is why they sometimes were called *deciduous,* as when leaves are shed from trees. There are 20 total primary teeth when the primary dentition period is completed, 10 per dental arch—as compared to 32 permanent teeth, with 16 per arch. The primary dentition includes the tooth types of incisors, canines, and molars (see Figures 15-1 and 15-3A). These are designated in the Universal Numbering System by the capital letters A through T. In the International Numbering System, the digits 5 through 8 are used for the first of two digits, numbering in a clockwise manner for the quadrants of the primary dentition. The digits 1 through 5 are used for the second digit, starting at the midline and numbering the teeth in a distal direction.

The primary molars are replaced by the permanent premolars; there are no premolars in the primary dentition like there are in the permanent dentition. The permanent molars erupt distal to the primary second molars.

Mineralization of the first primary teeth begin in utero at 13 to 16 weeks. By 18 to 20 weeks during prenatal development, all of the primary teeth have started to mineralize. There are usually no primary teeth visible in the oral cavity at birth. The first eruption of a primary tooth, a primary mandibular central incisor, occurs at an average age of 6 to 10 months with the further eruption of the rest of the primary dentition following (Table 18-1).

The primary dentition takes between 2 and 3 years to be completed, beginning with the initial mineralization of the primary mandibular central incisors, and later being completed with root formation in the primary maxillary second molar (see Figure 6-22, *A*). A 6-month

delay or acceleration is considered usual for an individual child. However, if a child patient is unusually early or late in getting their teeth, it is important to inquire about their related dental history concerning this issue.

The actual dates are not as important as the eruption sequence, because there can be a great deal of variation in the actual dates of eruption, which is noted in various texts. However, the sequence tends to be uniform (see Figure 20-5). In addition, the specific tooth types tend to erupt in pairs so that if there is any asymmetry noted within the primary dentition, a radiograph of the area may be required. Young women tend to shed their primary teeth and have the permanent teeth slightly earlier than young men, possibly reflecting the earlier overall physical maturation achieved.

Also, specific interproximal spaces between the primary teeth are present in most child patients because space is necessary for the proper alignment of the future permanent dentition. These important interproximal spaces still may concern the supervising adults, and they may need reassurance. These spaces are considered primate spaces, mainly involving spaces between the primary maxillary lateral incisor and canine, and also between the primary mandibular canine and first molar (see Figure 18-1 and **Chapter 20**).

Primary teeth are smaller overall than permanent teeth. However, the primary teeth should not be considered just "mini-mes" to the permanent teeth because there are important differences that occur in the structure as well as the size of primary teeth compared with that of permanent teeth (Figures 18-2 to 18-4).

The crown of any primary tooth is short in relation to its total length. The crowns are also more constricted, or narrower, at the cementoenamel junction (CEJ), making them appear bulbous in comparison to the thinner neck. The occlusal table on the primary is also narrower

FIGURE 18-1 Labial view of the primary dentition with the possible primate spaces of the primary dentition indicated *(arrows)*. Note the attrition of the masticatory surfaces, which is usually present, as well as a tendency for an end-to-end bite. (From Bird DL, Robinson DS: *Modern dental assisting*, ed 11, St Louis, 2015, Saunders/Elsevier.)

TABLE 18-1	Approximate Eruption and Shedding Ages for Primary Teeth	
TYPE OF TEETH	**ERUPTION, MEAN (RANGE)**	**SHEDDING, MEAN (RANGE)**
Maxillary Teeth		
Central incisor	10 (8-12 months)	6-7 years
Lateral incisor	11 (9-13 months)	7-8 years
Canine	19 (16-22 months)	10-12 years
First molar	16 (13-19 months, men; 14-19 months, women)	9-11 years
Second molar	29 (25-33 months)	10-12 years
Mandibular Teeth		
Central incisor	8 (6-10 months)	6-7 years
Lateral incisor	13 (10-16 months)	7-8 years
Canine	20 (17-23 months)	9-12 years
First molar	16 (14-18 months)	9-11 years
Second molar	27 (23-31 months, men; 24-30 months, women)	10-12 years

(All data from Nelson S: *Wheeler's dental anatomy, physiology and occlusion*, ed 10, St Louis, 2015, Saunders/Elsevier.)

than on the permanent counterpart. A prominent cervical ridge is present on both the labial and lingual surfaces of anterior teeth and on buccal surfaces of the molars, more than any similar structure on the even larger permanent molars (see Figure 18-4). The contacts are broad and flat within the primary dentition.

Roots of primary teeth are also narrower mesiodistally, and they are longer than the crown length (see Figures 18-2 to 18-4). Each crown-to-root ratio of primary teeth is smaller than those ratios of their permanent dentition counterparts. Molar roots flare more as they approach the apex, and the apical foramina may be larger with the accessory canals often larger and more numerous. Roots may also show partial resorption as the teeth begin to be shed, which can be noted radiographically (see Figure 6-27, *A*).

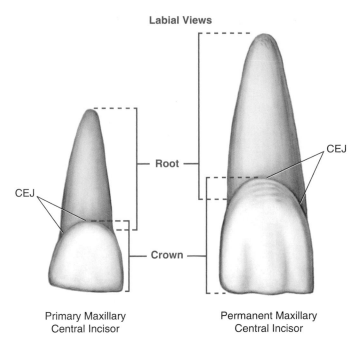

Labial Views

Primary Maxillary Central Incisor

Permanent Maxillary Central Incisor

FIGURE 18-2 Differences between the crowns of the primary and permanent teeth. Note the different crown/root ratios, as well as the differences at the cementoenamel junction.

The pulp cavity on primary teeth shows that both the pulp chambers and pulp horns are relatively large in proportion to those of the permanent teeth, especially the mesial pulp horns of the molars (Figure 18-5). However, great variation in both size and location exists in this dentition, but there is usually a pulp horn under each cusp. The pulp horns are also closer to the outer surface with the pulp chambers being shallow.

Overall, the dentin of the primary dentition is thinner than that of the permanent counterparts. However, the dentin thickness between the pulp chambers and the enamel can be greater especially in the primary mandibular second molar. The enamel is also relatively thin in comparison to permanent counterparts, but it has consistent thickness overlying the dentin of the crown. However, primary teeth also have whiter tone of enamel on their crowns than the permanent teeth because of the increased opacity of the enamel, which covers the underlying yellow dentin. Additionally, it needs to be noted that the enamel rods in the cervical area are directed occlusally.

Clinical Considerations for Primary Dentition

Child patients and supervising adults sometimes discount the importance of the teeth of the primary dentition because they believe they are temporary and soon replaced. It is true that a 70-year-old person will have spent 91% of his or her lifetime chewing with the permanent teeth but only 6% with the primary dentition. Thus, the primary dentition generally functions in esthetics, mastication, and speech for a child for only 5 to 12 years. However, these teeth also serve the important function of holding open the eruption arch space for the succedaneous permanent teeth, which will replace the primary teeth. Individually, each primary tooth also functions in the same way as its permanent counterpart when present.

In the past, many carious primary teeth were extracted instead of repaired, resulting in crowding and potential occlusal complications in the permanent dentition as it erupted (see **Chapter 20**). Worse still, many carious primary teeth were ignored, resulting in serious oral infections and discomfort for the child patient.

Mesial Views

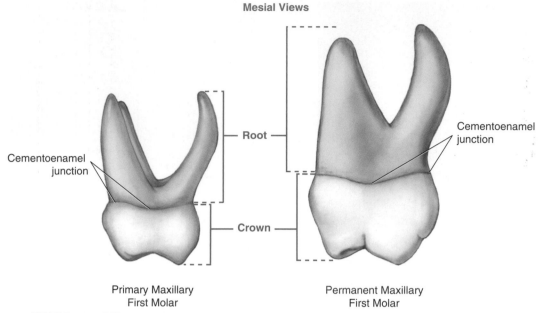

Cementoenamel junction

Root

Crown

Cementoenamel junction

Primary Maxillary
First Molar

Permanent Maxillary
First Molar

FIGURE 18-3 Differences between the crowns and roots of the primary and permanent teeth, especially the differences at the cementoenamel junction.

Whiter crown color

Smaller overall size

Prominent cervical ridge

Narrower roots

Primary

Permanent

Yellower crown color

Larger overall size

Wider roots

FIGURE 18-4 Extracted teeth showing the differences between the primary and permanent teeth. (Courtesy of Margaret J. Fehrenbach, RDH, MS.)

Mesiodistal Section

Pulp horns

Enamel

Dentin

Pulp cavity

Pulp horns

**Primary Mandibular
First Molar**

**Permanent Mandibular
First Molar**

FIGURE 18-5 Differences between the relatively large pulp chambers and pulp horns of the primary teeth and those of permanent teeth, which are relatively smaller.

FIGURE 18-6 Acute caries on the lingual surfaces of primary maxillary anterior teeth caused by early childhood caries, also called *baby bottle tooth decay*. (Courtesy of Margaret J. Fehrenbach, RDH, MS.)

The value of primary teeth is now more realistically appreciated and more are saved from caries because of early dental care. Still, the value of these teeth must be imparted to child patients and supervising adults. Supervision of homecare procedures must begin early, as soon as the first primary teeth erupt into the oral cavity, to prevent premature loss of the primary teeth. Because the enamel and dentin are thinner, the risk of endodontic complications is greater for the primary dentition.

In addition, since the pulp chamber and pulp horns are also larger on primary teeth, there is an increased risk of pulpal exposure during cavity preparation (see Figure 18-5 and **Chapter 13**). If a pulpotomy (partial removal) is performed on primary teeth, there may be perforations; a pulpectomy (complete removal) on primary molars has increased difficulty due to the more tortuous and irregular pulp canals.

For any extraction and other surgical procedures performed during the primary dentition period must be done with extreme caution due to the presence of the deeper developing tooth germs of the permanent dentition, especially with the primary second molars with the presence of the permanent premolars located between the roots (see Figures 6-27 and 6-28). The conical anterior roots facilitate easy surgical extraction but the flared roots of molars are more difficult to treat.

Bulging of the cervical ridge of primary teeth must also be taken into account when these teeth are involved in any restorative procedure as well as restoring the broad contacts (see Figure 18-4).

All of these complex factors are tied to the primary dentition along with the increased possibility of poor homecare in the young child patient, especially if lacking direction by supervising adults. Prolonged nighttime use of a baby bottle with a cavity-causing beverage or sugar on a pacifier must also be considered as an etiologic factor in a child patient with extensive acute caries of the primary teeth. This is known as early childhood caries (ECC), which is more commonly called *baby bottle tooth decay* (Figure 18-6).

A child's first dental appointment should occur within 6 months of the eruption of the first primary tooth and no later than 12 months of age. The intent of this recommendation is to provide information to the child's supervising adults, which will help to establish positive preventive behaviors, prevent serious dental problems, and allay concerns. This early initial visit affords the dental professional the opportunity to provide basic, timely information, and to do this in 6-month increments.

Early dental care is important not only for keeping the primary dentition healthy but also for assessing the need for any appropriate interceptive orthodontic therapy. This may include the use of space maintainers, retainers, and removal of any extraneous bulbous proximal crown width. Also, removal of retained primary teeth (or retained roots) as needed, may allow the correct eruption sequence and alignment of the permanent teeth later (see Figure 20-4).

Extraction procedures of primary teeth should always be performed with caution and with radiographic confirmation of a permanent replacement, especially with primary second molars. If the permanent teeth are missing due to partial anodontia, which can occur with second premolars, the extraction of the primary tooth (mainly the primary molar) must be avoided because retention is preferred and may cover many years of use (see Box 6-1, *B*). Extensive extrinsic staining of the primary teeth may be attributed to Nasmyth membrane (see Figure 6-29).

In addition, if severe periodontal inflammation and destruction in the primary and/or mixed dentition are found with evidence of little dental biofilm, either locally or generally, early aggressive periodontitis must be suspected (previously considered *juvenile periodontitis*). Early intervention with this severe yet uncommon periodontal disease can prevent further periodontal destruction. Thus, a periodontal probe should always be present on the dental tray during dental examinations with child patients.

PRIMARY INCISORS
GENERAL FEATURES

Each dental arch has four primary incisors. As in the permanent dentition, each quadrant has two incisor types: central incisor and lateral incisor. Both primary incisors resemble their permanent successor with some exceptions, such as a more prominent cervical ridge present on both the labial and lingual surfaces. Also, both have the same arch position, function, and general shape as the permanent counterpart, and they function as such for about 5 years.

Dental professionals sometimes note extensive wear or attrition of the incisal ridges of the primary incisors from bruxism (grinding) and the possible formation of an end-to-end bite between the arches. The significance of this finding and its possible relevance to later adult parafunctional habits are unknown (see Figure 18-1).

PRIMARY MAXILLARY CENTRAL INCISOR, E AND F (#51 AND 61)

Specific Features From the labial aspect, the crown of the primary maxillary central incisor (Figure 18-7) appears wider mesiodistally than incisocervically, which is the opposite of its permanent successor. In fact, it is the only anterior tooth of either dentition with this crown dimension. Additionally, its mesial and distal outlines are more rounded than the permanent central incisor as a result of the cervical constriction. The incisal outline is relatively straight from this view, but it slopes toward the distal with attrition.

Unlike their permanent successors, the primary maxillary central incisors have no mamelons, leaving the labial surface smooth. In addition, these teeth rarely have developmental depressions or imbrication lines, and no pits are evident on the lingual surface. However, the cingulum and marginal ridges on the lingual surface all are more prominent than on the permanent successor, and the lingual fossa is deeper.

Both proximal surfaces of the maxillary central incisor appear similar. Because of the short crown and its wide labiolingual measurement, the crown appears thick, even at the incisal third. The CEJ curves distinctly toward the incisal but not as much as on its permanent successor. This curvature is less distal than mesial, as in the

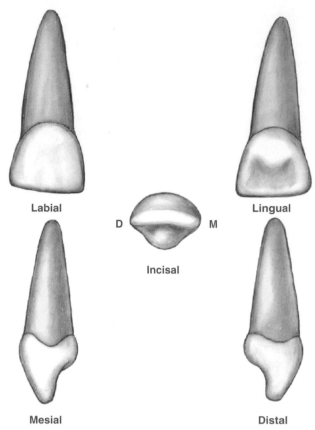

FIGURE 18-7 Views of the primary maxillary right central incisor.

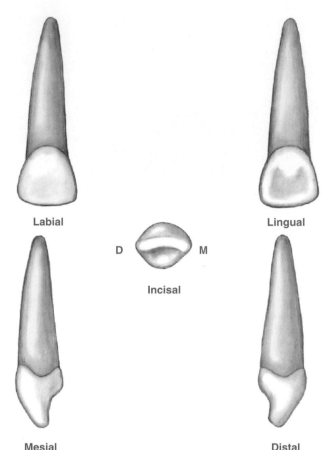

FIGURE 18-8 Views of the primary maxillary right lateral incisor.

permanent successor. From the incisal surface, the crown appears wider mesiodistally than labiolingually, and the incisal ridge appears nearly straight. The single root is generally round and tapers evenly to the apex, but it is longer, relative to crown length, than the permanent central incisor.

PRIMARY MAXILLARY LATERAL INCISOR, D AND G (#52 AND #62)

Specific Features The crown of the primary maxillary lateral incisor (Figure 18-8) is similar to the central incisor but is much smaller than the central in all dimensions. The lateral is also longer incisocervically than mesiodistally, which is exactly the opposite of the central. The incisal angles are also more rounded than the central. The root is also similar to that of the central, but the lateral's root is longer in proportion to its crown compared with the same proportions of the central, and its apex is sharper.

PRIMARY MANDIBULAR CENTRAL INCISOR, O AND P (#71 AND #81)

Specific Features The crown of the primary mandibular central incisor (Figure 18-9) looks more like the primary mandibular lateral incisor than its permanent successor or any other primary maxillary incisor. This tooth is also quite symmetrical, however, which is similar to its permanent successor. It is also not as constricted at the CEJ as the primary maxillary central incisor. From the labial aspect, the crown appears wide compared with its permanent successor. Its mesial and distal outlines from the labial aspect also show that the crown tapers evenly from the contact areas.

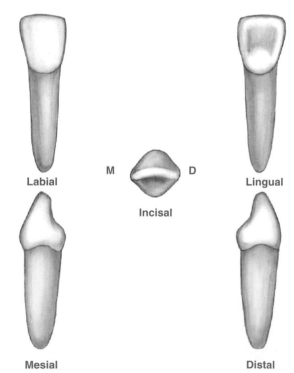

FIGURE 18-9 Views of the primary mandibular right central incisor.

The lingual surface of the primary mandibular central incisor appears smooth and tapers toward the prominent cingulum. The narginal ridges are less pronounced than those of the primary maxillary incisor; the lingual fossa is also shallow. Again, the CEJ curvature on the mesial surface is greater than on the distal. From the mesial aspect, this tooth is much wider labiolingually than its permanent successor.

The incisal ridge is centered over the root from both the proximal and incisal views and divides the labial and lingual into equal halves. The root is single, long, and slender. The labial and lingual surfaces of the root are both rounded, but the proximal surfaces are slightly flattened.

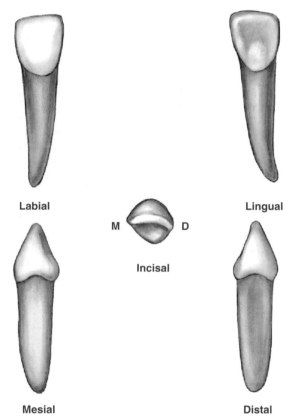

Labial   **Lingual**

M ⟷ D

Incisal

Mesial   **Distal**

FIGURE 18-10 Views of the primary mandibular right lateral incisor.

PRIMARY MANDIBULAR LATERAL INCISOR, Q AND N (#72 AND #82)

Specific Features The crown of the primary mandibular lateral incisor (Figure 18-10) is similar in form to the central incisor of the same arch, but the crown is wider and longer than that of the central. The cingulum is also more developed, and the lingual fossa is slightly deeper than that of the central incisor.

The incisal ridge slopes distally, and its distoincisal angle is more rounded, as is the distal margin. From the incisal aspect, the crown is not as symmetrical as is the central, because the cingulum is offset toward the distal, which has the same cingulum position as its permanent successor. The root may have a distal curvature in its apical third, and it usually has a distal longitudinal groove.

PRIMARY CANINES
GENERAL FEATURES

There are four primary canines, two in each dental arch, and one in each quadrant. These primary canines mainly resemble the outline of their permanent successors with some exceptions, a more prominent cervical ridge present on both the labial and lingual surfaces.

PRIMARY MAXILLARY CANINE, C AND H (#53 AND #63)

Specific Features The crown of the primary maxillary canine (Figure 18-11) has a relatively longer and sharper cusp than that of its permanent successor when first erupted. The mesial and distal outlines of the primary maxillary canine are both rounder, however, and greatly overhang the cervical line. The mesial cusp slope is longer than the distal cusp slope on this tooth, which is just the opposite of the primary mandibular canine and, also, is the opposite of its permanent counterpart.

On the lingual surface, the cingulum is well developed, as are the lingual ridge and marginal ridges. The lingual ridge extends from the cingulum to the cusp tip and divides the lingual surface into a shallow mesiolingual fossa and distolingual fossa. A tubercle is often present on the cingulum, extending from the cusp tip to the cingulum.

From the incisal aspect, the crown is diamond-shaped and the cusp tip is slightly offset to the distal. The root is twice as long as the

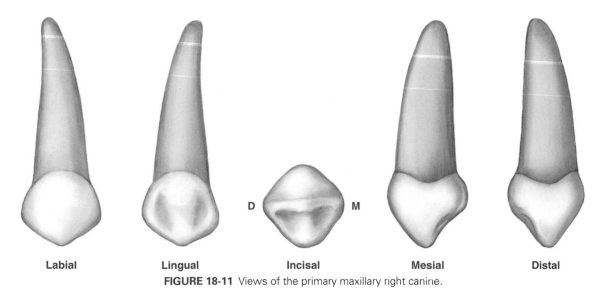

Labial   **Lingual**   **Incisal**   **Mesial**   **Distal**

D ⟷ M

FIGURE 18-11 Views of the primary maxillary right canine.

crown, more slender than that of its permanent successor, and it is inclined distally.

PRIMARY MANDIBULAR CANINE, M AND R (#73 AND #83)

Specific Features The crown of the primary mandibular canine (Figure 18-12) resembles that of the primary maxillary canine, although some dimensions are different. This tooth is much smaller labiolingually. The distal cusp slope is much longer than the mesial cusp slope, as is the case on its permanent counterpart.

The lingual surface is smoother than the primary maxillary canine and is marked by a shallow lingual fossa. The incisal ridge of the primary mandibular canine is straight and is centered over the crown labiolingually. The root is long, narrow, and almost twice the length of the crown, although it is shorter and more tapered than that of a primary maxillary canine.

PRIMARY MOLARS
GENERAL FEATURES

There are eight primary molars with two types: a first molar and second molar. One of each type is located in each quadrant of both dental arches. Both have the similar arch position, function, and general shape as the permanent counterpart, and they function as such for approximately 9 years. Primary molars are replaced by the permanent premolars when shed. However, none of the primary first molars resembles any other tooth in either dentition, but, instead, the crown of each primary second molar in both arches resembles the first molars

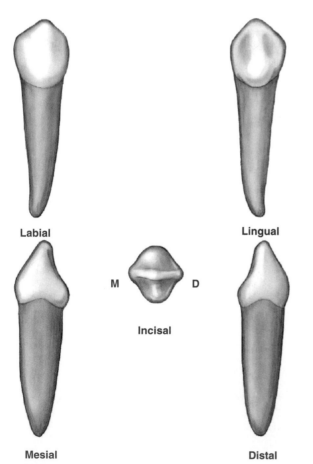

Labial   **Lingual**

M   D

Incisal

Mesial   **Distal**
FIGURE 18-12 Views of the primary mandibular right canine.

of the permanent dentition that will erupt distal to them. Each molar crown is shorter occlusocervically than mesiodistally (see Figure 18-4). A prominent cervical ridge is present on the buccal surfaces.

The occlusal table on a primary molar is more constricted buccolingually than with a permanent molar, rather like a rope around a corral (see Figure 18-13 for example). This constriction is due to both the buccal and lingual surfaces of a primary molar being flatter occlusal to the CEJ curvatures, thus narrowing the occlusal table. The occlusal anatomy of the cusps is also not as pronounced as on the permanent successors.

The roots of the molars are flared beyond the crown outlines, widely separating the roots (see Figure 18-4). Additional space is thus available between the roots for the deeper developing permanent premolar crowns. The primary molars each have a short root trunk, as with permanent posterior teeth; the roots branch a short distance from the base of the crown. Again, this arrangement creates more space for the developing permanent premolar crowns.

PRIMARY MAXILLARY FIRST MOLAR, B AND I (#54 AND #64)

Specific Features The crown of the primary maxillary first molar (Figure 18-13) does not resemble any other crown of either dentition. From the buccal aspect, both the mesial and distal outlines are rounded and constricted at the CEJ. The CEJ on the mesial half of the buccal surface curves around an extremely prominent buccal cervical ridge. The height of contour on the buccal is at the cervical one-third and for the lingual at the middle one-third.

The occlusal table on the maxillary first molar can have four cusps: mesiobuccal, mesiolingual, distobuccal, and distolingual with the two mesial cusps being the largest and the two distal cusps being quite small. It can also have only three cusps because the distolingual cusp may be absent. The occlusal table also has an extremely prominent transverse ridge. Additionally, an oblique ridge extends between the mesiolingual cusp and the distobuccal cusp; however, it is not as prominent as the one on its permanent counterpart.

The tooth also has an H-shaped groove pattern and three fossae: central, mesial triangular, and distal triangular. The central groove connects the central pit with the mesial pit and distal pit at each end of the occlusal table.

The buccal groove originates in the central pit and extends buccally, separating the mesiobuccal and distobuccal cusps. The distal triangular fossa contains the disto-occlusal groove, which extends obliquely and is parallel to the oblique ridge just distal to it. Both the buccal and disto-occlusal grooves remain located only at the occlusal table, which is unlike its permanent counterpart.

Primary maxillary first molars do have the same number and position of the roots as the permanent maxillary molars. The three root branches are thinner and have greater flare than on the permanent molar, and the root trunk is short. The mesiobuccal root is wider buccolingually than the distobuccal root and the lingual root is the longest and most divergent.

PRIMARY MAXILLARY SECOND MOLAR, A AND J (#55 AND #65)

Specific Features The primary maxillary second molar (Figure 18-14) is larger than the primary maxillary first molar. This tooth most closely resembles the form of the permanent maxillary first molar but is smaller in all dimensions. Thus, it usually has a cusp of Carabelli, the minor fifth cusp, as does its permanent counterpart.

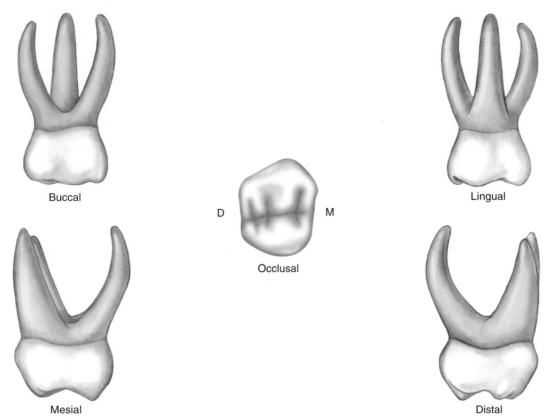

Buccal

Lingual

Occlusal

D   M

Mesial

Distal

FIGURE 18-13 Views of the primary maxillary first right molar.

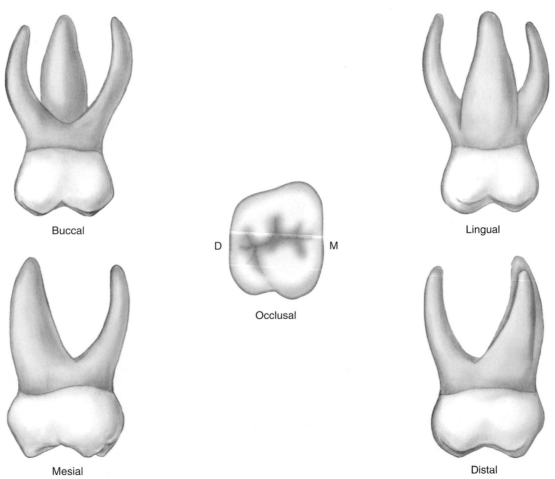

Buccal

Lingual

Occlusal

D   M

Mesial

Distal

FIGURE 18-14 Views of the primary maxillary right second molar.

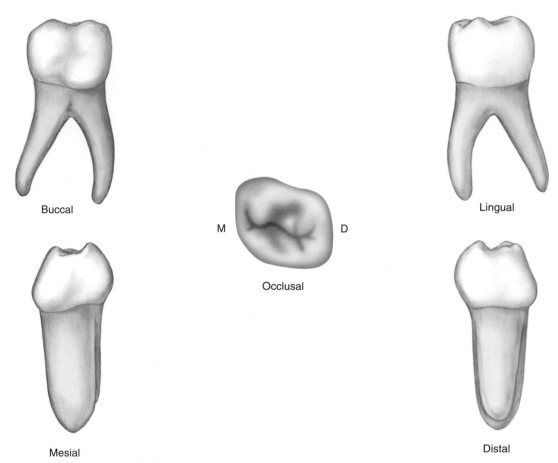

Buccal

Lingual

M   D

Occlusal

Mesial

Distal

FIGURE 18-15 Views of the primary mandibular right first molar.

PRIMARY MANDIBULAR FIRST MOLAR, L AND S (#74 AND #84)

Specific Features The primary mandibular first molar (Figure 18-15) has a crown unlike any other tooth of either dentition. The tooth does have a prominent buccal cervical ridge, which is also on the mesial half of the buccal surface, similar to other primary molars. The height of contour on the buccal is at the cervical one-third and for the lingual is in the middle one-third. The mesiolingual line angle of the crown is rounder than any other line angles.

The tooth has four cusps with the mesial cusps larger. The mesiolingual cusp is long, pointed, and angled in on the occlusal table. A transverse ridge passes between the mesiobuccal and mesiolingual cusps. The tooth does have two roots, which are positioned similarly to those of the permanent mandibular molars.

PRIMARY MANDIBULAR SECOND MOLAR, K AND T (#75 AND #85)

Specific Features The primary mandibular second molar (Figure 18-16) is larger than the primary mandibular first molar. The tooth most closely resembles the form of the permanent mandibular first molar that erupts distal to it, because it has five cusps. The three buccal cusps are nearly equal in size, however, and the primary mandibular second molar has an overall oval occlusal shape.

Clinical Considerations with Primary Molars

Child patients within the mixed dentition period and their supervising adults may not notice the presence of the newly erupted permanent first molar of either arch because, when it erupts, it appears similar to the larger primary second molar that is adjacent to it (Figure 18-17). These child patients and their supervising adults must be reminded that, to last a lifetime, these new posterior permanent teeth require diligent homecare and possibly enamel sealants applied to the occlusal surface.

The greater root spread of primary molars, along with their narrow shape and lack of root trunk, make primary molars susceptible to fracture during extraction procedures (see Figure 18-4). Dental professionals should also remember that shedding of primary teeth is an intermittent process with resorption of the dental tissue being followed by apposition. A loose primary tooth may tighten and thus may not be as ready as thought for extraction, a procedure which should always be considered with caution in these young patients (see earlier discussion and **Chapter 6**).

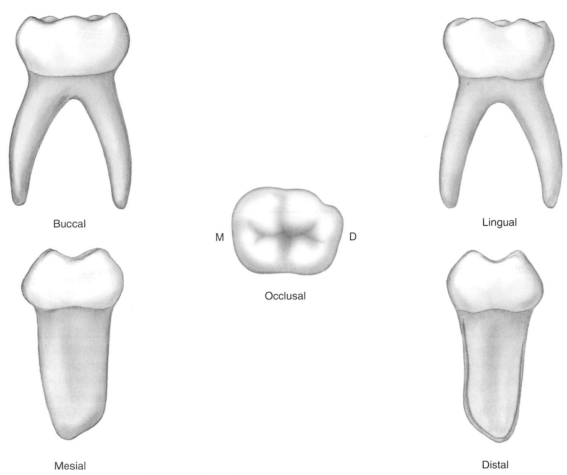

Buccal

M   D

Occlusal

Lingual

Mesial

Distal

FIGURE 18-16 Views of the primary mandibular right second molar.

Permanent mandibular first molar

Primary mandibular second molar

Primary mandibular first molar

Primary mandibular canine

Permanent mandibular incisors

FIGURE 18-17 The mixed dentition with the eruption of the permanent mandibular first molar distal to the primary mandibular second molar. Note that the newly erupted permanent first molar can be difficult to discern because it appears similar to the already erupted adjacent primary second molar. (Courtesy of Margaret J. Fehrenbach, RDH, MS.)

JOINT CAPSULE

A joint capsule completely encloses the TMJ (Figure 19-5; see Figures 19-1 and 19-3). To do this, the capsule wraps around the margin of the temporal bone's articular eminence and articular fossa superiorly. Inferiorly, the capsule wraps around the circumference of the mandibular condyle, at the level of the condyle's neck.

The joint capsule has two layers. The outer layer is a firm, fibrous connective tissue supported by the surrounding ligaments associated with the joint. The inner layer is a synovial (sy-no-vee-al) membrane, which consists of a thin connective tissue that contains nerves and blood vessels. The blood vessels in the synovial membrane produce synovial fluid. Synovial fluid is a thick substance that fills the joint, lubricates it, and provides nutrition to the avascular parts of the joint disc (discussed next).

JOINT DISC

A joint disc is located on each side between the temporal bone and mandibular condyle (Figure 19-6; see Figures 19-2 and 19-3). On cross section, each disc appears caplike on the mandibular condyle, with its superior aspect concavoconvex from anterior to posterior and its inferior aspect concave. As is shown, this shape of the disc conforms to the shape of the adjacent articulating two bones of the TMJ and is related to normal joint movements. Thus it functions as a deformable pad between the noncongruent articular surfaces of the bones of the joint.

The joint disc completely divides the TMJ into two compartments. These two compartments are synovial cavities, which consists of an upper and a lower synovial cavity. The synovial membrane lining the joint capsule produces the synovial fluid that fills these two cavities.

The joint disc is not free between the two bones but is attached to the lateral and medial poles of the mandibular condyle. However, the disc is not directly attached to the temporal bone anteriorly, but indirectly through the capsule. Posteriorly, the disc is divided into two areas. The upper division of the posterior part is attached to the temporal bone's postglenoid process, and the lower division is attached to the neck of the mandibular condyle. The disc blends with the capsule at these two points. This posterior area of attachment of the disc to the capsule is one of the regions where nerves and blood vessels from the periosteum of the two bones enter the joint.

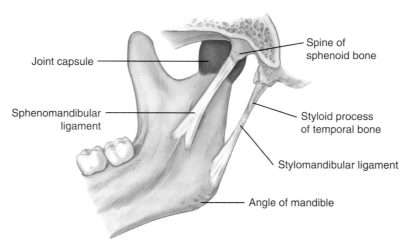

FIGURE 19-5 Joint capsule of the temporomandibular joint. (From Fehrenbach MJ, Herring SW: *Illustrated anatomy of the head and neck,* ed 4, St Louis, 2012, Saunders/Elsevier.)

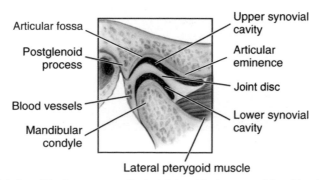

FIGURE 19-6 Joint disc of the temporomandibular joint and its two synovial cavities. (From Fehrenbach MJ, Herring SW: *Illustrated anatomy of the head and neck,* ed 4, St Louis, 2012, Saunders/Elsevier.)

The joint disc itself consists of dense connective tissue (Figure 19-7). Unlike other joint discs, it does not initially contain any cartilage. The central region of the disc is avascular and lacks innervation; in contrast, the peripheral region has both blood vessels and nerves. Few cells are present in the peripheral region, and include fibroblasts and white blood cells. The central region is also thinner but of denser consistency than the peripheral region, which is thicker but has a more cushioned consistency. The synovial fluid in the synovial cavities provides the nutrition for the avascular central region of the disc. With age, the entire disc thins and may undergo addition of cartilage in the central region, changes that may lead to impaired movement of the joint (discussed later).

JOINT MOVEMENT

Two basic types of movement of the mandible are performed by the TMJ and its associated **muscles of mastication** (mass-ti-**kay**-shin): a gliding movement and a rotational movement (Figures 19-8 and 19-9; Tables 19-1 and 19-2). These muscles are involved in mastication using these two movements.

The *gliding movement* of the TMJ occurs mainly between the disc and the articular eminence of the temporal bone in the upper synovial cavity, with the disc plus the mandibular condyle moving forward or backward, down and up the articular eminence. The gliding movement allows the lower jaw to move forward or backward. Bringing the lower jaw forward involves **protrusion** (pro-**troo**-zhin) **of the mandible** (see Figure 20-15). Bringing the lower jaw backward involves **retraction** (re-**trak**-shun) **of the mandible**.

The *rotational movement* of the TMJ occurs mainly between the disc and the mandibular condyle in the lower synovial cavity. The axis of rotation of the disc plus the mandibular condyle is transverse, and the movements accomplished are depression or elevation of the mandible. The **depression** (de-**presh**-in) **of the mandible** is the lowering of the lower jaw. The **elevation** (el-eh-**vay**-shun) **of the mandible** is the raising of the mandible.

With these two types of movements, gliding and rotation, and with the right and left TMJs working together, the finer movements of the jaw can be accomplished. These include opening and closing the jaws and shifting the lower jaw to one side.

Opening the jaws, which occurs during mastication, speech, and respiratory movements, involves both depression and protrusion of the mandible. When the jaws close, both elevation and retraction of the mandible occur. Thus, the natural opening and closing of the jaws involve a combination of gliding and rotational movements of the TMJs in their respective joint cavities. The disc plus the condyle glides on the articular fossa in the upper synovial cavity, moving forward or backward on the articular eminence. At approximately the same time, the mandibular condyle rotates on the disc in the lower synovial cavity.

Lateral deviation (de-vee-ay-shun) **of the mandible**, or lateral excursion, which involves shifting the lower jaw to one side, occurs during mastication (see Figure 20-13). Thus, lateral deviation involves both gliding and rotational movements of contralateral TMJs in their respective joint cavities. During lateral deviation, the ipsilateral disc plus the mandibular condyle glides forward and medially on the articular eminence in the upper synovial cavity, whereas the contralateral condyle and disc remain relatively stable in position in the articular fossa. These actions produce rotation around the more stable condyle.

During mastication, the power stroke (when the teeth crunch the food) involves a movement from a laterally deviated position back to the midline. If the food is on the right side of the mouth, the mandible is deviated to the right. The power stroke returns the mandible to the center, and thus the movement is to the left and involves retraction of the left side; the reverse situation occurs if the food is on the left.

Clinical Considerations for Joint Pathology

Patients may have pathology associated with one or both of their TMJs, or a **temporomandibular** (tem-poh-ro-man-**dib**-you-lar) **disorder (TMD)** (or dysfunction). It is the most common cause of facial pain after a toothache. Patients with TMD may experience chronic joint tenderness, swelling, and painful muscle spasms. They may also have difficulties in moving the joint, such as a limited or deviated mandibular opening. In a healthy joint, the surfaces in contact with one another (bone and cartilage) do not have any receptors to transmit the feeling of pain. The pain therefore originates from one of the surrounding soft tissue. When receptors from one of these areas are triggered, the pain causes a reflex to limit the mandible's movement. Furthermore, inflammation of the joints can cause constant pain, even without movement of the jaw.

Recognition of TMD includes palpation of the joint as the patient performs all the movements of the joint, as well as the associated muscles of mastication. The TMJ is palpated laterally at a depression inferior to the zygomatic arch and 1 to 2 cm anterior to the tragus. The posterior aspect of the joint is palpated through the external auditory canal. The joint should be palpated in both open and

FIGURE 19-7 Microscopic appearance of the temporomandibular joint from *(A)* an inferior section of the joint disc and *(B)* mandibular condyle. (From the personal collection of Major M. Ash, Jr.)

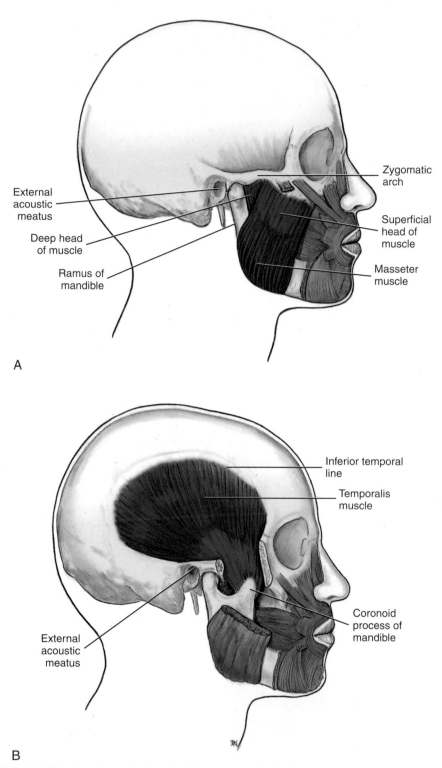

A

B

FIGURE 19-8 Muscles of mastication. **A,** Masseter muscle. **B,** Temporalis muscle. (**A** and **B,** From Fehrenbach MJ, Herring SW: *Illustrated anatomy of the head and neck,* ed 4, St Louis, 2012, Saunders/ Elsevier.)

Continued

closed positions and also both with the mandible moving laterally and posteriorly. While palpating, one should feel for muscle spasm, muscle or joint tenderness, and joint sound. The muscles palpated as a part of complete TMJ examination are masseter, temporalis, medial pterygoid, lateral pterygoid, and sternocleidomastoid. See the ***Workbook for Illustrated Dental Embryology, Histology, and***

Anatomy for a detailed explanation of an occlusal evaluation that includes an examination of the TMJ.

All signs and symptoms related to the TMD, such as the amount of mandibular opening and facial pain, should also be noted in the patient record, as should any parafunctional habits and related systemic diseases. To aid in diagnosis, a traditional skull radiograph

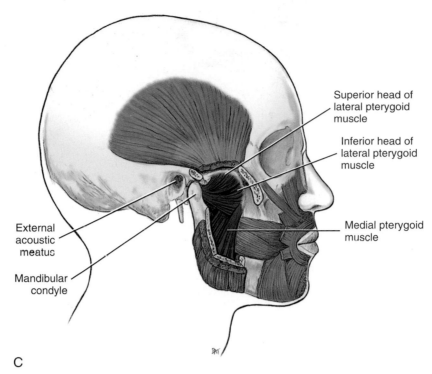

C

FIGURE 19-8, cont'd Muscles of mastication. **C,** Medical and lateral pterygoid muscles.

is taken, or magnetic resonance imaging (MRI) may be requested in more severe cases because this noninvasive procedure for imaging soft tissue uses no ionizing radiation but does deliver detailed sections (Figure 19-10).

Many controversies are associated with the etiology of these disorders. TMD is a heterogeneous, complex disorder involving many factors, such as behavioral stressors and parafunctional habits (clenching and/or bruxism [grinding]) (see **Chapter 20**). Trauma to the jaw may cause TMD, with the disc having adhesions to the bony surfaces; however, this is not the most common etiologic factor as are stressors and habits. Jaw thrusting (causing unusual speech and chewing habits) and excessive gum chewing or nail biting, as well as the size and hardness of food eaten, are other factors to be considered. Poor posture can also be an important factor in TMJ symptoms. For example, holding the head forward, while looking at a computer all day, strains the muscles of the face and neck.

Systemic diseases (such as osteoarthritis) may involve parts of the TMJ and contribute to TMD. Aging of the joint disc, which causes wear and hardening, may also be a factor in TMD; however, TMD does not usually become worse with age.

Not all patients with TMD have abnormalities in the joint disc or the joint itself; most symptoms seem to originate from the muscles. Muscle pain can sometimes be associated with muscle tissue trigger points, which is known as myofascial pain dysfunction syndrome. These trigger points can be localized by digital palpation, both intraorally and extraorally. Studies do not support the role of TMD in directly causing headaches, neck pain, back pain, or instability. However, cyclic episodes of TMD, and other incidents of chronic body pain, are commonly encountered in the population with TMD.

Joint sounds can occur because of disc derangement as the posterior part of the disc becomes caught between the condyle head and the articular eminence. Joint sounds are not a reliable indicator of TMD because they can change over time in a patient. The clicking, grinding, and popping sounds of the joint during movement, which

are commonly present with TMD, are also found in persons without TMD. In isolated cases of myofascial pain and dysfunction, joint tenderness and joint click are usually absent.

Many controversies surround the treatment of TMD, and fewer than half of patients with TMD seek treatment for their disorder. Most recent studies have determined that malocclusion and occlusal discrepancies are not involved in most cases of TMD, but lack of overbite may be an additive factor. Thus, occlusal adjustment, jaw repositioning, and orthodontic therapy are not the treatments of choice for all patients with TMD, nor do these treatments seem to prevent TMD.

Most cases of TMD improve over time with inexpensive and reversible treatments, including patient-based or prescription pain control, relaxation therapy, stress management, habit control, moderate home-based muscular exercises, and orofacial myology (see **Chapter 20**). Many of the homecare steps to treat TMJ problems can prevent such problems in the first place, for instance, by avoiding extreme jaw movements, learning relaxation techniques to reduce overall stress and muscle tension, and maintaining good posture, especially when working at a computer. Pausing often to change position, and resting hands and arms, can relieve stressed muscles. It is always important to use safety measures to reduce the risk of fractures and dislocations.

A flat-plane, full-coverage oral appliance, for instance, a non-repositioning stabilization splint, often is helpful to control bruxism and take stress off the TMJ, although some individuals may bite harder on it, thus worsening their condition. The anterior splint, with contact at the front teeth only, may then prove helpful if used short-term. Such inexpensive and reversible treatments (i.e., ones not causing permanent jaw or dentition changes) show the same success as more expensive and irreversible treatments, such as surgery. Thus, few patients with TMD require surgery or other extensive treatment. However, surgery of the TMJ can now make use of arthroscopy with an endoscope and lasers. Replacement of the jaw joint(s) or disc(s) with TMJ implants is considered as a treatment of last resort.

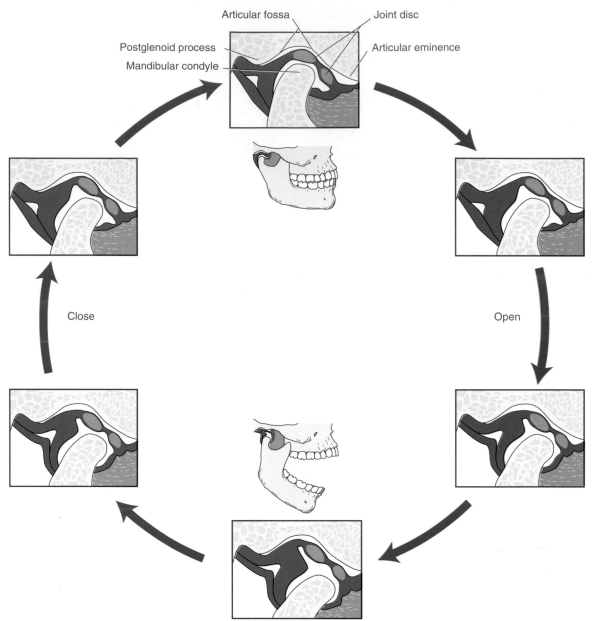

FIGURE 19-9 Movements of the mandible related to the temporomandibular joint to demonstrate what occurs during the opening and closing of the mouth.

An acute episode of TMD can occur when a patient opens too wide, causing maximal depression and protrusion of the mandible, as when yawning or receiving prolonged dental care. This causes **subluxation** (sub-luk-**say**-shun), or partial dislocation of both joints (Figure 19-11). Subluxation occurs when the head of each condyle moves too far anteriorly past the articular eminence. Then, when the patient tries to close and elevate the mandible, the condylar heads cannot move posteriorly because both the bony relationships prevent this, and the muscles have become spastic.

The patient now has **trismus** (**triz**-mus), or the inability to normally open the mouth.

Treatment of subluxation consists of relaxation of these muscles and careful movement of the mandible downward and back. The mandibular condylar heads can then assume the usual posterior position, in relation to the articular eminence, by the muscular action of the elevating muscles of mastication. Subsequently, these patients must refrain from extreme depression of the mandible, such as can occur with prolonged dental work.

TABLE 19-1	Origin and Insertion of Muscles of Mastication with Associated Movements of Mandible		
MUSCLES	**ORIGIN**	**INSERTION**	**ASSOCIATED MOVEMENTS OF MANDIBLE**
Masseter	Superficial head: Zygomatic process of maxilla and anterior two-thirds of the inferior border of the zygomatic arch	Superficial head: Angle of mandible	Elevation of mandible (during jaw closing)
	Deep head: Posterior one-third and medial surface of zygomatic arch	Deep head: Ramus of mandible	
Temporalis	Temporal fossa on temporal bone	Coronoid process and ramus of mandible	Elevation of mandible (during jaw closing) and retraction of mandible (lower jaw backward)
Medial pterygoid	Deep head: Medial surface of lateral pterygoid plate of sphenoid bone	Both heads: Medial surface of ramus and angle of mandible	Elevation of mandible (during jaw closing)
	Superficial head: Pyramidal process of palatine bone and maxillary tuberosity of maxilla		
Lateral pterygoid	Superior head: Greater wing of sphenoid bone	Superior head: Pterygoid fovea of mandible (mainly though fusion with inferior head) as well as temporomandibular joint disc and capsule	One muscle: Lateral deviation of mandible (shift lower jaw to contralateral side) Both muscles: Mainly protrusion of mandible (lower jaw forward), slight depression of mandible (during jaw opening)
	Inferior head: Lateral surface of lateral pterygoid plate of the sphenoid bone	Inferior head: Pterygoid fovea of mandible	

(From Fehrenbach MJ, Herring SW: *Illustrated anatomy of the head and neck,* ed 4, St Louis, 2012, Saunders/Elsevier.)

TABLE 19-2	Joint Movements
MANDIBULAR MOVEMENTS	**TEMPOROMANDIBULAR JOINT MOVEMENTS**
Protrusion of mandible, moving lower jaw forward	Gliding in both upper synovial cavities
Retraction of mandible, moving lower jaw backward	Gliding in both upper synovial cavities
Elevation and retraction of mandible, closing the jaws	Gliding in both upper synovial cavities and rotation in both lower synovial cavities
Depression and protrusion of the mandible, opening the jaws	Gliding in both upper synovial cavities and rotation in both lower synovial cavities
Lateral deviation of mandible, to shift lower jaw to the contralateral side	Gliding in one upper synovial cavity and rotation in the contralateral upper synovial cavity

(From Fehrenbach MJ, Herring SW: *Illustrated anatomy of the head and neck,* ed 4, St Louis, 2012, Saunders/Elsevier.)

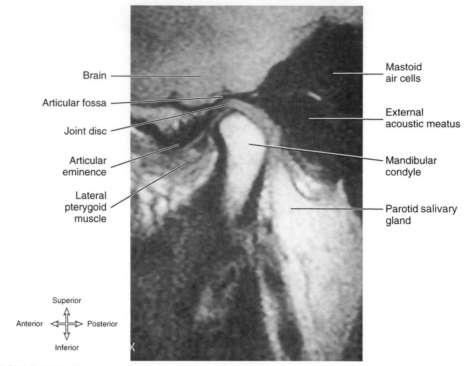

Brain

Articular fossa

Joint disc

Articular
eminence

Lateral
pterygoid
muscle

Mastoid
air cells

External
acoustic meatus

Mandibular
condyle

Parotid salivary
gland

Superior

Anterior ⟷ Posterior

Inferior

FIGURE 19-10 Coronal magnetic resonance imaging of the temporomandibular joint of an asymptomatic individual. (From Quinn PD: *Color atlas of temporomandibular joint surgery,* St Louis, 1998, Mosby/Elsevier.)

FIGURE 19-11 Lateral radiographic view of an individual with a dislocation of both the joints or subluxation. (From Reynolds PA, Abrahams PH: *McMinn's interactive clinical anatomy: head and neck,* ed 2, London, 2001, Mosby Ltd.)

CHAPTER 20

Occlusion

Additional resources and practice exercises are provided on the companion Evolve website for this book: http://evolve.elsevier.com/Fehrenbach/illustrated.

●●●LEARNING OBJECTIVES

1. Define and pronounce the key terms in this chapter.
2. Discuss occlusion and centric occlusion and its relationship to functional movements and patterns of the mandible.
3. Discuss arch form and the phases of arch development.
4. Describe dental curvatures and angulations.
5. Discuss centric relation, lateral and protrusive occlusions, and the mandibular rest position and how to achieve each of them on a skull, a dentition model, and a patient.
6. Demonstrate the movements of the mandible related to occlusion.
7. Discuss primary occlusion and the clinical considerations concerning it, integrating it into patient care.
8. Identify the key concepts of occlusion on a diagram, a dentition model, and a patient.
9. Discuss malocclusion and outline Angle classification and how it relates to patient care, including clinical considerations concerning parafunctional habits.
10. Identify on dentition models each division of Angle classification of malocclusion.
11. Demonstrate an initial occlusal evaluation on a patient and record findings.

OCCLUSION PROPERTIES

Occlusion (ah-kloo-zhun) is the contact relationship between the maxillary teeth and mandibular teeth when the jaws are in a fully closed (or occluded) position, as well as the relationship between the teeth in the same arch. Many patterns of tooth contact are possible; part of the reason for the variety is the substantial range of movement of the mandibular condyle within the temporomandibular joint (TMJ) (see Figure 19-9).

Occlusion develops in a child as the primary teeth erupt. During this time, oral motor behaviors develop and the masticatory skills are acquired. The deglutition skills to accommodate the mastication process begin to develop in utero and are modified on a developmental continuum as the primary dentition erupts. Occlusion of the erupting permanent dentition is dependent on the primary teeth shedding with the exception of the permanent molars, because these erupt distal to the primary dentition.

Interrelated factors, such as the associated musculature, neuromuscular patterns, TMJ functioning (see **Chapter 19**), tongue functioning and posturing, orofacial behaviors, and habit patterns are involved in the development of the occlusion. Thus, occlusion is only one aspect of an entire developing orofacial masticatory and deglutition system that includes many other factors and variables. The teeth, in proper alignment, are relatively self-cleansing by action of the cheek and lip musculature with the neutralizing flow of saliva over the tooth surfaces.

An ideal occlusion rarely exists, but this concept provides a basis for treatment. The optimum 138 occlusal contacts for the permanent dentition in the closure of 32 teeth are seldom, if ever, achieved. When occlusion is considered, the position of the dentition in centric occlusion serves as the basis for reference (discussed next). Thus, centric occlusion serves as the standard for describing an occlusion. Ideally, a centric resting posture of the tongue, lips, and mandible is also present (discussed later). To prevent occlusal disharmony, all patients should have an occlusal evaluation before and after completion of their dental treatment plan with reevaluation occurring on a regular basis; see the **Workbook for Illustrated Dental Embryology, Histology, and Anatomy** for guidelines and related techniques. Advanced digital imaging is also now available providing valuable three-dimensional views of the patient's occlusion, which can be used during orthodontic therapy as well as occlusal adjustments during periodontal therapy.

CENTRIC OCCLUSION

Centric occlusion (CO), or habitual occlusion, is the voluntary position of the dentition that allows the maximum contact when the teeth occlude (Figure 20-1). It is the centered contact position of the

FIGURE 20-1 Permanent dentition in centric occlusion (CO). **A,** Facial view. **B,** Buccal view. Dentition has the usual amount of overjet present, which is the horizontal overlap between the two arches. Also has the usual amount of overbite, which is the vertical overlap between the two arches. The use of three segments can be used to describe arch form: anterior, middle, and posterior. (Courtesy of Dona M. Seely, DDS, MSD, Orthodontics, Seattle and Bellevue, WA.)

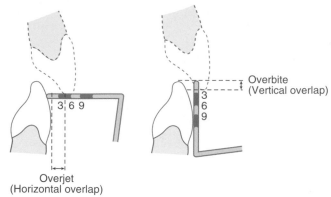

FIGURE 20-2 Comparison of overjet, the horizontal overlap between the two arches, and overbite, the vertical overlap between the two arches.

occlusal surfaces of mandibular teeth on the occlusal surface of the maxillary teeth. The position of CO is related to the functioning of the dentition. However, even when the teeth are in full closure, discrepancy between the relationships of the mandible, TMJs, and/or the maxilla may be significant (skeletal discrepancies are discussed later).

When the teeth are in the position of CO, each tooth of one arch is in occlusion with two others in the opposing arch, except for the mandibular central incisors and maxillary third molars. This structure serves to equalize the forces of impact in occlusion. Another benefit of this arrangement is that if a tooth is lost in one jaw, the alignment of the opposing jaw is not immediately disturbed or impaired. One antagonist remains until adequate restorative treatment can be performed.

If a tooth is lost for a longer period, the neighboring teeth usually tip in an effort to fill the edentulous space. The teeth become inclined, malaligned, and supereruption of the tooth opposing the space then occurs (see Figures 17-43 and 17-56). Thus, loss of one tooth disturbs the contact relationships in dhat area, as well as those teeth in the opposing arch, their antagonist(s), possibly causing changes in the

occlusion of the entire dentition. Patients must understand when discussing tooth replacement that teeth are like building blocks: Pull one out of the construction, and they all fall down, possibly resulting in occlusal disharmonies.

In addition to tooth loss, abnormal pressure or force of movement from the tongue (such as in tongue thrusting or an incorrect resting posture of the tongue) may create occlusal disharmony. An open mouth resting posture of the lips or chronic mouth breathing results in inadequate closure of the lips needed to maintain equilibrium between the lips and teeth as well as the surrounding orofacial structures. This most often leads to the teeth not being retained in the usual arch shape and thus malocclusion occurs (discussed later).

When the teeth usually occlude in CO, the maxillary arch horizontally overlaps the mandibular arch, which is referred to as **overjet** (Figure 20-2). The amount of horizontal overlap, usually 1 to 3 mm, between the anterior segment of the two arches associated with the overjet allows extensions in the movement of the **range of motion (ROM)** of the mandible, and assists in keeping the soft tissue of the oral cavity out of the way during mastication. The ROM is the maximum extent to which the parts of the TMJ can move when opening and closing as measured in degrees of a circle.

Overjet is measured in millimeters with the tip of a periodontal probe, once a patient is in CO. The probe is placed at 90° or right angle to the labial surface of a mandibular incisor at the base of the incisal ridge of a maxillary incisor. The measurement is taken from the labial surface of the mandibular incisor to the lingual surface of the maxillary incisor. Note that the labiolingual width of the maxillary incisor is not included in the measurement.

In CO, the maxillary arch also vertically overlaps the mandibular arch, which referred to as **overbite** (see Figure 20-2). The amount of vertical overlap, usually 2 to 5 mm between the anterior sextants of the two arches allows contact between the posterior teeth during mastication. It is usually expressed as a percentage at around 20% to 30%. Excessive amounts of either overjet or overbite are classified as a malocclusion (discussed later).

Overbite is measured in millimeters with the tip of a periodontal probe after a patient is placed in CO. The probe is placed on the incisal ridge of the maxillary incisor at 90° or at right angle to the mandibular incisor. As patients open their mouths or depress their jaws, the probe is then placed vertically against the mandibular incisor to measure the distance to the incisal ridge of the mandibular incisor.

Studies show that overjet measurements were equally distributed among women and men, but excessive overbite was noted more often in women than men. However, neither measurement was predictably associated with any particular craniofacial pattern. Both overjet and overbite tend to diminish with age, initially because of mandibular growth and later due to incisal wear. When the reverse is the case, and the mandibular arch extends forward beyond the maxillary arch, which is referred to as an **underbite** (or retrognathia) (see Figure 20-24, *A*).

There is a consensus on the amount of ROM of the mandible usually present. It is measured during **maximum mouth opening (MMO)**. MMO can be expressed either as interincisal distance or as corrected interincisal distance, which is determined by adding the amount of vertical overlap between the maxillary and mandibular incisors to the incisal distance. The interincisal opening range is 40 to 50 mm. The ability to position three fingers (index, middle, and ring finger of nondominant hand) in the mouth examination is a convenient index for assessing the usual amount of MMO. Most studies show that the maximum jaw ROM and MMO is related to body size and height; so men can usually open wider than women, taller people more than shorter people.

Within each dental arch, the teeth also create contact areas as they contact their same-arch neighbors at the proximal heights of contour; the exception is the last tooth in each arch of each dentition, which lacks a distal contact (see **Chapters 16 and 17**). When two teeth in the same arch come into contact, the curvatures next to the contact areas form spaces considered embrasures (see Figure 15-11). This contact between neighboring teeth and formation of embrasures serves two purposes: It protects the interdental papillae as well as stabilizing the position of each tooth in the dental arch.

Open contacts allow areas of food impaction from opposing cusps, called *plunging cusps,* resulting in trauma to the gingivosulcular area. Open contacts also do not allow mesiodistal stability between the teeth. Correct restorative treatment should not allow any open contacts, unless tooth position and tooth loss make this impossible. Although the practice is controversial, periodontal splints are often placed in the mouth lingually with tooth-colored resins and wires to simulate this stability needed for the teeth within the dental arch. All prosthetic treatment within the mouth, including the placement of bridges, implants, and removable dentures, is an attempt to simulate this stability.

Certain topics must be considered when studying CO: arch form and its development, dental curvatures and angulations, centric stops, centric relation, lateral and protrusive occlusion, mandibular rest position, and mastication patterns.

ARCH FORM

Each dental arch of the permanent dentition is divided into three segments when describing arch form: anterior, middle, and posterior (see Figure 20-1). The anterior segment includes the anterior teeth, the middle segment includes the premolars, and the posterior segment includes the molars. The concept of arch segments allows the arches to overlap slightly so that canines and first molars are cooperating in more than one segment. This arrangement serves to indicate that the canines and first molars function as anchor supports for both arches.

The anterior segment of each dental arch is curved and ends at the labial ridges of the canines. The middle segment is straight and extends from the distal part of the canines to the buccal cervical ridge of the mesiobuccal cusp of the first molar in each arch. The posterior segment creates a straight line, starting from the buccal cusps of the first molars and remaining in contact with the buccal surfaces of the second and third molars.

PHASES OF ARCH DEVELOPMENT

Each dental arch goes through phases of development as the permanent teeth erupt and the primary teeth are being shed (see Figure 6-22

FIGURE 20-3 Leeway space in the maxillary arch *(double-headed arrow)* during the mixed dentition period and phase three of the dental arch development. This space is due to the difference in size, mesiodistally, between primary molars and permanent premolars. (Courtesy of Margaret J. Fehrenbach, RDH, MS.)

for chronologic timetable). During this time, the ramus and body of the jaw develops and undergoes lengthening and horizontal growth to achieve its mature form and accommodate the larger permanent teeth.

Phase one occurs when the permanent first molars erupt (see Figure 18-17). These teeth add dramatically to chewing efficiency and jaw development during a period of rapid growth of the child. They help support the jaws while the primary anterior teeth are being shed and the other permanent teeth are erupting. The primate spaces in the primary dentition are still present to allow future space for the permanent teeth (see later discussion in this chapter and **Chapter 18**).

Phase two occurs with eruption of the permanent anterior teeth near the midline of the oral cavity. First, the permanent centrals, then the laterals generally erupt lingually to the primary anterior roots. However, shedding of the primary teeth and jaw growth finally place them labial to the position of the primary teeth they replaced (see Figures 6-26 and 18-17).

In addition, the permanent location of the permanent anterior teeth is not established until the development of the arch form is complete. Thus, some degree of transient anterior crowding may occur between 8 and 9 years of age and persist until the emergence of the permanent canines when the arch space for the teeth is adequate again. However, permanent incisor crowding that persists into a permanent dentition is considered a type of malocclusion (discussed later).

Phase three in the development of the form of the dental arches begins when the permanent premolars erupt anterior to the permanent molars (see Figures 6-27 and 6-28). Developmentally, this is quite significant because the premolars are so much smaller than the primary molars that they replace. This difference in size, mesiodistally between the two types of teeth, is called the **leeway space** (Figure 20-3). The contour of the alveolar process covering the narrower roots of the premolars, in addition to the state of flux of the bone formation in this area, furnishes adjustment for dental arch measurements, making the middle segment of the arches important architecturally. Thus, this arch space allows the future forward movement of the permanent molars, which is discussed later with regard to the occlusion of the primary teeth.

However, if there is early loss of the primary second molars and impaction of the second premolar, leeway space can become compromised. Also, if permanent second molars erupt before the premolars, the arch perimeter is significantly shortened and occlusal disharmony is likely to occur, as is malocclusion (discussed later) because the second premolar is also unable to erupt. A fixed or removable space maintainer may be used to save this leeway space from the shed primary molars for the permanent premolars (Figure 20-4).

Phase four begins when the permanent canines erupt and wedge themselves between the lateral incisors and the first premolars. Contact relations between the teeth are established, and the arch is complete from the permanent first molar forward. Simultaneously, the permanent second molars are due to emerge distally to the permanent first molars and support them during the wedging activity of the canines.

Phase five is the final phase of the development of the final dental arch form and consists of eruption of the third molars. Often the jaw length is not sufficient for eruption of these last teeth and dental treatment plan changes need to be considered (see **Chapter 17**).

Thus, the usual sequence for eruption of both the primary and permanent dentition is favorable to the development of the arches (Figures 20-5 and 20-6). Keeping this sequence in mind for each dentition is part of the treatment to prevent occlusal disruption in patients during the mixed dentition period. Disruption of this sequence, with overlong retention or too-early loss of primary teeth, may allow complications to occur with the eruption of the permanent dentition. Proper treatment of these cases of disruption in the eruption sequence and early orthodontic interceptive therapy increases the chances for a more ideal occlusion. A series of panoramic radiographs of the mixed dentition are important in order to monitor tooth eruption sequence and arch development (see Figure 6-27, *A*).

It is important to note that attrition of the proximal surfaces also reduces the mesial-distal dimensions of the teeth and significantly reduces arch length over a lifetime, which causes crowding or spacing challenges after age 40.

DENTAL CURVATURES AND ANGULATIONS

A common mistake is to assume that the forces of occlusion act on squared and flat teeth in straight lines or planes and that the axes of the teeth are at 90° or right angle to their masticatory surfaces. Many dental curvatures and angulations must be considered when studying occlusion.

If imaginary planes are placed on the masticatory surfaces of each dental arch, the arches do not conform to these flat planes; the maxillary arch is convex occlusally, and the mandibular arch is concave (Figure 20-7, *A*). Thus, when the maxillary and mandibular teeth come into CO, they align along anteroposterior and lateral curves.

FIGURE 20-5 Favorable sequence of eruption per dental arch of the primary dentition.

FIGURE 20-4 Removable maxillary space maintainer (sparkle variety) to hold the leeway space present from the shed primary second molar *(double-headed arrow)* to allow future eruption of the permanent second premolar. The permanent second molars have already erupted and may narrow the existing space in the premolar segment. Note that the permanent second premolar on the contralateral side is already fully erupted *(outlined)*, so leeway space does not need to be maintained any longer. (Courtesy of Margaret J. Fehrenbach, RDH, MS.)

FIGURE 20-6 Favorable sequence of eruption per dental arch of the permanent dentition.

This anteroposterior curvature is called the curve of Spee, which is produced by the curved alignment of all the teeth and is especially evident when viewing the posterior teeth from the buccal view.

Another curve of the dentition is the curve of Wilson (see Figure 20-7, *B*). This lateral curve results when a frontal section is visually compared to each set of maxillary and mandibular molars—the firsts, seconds, and then thirds. These imaginary dental curvatures are interesting, but it is important to note that modern dentistry does not use these curves often in practice because they have only a remote association with functional relationships. Both of these curves tend to be lost with age as a result of attrition (Figure 20-8). The composite of these curves created by the contact of the maxillary and mandibular teeth forms a line called the *occlusal plane.*

Individual teeth also exhibit some forms of curvature. Curves are found in the basic form of each tooth type. Every third of a tooth represents a curved surface, except where a tooth is worn or fractured. These curvatures of the teeth should be noted when studying the dentitions and especially when drawing them hoping to achieve lifelike drawings of each tooth. These curves also must be noted when restoring the teeth for proper function and esthetics.

When a tooth is bisected by its root axis line (RAL), the angulations related to each tooth's root(s) within the alveolar process are noted (Figure 20-9 and discussed per tooth type in **Chapters 16 and 17**). This angled arrangement of the teeth allows proper spacing between

the roots for blood and nerve supply and for securing anchorage of the roots in the jaws.

Each tooth is placed at the angle that best withstands the lines of forces brought against it while functioning during occlusion. The angle at which it is placed depends on the function that the tooth must perform. If the tooth is placed at a disadvantage because of misalignment in the dental arch or continued incorrect pressures against it from the tongue, lips, or cheeks, its functional efficiency is limited, and the permanence of its position is endangered. The anterior teeth seem to be placed at a disadvantage because they are more vertically situated in

FIGURE 20-8 Attrition or mechanical wear of the masticatory surfaces of the permanent teeth in this case is noted on a radiograph. The result is a loss of the curvatures of the teeth within the dental arches. (Courtesy of Margaret J. Fehrenbach, RDH, MS.)

FIGURE 20-7 Curves of the teeth noted within the permanent dental arches. **A,** Curve of Spee with the maxillary arch convex and the mandibular arch concave. **B,** Curve of Wilson is a concave curve that occurs when a frontal section is taken through each set of molars (one is shown). (**A** and **B,** Courtesy of Margaret J. Fehrenbach, RDH, MS.)

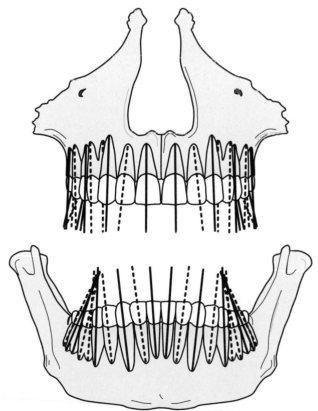

FIGURE 20-9 Each tooth of both arches of the permanent dentition is bisected by its root axis line, showing the angulations of the root within the alveolar process of each dental arch.

the alveolar process, but their function is only the momentary biting and cutting of food, not the full force of mastication that occurs in the posterior teeth, which usually have more angulation (see Table 15-4).

The masticatory surfaces of teeth do not have any flat planes, unless some are created over time by wear, traumatic accident, or orofacial myofunctional disorders (discussed later). Therefore, during occlusion, the curved surface of one tooth always comes into contact with the curved surfaces of another tooth. As the teeth come together in occlusion, the escapement spaces for the masticated food are provided for by each individual tooth's cusps, ridges, sulci, developmental grooves, and embrasures (see Figure 15-11). Thus these escapement spaces are necessary for efficient occlusion during mastication.

However, the location and form of the escapement spaces changes when the occlusal relation is changed, as with attrition, inappropriate functional patterning of the mandible, tongue thrusting, or even with restorative treatment. These changes can be related to loss of function of the teeth, tongue, lip, and mandibular function and the masticatory system. These changes can add up to an adverse functioning of the dentition and must be noted on the patient's chart. Additionally, knowing the angulation of the roots within the alveolar process is essential for the proper adaptation during the taking of radiographs and when performing instrumentation or restorative procedures. This measurement is also considered when evaluating a patient's smile.

CENTRIC STOPS

When the teeth are in CO, they should have maximal interdigitation with the locking of the two arch positions. The three areas of centric contacts, or **centric stops**, between the two arches are height of cusp contour, marginal ridges, and central fossae (Figure 20-10). Those cusps that function during CO are called the **supporting cusps** (kusps) and include the lingual cusps of the maxillary posterior teeth and the buccal cusps of the mandibular posterior teeth. The incisal ridges of the mandibular anterior teeth are usually included as supporting cusps.

These centric stops and supporting cusps are checked using articulating paper when restorative or prosthetic treatment is performed (Figure 20-11). An occlusal adjustment involving the removal of restorative, prosthetic, or natural tooth material may be necessary, depending on the results of the occlusal evaluation.

A dental manikin with unworn plastic teeth can show the ideal location of these centric stops and supporting cusps if articulating paper is used and mastication is simulated. However, the relationship of centric stops to the masticatory surfaces is not rigidly set and may in reality vary considerably among individuals. Centric stops are often in the central fossa and are related to the inner surface of the marginal ridges rather than the embrasure surfaces of the ridges, as indicated in an ideal mapping of centric stops.

These contact relationships change with wear of the dentition. With advancing attrition, the supporting cusps are seated closer and closer to the bottoms of the opposing fossae. This process continues until there is development of numerous flat surface contacts, which are the *wear facets*. This process can result in the loss of a definite locking of the two jaws in CO, in addition to creating an unstable occlusal environment.

The position of the centric stops helps determine the height of the lower one-third of the vertical dimension of the face when the teeth are in CO. This dimension cannot be exactly measured in patients with teeth, and thus its loss requires clinical judgment and is based on the Golden Proportion as it relates to the face. This dimension is involved in the proper functioning of the teeth and jaws and the

MAXILLARY ARCH

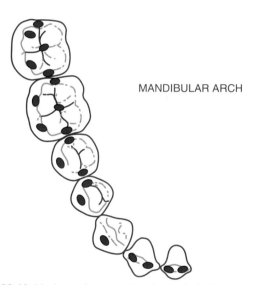

MANDIBULAR ARCH

FIGURE 20-10 Ideal centric stops showing articulation between the two arches of the permanent dentition are highlighted. Note that the stops include the height of cusps, incisal ridges, marginal ridges, or cingula, as well as any central fossae of the teeth.

esthetic appearance of a patient. Loss of this part of the vertical dimension is based on the resorption of the alveolar process and the attrition of the dentition (see Figure 14-22).

CENTRIC RELATION

Centric relation (CR) is the end point of closure of the mandible; the mandible is in the most retruded position to which it can be carried by the musculature and ligaments (see **Chapter 19**). Even though a patient is rarely in CR, except sometimes when swallowing, CR is a baseline measurement from which to evaluate a patient's occlusion because it can be easily repeated.

To attain CR, the mandible must undergo complete retraction (Figure 20-12). The position of CR must be determined by the clinician and without a patient's muscle participation. To do this, the clinician must gently establish the hinge movement of the mandible on the patient by

FIGURE 20-11 Articulating paper is used to check the centric stops during an occlusal evaluation or after restorative treatment. (Courtesy of Margaret J. Fehrenbach, RDH, MS.)

FIGURE 20-12 Attaining centric relation by establishing the hinge movement of the mandible. This is achieved by gently arching the mandible with the fingers in a closing and opening manner, several times. This is performed before attempting placement of the loosened jaw into centric relation —the end point of mandible closure in which the mandible is in the most retruded position. (Courtesy of Margaret J. Fehrenbach, RDH, MS.)

gently arcing the mandible with the fingers in a closing and opening manner several times, before attempting placement of the loosened jaw into CR. Researchers are currently exploring various ways of clinically relaxing patients' jaws to determine this position of the mandible more precisely in addition to promoting this during myofascial release and orofacial myofunctional therapy (discussed later).

Ideally, when the mandible is in CR, the dentition should be in CO thus centric relation equals centric occlusion, or CR = CO). The centric resting position also remains in a neutral pattern with an adequate freeway space maintained. Therefore, no major shift of the dentition from CR occlusion to CO should occur. However, the average

distance of shift or slide from a patient's occlusion in CR to CO is approximately 1 mm or less.

The position of CO can be attained by having a patient who is in CR clench his or her teeth together after achieving CR. The amount and direction of the shift in the dentition can then be recorded during the occlusal evaluation. One can easily simulate this procedure with their own dentition by putting the head back (CR) and then clench the teeth while bringing the head forward (CO).

However, if disorders such as those related to function (for instance, orofacial myofunctional disorders, discussed later) are present, striving to achieve CR in this manner may exacerbate the disorder. Clinicians should seat the patient in an upright position, inform the patient where the correct tongue placement is on the palate and having him or her bite the molars together (CO), followed by relaxing the mandible and allowing the maxillary and mandibular teeth to gently come apart until the masseter muscle is relaxed (CR is also the same as centric rest).

A slide or shift in the position of the dentition from CR to CO (centric relation does not equal centric occlusion or CR ≠ CO) should be noted. It is most often caused by premature contacts, where one or two teeth initially contact before the other teeth, or an orofacial myofunctional disorder (discussed later), as well as an incorrect habit pattern of the tongue and/or mandible, or deviation in the ROM patterning of the TMJ. The premature tooth contact, orofacial myofunctional disorder, and ROM deviation may contribute to occlusal disharmony. Additional slide between the teeth in CR to CO is also associated with tooth malalignment, improper intercuspation of the teeth, improper restorative treatment, and inherited arch lengths and relationships.

LATERAL AND PROTRUSIVE OCCLUSION

Masticatory movement entails not only the mandible going through elevation and depression but also deviations or excursions from side-to-side and forward during lateral and protrusion occlusion (see Figure 19-9). Therefore, other movements besides CO and its relationship to the teeth must be evaluated.

Evaluation of lateral occlusion is made by undergoing lateral deviation of the mandible or excursion by moving the mandible either to the right or to the left until the opposing canines on that side are in a edge-to-edge relationship (Figure 20-13).

Before the canines contact on each side, no other individual teeth should be contacting during lateral occlusion. The side to which the mandible has been moved is called the working side. Two working sides are noted in an occlusal evaluation: right lateral and left lateral. The side of the arch contralateral to the working side during lateral occlusion is called the balancing side or nonworking side.

During occlusion, the canine should be the only tooth in function during lateral occlusion; this is called canine (kay-nine) rise (or cuspid rise). Thus, the mandible is moved to the working side when checking lateral occlusion, until the opposing canines are edge-to-edge. If other teeth are involved in function during lateral occlusion, they must be noted; for example, the first molars (if in function) may present possible complications for the dentition.

If the canine rise does not exist on the working side because of cusp wear caused by parafunctional habits or tooth malalignment, it is acceptable that most of the entire posterior quadrant of each arch functions during lateral occlusion. This is called group function because all opposing posterior teeth are sharing the occlusal stress during function.

FIGURE 20-13 Undergoing lateral deviation, or excursion, to check the lateral occlusion on the working side (side to which the mandible has been moved) and balancing side (contralateral side of the arch from working side). Note that the mandible is being moved until the opposing canines are edge-to-edge during canine rise. (Courtesy of Margaret J. Fehrenbach, RDH, MS.)

FIGURE 20-15 Undergoing protrusion to evaluate protrusive occlusion. (Courtesy of Margaret J. Fehrenbach, RDH, MS.)

FIGURE 20-14 Using floss to confirm balancing interferences where teeth contact on the balancing side during lateral occlusion. (Courtesy of Margaret J. Fehrenbach, RDH, MS.)

No teeth should make contact on the contralateral balancing side during lateral occlusion. If teeth are in contact on the balancing side, this is called a balancing interference. Balancing interference can be involved in occlusal disharmonies. For further confirmation of any balancing interferences during lateral deviation, floss can be placed over the occlusal surfaces on the appropriate side (Figure 20-14).

With the mandible in protrusive occlusion, all eight of the most anterior teeth, the centrals and laterals of both arches are usually in contact as the mandible undergoes protrusion (Figure 20-15). If only one or two assume the stress of protrusion, occlusal disharmony may occur.

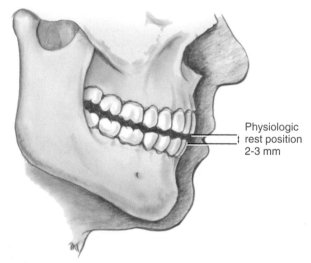

Physiologic rest position 2-3 mm

FIGURE 20-16 Physiologic rest position of the mandible, or interocclusal clearance of about 2 to 3 mm as shown in the permanent dentition.

MANDIBULAR REST POSITION

The physiologic rest position the mandible is achieved when the mandible is being held in a relaxed state and is not being used in mastication, speech, or respiratory movements (Figure 20-16). With this rest position, an average space of 2 to 3 mm is noted between the masticatory surfaces of the maxillary and mandibular teeth. This space or gap between the arches, when the mandible is at rest, is the interocclusal (in-ter- ah-kloo-zhal) clearance, or as more commonly called, *freeway space*.

This position of the mandible at rest is considered fairly stable, although it can be influenced by posture, fatigue, and tension. Thus failure to assume this position when the jaws are not at work ma mean that the patient is temporarily tense or has parafunctional habits, such as clenching or grinding (bruxism) which may be involved in occlusal difficulties (discussed later).

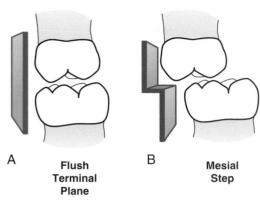

A Flush Terminal Plane **B** Mesial Step

FIGURE 20-17 Evaluation of the primary dentition from buccal view of right side. **A,** Flush terminal plane, in which the primary maxillary and mandibular second molars are in an end-to-end relationship. This allows the usual molar relationship to occur in the permanent dentition. **B,** Mesial step in which the mandibular second molar is mesial to the maxillary molar. This will most likely allow the usual molar relationship to occur in the permanent dentition.

Overall, **resting posture** is the usual physiologic position of the tongue, lips, and mandible when not functioning during mastication swallowing, or speech (see earlier discussions). Correct resting posture is achieved when the tongue is resting on the palate, the teeth are not in occlusion, and the lips are gently closed without any signs of facial grimacing. In addition, an **interlabial** (in-ter-**lay**-be-al) gap is the distance between the inferior border of the upper lip and the superior border of the lower lip when the mandible is in a physiologic resting position.

PRIMARY OCCLUSION

Similar to the permanent dentition, the primary dentition also has an ideal form (Figure 20-17). The canine relationship between the arches in primary teeth is the same as that of the permanent dentition. The ideal molar relationship within the primary dentition, when in CO, is referred to as the **terminal plane**. This can involve either a **flush terminal plane**, in which the primary maxillary and mandibular second molars are in an end-to-end relationship, or a **mesial** (me-ze-il) **step**, in which the primary mandibular second molar is mesial to the maxillary molar.

A **distal** (dis-tl) **step** relationship, in which the primary mandibular second molar is distal to the maxillary second molar, is not an ideal molar relationship in the primary dentition and thus is not a type of terminal plane relationship (Figure 20-18). With the presence of a mesial step, an ideal permanent molar relationship most likely occurs after the eruption of the permanent dentition. An ideal molar relationship in the permanent dentition may still occur with a flush terminal plane, but rarely with the presence of a distal step relationship.

Within a primary dentition, primate spaces may be present between the primary teeth; a space can be noted between the maxillary lateral incisor and the canine, and between the mandibular first molar and canine (see Figure 18-1). If primate spacing exists in the primary mandibular arch, after the eruption of the permanent first molar, the permanent first molar puts pressure on the primary second and first molars, causing forward movement of the primary mandibular canine and first molar (discussed earlier with regard to arch development). Thus, this primate space actually allows for this movement, which then facilitates the development of an ideal permanent molar relationship, along with the presence of a mesial step relationship.

When the child patient enters the mixed dentition period, analysis of arch space is performed so as to allow for early interceptive

Distal Step

FIGURE 20-18 Primary dentition from buccal view of right side in which distal step relationship exists with the primary mandibular second molar distal to the maxillary second molar. This is not a beneficial molar relationship because it will not usually result in the usual molar relationship in the permanent dentition when molar eruption occurs and the primary teeth are shed.

orthodontic therapy (see Figures 15-4 and 18-17). This analysis can range from a general examination to a specific arch length analysis by radiographs, size of erupted permanent mandibular incisors, and prediction scheme by orthodontists. This analysis is performed during this period because there is no appreciable growth of the jaws anterior to the permanent first molars after age 7 or 8 without intervention.

Clinical Considerations with Occlusion

When the teeth in the dentition are not aligned properly or there are orofacial myofunctional imbalances and/or parafunctional habit patterns present, they lose the ability to self-cleanse. More importantly, when teeth of either dentition are not occluding properly, the teeth and periodontium may not be able to perform the functions for which they were designed. Unnatural occlusal stress is then placed on the dentition, which often results in occlusal disharmony. Occlusal disharmony may then lead to **occlusal** (ah-**klooz**-l) **trauma**. The dentition and the periodontium are usually able to withstand many of these daily stresses; however, these stresses can become excessive, such as with incorrect tongue, lip, and/or mandibular resting posture patterns and/or parafunctional habits (discussed later). Structural changes within the periodontium can occur with occlusal trauma (see Figures 14-33 and 14-34).

Dental professionals must remember that occlusal trauma does not directly cause pathogen-based periodontal disease, but it may create an overriding adverse force factor in initiating or contributing to an already weakened and diseased periodontium. It also may be associated on an acute basis, with the production of a cracked tooth from masticatory impact on a hard object, and fracture of the restoration margin may also occur. Occlusal trauma can usually be halted if the etiologic factors are eliminated, or if the involved teeth are protected from these stresses.

Unfortunately, the effects of occlusal trauma are often irreversible if not intercepted early enough. These occlusal disharmonies, orofacial myofunctional patterns, and parafunctional habits should be controlled or eliminated during dental treatment and preventive maintenance therapy before initiating occlusal therapy (see later discussion). Signs or symptoms indicating abnormal patterns and habits must be addressed to eliminate the harmful occlusal disharmonies on a long-term basis. The effects on a patient's occlusion must also be kept in mind during all phases of dental treatment, especially during restorative treatment or when treating a temporomandibular disorder (TMD) (see **Chapter 19**).

MALOCCLUSION

Malocclusion (mal-ah-kloo-zhun) is related to lack of an overall ideal form in the dentition while in CO. Rarely, malocclusion is directly associated with severe occlusal trauma. Malocclusion may affect patients by having a negative impact on their appearance and increasing their difficulty with homecare procedures. Poor homecare favors dental biofilm retention and increases the possibility that periodontal disease or caries will affect the dentition with a malocclusion. Many malocclusions stem from hereditary factors.

An orthodontist working with other specialists, such as an orofacial myologist or speech therapist, can correct many malocclusions related to the teeth and possibly the rest of the masticatory system (see Figure 14-20). Thus, when correcting a malocclusion to achieve a more ideal form for the dentition, the occlusal functioning of the dentition also must be considered. Early intervention in the primary and mixed dentitions can prevent many malocclusions from occurring.

Approximately 80% of children and teenagers show some degree of malocclusion. The most common occlusal difficulties are crowding, which is a type of malocclusion that affects 40% of children and 80% of teenagers. The second most common type of malocclusion is excessive overjet of the maxillary incisors, which affects approximately 15% of children and teenagers.

Other factors are also involved in the consideration of smile design, such as gender, symmetry of color or shape, and position of teeth in relationship to the midline. A negative space (dark area) is also a consideration within an ideal smile and highlights the rest of the smile. The back of the mouth is considered a desired negative space because no light enters when standing. An example of an undesirable negative space is anterior or lateral crowded teeth creating shadows, a diastema, or even a loss of a prominent tooth that stands out from the whiteness of the rest of the teeth.

For a long time, clinicians have used the Angle classification of malocclusion because it has not been adequately replaced by another system (Table 20-1). Although the Angle system has many inadequacies, it does serve to initially and simply address malocclusion. However, many malocclusions do not fit neatly into the Angle system, but this classification system of malocclusion does give clinicians a starting point in describing a particular case.

TABLE 20-1	Angle Classification of Malocclusion*		
CLASS	**MODEL**	**ARCH RELATIONSHIPS**	**FEATURES**
Class I		Molar: MB cusp of the maxillary first occluding with the MB groove of the mandibular first molar Canines: Maxillary occluding with the distal half of the mandibular canine and the mesial half of the mandibular first premolar	Dental malalignment(s) present (see text), such as crowding or spacing; mesognathic profile
Class II	\n\nDivision I	Molar: MB cusp of the maxillary first occluding (by more than the width of a premolar) mesial to the MB groove of the mandibular first molar	Division I: Maxillary anterior teeth protruding facially from the mandibular anterior teeth with severe overbite; retrognathic profile
	\n\nDivision II	Canines: Distal surface of the mandibular canine distal to the mesial surface of the maxillary canine by at least the width of a premolar	Division II: Maxillary central incisors either upright or retruded, and lateral incisors either tipped labially or overlapping the central incisors with severe overbite; mesognathic profile
Class III		Molar: MB cusp of the maxillary first occluding (by more than the width of a premolar) distal to the MB groove of the mandibular first molar Canines: Distal surface of the mandibular mesial to the mesial surface of the maxillary by at least the width of a premolar	Mandibular incisors in complete crossbite; prognathic profile

*Note that this system deals with the classification of the permanent dentition.
MB, Mesiobuccal

MALOCCLUSION CLASSIFICATION

The Angle classification of malocclusion does *not* describe the occlusion usually present or even ideal occlusion, only malocclusion of the molars and canines. The basis of the Angle classification system was the simple hypothesis that the permanent maxillary first molar was the key to occlusion. Later, the relationship of the opposing canines was also evaluated. Therefore, the Angle system does not describe lateral or protrusive discrepancies, only those that are mesiodistally placed as related to the molars or canines.

The Angle system also assumes that a patient is occluding in a position of CO; thus it does not address the potential functional discrepancies between CR and CO. Additional information is needed to more fully evaluate a patient's occlusion than just a basic classification system. It was also assumed that patients in malocclusion had all their permanent teeth. Thus, this classification system does not describe primary or mixed dentition malocclusions, although there are specific ways to classify the relationships of canines and molars in a primary dentition (discussed earlier).

In the Angle classification, most cases of malocclusion are grouped into three main classes, according to the position of the permanent maxillary first molar to the mandibular first molar. This classification system is based on the relationship of the teeth and *not* the skeletal considerations that are due to the disproportionate size or position of the jaws (discussed later). These three main classes are designated by Roman numerals (I to III), and they assume that both sides of the dentition are affected equally, unless specifically noted. Separate defining classifications can be made, depending on which side is affected. Placement into the Angle system is only an initial baseline classification and *not* a complete diagnosis of a complex occlusal situation that may be present.

CLASS I MALOCCLUSION

All cases in a **Class I malocclusion** (neutroclusion) in a permanent dentition are characterized by an ideal mesiodistal relationship of the jaws and dental arches (Figure 20-19). Thus in these cases, the mesiobuccal cusp of the maxillary first molar occludes with the mesiobuccal

FIGURE 20-19 Class I malocclusion in a permanent dentition. **A,** Buccal view. **B,** Facial view. **C,** Facial profile. Mesiobuccal cusp of the maxillary first molar occludes with the mesiobuccal groove of the mandibular first molar, and the maxillary canine occludes with the distal half of the mandibular canine and the mesial half of the mandibular first premolar. Malocclusion in this case is due to dental malalignments, such as anterior crowding with a mesognathic profile (see completed orthodontic therapy case in Figure 20-1). (Courtesy of Dona M. Seely, DDS, MSD, Orthodontics, Bellevue, WA.)

groove of the mandibular first molar. In relation to the opposing canines, the maxillary canine occludes with the distal half of the mandibular canine and the mesial half of the mandibular first premolar.

Class I malocclusion is due to dental malalignments, such as crowding (or "crooked teeth") or irregular spacing within the jaws. These patients usually have a facial profile as described by many clinicians with the older term **mesognathic** (me-so-**nath**-ik). This facial profile in CO has slightly protruded jaws, giving the facial outline a relatively flat appearance or straight profile (Figure 20-20) (see the discussion of later cases for the differing facial profiles). Each type of facial profile present can be measured by the **gnathic (nath-ick) index** (or alveolar index), that is, the ratio of the distance from the middle of the nasion to the basion. This measurement gives the degree of prominence of the maxilla as opposed to the mandible.

Complications from crowding, in which the teeth are out of line within the dental arch, occur because of a disproportion between the size of the teeth and arch size. Spacing challenges occur within an arch where the teeth are small relative to the size of the arch or where teeth are missing. Included in this class of malocclusion is crowding that occurs because of mesial drift as the dentition ages (Figure 20-21; see also **Chapter 14**). Mesial drift, or physiologic drift, is the movement phenomenon in which all the teeth move slightly toward the midline of the oral cavity over time. This can cause crowding of a once-perfect dentition late in life. It occurs rather slowly, depending mostly on the degree of wear of the contact points between adjacent teeth and on the number of missing teeth. Overall, drift distances usually total no more than 1 cm over a lifetime. However, even this small amount may eventually lead to poor homecare and esthetics in the area of crowding.

Class I cases frequently have some protrusive or retrusive discrepancies in the anterior teeth, but other classes can also have these discrepancies (Figure 20-22). Within this grouping, overbites may be slight, moderate, or severe. Certain Class I cases have an **open bite**, in which the anterior teeth do not occlude (see Figures 16-8, *A* and Figure 14-3). In addition, Class I cases may have an **end-to-end bite** (or edge-to-edge bite) in which the teeth occlude without the maxillary teeth overlapping the mandibular teeth. With this type of occlusion, the anterior teeth of both jaws meet along their incisal ridges when the teeth are in CO. An end-to-end bite can occur both anteriorly and posteriorly, unilaterally or bilaterally.

Class I cases can also include a **crossbite**, which occurs when a mandibular tooth or teeth are placed facially to a maxillary tooth or teeth (see Figure 14-3) (for other class crossbite involvement, see Figure 20-26, *A* and *B*). A crossbite can occur either anteriorly or posteriorly, unilaterally or bilaterally. Individual teeth may be slightly deviated labially or lingually relative to the adjoining teeth in the same arch; they may be in labioversion or linguoversion.

CLASS II MALOCCLUSION

All cases in **Class II malocclusion** (distoclusion) in the permanent dentition are characterized by the mesiobuccal cusp of the maxillary first molar occluding (by more than the width of a premolar) mesial to the mesiobuccal groove of the mandibular first molar (Figure 20-23). The distal surface of the mandibular canine is distal to the mesial surface of the maxillary canine by at least the width of a premolar. A tendency to this type of malocclusion (less than the width of a premolar) can be noted. The major group of Class II malocclusion has two subgroups, a division I and a division II, based on the position of the anterior teeth, shape of the palate, and resulting facial profile.

In **Class II malocclusion, division I**, in the permanent dentition, the maxillary anterior teeth protrude facially from the mandibular

Mesognathic

Retrognathic

Prognathic

FIGURE 20-20 Three facial profiles: mesognathic, retrognathic, and prognathic, which can be measured by the gnathic index (or alveolar index), that is, the ratio of the distance from the middle of the nasion (intersection of frontal bone and two nasal bones) to the basion (midpoint on anterior margin of the foramen magnum on the occipital bone). This measurement gives the degree of prominence of the maxilla as opposed to the mandible. Note that an index below 98 is retrognathic, from 98 to 103 is mesognathic, and above 103 is prognathic.

anterior teeth (Figure 20-24). The mandibular incisors usually "over-erupt," causing a severe overbite (or deep overbite). The palate is often narrow and V-shaped. The facial profile shows an underbite, protruding upper lip, or recessive mandible and chin, or convex profile. The older term for describing the facial profile in Class II, division I, is retrognathic (ret-row-nath-ik) (see Figure 20-20).

In Class II malocclusion, division II, in a permanent dentition, the molars are in the same position as division I, but rather than having protrusive maxillary anterior teeth, the maxillary central incisors are either upright or retruded (Figure 20-25). The maxillary lateral incisors are either tipped labially or overlap the central incisors. Overbite is severe (or deep overbite), yet the palate is the usual width or

wider compared with division I. The facial profile for Class II, division II, is usually a mesognathic profile, often with a rather prominent chin (see Figure 20-20).

CLASS III MALOCCLUSION

All cases of a Class III malocclusion (mesioclusion) in a permanent dentition are characterized by the mesiobuccal cusp of the maxillary first molar occluding (by more than the width of a premolar) distal to the mesiobuccal groove of the mandibular first molar (Figure 20-26).

FIGURE 20-23 Class II malocclusion in a permanent dentition from buccal view. Mesiobuccal cusp of the maxillary first molar is occluding (by more than the width of a premolar) mesial to the mesiobuccal groove of the mandibular first molar, and the distal surface of the mandibular canine is distal to the mesial surface of the maxillary canine by at least the width of a premolar. (Courtesy of Dona M. Seely, DDS, MSD, Orthodontics, Bellevue, WA.)

FIGURE 20-21 Mesial drift is the movement phenomenon in the permanent dentition in which all the teeth move slightly toward the midline of the oral cavity over time. It can cause crowding, late in life, of a once-perfect dentition and may lead to poor homecare in the area of crowding, as the presence of calculus demonstrates. (Courtesy of Margaret J. Fehrenbach, RDH, MS.)

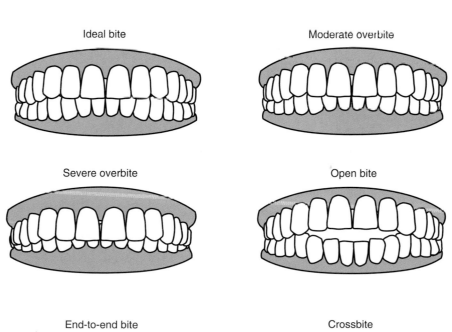

Ideal bite   Moderate overbite

Severe overbite   Open bite

End-to-end bite   Crossbite

Anterior   Posterior   Anterior   Posterior (bilateral)

FIGURE 20-22 Moderate and severe overbites contrasting with the ideal bite; open bite, end-to-end bites, and crossbites noted within the permanent dentition.

FIGURE 20-24 Class II malocclusion, division I, in a permanent dentition. **A,** Facial view. **B,** Facial profile. Maxillary anterior teeth also protrude facially from the mandibular anterior teeth, causing a severe overbite, and the facial profile is convex, or retrognathic. (Courtesy of Dona M. Seely, DDS, MSD, Orthodontics, Bellevue, WA.)

FIGURE 20-25 Class II malocclusion, division II, in a permanent dentition. **A,** Facial view. **B,** Facial profile. Central incisors are in a retruded position, and the lateral incisors are tipped labially with a severe overbite, but the facial profile is mesognathic. (Courtesy of Dona M. Seely, DDS, MSD, Orthodontics, Bellevue, WA.)

The distal surface of the mandibular canine is mesial to the mesial surface of the maxillary canine by at least the width of a premolar.

In comparison with Class II, division I, in which the maxillary incisors are flared mesially, the mandibular incisors are usually in complete crossbite. In most cases, the mandibular incisors are also inclined lingually despite the crossbite. The facial profile usually shows a rather prominent mandible and possibly a retrusive maxilla, thus a concave profile. The older term that describes the facial profile with a Class III malocclusion is prognathic (prog-nath-ik) (see Figure 20-20). A tendency to this type of malocclusion (less than the width of a premolar) can be noted.

MALOCCLUSION SUBDIVISIONS

As was noted, the Angle system of malocclusion does recognize that a case of malocclusion did occasionally have differing classifications on each side of the dentition. These asymmetrical cases are labeled *subdivisions* and usually demonstrate the main characteristics of the main class and division.

Thus, the Angle classification of malocclusion allows for a Class II malocclusion, division I subdivision in which the patient has both a Class II and Class I malocclusion, showing a division I anterior pattern. Another situation that may present is a Class II malocclusion,

FIGURE 20-26 Class III malocclusion in a permanent dentition. **A,** Buccal view. **B,** Facial view. **C,** Facial profile. Mesiobuccal cusp of the maxillary first molar is occluding (by more than the width of a premolar) distal to the buccal groove of the mandibular first molar, and the distal surface of the mandibular canine is mesial to the mesial surface of the maxillary canine by at least the width of a premolar. Mandibular incisors are also in crossbite, as are other teeth, and the facial profile is concave, or prognathic. (Courtesy of Dona M. Seely, DDS, MSD, Orthodontics, Bellevue, WA.)

division II subdivision, in which a patient has both a Class II and Class I, showing a division II anterior pattern. Finally, yet another situation that may present is a Class III malocclusion subdivision, in which a patient has both a Class III and Class I malocclusion on each side of the dentition.

Clinical Considerations with Skeletal Discrepancies

Many malocclusions are linked not only to the teeth, such as in the Angle classification of malocclusion, but also to discrepancies between the maxilla and mandible, which then affect the occlusion of the teeth. An oral and maxillofacial surgeon when working along with an orthodontist can correct skeletal discrepancies of the jaws; orthodontic therapy with tooth movement alone is not effective. However in many cases, timely orthodontic intervention in young children, using certain orthodontic appliances, can direct bone growth of the jaws by arch expansion and by increasing arch length and level. These interventions may prevent the need for surgical intervention. In contrast, adults and those patients whose jaw bone growth is complete, orthognathic surgery may be the only remedy for jaw discrepancies, because orthodontic appliances do not in themselves produce ideal results.

Generally, orthodontic patients requiring orthognathic surgical intervention undergo an initial period of orthodontic therapy before surgery so that the teeth occlude properly after surgery. Any orthodontic appliances used to align the teeth before surgery are left in place during the surgical procedure to stabilize the teeth and jaws. After surgery, a period of follow-up orthodontic therapy helps achieve the final alignment of the teeth.

In addition to aligning the jaws, the most commonly corrected difficulties include a protruding or retruding chin, unsightly display of gingiva superior to the maxillary anterior teeth ("gummy smile"), an inability to achieve resting lip closure (also considered lip incompetence), and an overall elongation of the face. Associated TMDs may also be minimized with surgery in severe cases (see **Chapter 19**).

Three basic spatial planes are involved in the classification of skeletal malocclusions: horizontal, vertical, and transverse. Horizontal malocclusions are further classified as either Class II or Class III malocclusions, similar to the Angle classification of malocclusion system. Vertical malocclusions include open bites and severe overbites. Transverse malocclusions include crossbites. Most patients undergoing orthognathic surgery have a combination of these types of skeletal malocclusions.

The use of computerized treatment planning can now minimize treatment times, recovery periods and the overall surgical efficacy as well as use of titanium plates and miniature screws that provide stability, strength and predictability to the treatment. These advances in technology, procedures, and equipment reduce postsurgical recovery time, thus allowing patients to return to their usual routines soon after the surgery.

Clinical Considerations for Parafunctional Habits

Parafunctional (pare-ah-funk-shun-al) habits are those movements of the mandible that are *not* within the usual ROM associated with mastication, speech, or respiratory movements. Thus, these movement habits occur more commonly and in longer duration than motions usually associated with functioning.

Parafunctional habits include clenching the teeth in CO or a pattern deviation for long periods, without breaking into a mandibular rest position or interocclusal clearance. Grinding the teeth, or bruxism (bruk-sizm), is also a parafunctional habit. Grinding the teeth involves forceful meshing of the teeth, often causing audible noises. Attrition of the masticatory surfaces of differing levels is evident in cases of grinding, causing *wear facets,* especially on the canines' cusp tips (see Figure 20-8; **Chapters 16 and 17**).

Parafunctional habits can be related to gingival recession and abfraction including a shearing or flaking of the enamel surface (see **Chapter 10** and Figure 12-1, *B*). Also, in many cases of parafunctional habits, a larger area of the buccal mucosa than just the linea alba can become hyperkeratinized (see Figure 9-7).

These parafunctional habits are often subconscious and occur when a person is sleeping or concentrating deeply, such as when driving, reading, watching television, or using the computer. Usually, around 20 to 30 pounds per square inch are exerted on molars during mastication, but grinders, especially at night without restraint, can exert as much as 200 pounds per square inch on their teeth. A person with these habits may have overdeveloped masseter muscles and facial and masticatory tension is considered the norm for them (Figure 20-27). Stress may be a factor in the etiology of these habits, although it is not always present. Parafunctional habits may be linked to the individual ways a person processes neurologic impulses; about 10% to 15% of adults grind their teeth moderately to severely.

Patients who grind their teeth can wear a professionally made flat-plane, non-repositioning oral splint, or mouthguard during waking hours or when sleeping. This oral splint consists of a removable hard plastic, acrylic or silicone appliance(s) that covers the dental arch (or arches). These types of devices can protect the teeth from further damage, such as attrition or recession from abfraction, and can reduce the occlusal stress of the habit throughout the dentition. In contrast, individuals who clench need a mouthguard made of a softer material in order to provide a cushion to the teeth. An oromotor chewing appliance also can be used to cushion and protect the buccal, lingual, and occlusal surfaces of the teeth.

Another consideration when discussing parafunctional habits and occlusion is orofacial myology (my-ol-oh-je) (OM), a specialized professional discipline that evaluates and treats a variety of orofacial muscle postural and functional disorders as well as habit patterns that may contribute to the disruption of dental development and be involved in orofacial esthetic challenges. Each of these disorders is considered an orofacial myofunctional (my-oh-funk-shun-al) disorder (OMD). OMDs involve behaviors and patterns created by inappropriate muscle function and incorrect habits involving tongue, lips, and jaws, as well as the face. Functional difficulties in speech may be associated with OMDs. Importantly, studies have found a prevalence of OMDs of around 38% in the general population to 81% in children exhibiting speech difficulties.

Treatment for an OMD is through the use of orofacial myofunctional therapy (OMT), a program used to retrain the patterning of the oral and facial muscles that is established by a certified orofacial myologist (COM). Individuals practicing in this specialty area may also be licensed in a dental discipline or speech pathology. Orofacial myologists work in a collaborative and team approach with other dental professionals, especially orthodontists, periodontists, and oral and maxillofacial surgeons as well as other healthcare professionals, such as speech pathologists, physical therapists, and occupational therapists.

With OMT, a variety of facial and tongue exercises and behavior modification techniques are included that work with functional head and neck postures, basing it all on individual evaluation and treatment protocols. The treatment goals for OMT include the improvement of muscle tonicity and establishing correct functional activities of the tongue, lips, and mandible so that growth and development can take place or progress in a stable homeostatic oral environment. Studies have shown that OMT can be 80% to 90% effective in correcting swallowing and rest posture function and that these corrections are retained years after completing therapy. The most recent studies show that OMT with orthodontic therapy was effective in closing and maintaining closure of open bites in Angle Class I and Class II malocclusions, and it reduced the relapse of open bites in patients with improper tongue movement and position.

Thus the most common OMD cited by many orofacial mycologists relative to occlusion is incorrect patterning during tongue function, which is commonly called tongue thrust (Figure 20-28). During the act of swallowing, and/or during the rest posture, an incorrect positioning of the tongue may contribute to improper orofacial development

FIGURE 20-27 Overdevelopment of the masseter muscles with bilateral enlargement. Patient has a history of the parafunctional habit of bruxism (grinding). (From Fehrenbach MJ, Herring SW: *Illustrated anatomy of the head and neck,* ed 4, St Louis, 2012, Saunders/Elsevier.)

FIGURE 20-28 Anterior open bite resulting from a tongue thrust swallowing pattern. (From Dean JA, McDonald RE, Avery DR: *McDonald and Avery's dentistry for the child and adolescent,* ed 9, St Louis, 2011, Mosby/Elsevier.)

and maintenance of the misalignment of the teeth from this parafunctional habit. The tongue should naturally rest against the palate during swallowing as well as during the rest posture. The current view in OM is that a tongue thrust and forward interdental resting posture of the tongue serve as clues that there is likely a retained sucking habit or unresolved airway issue. Such patients are also in need of referral to pediatricians, family physicians, allergists, or ear, nose, and throat (ENT) specialists for definitive evaluation of the airway as appropriate.

A prime example of an OMD, familiar to all pediatricians and dental professionals, is a retained sucking habit past age 4 or 5, through digit sucking as well as excessive use of a pacifier or "sippy" cup (Figure 20-29). While it is tempting to ignore such habits because some children do outgrow them, many children do not spontaneously discontinue noxious habits (such as sucking) and will need help in eliminating the habits. A range of malocclusion in a developing dentition is associated with a retained sucking habit, such as overbite and open bite, as well as a posterior crossbite. The behavioral approaches of the orofacial myologists may be effective in eliminating thumb and finger and other associated sucking habits (Figure 20-30).

Another OMD cited by many orofacial myologists is an open mouth, with lips apart, at the resting posture. This is often referred to as lip incompetence (Figure 20-31). The patient's lips should be in repose during the examination to obtain a clear indication of this OMD; patients frequently mask lip incompetence by forcing their lips together. This open mouth habit can distract from an esthetic facial appearance as well as compromising the beneficial influence that closed lips (considered a lip seal) have on the development and maintenance of correct dental arch form (see earlier discussion). A chronic open mouth rest posture may contribute to an increased vertical height of the face, a retrognathic profile with a downward and backward growth of the lower one-third of the face (rather than downward and forward), and hypotonic (or flaccid) lips.

Less than optimal nasal breathing may be associated with lip incompetence, so referral again may be necessary because nasal breathing must at all times be facilitated. At birth, infants instinctively are all nasal breathers with many benefits, such as filtering and warming air, increasing the ability to absorb oxygen, reducing pulse rate, and aiding in correcting tongue thrust habit as well as reducing snoring by helping maintain airflow. Instead, there may be mouth breathing associated with open lip posture, which may be associated with nasal airway obstruction, such as enlarged palatal tonsils and adenoids, a deviated septum, and persistent allergies as well as a restricted labial frenum.

Mouth breathers may have a low forward tongue posture with the tongue no longer providing support for the upper jaw, thus affecting

FIGURE 20-29 Occlusion of three children with differing patterns of a retained (digit) sucking habit and the open bites that can result from this orofacial myofunctional disorder. (From Dean JA, McDonald RE, Avery DR: *McDonald and Avery's dentistry for the child and adolescent,* ed 9, St Louis, 2011, Mosby/Elsevier.)

FIGURE 20-30 A, Open bite in the mixed dentition of an 8-year-old child associated with the orofacial myofunctional disorder of a retained (digit) sucking habit. **B,** Bite improved after orofacial myofunctional therapy 1 year later at age 9. (From Dean JA, McDonald RE, Avery DR: *McDonald and Avery's dentistry for the child and adolescent,* ed 9, St Louis, 2011, Mosby/Elsevier.)

FIGURE 20-31 Young patient has lip incompetence. She also has a hyperactive mentalis muscle, which is commonly associated with this orofacial myofunctional disorder as shown here during forced lip closure. (From Dean JA, McDonald RE, Avery DR: *McDonald and Avery's dentistry for the child and adolescent,* ed 9, St Louis, 2011, Mosby/Elsevier.)

the palatal vault as well as other bones of the skull. Dry mouth (or xerostomia) and lack of air filtering are also noted. Mouth breathers often carry the head forward in order to open their airway.

In many instances, therapy to achieve a resting lip seal can avoid the need for any further tongue therapy and can also lead to a functioning freeway space dimension. Thus the concept of the freeway space is an important component associated with OMDs. This importance of the freeway space with the development of OMDs distinguishes the focus of orofacial myologists from orthodontists and other forms of dental treatment that mainly deal with a closed mouth and the role of occlusion. A primary goal of orofacial myologists is to recapture or establish a more functional level of freeway space.

Another issue for occlusal harmony can be the length of the lingual frenulum. If the lingual frenum is restricted as with ankyloglossia, it limits the possibility of creating appropriate pressure against the maxillary arch for usual level of expansion, where it may cause low and forward tongue resting posture (see Figure 5-10). Thus it may be associated with an anterior open bite (see Figure 16-8). It may also contribute to the developing shape of the palate. This is because the tongue cannot move up to rest properly on the palate, and a crossbite often develops. It also increases the risk factors of having incorrect functional speech patterns and articulation difficulties as well as challenges with feeding by the infant. Surgery is now considered after OMT, which in many cases can help lengthen the shorter lingual frenum.

Early identification and treatment of an OMD by an orofacial myologist with an OMT program has its advantages, as does early intervention orthodontic therapy, but individuals at any age can benefit from either therapy. However, the general rule in dentistry, and affirmed in pediatric medicine, is that orofacial parafunctional habits should be addressed and eliminated prior to the eruption of the permanent incisors, or by age 6. Individuals with special needs and syndromes also may benefit significantly from including an OMT program into their medical treatment plan. Thus, an initial OM examination and parafunctional habit pattern assessment should be incorporated into the examination procedure by dental professionals and speech pathologists as well as medical personnel to allow the patient to benefit from this area of specialized treatment.

Bibliography

Guidelines

American Academy of Pediatric Dentistry Clinical Affairs Committee Developing Dentition Subcommittee: Guideline on management of the developing dentition and occlusion in pediatric dentistry, *Pediatr Dent* 30(7 Suppl):184–195, 2009.

American Academy of Periodontology: Comprehensive periodontal therapy: a statement by the American Academy of Periodontology, *J Periodontol* 82(7):943–949, 2011.

Rethman MP, Beltrán-Aguilar ED, Billings RJ, et al: Nonfluoride caries-preventive agents: executive summary of evidence-based clinical recommendations, *J Am Dent Assoc* 142(9):1065–1071, 2011.

Rozier RG, Adair S, Graham F, et al: Evidence-based clinical recommendations on the prescription of dietary fluoride supplements for caries prevention: a report of the American Dental Association Council on Scientific Affairs, *J Am Dent Assoc* 141(12):1480–1489, 2010.

Journal Articles

Arambawatta K, Peiris R, Nanayakkara D: Morphology of the cemento-enamel junction in premolar teeth, *J Oral Sci* 51(4):623–627, 2009.

Asikainen P, Ruotsalainen TJ, Mikkonen JJ, et al: The defence architecture of the superficial cells of the oral mucosa, *Med Hypotheses* 78(6):790–792, 2012.

Bala R, Pawar P, Khanna S, et al: Orally dissolving strips: a new approach to oral drug delivery system, *Int J Pharm Investig* 3(2):67–76, 2013.

Bosshardt DD, Lang NP: The junctional epithelium: from health to disease, *J Dent Res* 84(1):9–20, 2005.

Brocklehurst PR, Baker SR, Speight PM. Oral cancer screening: what have we learnt and what is there still to achieve? *Future Oncol* 6(2):299–304, 2010.

Bullon P, Cordero MD, Quiles JL, et al: Mitochondrial dysfunction promoted by Porphyromonas gingivalis lipopolysaccharide as a possible link between cardiovascular disease and periodontitis, *Free Radic Biol Med* 50(10):1336–1343, 2011.

Checchi L, Montevecchi M, Checchi V, et al: The relationship between bleeding on probing and subgingival deposits: an endoscopical evaluation, *Open Dent J* 28(3):154–160, 2009.

Chung G, Jung SJ, Oh SB: Cellular and molecular mechanisms of dental nociception, *J Dent Res* 92(11):948–955, 2013.

Cogulu D, Becerik S, Emingil G, et al: Oral rehabilitation of a patient with amelogenesis imperfecta, *Pediatr Dent* 31(7):523–527, 2009.

Coppe C, Zhang Y, Den Besten PK: Characterization of primary dental pulp cells in vitro, *Pediatr Dent* 31(7):467–471, 2009.

Dahlström L, Carlsson GE: Temporomandibular disorders and oral health-related quality of life: a systematic review, *Acta Odontol Scand* 68(2):80–85, 2010.

Dimitriu B, Vârlan C, Suciu I, et al: Current considerations concerning endodontically treated teeth: alteration of hard dental tissues and biomechanical properties following endodontic therapy, *J Med Life* 2(1):60–65, 2009.

Enoch S, Peake MA, Wall I, et al: 'Young' oral fibroblasts are geno/phenotypically distinct, *J Dent Res* 89(12):1407–1413, 2010.

Finoti LS, Anovazzi G, Pigossi SC, et al: Periodontopathogens levels and clinical response to periodontal therapy in individuals with the interleukin-4 haplotype associated with susceptibility to chronic periodontitis, *Eur J Clin Microbiol Infect Dis* 32(12):1501–1509, 2013.

Fleischmannova J, Matalova E, Sharpe PT, et al: Formation of the tooth-bone interface, *J Dent Res* 89(2):108–815, 2010.

Ghaname ES, Ritter AV, Heymann HO, et al: Correlation between laser fluorescence readings and volume of tooth preparation in incipient occlusal caries in vitro, *J Esthet Restor Dent* 22(1):31–39, 2010.

Gordan VV, Bader JD, Garvan CW, et al: Restorative treatment thresholds for occlusal primary caries among dentists in the dental practice-based research network, *J Am Dent Assoc* 141(2):171–184, 2010.

Gutmann JL: Bernhard Gottlieb's impact on contemporary endodontology, *J Hist Dent* 61(2):85–106, 2013.

Hinz B: Matrix mechanics and regulation of the fibroblast phenotype, *Periodontol 2000* 63(1):14–28, 2013.

Hong L, Levy SM, Warren JJ, et al: Amoxicillin use during early childhood and fluorosis of later developing tooth zones, *J Public Health Dent* 71(3):229–235, 2009.

Huang GT: Pulp and dentin tissue engineering and regeneration: current progress, *Regen Med* 4(5):697–707, 2009.

Iorgulescu G: Saliva between normal and pathological: important factors in determining systemic and oral health, *J Med Life* 2(3):303–307, 2009.

Jiang R, Bush JO, Lidral AC: Development of the upper lip: morphogenetic and molecular mechanisms, *Dev Dyn* 235(5):1152–1166, 2006.

Lam JK, Xu Y, Worsley A, et al: Oral transmucosal drug delivery for pediatric use, *Adv Drug Deliv Rev*, 2013. S0169–409X(13)00194-4 [Epub].

Magloire H, Maurin JC, Couble ML, et al: Topical review: dental pain and odontoblasts: facts and hypotheses, *J Orofac Pain* 24(4):335–349, 2010.

Martin-Biedma B, Gonzalez-Gonzalez T, Lopes M, et al: Colorimeter and scanning electron microscopy analysis of teeth submitted to internal bleaching, *J Endod* 36(2):334–337, 2010.

Martinez EF, da Silva LA, Furuse C, et al: Dentin matrix protein 1 (DMP1) expression in developing human teeth, *Braz Dent J* 20(5):365–369, 2009.

Mason RM: A retrospective and prospective view of orofacial myology, *Int J Orofac Myol* 34:5–14, 2008.

Miller JR, Mancl L: Risk factors for the occurrence and prevention of temporomandibular joint and muscle disorders: lessons from 2 recent studies, *Am J Orthod Dentofac Orthop* 134(4):537–542, 2008.

Moharamzadeh K, Colley H, Murdoch C, et al: Tissue-engineered oral mucosa, *J Dent Res* 91(7):642–650, 2012.

Patil MS, Patil SB, Acharya AB: Palatine rugae and their significance in clinical dentistry: a review of the literature, *J Am Dent Assoc* 139(11):1471–1478, 2008.

Pessoa RS, Oliveira SR, Menezes HH, et al: Effects of platelet-rich plasma on healing of alveolar socket: split-mouth histological and histometric evaluation in Cebus apella monkeys, *Indian J Dent Res* 20(4):442–447, 2009.

Ponsford MW, Stella JP: Algorithm for the differential diagnosis of posterior open bites: two illustrative cases, *J Oral Maxillofac Surg* 71(1):110–127, 2013.

Rath-Deschner B, Daratsianos N, Dühr S, et al: The significance of RUNX2 in postnatal development of the mandibular condyle, *J Orofac Orthop* 71(1):17–31, 2010.

Rinaldi JC, Arana-Chavez VE: Ultrastructure of the interface between periodontal tissues and titanium mini-implants, *Angle Orthod* 80(3):459–465, 2010.

Ricucci D, Lin LM, Spangberg LS: Wound healing of apical tissues after root canal therapy: a long-term clinical, radiographic, and histopathologic observation study, *Oral Surg Oral Med Oral Pathol Oral Radiol Endod* 108(4):609–621, 2009.

Saccomanno S, Antonini G, D'Alatri L, et al: Causal relationship between malocclusion and oral muscles dysfunction: a model of approach, *Eur J Paediatr Dent* 13(4):321–323, 2012.

Sapna G, Gokul S, Bagri-Manjrekar K: Matrix metalloproteinases and periodontal diseases, *Oral Dis* 20(6):529–632, 2013.

Saussez S, De Maesschalk T, Mahillon V, et al: Second branchial cyst in the parapharyngealspace: a case report, *Auris Nasus Larynx* 36(3):376–379, 2009.

Shashikiran ND, Babaji P, Reddy VV: Double facial and a lingual trace talon cusps: a case report, *J Indian Soc Pedod Prev Dent* 23(2):89–91, 2005.

Sierant ML, Bartlett JD: Stress response pathways in ameloblasts: implications for amelogenesis and dental fluorosis, *Cells* 1(3):631–645, 2012.

Terrer E, Raskin A, Koubi S, et al: A new concept in restorative dentistry: LIFEDT-light-induced fluorescence evaluator for diagnosis and treatment: part 2—treatment of dentinal caries, *J Contemp Dent Pract* 11(1):E095–E102, 2010.

Vidal R, Greenwell H, Hill M, et al: Success rate of immediate implants placed and restored by novice operators, *Implant Dent* 19(1):81–90, 2010.

Villar CC, Cochran DL: Regeneration of periodontal tissues: guided tissue regeneration, *Dent Clin North Am* 54(1):73–92, 2010.

Wenzel A, Møystad A: Work flow with digital intraoral radiography: a systematic review, *Acta Odontol Scand* 68(2):106–114, 2010.

Yoithapprabhunath TR, Maheswaran T, Dineshshankar J, et al: Pathogenesis and therapeutic intervention of oral submucous fibrosis, *J Pharm Bioallied Sci* 5(Suppl 1):S85–S88, 2013.

Textbooks

Fehrenbach MJ, et al: *Mosby's dental dictionary*, ed 3, St Louis, 2014, Mosby/Elsevier.

Fehrenbach MJ, Herring SW: *Illustrated anatomy of the head and neck*, ed 4, St Louis, 2012, Saunders/Elsevier.

Ibsen OAC, Phelan JA: *Oral pathology for the dental hygienist*, ed 6, St Louis, 2014, Saunders/Elsevier.

Moore KL, Persaud TVN, Torchia MG: *The developing human: clinically oriented embryology*, ed 10, Philadelphia, 2015, Saunders/Elsevier.

Nanci A: *Ten Cate's oral histology*, ed 8, St Louis, 2013, Mosby/Elsevier.

Nelson SJ, Ash MM: *Wheeler's dental anatomy, physiology, and occlusion*, ed 10, St Louis, 2015, Saunders/Elsevier.

Newman MG, Takei HH, Klokkevold PR: *Carranza's clinical periodontology*, ed 12, St Louis, 2015, Saunders/Elsevier.

Okeson JP: *Management of temporomandibular disorders and occlusion*, ed 7, St Louis, 2013, Mosby/Elsevier.

Perry DA, Beemsterboer PL, Essex G: *Periodontology for the dental hygienist*, ed 4, St Louis, 2014, Saunders/Elsevier.

Stevens A, Lowe J: *Human histology*, ed 4, St Louis, 2015, Mosby/Elsevier.

Young B, Lowe JS, Stevens A, et al: *Wheater's functional histology: a text and colour atlas*, ed 5, London, 2006, Churchill Livingstone/Elsevier.

A

Abfraction (ab-frak-shen) Hard tooth tissue loss from tensile and compressive forces during tooth flexure.

Abrasion (uh-brey-zhun) Hard tooth tissue loss caused by friction from toothbrushing and/or toothpaste.

Accessory canals Extra openings located on lateral parts of roots.

Accessory root Extra root on tooth.

Acellular cementum (see-men-tum) First layers of cementum deposited without embedded cementocytes.

Acinus (plural, acini) (as-i-nus, as-i-ny) Group(s) of secretory cells of salivary gland.

Active eruption Vertical tooth movement through oral tissue.

Adipose (ad-i-pose) connective tissue Specialized connective tissue composed of fat, little matrix, adipocytes.

Afferent (af-er-int) vessels Lymphatic vessels that allow flow of lymph into lymph node.

Ala (plural, alae) (ah-lah, ah-lay) Winglike cartilaginous structure(s) bounding nares laterally.

Alveolar (al-vee-o-lar) bone proper (ABP) Bone lining alveolus.

Alveolar crest Most cervical rim of alveolar bone proper.

Alveolar crest group Alveodental ligament subgroup originating in alveolar crest to insert into cervical cementum.

Alveolar mucosa (mu-ko-sah) Oral mucosa immediately apical to mucogingival junction.

Alveolar process Dental arch or tooth-bearing part of each jaw that contains alveoli.

Alveolodental (al-vee-o-lo-dent-al) ligament Main principal fiber group with subgroups: alveolar crest, horizontal, oblique, apical, and interradicular.

Alveolus (plural, alveoli) (al-vee-oh-lus, al-vee-oh-lie) Socket(s) of tooth.

Ameloblasts (ah-mel-oh-blasts) Cells that differentiate from preameloblasts to form enamel during amelogenesis.

Amelogenesis (ah-mel-oh-jen-i-sis) Apposition of enamel matrix by ameloblasts.

Amelogenesis imperfecta (im-per-fek-tah) Hereditary enamel dysplasia with absent or thin enamel.

Amniocentesis (am-nee-o-sen-tee-sis) Prenatal diagnostic procedure sampling amniotic fluid.

Amniotic (am-nee-ot-ik) cavity Fluid-filled cavity facing epiblast layer.

Anaphase (an-ah-faze) Third phase of mitosis with separation of two chromatids of each chromosome and migration.

Anatomic crown Part of crown covered by enamel.

Anatomic root Part of root covered by cementum.

Anchoring collagen (kol-ah-jen) fibers Fibers from connective tissue involved in basement membrane.

Angle of the mandible (man-di-bl) Thickened area on posterior-inferior border of mandibular ramus.

Angle classification of malocclusion (mal-ah-kloo-zhun) System used to initially classify malocclusion.

Ankyloglossia (ang-kel-lo-gloss-ee-ah) Lingual frenum with abnormally short attachment.

Anodontia (an-ah-don-she-ah) Absence of single tooth or multiple teeth owing to lack of initiation.

Anterior faucial (faw-shawl) pillar Anterior lateral folds of tissue in pharynx created by underlying muscle forming the fauces.

Anterior teeth Incisors and canines at front of the oral cavity.

Apex of the nose Tip of nose.

Apex of the tongue Tip of tongue.

Apical foramen (ay-pi-kl for-ay-men) Opening from pulp near apex of tooth.

Apical group Alveolodental ligament subgroup radiating apically from cementum to insert into alveolar bone proper.

Appositional (ap-oh-zish-in-al) growth Growth by addition of layers to outside of tissue mass such as that occurs to firm or hard tissue such as cartilage, bone, enamel, dentin, and/or cementum.

Arrest lines Smooth, stained microscopic lines caused by appositional growth in cartilage, bone, and/or cementum.

Articular (ar-tik-you-ler) eminence Rounded protuberance on inferior aspect of zygomatic process for articulation of temporomandibular joint.

Articular fossa Depression on inferior aspect of temporal bone for articulation of temporomandibular joint.

Articulating (ar-tik-you-late-ing) surface of the condyle (kon-dyl) Head of mandibular condyle within the temporomandibular joint.

Attached gingiva (jin-ji-vah) Gingiva that tightly adheres to alveolar process around the roots of teeth.

Attrition (ah-trish-un) Hard tooth tissue loss caused by tooth-to-tooth contact during mastication or parafunctional habits.

Avulsion (ah-vul-shin) Complete tooth displacement from socket due to extensive trauma.

Axon (ax-on) Process that conducts impulses away from the cell body.

B

B cell Lymphocyte that matures in lymph nodes and works during humoral immune response.

Balancing interference Teeth in contact on balancing side during lateral occlusion.

Balancing side Other side of the arch from the working side during lateral occlusion.

Basal (bay-sal) bone Part of jaws that forms the body of the maxilla or mandible.

Basal lamina (lam-i-nah) Superficial part of basement membrane within the dentogingival junction, which has both an external and internal basal lamina surrounding the junctional epithelium.

Basal layer Single layer of cuboidal epithelial cells overlying basement membrane.

Base of the tongue Most posterior part of tongue.

Basement membrane Extracellular material consisting of basal and reticular lamina produced by either epithelium or connective tissue.

Basophil (bay-sah-fil) White blood cell containing granules of histamine.

Bell stage Fourth stage of odontogenesis with enamel organ assuming bell shape.

Bifurcated (bi-fer-kay-ted) Tooth having two root branches.

Bilaminar embryonic (by-lam-i-nar em-bre-on-ik) disc Circular plate of bilayered cells developed from blastocyst.

Bilateral symmetry (sim-me-try) Each half of embryo mirrors the other half.

Black hairy tongue Tongue lesion marked by dead cells and keratin buildup that becomes extrinsically stained.

Blastocyst (blas-tah-sist) Structure formed during prenatal development consisting of trophoblast cells and inner mass of cells that develop into embryo.

Blood Fluid connective tissue containing cells and plasma.

Body of the mandible (man-di-bl) Horizontal part of lower jaw inferior to teeth.

Body of the maxilla (mak-sil-ah) Horizontal part of upper jaw superior to teeth.

Body of the tongue Anterior part of the tongue.

Bone Rigid connective tissue.

Bone marrow (mar-oh) Innermost part of bone in medullary cavity.

Branchial apparatus (brang-ke-al ap-pah-ra-tis) Group that includes branchial arches, branchial grooves and membranes, and pharyngeal pouches.

Branchial arches Six stacked bilateral swellings of tissue that appear inferior to stomodeum, including mandibular arch.

Branchial cleft cyst Developmental cervical cyst due to obliteration failure of second branchial groove.

Branchial grooves Grooves between neighboring branchial arches on each side of the embryo.

Bruxism (bruk-sizm) Parafunctional habit of tooth grinding.

Buccal (buk-al) Structures or facial surface of tooth close to inner cheek.

Buccal fat pad Pad of underlying adipose connective tissue in vestibules.

Buccal mucosa Mucosa that lines inner cheek.

Buccal region Region of face composed of the soft tissue of cheek.

Bud stage Second stage of tooth development marked by growth of dental lamina into buds.

C

Calcium hydroxyapatite (hy-drox-see-ap-ah-tite) Main inorganic crystal with chemical formula of $Ca_{10}(PO_4)_6(OH)_2$ in enamel, alveolar bone, dentin, and cementum.

Canaliculi (kan-ah-lik-u-lie) Tubular canals in both bone and cementum.

Cancellous (kan-sel-us) bone Spongy bone within compact bone with trabeculae instead of Haversian system.

Canine eminence (kay-nine em-i-nins) Vertically oriented and labially placed bony ridge of alveolar process.

Canine rise Contralateral canine should be only tooth in function during lateral occlusion.

Canines Anterior teeth that are the third from midline in each quadrant.

Cap stage Third stage of tooth development with dental lamina growing into cap shape.

Capillary (cap-ih-lary) plexus Capillaries located between papillary layer and deeper layers of lamina propria.

Capsule (kap-sule) Connective tissue that surrounds outer part of entire gland or lesion.

Cartilage (kar-ti-lij) Firm, non-mineralized connective tissue.

Caudal (kaw-dal) end Tail end of structure.

Cell Smallest unit of organization in the body.

Cell membrane Membrane that completely surrounds a cell.

Cellular cementum (see-men-tum) Outer layers of cementum that contain embedded cementocytes.

Cemental (see-men-tal) caries Shallow carious lesion of cementum.

Cemental spurs Symmetrical spheres of cementum attached to the root surface.

Cementicles (see-men-ti-kuls) Mineralized bodies of cementum either attached to root or free in periodontal ligament.

Cementoblasts (see-men-tah-blasts) Cells that form cementoid and are differentiated from the dental sac.

Cementocytes (see-men-toe-sites) Cementoblasts entrapped by the cementum they produce.

Cementoenamel (see-men-to-ih-nam-l) junction (CEJ) Tooth anatomy where crown enamel and the root cementum are close.

Cementogenesis (see-men-toe-jen-i-sis) Appositional growth of cementum in the root area.

Cementoid (see-men-toyd) Cementum matrix laid down by cementoblasts.

Cementum (see-men-tum) Outermost layer of the root of a tooth.

Central cells of the dental papilla (pah-pil-ah) Primordium of the pulp.

Central fossa (fos-ah) Fossa located at convergence of cusp ridges in a central point on occlusal surface of the posterior teeth.

Central groove Most prominent developmental groove on the posterior teeth, traveling mesiodistally to separate occlusal table buccolingually.

Centric occlusion (ah-kloo-zhun) (CO) Voluntary position of dentition that allows maximal contact when teeth occlude.

Centric relation (CR) End point of closure of mandible in which the mandible is in most retruded position.

Centric stops Centric contacts between the two arches that includes height of cusp contour, marginal ridges, and central fossae.

Centrioles (sen-tree-ols) Pair of cylindrical structures in centrosome.

Centromere (sen-tro-mere) Clear constricted area where two chromatids of chromosome are joined.

Centrosome (sen-tro-some) Organelle associated with centrioles.

Cephalic (se-fal-ik) end Head end of structure.

Cervical loop Most cervical part of enamel organ responsible for root development.

Cervical ridge Ridge running mesiodistally in cervical one-third of buccal crown surface on primary dentition and permanent molars.

Chondroblasts (kon-dro-blasts) Cells that produce cartilage tissue.

Chondrocytes (kon-dro-sites**)** Mature chondroblasts.

Chromatids (kro-mah-tids**)** Two filamentous daughter chromosomes joined at a centromere during cell division.

Chromatin (kro-mah-tin**)** Chief nucleoprotein in the nondividing nucleoplasm.

Chromosomes (kro-mah-somes**)** Separate concentrations of chromatin in a dividing nucleus of a cell.

Cingulum (sin-gu-lum**)** Raised and rounded area on the cervical third of the lingual surface on the anterior teeth.

Circumpulpal (serk-um-pul**-**pal**) dentin** Layer of dentin around the outer pulpal wall.

Circumvallate (serk-um-val**-**ate**) lingual papillae (pah-**pil**-ay)** Larger mushroom-shaped lingual papillae that line up along the anterior side of the sulcus terminalis on the tongue.

Class I malocclusion (mal-ah-kloo**-zhun)** Malocclusion characterized by ideal mesiodistal relationship of jaws and dental arches with minor dental malalignments.

Class II malocclusion Malocclusion with mesiobuccal cusp of the maxillary first molar occluding by more than the width of a premolar mesial to the mesiobuccal groove of the mandibular first molar.

Class II malocclusion, division I Class II malocclusion with permanent maxillary anterior teeth protruding facially.

Class II malocclusion, division II Class II malocclusion with maxillary central incisors either upright or retruded.

Class III malocclusion Malocclusion with mesiobuccal cusp of maxillary first molar occluding by more than width of a premolar distal to mesiobuccal groove of mandibular first molar.

Cleavage (kleve-ij**)** Process during prenatal development when mitosis converts a zygote to a blastocyst.

Cleft (kleft) lip Developmental disturbance of upper lip from failure of fusion of maxillary processes with medial nasal process.

Cleft palate (pal-it**)** Developmental disturbance from failure of fusion of palatal shelves with primary palate or with each other.

Cleft uvula (u-vu-lah**)** Mildest form of cleft palate.

Clenching Parafunctional habit with teeth held in centric occlusion for long periods without interocclusal clearance.

Clinical crown Part of anatomic crown visible in the oral cavity and not covered by gingival tissue.

Clinical root Part of anatomic root visible in the oral cavity and not covered by gingival tissue.

Cloacal (klo-ay**-**kal**) membrane** Membrane at caudal end of embryo that is the location of future anus.

Col (kohl) Interdental gingiva apical to contact area assumes nonvisible concave form between facial and lingual gingival surfaces.

Collagen (kol-ah-jen**) fibers** Main protein fiber.

Colloid (kol-oid**)** Material in follicles of thyroid reserved for production of thyroxine.

Compact (kom-pak**) bone** Bone deep to periosteum with Haversian system of bone with lamellae.

Concrescence (kahn-kres**-**ens**)** Union of root structure of two or more teeth through cementum only.

Congenital malformations (kon-jen**-i-til mal-for-**may**-shins)** Birth defects or developmental problems evident at birth.

Connective tissue Basic tissue mainly composed of cells and matrix.

Connective tissue papillae (pah-pil**-ay)** Interdigitation of loose connective tissue with epithelium.

Connective tissue proper Two adjacent layers consisting of loose and dense connective tissue.

Contact area Tooth anatomy where adjacent tooth crowns in same arch touch on each proximal surface.

Contour lines of Owen Adjoining imbrication lines in dentin that demonstrate disturbance in body metabolism.

Copula (kop-u-lah**)** Posterior swelling formed from the third and fourth branchial arches that overgrows the second arches to form the tongue base.

Coronal pulp Pulp located in tooth crown.

Coronoid (kor-ah-noid**) notch** Main part of anterior border of mandibular ramus.

Coronoid process Bony projection at anterior border of mandibular ramus.

Cortical (kor-ti-kal**) bone** Plates of compact bone on facial and lingual surfaces of alveolar process.

Crossbite Malocclusion in which mandibular tooth or teeth are placed facially to maxillary tooth or teeth.

Crown Part of tooth composed of dentin and pulp covered by enamel.

Curve of Spee Anteroposterior curvature produced by planes placed on masticatory surfaces of each dental arch.

Curve of Wilson Concave curve produced when frontal section is taken through maxillary and mandibular molars.

Cusp (kusp) One or more major elevations on the masticatory surface of the canine and posterior teeth.

Cusp of Carabelli (kare-ah-**bell**-ee)** Small cusp on the permanent maxillary first and second molar in some cases.

Cusp of Carabelli groove Groove associated with a cusp of Carabelli.

Cusp ridge Ridge that descends from each cusp tip on the posterior teeth.

Cusp slope Two ridges on the incisal edge of the canine teeth divided by cusp tip.

Cusp tip Tip of cusp on incisal surface of the canine teeth and occlusal table of the posterior teeth.

Cytodifferentiation (site-oh-dif-er-en-she-ay**-shin)** Development of different cell types.

Cytoplasm (cy-to-plazm) Fluid part contained within the cell membrane.

Cytoskeleton (sigh-toh-skel**-eh-ton) (CSK)** Three-dimensional system of support within cell.

D

D-A-Q-T System System to designate teeth: *D* for dentition, *A* for arch, *Q* for quadrant, and *T* for tooth type.

Dens in dente (denz in den-tay**)** Developmental disturbance caused by invagination of enamel organ into dental papilla.

Dense connective tissue Deepest layers of dermis or lamina propria.

Dense layer Dense connective tissue in the dermis and lamina propria.

Dental anatomy Area of dental sciences dealing with tooth morphology.

Dental arch Alveolar process or tooth-bearing part of each jaw in either maxillary or mandibular arch.

Dental lamina (lam-i-nah**)** Growth from oral epithelium giving rise to tooth buds.

Dental papilla (pah-pil**-ah)** Inner mass of ectomesenchyme of tooth germ that produces dentin and pulp.

Dental sac Tooth germ part consisting of ectomesenchyme surrounding outside of enamel organ.

Dentigerous (den-ti**-jer-os) cyst** Odontogenic cyst that forms from reduced enamel epithelium.

Dentin (den-tin**)** Hard inner layer of tooth crown overlying pulp.

Dentin dysplasia (dis-play**-ze-ah)** Faulty development of dentin.

Dentinal (den-tin-al**) caries** Carious lesion gone beyond dentinoenamel junction from enamel invasion.

Dentinal fluid Fluid within dentinal tubule in dentin.

Dentinal hypersensitivity (hi-per-**sen**-si-**tiv**-it-ee) Exposed dentin sensitive to various stimuli.

Dentinal tubules Long tubes in dentin.

Dentinocemental (**den**-tih-no-see-men-tal) **junction (DCJ)** Junction between dentin and cementum formed during root development.

Dentinoenamel (**den**-tih-no-ih-nam-l) **junction (DEJ)** Junction between dentin and enamel formed by mineralization of disintegrating basement membrane.

Dentinogenesis (den-tin-oh-**jen**-i-sis) Appositional growth of predentin by odontoblasts.

Dentinogenesis imperfecta (im-per-**fek**-tah) Dentin dysplasia with hereditary basis and blue-gray or brown teeth with opalescent sheen.

Dentition (den-**tish**-in) Natural teeth in jaws of either primary and permanent or mixed grouping of teeth.

Dentition periods Three periods that occur throughout lifetime: primary, mixed, and permanent.

Dentogingival (den-to-jin-**ji**-val) **junction** Junction between tooth surface and gingival tissue.

Dentogingival junctional tissue Tissue that includes sulcular epithelium and junctional epithelium.

Depression (de-**presh**-in) **of the mandible** Lowering of lower jaw.

Dermis (**der**-mis) Connective tissue proper in the skin.

Desmosome (**des**-mo-some) Intercellular junction between cells.

Developmental depression Depression usually evident in specific tooth area.

Developmental groove Primary groove that marks junction among developmental lobes on lingual surface of the anterior teeth or occlusal table of the posterior teeth.

Developmental pits Pits on the lingual surface of the anterior teeth or on occlusal table and buccal, and lingual surface of the posterior teeth.

Diastema (di-ah-**ste**-mah) Open contact that can exist between permanent maxillary central incisors.

Differentiation (dif-er-en-she-**ay**-shin) Change in embryonic cells to become quite distinct structurally and functionally.

Dilaceration (die-las-er-**ay**-shun) Crown or root(s) showing angular distortion.

Distal (**dis**-tl) Surface of tooth farthest away from midline.

Distal step No terminal plane relationship exists because the primary mandibular second molar is distal to the maxillary second molar.

Dorsal surface of the tongue Top surface of tongue.

Down syndrome Developmental disturbance that involves trisomy of chromosome number 21.

Duct Passageway that allows glandular secretion to be directly emptied.

E

Early childhood caries (ECC) Extensive acute caries of primary teeth.

Ectoderm (**ek**-toe-derm) Layer in trilaminar embryonic disc derived from epiblast layer and lining stomodeum.

Ectodermal dysplasia (**ek**-toe-derm-al dis-**play**-ze-ah) Syndrome involving abnormal development of one or more ectodermal structures including anodontia.

Ectomesenchyme (**ek**-toe-mes-eng-kime) Mesenchyme from ectoderm influenced by neural crest cells.

Ectopic (ek-**top**-ik) **pregnancy** Implantation occurring outside the uterus.

Edentulous (e-**den**-tu-lus) Dentition with either partial or complete loss of teeth.

Efferent (**ef**-er-ent) **vessel** Lymphatic vessel in which lymph flows out of lymph node.

Elastic cartilage (e-**las**-tik **kar**-ti-lij) Cartilage found in ear and epiglottis.

Elastic connective tissue Specialized connective tissue with mostly elastic fibers.

Elastic fiber Protein fiber in connective tissue composed of microfilaments.

Elevation (el-eh-**vay**-shun) **of the mandible** Raising of lower jaw.

Embrasures (em-**bray**-zhers) Spaces from curvatures where two teeth in same arch contact.

Embryo (**em**-bre-oh) Structure derived from implanted blastocyst.

Embryoblast (**em**-bre-oh-blast) **layer** Small inner mass of embryonic cells in blastocyst.

Embryology (em-bre-**ol**-ah-jee) Study of prenatal development.

Embryonic (em-bre-**on**-ik) **cell layers** Germ layers derived from increased number of embryonic cells.

Embryonic folding Embryonic folding of embryo placing tissue in proper position.

Embryonic period Prenatal developmental time period for embryo from second to eighth week.

Enamel (ih-**nam**-l) Hard outer layer of tooth crown.

Enamel caries Carious lesion invaded through enamel either by pits and grooves or through smooth surface.

Enamel dysplasia (dis-**play**-ze-ah) Faulty development of enamel.

Enamel knot Region noted in molars' enamel organ involved in crown form.

Enamel lamellae (lah-**mel**-ay) Partially mineralized vertical sheets of enamel matrix.

Enamel matrix (**may**-triks) Matrix of enamel formed during amelogenesis by the ameloblasts.

Enamel organ Cap or bell-shaped part of tooth germ that produces enamel.

Enamel pearl Small spherical enamel projections on tooth surface.

Enamel rod Crystalline structural unit of enamel.

Enamel spindles Microscopic feature present in mature enamel as short dentinal tubules near dentinoenamel junction.

Enamel tufts Microscopic feature in mature enamel of small dark brushes near dentinoenamel junction.

Endochondral ossification (en-do-**kon**-dril os-i-fi-**kay**-shun) Formation of osteoid within cartilage model.

Endocrine (en-**dah**-krin) **gland** Ductless gland that secretes directly into the blood.

Endocytosis (en-do-sigh-**toe**-sis) Uptake of materials from extracellular environment into cell.

Endoderm (en-**doe**-derm) Layer in trilaminar embryonic disc derived from hypoblast layer.

Endoplasmic reticulum (en-do-**plas**-mik rey-**tik**-u-lum) **(ER)** Membrane-bound organelle with channels that is either rough or smooth.

Endosteum (en-**dos**-te-um) Lining of medullary cavity of bone.

Endothelium (en-do-**thee**-lee-um) Unstratified squamous epithelium lining vessels and serous cavities.

End-to-end bite Teeth that occlude without maxillary teeth overlapping mandibular teeth.

Eosinophil (e-ah-**sin**-ah-fil) White blood cell involved in parasitic diseases because primary function is phagocytosis of immune complexes.

Epiblast (**ep**-i-blast) **layer** Superior layer in bilaminar disc.

Epidermis (ep-i-**der**-mis) Superficial layers of skin.

Epiglottic (ep-ee-**glot**-ik) **swelling** Posterior swelling that develops from fourth branchial arches marking the development of future epiglottis.

Epithelial (ep-ee-thee-lee-al) attachment (EA) Device that attaches junctional epithelium to tooth surface.

Epithelial rests of Malassez (mal-ah-say) (ERM) Epithelial cell groups in periodontal ligament after disintegration of Hertwig epithelial root sheath.

Epithelium (plural, epithelia) (ep-ee-thee-lee-um, ep-ee-thee-lee-uh) Basic tissue that covers and lines external and internal body surfaces.

Erectile (e-rek-tile) tissue Thin-walled vessels in nasal cavity capable of considerable engorgement.

Erosion (e-ro-zhun) Hard tooth tissue loss through chemical means not involving bacteria.

Excretory (ex-kreh-tor-ee) duct Duct of salivary gland through which saliva exits into the oral cavity.

Exocrine (ek-sah-krin) gland Gland having ducts associated with it.

Exocytosis (ek-so-sigh-toe-sis) Active transport of material from vesicle out into extracellular environment.

Exostoses (eks-ox-toe-seez) Small localized bone growths noted usually on facial surface of alveolar process of maxilla.

External basal lamina (bay-sal lam-i-nah) Basal lamina between the junctional epithelium and the lamina propria.

External nose Surface of the nose in the nasal region.

F

Facial (fay-shal) Structure or tooth surface closest to the outer face.

Fauces (faw-seez) Opening posteriorly from the oral cavity proper into pharynx.

Fertilization (fur-til-uh-zay-shun) Process by which sperm penetrates ovum during preimplantation period.

Fetal (fete-il) alcohol syndrome (FAS) Syndrome in infant during embryonic period resulting from ethanol ingested by pregnant woman.

Fetal period Prenatal development period for fetus from third to ninth month.

Fetus (fete-is) Structure of fetal period of prenatal development derived from enlarged embryo.

Fibroblast (fi-bro-blast) Cell that synthesizes protein fibers and intercellular substance.

Fibrocartilage (fi-bro-kar-ti-lij) Cartilage of parallel, thick, compact collagenous bundles.

Fifth branchial (brang-ke-al) arch(es) Rudimentary embryonic branchial arch(es) that is absent or included with fourth branchial arch(es).

Filiform (fil-i-form) lingual papillae (pah-pil-ay) Slender thread-like lingual papillae giving dorsal surface of tongue its velvety texture.

First branchial (brang-ke-al) arch(es) Mandibular arch(es) in embryo.

Floor of the mouth Area of oral cavity proper underneath the ventral surface of tongue and bordered by the mandibular arch.

Flush terminal plane Terminal plane relationship where primary maxillary and mandibular second molars are in an end-to-end relationship.

Fluting Elongated developmental depression on the surface root branches.

Foliate (fo-le-ate) lingual papillae (pah-pil-ay) Vertical ridges of lingual papillae on lateral tongue surface.

Follicles (fol-i-kls) Masses embedded in meshwork of reticular fibers within lobules of thyroid.

Foramen cecum (for-ay-men se-kum) Small pitlike depression located where sulcus terminalis points backward toward the pharynx.

Fordyce (for-dice) spots Small yellowish elevations of sebaceous glands on oral mucosa.

Foregut (fore-gut) Anterior part of future digestive tract or primitive pharynx that forms oropharynx.

Fossa (plural, fossae) (fos-ah, fos-ay) Shallow, wide depression(s) on the lingual surface of the anterior teeth or the occlusal table of the posterior teeth.

Fourth branchial (brang-ke-al) arch(es) Branchial arch(es) in embryo that participates in formation of laryngeal cartilages.

Free gingival (jin-ji-val) crest Most coronal part of marginal gingiva.

Free gingival groove Groove that separates attached gingiva from marginal gingiva.

Frontal (frun-tal) region Region of face that includes forehead and area above the eyes.

Frontonasal (frun-to-nay-zil) process Prominence in upper facial area at cephalic end of embryo.

Fungiform (fun-ji-form) lingual papillae (pah-pil-ay) Smaller mushroom-shaped lingual papillae on the dorsal tongue surface.

Furcation (fer-kay-shin) Area between two or more root branches before division from root trunk.

Furcation crotches Spaces between roots at the furcation.

Fusion (fu-zhin) Joining of embryonic tissue of two separate surfaces, elimination of a furrow between two adjacent swellings, or developmental disturbance in which adjacent tooth germs unite to form large tooth.

G

Gemination (jem-i-nay-shin) Developmental disturbance with single tooth germ trying to divide forming large single-rooted tooth.

Generalized resorption (re-sorp-shun) Resorption of hard tissue or entire skeleton of bone in varying amounts, resulting from endocrine activity.

Geographic tongue Lesion that appears as red and then paler pink to white patches on the tongue body.

Germinal (jurm-i-nil) center Center region of lymphatic nodule of a lymph node where lymphocytes mature.

Gingiva (jin-ji-vah) Gum tissue composed of mucosa surrounding the maxillary and mandibular teeth while covering the alveolar processes.

Gingival crevicular (jin-ji-val kre-vik-koo-ler) fluid (GCF) Fluid in gingival sulcus.

Gingival fiber group Fiber groups within gingiva that have no bony attachments.

Gingival hyperplasia (hi-per-play-ze-ah) Overgrowth of mainly interproximal gingiva.

Gingival recession (re-sesh-un) Inferiorly placed margin of the free gingival crest.

Gingival sulcus (sul-kus) Space facing the sulcular gingiva.

Gingivitis (jin-ji-vie-tis) Periodontal disease of the gingival tissue.

Gland Structure that produces secretion necessary for normal body functioning.

Globular (glob-u-lar) dentin Dentin with both primary and secondary mineralization.

Gnathic (nath-ick) index Measurement that gives degree of maxillary arch prominence.

Goblet cells Cells in respiratory mucosa that produce mucus for moisture.

Goiter (goy-ter) Enlarged thyroid.

Golden Proportions Principle that provides guide for esthetically pleasing proportion.

Golgi (gol-jee) complex Organelle of cell involved in protein segregation, packaging, and transport.

Granular layer Layer superficial to prickle layer in some forms of keratinized epithelium.

Granulation (gran-yoo-lay-shin) tissue Immature connective tissue formed during initial repair.

Group function Entire posterior quadrant functions during lateral occlusion.

H

Hard palate (pal-it) Anterior part of palate.

Haversian (hah-ver-zi-an) canal Vascular tissue space in osteon.

Haversian system Organized arrangement of lamellae and canals in compact bone.

Height of contour Crest of curvature that is the greatest elevation of the tooth crown either incisocervically or occlusocervically.

Hemidesmosome (hem-eye-des-mo-some) Forms intercellular junction involving attachment of cell to nearby noncellular surface.

Hertwig (hirt-wig) epithelial root sheath (HERS) Part of cervical loop that functions to shape the root(s) and induce root dentin formation.

Hilus (hi-lus) Depression on one side of a lymph node.

Hindgut (hinde-gut) Posterior part of future digestive tract.

Histodifferentiation (his-toe-dif-er-en-she-ay-shun) Development of different tissue types.

Histology (his-tol-oh-jee) Study of microscopic structure and function of tissue.

Horizontal group Alveodental ligament subgroup originating in alveolar bone proper to insert horizontally into cementum.

Howship lacuna (how-ship lah-ku-nah) Large shallow pit in bone created by osteoclast.

Hunter-Schreger (hun-ter-shray-ger) bands (HSB) Alternating light to dark lines noted in certain sections of enamel using reflected rather than transmitted light.

Hutchinson incisors (hutch-in-sun in-sigh-zers) Developmental disturbance in permanent incisors with screwdriver-shaped crowns caused by congenital syphilis.

Hyaline cartilage (hi-ah-line kar-ti-lij) Cartilage that contains no nerves or blood vessels and serves as growth center in the temporomandibular joint.

Hyoid (hi-oid) arch(es) Second branchial arch(es) that lies inferiorly to mandibular arch(es) in embryo.

Hyoid bone Bone suspended in anterior midline of neck that has many muscle attachments.

Hypercementosis (hi-per-see-men-toe-sis) Excessive production of cellular cementum.

Hyperkeratinization (hi-per-ker-ah-tin-zay-shun) Excessive production of keratin.

Hypoblast (hi-po-blast) layer Inferior layer in bilaminar disc.

Hypodermis (hi-poh-der-mis) Deeper to the dermis.

Hyposalivation (hi-po-sal-i-vay-shen) Decreased production of saliva.

I

Imbrication (im-bri-kay-shun) lines Slight ridges that extend mesiodistally in cervical third associated with lines of Retzius in enamel.

Imbrication lines of von Ebner (von eeb-ner) Incremental lines in mature dentin.

Immunogen (im-un-ah-jen) Antigen treated as foreign capable of triggering immune response.

Immunoglobulin (im-u-nah-glob-ul-in) (Ig) Blood protein or antibody produced by plasma cells during immune response.

Impacted (im-pak-ted) Unerupted or partially erupted tooth positioned against another tooth, bone, or soft tissue preventing eruption.

Implantation (im-plan-tay-shin) Embedding of blastocyst in endometrium.

Incisal (in-sigh-zl) angles Two angles on permanent incisors formed from incisal ridge or edge and each proximal surface.

Incisal edge Flattened incisal ridge on permanent incisors due to attrition after eruption.

Incisal ridge Linear elevation on incisal or masticatory surface of incisors when newly erupted.

Incisal surface Masticatory surface for anterior teeth.

Incisive papilla (in-sy-ziv pah-pil-ah) Small bulge of tissue at anterior hard palate.

Incisors (in-sigh-zers) First and second anterior teeth from midline: centrals and laterals.

Inclined cuspal (kusp-al) planes Sloping planes located between cusp ridges on the posterior teeth.

Inclusions (in-kloo-zhins) Metabolically inert substances or transient structures within cell.

Induction (in-duk-shin) Action of one group of cells on another leading to developmental pathway in responding tissue.

Infraorbital (in-frah-or-bit-al) region Facial region located both inferior to orbital region and lateral to nasal region.

Initiation stage First stage of tooth development.

Inner enamel epithelium (ih-nam-l ep-ee-thee-lee-um) (IEE) Innermost cells of enamel organ that form ameloblasts.

Intercalated (in-turk-ah-lay-ted) duct Duct associated with acinus or terminal part of salivary gland.

Intercellular junctions Mechanical attachments between cells or between cells and nearby noncellular surfaces.

Intercellular substance Transparent substance that fills in spaces between tissue cells.

Interdental gingiva (in-ter-den-tal jin-ji-vah) The interdental gingiva is the gingival tissue between adjacent teeth adjoining attached gingiva.

Interdental ligament Principal fiber subgroup that inserts interdentally into cervical cementum of neighboring teeth.

Interdental papilla (plural, papillae) (pah-pil-ah, pah-pil-ay) Extension(s) of the interdental gingiva between adjacent teeth adjoining attached gingiva.

Interdental septum Alveolar process between two neighboring teeth.

Interglobular (in-ter-glob-u-lar) dentin Dentin with only primary mineralization.

Interlabial (in-ter-lay-be-al) gap Distance between inferior border of upper lip and superior border of lower lip when at physiologic resting position.

Intermaxillary (in-ter-mak-si-lare-ee) segment Growth from paired medial nasal processes on inside of stomodeum.

Intermediate filaments (fil-ah-ments) Components of cytoskeleton.

Intermediate layer Layer of epithelium superficial to basal layer in nonkeratinized epithelium.

Internal basal lamina (bay-sal lam-i-nah) Basal lamina that is part of the epithelial attachment to the tooth surface.

International Numbering System (INS) International system for tooth designation using a two-digit code.

Interocclusal (in-ter-ah-kloo-zhal) clearance Space between dental arches when mandible is at rest.

Interphase (in-ter-faze) Period when cell is between divisions but is growing and functioning.

Interproximal (in-ter-prok-si-mal) space Area between adjacent tooth surfaces.

Interradicular (in-ter-rah-dik-u-lar) group Alveolodental ligament subgroup on multirooted teeth inserted on cementum of one root to cementum of other root(s).

Interradicular septum Alveolar process between the roots of same tooth.

Interrod enamel (ih-nam-l) Outer enamel surrounding each enamel rod core, creating an interprismatic region.

Interstitial (in-ter-stish-il) growth Growth from deep within tissue or organ.

Intertubular (in-ter-tube-u-lar) dentin Dentin between dentinal tubules.

Intramembranous ossification (in-trah-mem-bran-us os-i-fi-kay-shun) Formation of osteoid within dense connective tissue.

J

Joint capsule Two-layered connective tissue that completely encloses temporomandibular joint.

Joint disc Disc of temporomandibular joint located between temporal bone and mandibular condyle.

Junctional epithelium (jungk-shun-al ep-ce-thee-lee-um) (JE) Deeper extension of sulcular epithelium.

K

Karyotype (kare-e oh-tipe) Photographic analysis of chromosomes.

Keratin (ker-ah-tin) Intermediate protein filament found in calloused epithelium consisting of opaque waterproof substance.

Keratin layer Most superficial layer in keratinized epithelium.

Keratohyaline (ker-ah-toe-hi-ah-lene) granules Prominent granules in cytoplasm of epithelial cells that form keratin chemical precursor.

L

Labial (lay-be-al) Structures or facial surface of the teeth close to the lips.

Labial commissure (kom-i-shoor) Corner of the mouth where the upper and lower lips meet.

Labial frenum (plural, frena) (free-num, free-nah) Fold(s) of tissue located at midline between labial mucosa and alveolar mucosa on the dental arch(es).

Labial mucosa (mu-ko-sah) Mucosal lining of inner parts of the lips.

Labial ridge Central ridge on labial surface of canines from greater development of middle labial developmental lobe.

Lacuna (plural, lacunae) (lah-ku-nah, lah-ku-nay) Small space(s) that surrounds chondrocyte or osteocyte within cartilage matrix or bone.

Lamellae (lah-mel-ay) Closely apposed sheets of bone tissue in compact bone.

Lamina dura (lam-i-nah dur-ah) Radiopaque line representing alveolar bone proper.

Lamina propria (pro-pree-ah) Connective tissue proper region of oral mucosa.

Laryngopharynx (lah-ring-gah-fare-inks) Most inferior part of pharynx close to laryngeal opening.

Larynx (lare-inks) Voice box in midline of neck.

Lateral deviation (de-vee-ay-shun) of the mandible Shifting lower jaw to one side.

Lateral lingual swellings Parts of developing tongue that form on each side of tuberculum impar.

Lateral nasal process(es) Tissue on outer part of nasal pits that forms nasal alae.

Lateral occlusion (ah-kloozh-n) Movement that occurs when mandible moves to the side until the canines are in a cusp-to-cusp relationship.

Lateral surface of the tongue Side of tongue.

Leeway space Space created when primary molars are shed to make room for smaller mesiodistal permanent premolars.

Lens placodes (plak-odz) Placodes forming eyes and related tissue.

Line angle Line formed by junction of two crown surfaces.

Linea alba (lin-ee-ah al-bah) White ridge of keratinized epithelium on buccal mucosa at the level where teeth occlude.

Lines of Retzius (ret-zee-us) Incremental lines in mature enamel.

Lingual (ling-gwal) Structures or tooth surface closest to tongue..

Lingual frenum (free-num) Midline fold of tissue between the ventral surface of tongue and the floor of the mouth.

Lingual papillae (pah-pil-ay) Small elevated structures of specialized mucosa on the tongue.

Lingual ridge Vertically oriented and centrally placed ridge that extends from cusp tip to cingulum on the lingual surface of the canine teeth.

Lingual tonsil (ton-sil) Irregular mass of tonsillar tissue located posteriorly on the dorsal surface of the tongue.

Lining mucosa (mu-ko-sah) Mucosa associated with nonkeratinized stratified squamous epithelium.

Lip incompetence Open mouth, with lips apart, at resting posture.

Lobes Large inner parts of glands or regions of tooth during development.

Lobules (lob-ules) Smaller inner parts of glands.

Localized resorption (re-sorp-shun) Resorption of bone or other hard tissue that occurs in specific area.

Loose connective tissue Superficial layer of dermis of the skin or lamina propria of the oral mucosa.

Lumen (loo-men) Central opening where saliva is deposited into duct after production by secretory cells.

Lymph (limf) Tissue fluid that drains from surrounding region into lymphatic vessels.

Lymph nodes Bean-shaped filtering bodies grouped in clusters along connecting lymphatic vessels.

Lymphadenopathy (lim-fad-uh-nop-ah-thee) Enlarged and palpable lymph nodes.

Lymphatic(s) (lim-fat-ik[s]) Network of lymphatic vessels that collect and transport lymph, linking lymph nodes.

Lymphatic ducts Ducts that smaller lymphatic vessels containing lymph converge into and then empty into the venous system.

Lymphatic nodules (nah-jools) Masses of lymphocytes in lymph node

Lymphatic vessels System of endothelium-lined channels that carry lymph.

Lymphocyte (lim-fo-site) Second most common white blood cell in the blood involved in immune response.

Lysosomes (li-sah-somes) Organelles of cell functioning in both intracellular and extracellular digestion.

M

Macrodontia (mak-roe-don-she-ah) Abnormally large teeth.

Macrophage (mak-rah-faje) Most common white blood cell in connective tissue proper or *monocyte* before migration from blood.

Major salivary (sal-i-ver-ee**) glands** Large paired glands that have named associated ducts.

Malocclusion (mal-ah-**kloo**-zhun**)** Failure to have overall ideal form to the dentition while in centric occlusion.

Mamelons (mam-ah-lons**)** Rounded enamel extensions on the incisal ridge of the anterior teeth.

Mandible (man-di-bl**)** Lower jaw.

Mandibular (man-**dib**-you-lar**) arch(es)** Lower dental arch(es) with mandibular teeth, or the first branchial arch(es) in embryo.

Mandibular condyle (kon-dyl**)** Bony projection off posterior and superior border of mandibular ramus.

Mandibular notch Depression between coronoid process and condyle.

Mandibular processes Processes of first branchial arches that fuse at midline to form the mandibular arch.

Mandibular symphysis (sim-fi-sis**)** Midline area of mandible marking fusion of the two mandibular processes.

Mandibular teeth Teeth in mandibular arch of lower jaw or mandible.

Mandibular torus (plural, tori) (tore-us, **tore**-eye**)** Bone growth(s) noted on lingual aspect(s) of mandibular arch.

Mantle dentin Outermost layer of dentin found in crown region adjacent to the dentinoenamel junction.

Marginal gingiva (jin-ji-vah**)** Gingiva at the gingival margin of each tooth.

Marginal grooves Developmental grooves that cross either marginal ridge.

Marginal ridges Rounded raised borders on mesial and distal parts of the lingual surface of the anterior teeth or the occlusal table of the posterior teeth.

Masseter (mass-et-er**) muscle** Powerful bilateral muscle of mastication.

Mast cell White blood cell similar to basophil due to involvement in allergic responses.

Mastication (mass-ti-**kay**-shin**)** Chewing process.

Masticatory mucosa (mass-ti-ka-tor-ee mu-**ko**-sah**)** Mucosa associated with keratinized stratified squamous epithelium.

Masticatory surface Chewing tooth surface on crown.

Matrix (may-triks**)** Extracellular substance or surrounding medium; in connective tissue composed of intercellular substance and fibers; or one that is partially mineralized and serves as a framework for later mineralization for hard dental tissue.

Maturation (ma-cher-**ray**-shin**)** Attainment of adult size as well as adult form and function.

Maturation stage Final stage of odontogenesis when matrices of hard dental tissue types fully mineralize.

Maxilla (mak-**sil**-ah**)** Upper jaw.

Maxillary (mak-si-lare-ee**) arch** Upper dental arch with maxillary teeth.

Maxillary process Prominence from mandibular arch that grows superiorly and anteriorly on each side of stomodeum.

Maxillary sinus (sy-nus**)** Paranasal sinus within maxilla.

Maxillary teeth Teeth in maxillary arch or maxilla or upper jaw.

Maxillary tuberosity (too-beh-**ros**-i-tee**)** Tissue-covered bony elevation just distal to last tooth of maxillary arch.

Maximum mouth opening (MMO) The greatest amount of interincisal opening of the mouth.

Meckel cartilage (mek-el kar-ti-lij**)** Cartilage that forms within each side of the mandibular arch(es) and that disappears as bony mandible forms.

Medial nasal process(es) Middle part of the tissue growing around nasal placodes located between the two nasal pits.

Median lingual sulcus (ling-gwal **sul**-kus**)** Midline depression on dorsal surface of tongue.

Median palatine raphe (pal-ah-tine **ra**-fee**)** Midline ridge of tissue on hard palate that overlies bony fusion marked by median palatine suture.

Meiosis (my-**oh**-sis**)** Process of reproductive cell production that ensures correct number of chromosomes.

Melanin (mel-a-nin**) pigmentation** Localized macules of pigmentation caused by presence of melanin.

Melanocytes (meh-lah-no-sites**)** Cells that form pigment of melanin.

Mental (men-tal**) region** Region of the face with the chin as the major feature.

Mesenchyme (mes-eng-kime**)** Embryonic connective tissue.

Mesial (me-ze-il**)** Surface of tooth closest to midline.

Mesial drift Natural movement of teeth over time toward the midline of the oral cavity.

Mesial step Terminal plane relationship with primary mandibular second molar is mesial to maxillary molar.

Mesiodens (me-ze-oh-denz**)** Supernumerary tooth between two permanent maxillary central incisors.

Mesoderm (mes-oh-derm**)** Embryonic layer located between ectoderm and endoderm.

Mesognathic (me-so-**nath**-ik**)** Facial profile in centric occlusion with slightly protruded jaws, giving facial outline a relatively flat appearance or straight profile.

Metaphase (met-ah-faze**)** Second phase of mitosis in which chromosomes are aligned into equatorial position.

Microdontia (mi-kro-**don**-she-ah**)** Abnormally small teeth.

Microfilaments (my-kroh-**fil**-ah-ments**)** Components of cytoskeleton that are delicate and threadlike.

Microplicae (my-kro-**plee**-kay**) (MPL)** Ridgelike folds on the surface of superficial cells of all types of oral epithelium.

Microtubules (my-kroh-**too**-bules**)** Components of the cytoskeleton that are slender tubular microscopic structures.

Midgut (mid-gut**)** Middle part of future digestive tract.

Minor salivary (sal-i-ver-ee**) glands** Small salivary glands with short unnamed ducts.

Mitochondria (mite-ah-**kon**-dree-ah**)** Organelles associated with manufacture of energy for cell.

Mitosis (my-**toe**-sis**)** Cell division that occurs in phases and results in two daughter cells.

Mixed dentition (den-**tish**-in**)** Dentition with both primary and permanent teeth present.

Mixed dentition period Transitional stage involving the dentition when both primary and permanent teeth are present.

Molars (mo-lerz**)** Most posterior teeth with firsts, seconds, and thirds.

Monocyte (mon-ah-site**)** White blood cell that becomes macrophage after migration from the blood into the tissue.

Morphodifferentiation (mor-foe-dif-er-en-she-**ay**-shin**)** Development of the differing form that creates a specific structure.

Morphogenesis (mor-fo-**jen**-is-is**)** Process of development of specific tissue morphology.

Morphology (mor-**fol**-ah-je**)** Form of structure.

Mucobuccal (mu-ko-**buk**-al**) fold** Area within vestibule where labial mucosa or buccal mucosa meets alveolar mucosa.

Mucocele (mu-kah-sele**)** Lesion due to retention of saliva in minor salivary gland.

Mucocutaneous (moo-ko-ku-tay-nee-us**) junction** Transition zone at the vermilion border outlining the lips from the surrounding skin.

Mucogingival (mu-ko-**jin**-ji-val**) junction** Line of demarcation between attached gingiva and alveolar mucosa.

Mucoperiosteum (mu-ko-per-ee-**os**-te-um**)** Combined structure consisting of a mucous membrane, in the case of the oral cavity, the epithelium and lamina propria of the oral mucosa, with the periosteum of bone.

Mucous acini (mu-kis **as-**i-ny) Group of mucous cells producing mucous secretory product.

Mucous cells Secretory cells that produce mucous secretory product.

Mulberry molars (mull-bare-ee **mo-**lers) Developmental disturbance resulting from congenital syphilis forming enamel nodules on the molars' occlusal surface.

Multirooted Teeth with two or more root branches.

Muscle Fibrous tissue bundle that can contract to produce movement in or maintaining the position of parts of the body.

Muscles of mastication (mass-ti-**kay-**shin) Muscles involved in mastication: masseter, temporalis, and medial and lateral pterygoid.

Myoepithelial (my-oh-ep-ee-**thee-**lee-al) **cells** Contractile epithelial cells on acini that facilitate the flow of saliva out of each lumen into connecting ducts.

N

Naris (plural, nares) (nay-ris, **nay-**rees) Nostril(s) of nose.

Nasal cavity (kav-it-ee) Inner space of nose.

Nasal conchae (kong-kay) Projecting structures that extend inward from each lateral wall of the nasal cavity.

Nasal pits Depressions in center of each nasal placode that evolve into the nasal cavities.

Nasal placodes (plak-odz) Placodes that develop into olfactory organ for the sensation of smell located in mature nose.

Nasal region Region of the face occupied by external nose.

Nasal septum (sep-tum) Midline part of the nose that separates the nares.

Nasmyth (nas-mith) **membrane** Residue on newly erupted teeth that may become extrinsically stained.

Nasopharynx (nay-zo-**fare-**inks) Division of pharynx superior to level of soft palate.

Natural killer (NK) cell Large lymphocyte involved in first line of defense.

Neonatal (ne-oh-**nate-**l) **line** Accentuated incremental line of Retzius in enamel or contour line of Owen in dentin from birth process.

Nerve Bundle of neural processes outside the central nervous system.

Neural (noor-al) **crest cells (NCCs)** Specialized group of cells developed from neuroectoderm that migrate from the crests of the neural folds and disperse to specific sites within the mesenchyme.

Neural folds Raised ridges in the neural plate that surround deepening neural groove.

Neural groove Groove from further growth and thickening of neural plate.

Neural plate Centralized band of cells that extends length of embryo.

Neural tube Tube formed when neural folds meet and fuse superior to neural groove.

Neuroectoderm (noor-oh-**ek-**toe-derm) Specialized group of cells that differentiates from ectoderm.

Neuron (noor-on) Functional cellular component of nervous system.

Nicotinic stomatitis (nik-ah-**tin-**ik sto-mah-**ti-**tis) Whitish lesion on hard palate caused by heat from smoking or hot liquid consumption.

Nonkeratinized stratified squamous epithelium (non-**ker-**ah-tin-izd **strat-**i-fide **skway-**mus ep-ee-**thee-**lee-um) Epithelium in superficial layers of lining mucosa.

Nonsuccedaneous (non-suk-seh-**dane-**ee-us) Permanent teeth without primary predecessors, namely the molars.

Nuclear (noo-kle-er) **envelope** Double membrane completely surrounding nucleus.

Nuclear pores Avenues of communication between inner nucleoplasm and outer cytoplasm.

Nucleolus (noo-kle-oh-lis) Rounded nuclear organelle centrally placed in nucleoplasm.

Nucleoplasm (noo-kle-ah-plazm) Semifluid part within nucleus.

Nucleus (plural, nuclei) (noo-kle-is, **noo-**kle-eye) Largest, densest, most conspicuous organelle(s) in cell.

O

Oblique (o-bleek) group Alveolodental ligament subgroup originating in alveolar bone proper to extend apically and obliquely to insert into cementum.

Oblique ridge Transverse ridge that crosses occlusal table obliquely from mesiolingual to distobuccal on most maxillary molars.

Occlusal (ah-**klooz-**l) **pits** Sharp pinpoint depression in fossae on occlusal table of the posterior teeth.

Occlusal surface Masticatory surface of the posterior teeth.

Occlusal table Part of the occlusal surface of the posterior teeth bordered by marginal ridges.

Occlusal trauma Trauma to periodontium from occlusal disharmony.

Occlusion (ah-**kloo-**zhun) Anatomic alignment of teeth and relationship to masticatory system.

Odontoblastic (oh-don-toe-**blast-**ik) **process** Attached cellular extension of odontoblast within dentinal tubule.

Odontoblasts (oh-**don-**toe-blasts) Cells that produce dentin and differentiate from outer cells of the dental papilla.

Odontoclasts (oh-**don-**toe-klasts) Cells that resorb dentin, cementum, and enamel.

Odontogenesis (oh-don-to-**jen-**eh-sis) Process of tooth development.

Olfactory mucosa (ol-**fak-**tor-e mu-**ko-**sah) Mucosa in the roof of each part of the nasal cavity that carries sense of smell receptors.

Open bite Malocclusion due to the anterior teeth of both dental arches not occluding.

Oral cavity proper Inside of mouth.

Oral epithelium (ep-ee-**thee-**lee-um) Embryonic lining of oral cavity derived from ectoderm.

Oral mucosa (mu-**ko-**sah) Mucosa or mucous membrane lining oral cavity.

Oral region Region of face that contains the lips and oral cavity.

Orbit (or-bit) Bony socket that contains eyeball.

Orbital (or-bit-al) **region** Facial region that includes bony orbit and eyeball.

Organ Somewhat independent body part formed from tissue that performs specific function or functions.

Organelles (or-gan-**eels**) Specialized structures within cell that are permanent and metabolically active.

Orofacial myofunctional (my-oh-**funk-**shun-al) **disorder (OMD)** Behaviors and patterns created by inappropriate muscle function and incorrect habits involving tongue, lips, jaws, and face.

Orofacial myofunctional therapy (OMT) Variety of exercises are involved that are based on individual evaluation and treatment protocols to eliminate orofacial myofunctional disorders.

Orofacial myology (my-ol-oh-je) **(OM)** Discipline that evaluates and treats a variety of orofacial muscle postural and functional disorders as well as habit patterns.

Oronasal (or-oh-**nay-**zil) **membrane** Embryonic membrane that disintegrates to bring the nasal and oral cavities into communication.

Oropharyngeal (or-oh-fah-**rin-**je-al) **membrane** Membrane at cephalic end of embryo.

Oropharynx (or-o-**fare-**inks) Oral division of pharynx.

Orthokeratinized stratified squamous epithelium (or-tho-**ker-**ah-tin-izd **strat-**i-fide **skway-**mus ep-ee-**thee-**lee-um) Epithelium that demonstrates keratinization of epithelial cells.

Ossification (os-i-fi-**kay**-shun) Bone formation.

Osteoblasts (**os**-te-oh-blasts) Bone-forming cells.

Osteoclast (**os**-te-oh-klast) Cell that functions in resorption of bone.

Osteocytes (**os**-tee-oh-sites) Mature osteoblasts entrapped in bone matrix.

Osteoid (**os**-te-oid) Initially formed bone matrix.

Osteons (**os**-te-onz) Concentric layers of lamellae in compact bone.

Otic placodes (**o**-tik **plak**-odz) Placodes in embryo forming future internal ear.

Outer cells of the dental papilla (pah-**pil**-ah) Cells of dental papilla tissue that differentiate into odontoblasts.

Outer enamel epithelium (ih-**nam**-l ep-ee-**thee**-lee-um) (OEE) Outer cells of enamel organ that serve as protective barrier.

Overbite Maxillary arch vertically overlaps mandibular arch.

Overjet Maxillary arch horizontally overlaps mandibular arch.

Ovum (**oh**-vum) Female reproductive cell or egg that can be fertilized.

P

Palatal (**pal**-ah-tal) Lingual structures or tooth surface closest to palate.

Palatal shelves Two processes derived from maxillary processes during prenatal development.

Palatal torus (**tore**-us) Normal variation of bone growth noted on midline of hard palate.

Palate (**pal**-it) Roof of mouth.

Palatine rugae (**pal**-ah-tine **ru**-gee) Firm, irregular ridges of tissue directly posterior to incisive papilla.

Palatine tonsils (**ton**-sils) Tonsillar tissue located between faucial pillars.

Palmer Notation Method System of tooth designation commonly used in orthodontics; when oral cavity is divided into quadrants and each tooth is designated by a numeral 1 to 8.

Papillary (**pap**-i-lar-ee) **layer** Layer of loose connective tissue of dermis or lamina propria.

Parafunctional (pare-ah-**funk**-shun-al) **habits** Mandible movements not within normal motions associated with mastication, speech, or respiratory movements.

Parakeratinized stratified squamous epithelium (pare-ah-**ker**-ah-tin-izd **strat**-i-fide **skway**-mus ep-ee-**thee**-lee-um) Keratinized epithelium associated with masticatory mucosa of attached gingiva.

Paranasal sinuses (pare-ah-**na**-zil **sy**-nuses) Paired air-filled cavities in bone.

Parathyroid (par-ah-**thy**-roid) **glands** Endocrine glands along posterior aspects of thyroid.

Parotid (pah-**rot**-id) **duct** Duct associated with parotid.

Parotid papilla (pah-**pil**-ah) Small elevation of tissue on inner part of the buccal mucosa that protects parotid duct.

Parotid salivary gland Major salivary gland located irregularly from zygomatic arch to posterior border of the mandible.

Passive eruption Eruption that takes place when gingiva recedes with no actual tooth movement.

Peg lateral Lateral incisor crown that is smaller from partial microdontia.

Peg molars (**mo**-lers) Microdontia usually of the third molar.

Perichondrium (per-ee-**kon**-dre-um) Outermost connective tissue layer surrounding most cartilage.

Perikymata (per-ee-ki-**maht**-ah) Grooves evident on teeth associated with the lines of Retzius in enamel.

Periodontal (pare-ee-o-**don**-tal) **ligament (PDL)** Ligament surrounding the teeth that supports and attaches them to alveoli bony surface.

Periodontal ligament (PDL) space Radiolucent area representing periodontal ligament on radiographs.

Periodontal pocket Deepened gingival sulcus from periodontitis that is lined by pocket epithelium.

Periodontitis (pare-e-oh-don-**tie**-tis) Periodontal disease involving the periodontium.

Periodontium (per-e-o-**don**-she-um) Supporting hard and soft dental tissue between and including parts of tooth and alveolar process.

Periosteum (per-ee-**os**-te-im) Dense connective tissue layer on outer part of bone.

Peritubular (pare-i-**tube**-u-lar) **dentin** Dentin that creates wall of dentinal tubule.

Permanent dentition (den-**tish**-in) Second and final dentition with all the permanent teeth or adult teeth present. Also called *permanent teeth.*

Permanent dentition period Final stage in the dentition with all the permanent teeth present.

Permanent teeth *See* permanent dentition.

Phagocytosis (fag-oh-sigh-**toe**-sis) Engulfing and then digesting of solid waste or foreign material by cell.

Pharyngeal (fah-**rin**-je-il) **pouches** Four pairs of evaginations lining the pharynx between branchial arches.

Pharyngeal tonsils Located on superior and posterior walls of nasopharynx.

Pharynx (**fare**-inks) Muscular tube of neck or throat.

Philtrum (**fil**-trum) Vertical groove on midline of upper lip.

Pit and groove patterns Patterns formed from pits and grooves on the lingual surface of the permanent anterior teeth or the occlusal surface of the permanent posterior teeth.

Placenta (pla-**sen**-tuh) Temporary prenatal organ that provides support to the developing embryo.

Plasma (**plaz**-mah) Fluid substance in the blood vessels that carries blood cells and metabolites.

Plasma cells White blood cells derived from B-cell lymphocytes to form immunoglobulins or antibodies.

Platelets (**plate**-lits) Blood cell fragments functioning in clotting mechanism.

Plica fimbriata (plural, plicae fimbriatae) (**pli**-kah fim-bree-**ay**-tah, **pli**-kay fim-bree-ay-tay) Fold(s) with fringelike projections on ventral surface of the tongue.

Pocket epithelium (ep-ee-**thee**-lee-um) (PE) Epithelium lining periodontal pocket.

Point angle Imaginary line formed by junction of three crown surfaces.

Polymorphonuclear leukocyte (pol-ee-mor-fah-**noo**-klee-er **loo**-ko-site) (PMN) Most common white blood cell involved in inflammatory response or neutrophil.

Posterior faucial (**faw**-shawl) **pillar** Posterior lateral folds of tissue in pharynx created by underlying muscle forming the fauces.

Posterior teeth Molars (and premolars if present) in the back of the mouth.

Postglenoid (post-**glen**-oid) **process** Sharp ridge posterior to articular fossa.

Preameloblasts (pre-ah-**mel**-oh-blasts) Cells from inner enamel epithelium of enamel organ that differentiate into ameloblasts.

Predentin Dentin matrix laid down by appositional growth by odontoblasts.

Preimplantation (pre-im-plan-**tay**-shin) **period** Period of unattached conceptus taking place during first week of prenatal development.

Premature contacts Situation in which one or two teeth initially contact before other teeth.

Premolars (pre-mo-lerz) Fourth and fifth posterior teeth from midline in permanent dentition, including firsts and seconds or bicuspids.

Prenatal (pre-nay-tal) development Processes that occur from start of pregnancy to birth.

Prickle layer Layer that is superficial to basal layer in keratinized epithelium.

Primary bone First bone to be produced by either ossification method.

Primary dentin Dentin formed before completion of apical foramen.

Primary dentition (den-tish-in) First stage in the dentition when all the primary or deciduous teeth are present. Also called *primary teeth*.

Primary dentition period Only primary teeth are present with this dentition.

Primary palate (pal-it) Anterior part of final palate derived from intermaxillary segment during prenatal development.

Primary teeth First teeth present or deciduous teeth. Also called *primary dentition*.

Primate spaces Developmental spaces between primary teeth.

Primitive pharynx (fare-inks) Cranial part of foregut that forms oropharynx.

Primitive streak Furrowed, rod-shaped thickening in middle of embryonic disc.

Primordium (pry-more-de-um) Earliest indication of part or organ during prenatal development.

Principal fibers Collagen fibers organized into groups on the basis of orientation to tooth and related function.

Prognathic (prog-nath-ik) Facial profile with rather prominent mandible and possibly normal or even retrusive maxilla, or concave profile.

Proliferation (pro-lif-er-ay-shin) Controlled cellular growth such us that which occurs in prenatal development or tooth development.

Prophase (pro-faze) First phase of mitosis with chromatin condensing into chromosomes.

Protrusion (pro-troo-zhin) of the mandible Moving lower jaw forward.

Protrusive occlusion (ah-kloo-zhun) Occlusion when mandible undergoes protrusion.

Proximal Mesial and distal surface between adjacent teeth.

Pseudostratified (soo-doh-strat-i-fide) columnar epithelium Simple epithelium that falsely appears as multiple cell layers.

Pterygomandibular (teh-ri-go-man-dib-you-lar) fold Tissue fold that extends from junction of hard and soft palates down to mandible.

Pulp Soft innermost connective tissue in both crown and root.

Pulp chamber Part of the tooth containing mass of pulp.

Pulp horns Extensions of coronal pulp into cusps of the posterior teeth.

Pulp stones Masses of mineralized dentin in pulp.

Pulpitis (pul-pie-tis) Inflammation of pulp.

Q

Quadrants (kwod-rints) Division of each dental arch into two parts with four quadrants in oral cavity.

R

Radicular (rah-dik-u-lar) pulp Pulp located in the root area of tooth.

Ramus (plural, rami) (ray-mus, rame-eye) Mandibular plate(s) that extend(s) upward and backward from the body on each side.

Range of motion (ROM) Normal physiologic and functional reciprocal range of motion/movement for mandibular opening or closure.

Ranula (ran-u-lah) Lesion from retention of saliva usually in submandibular salivary gland.

Red blood cell (RBC) Blood cell whose cytoplasm contains hemoglobin that binds and then transports the oxygen.

Reduced enamel epithelium (ih-nam-l ep-ee-thee-lee-um) (REE) Layers of flattened cells overlying enamel surface from compressed enamel organ.

Regeneration Renewal of a tissue and possibly even an organ.

Regions of the face Facial surface areas: frontal, orbital, nasal, infraorbital, zygomatic, buccal, oral, and mental.

Regions of the neck Areas that extend from the skull and mandible inferior to clavicles and sternum.

Reichert cartilage (rike-ert kar-ti-lij) Cartilage in second branchial arch(es) that eventually disappears.

Remodeling Process by which bone is replaced over time.

Repolarization (re-po-ler-i za-shun) Process that occurs in cell with nucleus moving away from the center to a position farthest away from basement membrane.

Respiratory mucosa (mu-ko-sah) Mucosa that consists of pseudostratified ciliated columnar epithelium.

Resting posture Normal physiologic position of tongue, lips, and mandible when not in function of chewing, swallowing, or speech.

Retained sucking habit Parafunctional habit includes digit and pacifier use past the age of 2.

Rete (ree-tee) ridges Interdigitation of epithelium into connective tissue.

Reticular (re-tik-u-ler) connective tissue Delicate network of interwoven reticular fibers.

Reticular fibers Fibers in embryonic tissue.

Reticular lamina (lam-i-nah) Deeper part of basement membrane.

Retraction (re trak-shun) of the mandible Moving lower jaw backward.

Retrognathic (re-tro-nath-ik) Facial profile with protruding upper lip with recessive mandible and chin and convex profile.

Retromolar (re-tro-mo-ler) pad Dense pad of tissue just distal to last tooth of mandibular arch.

Reversal lines Stained, scalloped microscopic lines caused by resorption in cartilage, bone, and cementum.

Ribosomes (ry-bo-somes) Organelles of cell associated with protein production.

Ridges Linear elevations on masticatory surface of either anterior or posterior teeth.

Root(s) Part of a tooth composed of dentin covered by cementum.

Root axis line (RAL) Imaginary line representing long axis line of tooth drawn to bisect cervical line.

Root concavities Indentations on the surface of the root.

Root fusion Developmental disturbance that creates deep developmental grooves with root fusion.

Root of the nose Nose located between the eyes.

Root trunk Root of multirooted teeth where the root originates from crown.

Rubella (roo-bell-ah) Viral infection that can serve as teratogen transmitted by way of placenta to embryo.

S

Saliva (sah-li-vah) Secretion from salivary glands that lubricates and cleanses the oral cavity and helps in digestion.

Salivary (sal-i-ver-ee) glands Glands that produce saliva.

Second branchial (brang-ke-al) **arch(es)** Branchial arch(es) inferior to mandibular arch(es) in embryo, or hyoid arch(es).

Secondary bone Mature bone tissue that replaces immature bone.

Secondary dentin Dentin that is formed after completion of apical foramen.

Secondary palate (pal-it) Posterior part of final palate formed by fusion of two palatal shelves.

Secretory (sek-kre-tory) **cells** Epithelial cells that produce saliva.

Septum (plural, septa) (sep-tum, **sep-**tah) Connective tissue divides inner part of glands.

Serous acini (sere-us **as-**i-ny) Group of serous cells producing serous secretory product.

Serous cells Secretory cells that produce serous secretory product.

Serous demilune (dem-ee-lune) Serous cells superficial to mucous secretory cells in mucoserous acinus.

Sextants (sex-tants) Dental arch division into three parts based on relationship to midline.

Sharpey (shar-pee) **fibers** Collagen fibers from periodontal ligament partially inserted into both cementum and bone.

Simple epithelium (ep-ee-**thee-**lee-um) Epithelium that consists of a single layer of cells.

Sinusitis (sy-nu-si-tis) Inflamed mucosal tissue in paranasal sinus.

Sixth branchial (brang-ke-al) **arch(es)** Branchial arch(es) in embryo that fuses with fourth branchial arch(es) to participate in formation of laryngeal cartilages.

Skeletal muscle Striated muscles under the voluntary control of the central and peripheral nervous systems.

Soft palate (pal-it) Posterior part of palate.

Somites (so-mites) Paired cuboidal aggregates of cells differentiated from mesoderm.

Specialized mucosa (mu-ko-sah) Mucosa found on dorsal and lateral surface of tongue in the form of the lingual papillae.

Sperm Cell containing male contribution of chromosomal information that fertilizes female ovum.

Spina bifida (spi-nah **bif-**ah-dah) Neural tube defect affecting vertebral arches.

Squames (skwaymz) Flattened platelike epithelial cells.

Stellate reticulum (stel-ate reh-**tik-**u-lum) Star-shaped cell layer between outer and inner enamel epithelium of enamel organ.

Sternocleidomastoid (stir-no-klii-do-**mass-**toid) **muscle** Large strap muscle of neck.

Stippling Pin-point depressions present on surface of attached gingiva.

Stomodeum (sto-mo-**de-**um) Primitive mouth in embryo.

Stratified (strat-i-fide) **epithelium (ep-ee-thee-**lee-um) Epithelium consisting of two or more layers.

Stratified squamous (skway-mus) **epithelium** Epithelium of skin and oral mucosa.

Stratum intermedium (stra-tum in-ter-**mede-**ee-um) Compressed layer between outer and inner enamel epithelium of enamel organ.

Striated (stri-ate-ed) **duct** Larger duct connecting lobules of salivary gland.

Sublingual caruncle (sub-ling-gwal **kar-**unk-kl) Small papilla at anterior end of each sublingual fold.

Sublingual duct Short duct associated with sublingual gland.

Sublingual fold Ridge of tissue on each side of the floor of the mouth.

Sublingual salivary gland Major salivary gland located in neck.

Subluxation (sub-luk-say-shun) Partial dislocation of both temporomandibular joints.

Submandibular (sub-man-dib-you-lar) **duct** Duct associated with submandibular gland.

Submandibular salivary gland Major salivary gland located in neck.

Submucosa (sub-mu-ko-sah) Tissue deep to oral mucosa composed of loose connective tissue.

Succedaneous (suk-seh-dane-ee-us) Permanent teeth with primary predecessors: anterior teeth and premolars.

Successional (suk-sesh-shun-al) **dental lamina** Extension of dental lamina into ectomesenchyme forming succedaneous permanent teeth.

Sulcular epithelium (sul-ku-lar ep-ee-**thee-**lee-um) **(SE)** Epithelium that stands away from the tooth creating gingival sulcus.

Sulcus terminalis (sul-kus **ter-**mi-nal-is) Groove located posteriorly on dorsal tongue surface.

Superficial layer Most superficial layer in nonkeratinized epithelium.

Supernumerary (soo-per-nu-mer-air-ee) **teeth** Developmental disturbance characterized by one or more extra teeth.

Supplemental groove Secondary groove on the lingual surface of the anterior teeth and the occlusal table on the posterior teeth.

Supporting alveolar bone (SAB) Consists of both cortical bone and trabecular bone.

Supporting cusps (kusps) Cusps that function during centric occlusion: lingual cusps of the maxillary posterior teeth, buccal cusps of the mandibular posterior teeth, and incisal edges of the mandibular anterior teeth.

Synapse (sin-aps) Junction between two neurons or between neuron and effector organ where neural impulses transmit.

Synovial (sy-no-vee-al) **cavities** Upper and lower compartments divided by disc of temporomandibular joint.

Synovial fluid Fluid in the joint capsule that fills and lubricates temporomandibular joint.

Synovial membrane Inner layer of temporomandibular joint capsule producing synovial fluid.

Syphilis (sif-i-lis) Infective teratogen spirochete *Treponema pallidum* that can produce dental anomalies and other defects.

System Group of organs functioning together.

T

T cell Lymphocyte that matures in thymus working during cell-mediated immune response.

Taste buds Barrel-shaped organs of taste associated with lingual papillae.

Taste pore Opening in taste bud.

Telophase (tel-oh-faze) Final phase of mitosis with division into two daughter cells and reappearance of nuclear membrane.

Temporomandibular (tem-poh-ro-man-dib-you-lar) **disorder (TMD)** Disorder associated with one or both temporomandibular joints.

Temporomandibular joint (TMJ) Joint where temporal bone of the skull articulates with mandible.

Teratogens (ter-ah-to-jens) Environmental agents or factors (such as, infections, drugs, or radiation) causing malformations.

Terminal plane Ideal molar relationship in primary dentition when in centric occlusion.

Tertiary dentin Dentin formed in response to localized injury to exposed dentin.

Tetracycline (tet-rah-si-kleen) **stain** Intrinsic tooth stain from ingestion of antibiotic tetracycline during tooth development.

Third branchial (brang-ke-al) **arch(es)** Branchial arch(es) in embryo responsible for formation of parts of hyoid bone.

Thirds Crown surface or root division into three parts: crown horizontally and vertically and root horizontally.

Thyroglossal (thy-ro-gloss-al) duct Temporary tube that connects thyroid with tongue base during prenatal development.

hyroid (thy-roid kar-ti-lij) cartilage Midline prominence of larynx.

Thyroid gland Endocrine gland in neck.

Thyroxine (thy-rok-sin) Hormone from thyroid gland that stimulates the metabolic rate.

Tissue Structure formed by grouping of cells with similar characteristics of shape and function.

Tissue fluid Interstitial body fluid.

Tomes (tomes) granular layer Dentin beneath cementum and adjacent to dentinocemental junction that looks granular.

Tomes process Secretory surface of each ameloblast.

Tongue Oral cavity structure consisting of muscle and covered by oral mucosa.

Tongue thrust Incorrect patterning during tongue function resulting in parafunctional habit.

Tonofilaments (ton-oh-fil-ah-ments) Intermediate filaments having major role in intercellular junctions.

Tonsillar tissue Nonencapsulated masses of lymphoid tissue.

Tooth fairy Mythological creature that takes children's shed primary teeth from under their pillow and leaves a sum of cash during the night; helpers are always appreciated.

Tooth germ Primordium of tooth consisting of enamel organ, dental papilla, and dental sac.

Trabeculae (trah-bek-u-lay) Joined matrix pieces forming lattice in cancellous bone or bands of connective tissue in lymph node that separate lymphatic nodules.

Trabecular (trah-bek-u-lar) bone Cancellous bone between alveolar bone proper and places of cortical bone.

Transverse (trans-vers) ridge Ridge formed by joining of two triangular ridges crossing occlusal table transversely or from labial to lingual outline.

Treacher Collins (tree-chur kol-inz) syndrome (TCS) Developmental disturbance with wide ranging implications due to migration failure of neural crest cells to facial region.

Triangular fossa (fos-ah) Fossa that has triangular shape where triangular grooves terminate.

Triangular groove Groove that separates a marginal ridge from the triangular ridge of cusp and forms triangular fossae at the termination of the ridges.

Triangular ridge Cusp ridge that descends from the cusp tips toward the central part of occlusal table.

Trifurcated (try-fer-kay-ted) Tooth having three root branches.

Trilaminar embryonic (try-lam-i-nar em-bre-on-ik) disc Embryonic disc with three layers: ectoderm, mesoderm, and endoderm.

Trismus (triz-mus) Inability to normally open the mouth.

Trophoblast (trof-oh-blast) layer Layer of peripheral cells of blastocyst.

Tubercle (too-ber-kl) of the upper lip Midline thickening of upper lip.

Tubercles Accessory cusps on cingulum of the anterior teeth or occlusal tables of the permanent molars.

Tuberculum impar (too-ber-ku-lum im-par) Initial part of developing tongue located in midline.

Turnover time Time that it takes for newly divided cells to be completely replaced throughout entire tissue.

U

Underbite When lower jaw extends forward beyond upper jaw.

Universal Numbering System (UNS) Numbering system for permanent teeth by using Arabic numerals #1 through #32 and for primary teeth by using capital letters A through T.

Uvula (u-vu-lah) Midline muscular structure hanging down from posterior margin of soft palate.

V

Vacuoles (vak-you-oles) Spaces or cavities within cytoplasm.

Ventral surface of the tongue Underside of tongue.

Vermilion (ver-mil-yon) zone Darker appearance of the lips with its outlining mucocutaneous junction at the vermilion border as compared with surrounding skin.

Vertical dimension of the face Dividing face into three horizontal parts.

Vestibular fornix (ves-tib-u-lar fore-niks) Deepest recess of each vestibule.

Vestibules (ves-ti-bules) Maxillary and mandibular spaces between the lips and cheeks anteriorly and laterally—and the teeth and gingiva medially and posteriorly.

Volkmann (volk-man) canals Vascular canals in compact bone other than Haversian canals.

von Ebner salivary (von eeb-ner sal-i-ver-ee) glands Serous minor salivary glands associated with circumvallate lingual papillae.

W

White blood cell (WBC) Blood cells from bone marrow's stem cells that mature there or in other lymphatic tissue.

Working side Side to which mandible has been moved during lateral occlusion.

X

Xerostomia (zer-oh-sto-me-ah) Dry mouth.

Y

Yolk sac Fluid-filled cavity that faces hypoblast layer.

Z

Zygomatic (zy-go-mat-ik) arch Bony support for cheek.

Zygomatic region Facial region that overlies zygomatic arch.

Zygote (zy-gote) Fertilized egg from union of ovum and sperm.

Anatomic Position

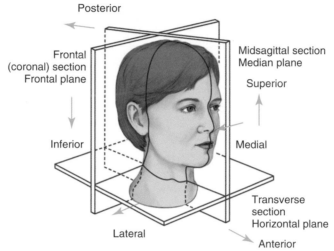

FIGURE A-1 Head and neck in anatomic position showing the midsagittal, transverse, and frontal sections. (Adapted from Fehrenbach MJ, Herring SW: *Illustrated anatomy of the head and neck*, ed 4, St Louis, 2012, Saunders/Elsevier.)

Units of Measure

UNIT	ABBREVIATION	EQUIVALENT	MEASUREMENT APPLICATION
Centimeter	cm	0.4 inch	Naked eye: Pathologic lesions
Millimeter	mm	0.1 cm	Naked eye: Extremely large human cells (muscle, liver), periodontal pockets
Micrometer	mm	0.001 mm	Light microscopy: Most human cells, large organelles, bacteria, ameloblasts
Nanometer	nm	0.001 µm	Electron microscopy: Smaller organelles, largest of macromolecules, dental tissue units

Tooth Measurements*

TABLE C-1								
Measurements of the Permanent Incisors (in Millimeters)								
	CERVICOINCISAL LENGTH OF CROWN	LENGTH OF ROOT	MESIODISTAL DIAMETER OF CROWN	MESIODISTAL DIAMETER OF CROWN AT CERVIX	LABIOLINGUAL DIAMETER OF CROWN	LABIOLINGUAL DIAMETER OF CROWN AT CERVIX	CURVATURE OF CERVICAL LINE: MESIAL	CURVATURE OF CERVICAL LINE: DISTAL
Maxillary central incisor	10.5	13.0	8.5	7.0	7.0	6.0	3.5	2.5
Maxillary lateral incisor	9.0	13.0	6.5	5.0	6.0	5.0	3.0	2.0
Mandibular central incisor	9.0	12.5	5.0	3.5	6.0	5.3	3.0	2.0
Mandibular lateral incisor	9.5	14.0	5.5	4.0	6.5	5.8	3.0	2.0

TABLE C-2								
Measurements of the Permanent Canines (in Millimeters)								
	CERVICOINCISAL LENGTH OF CROWN	LENGTH OF ROOT	MESIODISTAL DIAMETER OF CROWN	MESIODISTAL DIAMETER OF CROWN AT CERVIX	LABIOLINGUAL DIAMETER OF CROWN	LABIOLINGUAL DIAMETER OF CROWN AT CERVIX	CURVATURE OF CERVICAL LINE: MESIAL	CURVATURE OF CERVICAL LINE: DISTAL
Maxillary canine	10.0	17.0	7.5	5.5	8.0	7.0	2.5	1.5
Mandibular canine	11.0	16.0	7.0	5.5	7.5	7.0	2.5	1.0

*All data from Nelson S: *Wheeler's dental anatomy, physiology, and occlusion,* ed 9, St Louis, 2009, Saunders/Elsevier.

TABLE C-3	Measurements of the Permanent Premolars (in Millimeters)

	CERVICO-OCCLUSAL LENGTH OF CROWN	LENGTH OF ROOT	MESIODISTAL DIAMETER OF CROWN	MESIODISTAL DIAMETER OF CROWN AT CERVIX	BUCCOLINGUAL DIAMETER OF CROWN	BUCCOLINGUAL DIAMETER OF CERVIX	CURVATURE OF CERVICAL LINE: MESIAL	CURVATURE OF CERVICAL LINE: DISTAL
Maxillary first premolar	8.5	14.0	7.0	5.0	9.0	8.0	1.0	0.0
Maxillary second premolar	8.5	14.0	7.0	5.0	9.0	8.0	1.0	0.0
Mandibular first premolar	8.5	14.0	7.0	5.0	7.5	6.5	1.0	0.0
Mandibular second premolar	8.0	14.5	7.0	5.0	8.0	7.0	1.0	0.0

TABLE C-4	Measurements of the Permanent Maxillary Molars (in Millimeters)

	CERVICO-OCCLUSAL LENGTH OF CROWN	LENGTH OF ROOT	MESIODISTAL DIAMETER OF CROWN	MESIODISTAL DIAMETER OF CROWN AT CERVIX	BUCCOLINGUAL DIAMETER OF CROWN	BUCCOLINGUAL DIAMETER AT CERVIX	CURVATURE OF CERVICAL LINE: MESIAL	CURVATURE OF CERVICAL LINE: DISTAL
Maxillary first molar	7.5	Buccal = 12.0 Lingual = 13.0	10.0	8.0	11.0	10.0	1.0	0.0
Maxillary second molar	7.0	Buccal = 11.0 Lingual = 12.0	9.0	7.0	11.0	10.0	1.0	0.0
Maxillary third molar	6.5	11.0	8.5	6.5	10.0	9.5	1.0	0.0

TABLE C-5	Measurements of the Permanent Mandibular Molars (in Millimeters)

	CERVICO-OCCLUSAL LENGTH OF CROWN	LENGTH OF ROOT	MESIODISTAL DIAMETER OF CROWN	MESIODISTAL DIAMETER OF CROWN AT CERVIX	BUCCOLINGUAL DIAMETER OF CROWN	BUCCOLINGUAL DIAMETER AT CERVIX	CURVATURE OF CERVICAL LINE: MESIAL	CURVATURE OF CERVICAL LINE: DISTAL
Mandibular first molar	7.5	14.0	11.0	9.0	10.5	9.0	1.0	0.0
Mandibular second molar	7.0	13.0	10.5	8.0	10.0	9.0	1.0	0.0
Mandibular third molar	7.0	11.0	10.0	7.5	9.5	9.0	1.0	0.0

TABLE C-6	Measurements of the Primary Teeth (in Millimeters)						
	LENGTH OVERALL	**LENGTH OF CROWN**	**LENGTH OF ROOT**	**MESIODISTAL DIAMETER OF CROWN**	**MESIODISTAL DIAMETER AT CERVIX**	**FACIAL-LINGUAL DIAMETER OF CROWN**	**FACIAL-LINGUAL DIAMETER AT CERVIX**
Maxillary Teeth							
Central incisor	16.0	6.0	10.0	6.5	4.5	5.0	4.0
Lateral incisor	15.8	5.6	11.4	5.1	3.7	4.8	3.7
Canine	19.0	6.5	13.5	7.0	5.1	7.0	5.5
First molar	15.2	5.1	10.0	7.3	5.2	8.5	6.9
Second molar	17.5	5.7	11.7	8.2	6.4	10.0	8.3
Mandibular Teeth							
Central incisor	14.0	5.0	9.0	4.2	3.0	4.0	3.5
Lateral incisor	15.0	5.2	10.0	4.1	3.0	4.0	3.5
Canine	17.0	6.0	11.5	5.0	3.7	4.8	4.0
First molar	15.8	6.0	9.8	7.7	6.5	7.0	5.3
Second molar	18.8	5.5	11.3	9.9	7.2	8.7	6.4

Tooth Development*

TABLE D 1	Development of Permanent Incisors			
	MAXILLARY CENTRAL INCISOR	**MAXILLARY LATERAL INCISOR**	**MANDIBULAR CENTRAL INCISOR**	**MANDIBULAR LATERAL INCISOR**
Number of lobes		Four lobes		
First evidence of calcification	3–4 months	1 year	3–4 months	3–4 months
Completion of enamel	4–5 years	4–5 years	4–5 years	4–5 years
Eruption date	7–8 years	8–9 years	6–7 years	7–8 years
Completion of root	10 years	11 years	9 years	10 years

TABLE D-2	Development of Permanent Canines	
	MAXILLARY CANINE	**MANDIBULAR CANINE**
Number of lobes	Four lobes	
First evidence of calcification	4–5 months	4–5 months
Completion of enamel	6–7 years	6–7 years
Eruption date	11–12 years	9–10 years
Completion of root	13–15 years	12–14 years

TABLE D-3	Development of Permanent Premolars			
SPECIFIC TEETH	**MAXILLARY FIRST PREMOLAR**	**MAXILLARY SECOND PREMOLAR**	**MANDIBULAR FIRST PREMOLAR**	**MANDIBULAR SECOND PREMOLAR**
Number of lobes		Four lobes		Four or five lobes
First evidence of calcification	1½–1¾ years	2–2½ years	1¾–2 years	2¼–2½ years
Completion of enamel	5–6 years	6–7 years	5–6 years	6–7 years
Eruption date	10–11 years	10–12 years	10–12 years	11–12 years
Completion of root(s)	12–13 years	12–14 years	12–13 years	13–14 years

*All data from Nelson S: *Wheeler's dental anatomy, physiology, and occlusion,* ed 9, Philadelphia, 2009, Saunders/Elsevier.

TABLE D-4	**Development of Permanent Maxillary Molars**		
	MAXILLARY FIRST MOLAR	**MAXILLARY SECOND MOLAR**	**MAXILLARY THIRD MOLAR**
Number of lobes	Five lobes	Four lobes	
First evidence of calcification	Birth	2½ years	7–9 years
Completion of enamel	3–4 years	7–8 years	12–16 years
Eruption date	6–7 years	12–13 years	17–21 years
Completion of root(s)	9–10 years	14–16 years	18–25 years

TABLE D-5	**Development of Permanent Mandibular Molars**		
	MANDIBULAR FIRST MOLAR	**MANDIBULAR SECOND MOLAR**	**MANDIBULAR THIRD MOLAR**
Number of lobes	Five lobes	Four lobes	
First evidence of calcification	Birth	2½–3 years	8–10 years
Completion of enamel	2½–3 years	7–8 years	12–16 years
Eruption date	6–7 years	11–13 years	17–21 years
Completion of roots(s)	9–10 years	14–15 years	18–25 years

Index

A

Abfraction, 148–149, 149f
Abrasion, 148
Accessory canals, 168
Accessory roots, 68
Acellular cementum
  cementotypes, absence, 177f
  components, 175
Acid etching, 156
  demineralization, 156–157
Acinus (acini), 134–136
  lobule, microscopic section, 134f
  mucous acini, 135
  serous acini, 135
Active eruption, 68–69
Adipose connective tissue, 93
  presence, 115f
Adult face, facial processes (embryonic derivatives), 34f
Adult palate, derivative developmental structures (diagram), 47f
Adult teeth (permanent teeth), 12–13, 193
Afferent nerve (sensory nerve), 102, 187
Afferent vessels, 143
Aggregatibacter actinomycetemcomitans (Aa), 131
Aging dentin, 167
Aging pulp, 170–171
Ala (alae), 1–2
Alveolar bone, 10
  supporting alveolar bone (SAB), 180
Alveolar bone proper (ABP), 180
  photomicrograph, 183f
Alveolar crest, 180, 189
  photomicrograph, 183f
Alveolar mucosa, 10, 111
  clinical appearance, 111
  histologic features, 111
Alveolar processes, 10–17, 68, 179
  alveolar bone, 10
  anatomy, 181f
  bilateral cleft, 48f
  cementum, relationship, 173f
  changes, edentulous states (impact), 185f
  clinical considerations, 13
  density, 187

Alveolar processes *(Continued)*
  diagram, 12f
  formation, clinical considerations, 180
  loss, 183–184
  microscopic components, 179f
  occlusal drift (supereruption), 183
  procedures/pathology, clinical considerations, 182–187
  properties, 179–187
  radiographic landmarks, 182f
  resorption, 183
  root, angulations, 285f
Alveolodental ligament, 188–190, 191f
  fiber subgroups, 188–189, 189t
    identification, 188f
    spoke-like arrangement, 189f
Alveologingival ligament, alveolar crest origin, 190
Alveolus (alveoli), 10
Ameloblasts
  close-up view, 149f
  differentiation, 63
  formation, 63–66
    photomicrographs, 65f
  impact, 153f
Amelogenesis imperfecta, 65–66
Amniocentesis, 18
Amniotic cavity, 24
Anaphase, 81, 82t
Anatomical crown, 199
  presence, 199f
Anatomical root, 199
Anchoring collagen fibers, 89
Ankyloglossia, 50
  result, 50f
Anodontia
  anomaly, 183
  production, 54
Anterior faucial pillar, 14–15
Anterior open bite, result, 296f
Anterior teeth, 12–13
  anatomical crown/root, presence, 199f
  clinical considerations, 208
  contour height, 201f

Anterior teeth *(Continued)*
  crown
    line angles, designation, 202f
    point angles, designation, 202f
    third, identification, 203f
  dental tissue, involvement, 199f
  identification, 198f
  incisal surface, 200
  permanent anterior teeth, identification, 208f
  restoration, 208
  root thirds, identification, 203f
Antibodies (immunoglobulins), 101t
Apical foramen, 168
  obliteration, 170
Apical group, 189
Appositional growth, 22
Apposition stage, 62–66
  disturbances, clinical considerations, 64–66
  photomicrograph, 64f
Arches. *See* Dental arches
  articulation, centric stops, 286f
  development, phases, 283–284
  form, 283–284
  horizontal overlap, 282f
  permanent dentition, 285f
Arrest lines, 98, 179f
  cementum, 177f
Articular eminence, 272
Articulating paper, usage, 287f
Attached gingiva, 13, 112–113
  clinical appearance, 112–113
  edema, 129f
  histologic features, 113
  keratinized attached gingiva, nonkeratinized alveolar mucosa (junction), 115f
  lamina propia, 113, 126f
  masticatory mucosa, 123
  photomicrograph, 114f, 120f
  pigmentation, 119f
Attachment plaques, 90f
Attrition, 148
Autonomic nervous system (ANS), 103
Avulsion, 215
Axons, 101, 102f

Page numbers followed by *f* indicate figures; *t*, tables; *b*, boxes.

B

Baby bottle tooth decay, 265f
Baby teeth (primary teeth), 12, 193
Balancing interferences, 288
    confirmation, floss (usage), 288f
Balancing side, 287
Basal bone, 180
Basal lamina
    external basal lamina, 128
    schematic diagram, 90f
Basal layer (stratum basale), 107–108
Basement membrane, 89
    direct relationship, 88f
    histology, 89
    location, 87f
    properties, 89
    schematic diagram, 90f
Basophil, 99
B cells, 99
Bell stage, 60–62
    outer to inner, 61t
    photomicrograph, 61f
    transition, 60f
Bifurcated teeth, 230
    pulp cavity, 234
Bilaminar embryonic disc, 23
    epiblast layer cells, migration, 25f
    formation, blastocyst (impact), 23f
    primitive streak, 24f
        formation, 24
Bilateral cleft, 48f
    lip deformities, types, 38f
Bilateral mandibular tori, variation,
    13f
Bilateral symmetry, 24
Black hairy tongue, 118, 119f
Blastocyst
    components, 21f
    impact, 23f
    implantation, 21
    photomicrograph, 21f
Bleaching (vital whitening), 159
Bleeding after probing (BoP), 130
Blood, 98
    blood-related situations, clinical
        considerations, 99–100
    cells
        development, flowchart, 99f
        tissue cells, relationship, 100t
    components, 98–100
        types, 98t
    properties, 98–100
Body
    components/examples, 79t
    regeneration, 85
Bones, 94
    anatomy, 94f
    cells, presence, 95f
    development, 96
        stages, 97f
    endochondral transformation, 273f
    grafting, inclusion, 186
    histology, 95–96
    loss
        evidence, 186
        periodontal disease, impact, 186f
    marrow, 95
    properties, 94–98

Bones *(Continued)*
    remodeling/repair/aging, 96–98
    resorption, close-up view, 186f
    tissue, clinical considerations, 98–99
Bony components, temporomandibular joints
    (association), 273f
Branchial apparatus, 38
    development, clinical considerations,
        41–42
    formation, 38–42
Branchial arches, 38
    derivations, 49f
    derivative structures, 41t
    fifth branchial arch, 38
    first branchial arch, 38
    fourth branchial arch, 41
    second branchial arch, 38
    sixth branchial arch, 41
    third branchial arch, 41
Branchial cleft cyst, 42, 42f
Branchial grooves, 41
Bruxism (grinding), 288, 296
Buccal cervical ridge, 256
Buccal cusp ridge, 236
Buccal fat pad, 10
Buccal mucosa, 9–10, 110
    clinical appearance, 110
    histologic features, 110
    hyperkeratinization, 109f
    photomicrograph, 111f
    variations, 11f
Buccal ridge, 232
Buccal root features, 230f
Buccal triangular ridge, 236
Bud stage, 54
    disturbances, clinical
        considerations, 54
Bundle bone, 180

C

Calcium hydroxyapatite, 95
    chemical formula, 172
Calculus, embedding, 174f
Canaliculi, 95
    orientation, 175f
    presence, 174–175
Cancellous bone, 94
    close-up view, 94f
Canines, 12
    clinical considerations, 222–223
    eminence, 10, 222
    features, 220–223
    morphological consideration, 203
    permanent canines, 220–227
    permanent maxillary canines,
        223–225
    primary canines, 267–268
    rise, 287
Capillary plexus, 108–109
Cap stage, 54–60
    disturbances, clinical considerations, 60
    fusion, 60
    gemination, 60
    photomicrograph, 59f
    tooth germ, 59t
    transition, 60f
Capsule, 134

Caries, 148
    groove caries, 151
    pit caries, 151
    smooth surface caries, 151f
    types, demonstration, 151f
Cartilage, 93
    cells, presence, 93f
    condylar cartilage, appearance, 180
    development, 94
    disintegration, osteoblast penetration,
        97f
    elastic cartilage, 94
    fibrocartilage, 94
    growth, 273
    histology, 93–94
    hyaline cartilage, 93–94
    properties, 93–94
    repair/aging, 94
Casein phosphopeptide-amorphous calcium
    phosphate (CPP-ACP), 152
Caudal ends, 25–26, 25f
Cell-free zone, 169
Cells
    adhesion, 83f
    anatomy, 77–79
    body, 102f
    cycle, 82t
    data bank, 79
    division (mitosis), 81
    electron micrograph, 78f
    inclusions, 81
    intercellular junctions, 83, 83f
    interphase process, 81, 82t
    membrane (plasma membrane),
        77–79
        electron micrograph, 78f
        schematic, 78f
    nucleus, electron micrograph, 78f
    organelles, 78f
    properties, 77–81
Cellular cementum, 175
    cementotypes, embedding, 177f
    microscopic appearance, 175f
    width, change, 175
Cellular repolarization, 62
Cemental caries
    dentin invasion, 174f
    risk, increase, 173
Cemental root surface, subgingival dental
    biofilm (scanning electron micrograph),
        174f
Cemental spurs, 178
Cementicle
    attachment, 178f
    mineralization, 177
Cementoblasts, 66
Cementocytes, 66
    absence, 177f
    embedding, 177f
    lacunae/canaliculi, orientation, 175f
Cementoenamel junction (CEJ), 127f
    cementum, thinness, 172
    distal furcation, 249
    interfaces, 176f
    phase-contrast image, 175f
Cementogenesis, process, 66
Cementoid, 66
    thickness, attainment, 174

Cementum, 10–12, 127f
  appositional growth, root area, 68f
  arrest lines, 177f
  calculus, embedding, 174f
  cellular cementum, microscopic appearance, 175f
  dental sac development, 174
  development, 174
  formation, 66–67
    disturbances, clinical considerations, 66–67
    excess, 66–67
  histology, 174–175
  matrix, 66
  overlap, 176f
  pathology, clinical considerations, 177–178
  primary cementum, 175
  properties, 172–178
  repair, 175–178
  reversal lines, 177f
  root surface types, 177f
  secondary cementum, 175
  structure, clinical considerations, 173
  teeth
    alveolar process, relationship, 173f
    cross section, microscopic view, 189f
    types, 175, 177t
Central canal (Haversian canal), 96
Central fossa, 228–229
Central fused tissue, disintegration, 72f
Central groove, 229
Central incisors, retrusion, 294f
Central nervous system (CNS), 103
Centric occlusion (CO), 281–289
  permanent dentition, 282f
Centric relation (CR), 286–287
  attainment, 286–287
    mandible, hinge movement (establishment), 287f
Centric stops, 286
  arch articulation, 286f
  checking, articulating paper (usage), 287f
Centrioles, 81
Centromere, 79
Centrosome, 81
Cephalic ends (head end), 25–26, 25f
Cervical loop, 66
  horizontal extensions, 69f
Cervical ridge, bulging, 265
Chondroblasts, 93
  presence, 93f
Chondrocytes, 93
  presence, 93f
Chromatids, 79
Chromatin, 79f
  form, 79
Chromosomes, 79
  chromosome 21, impact, 21f
  photographic analysis, 20f
Cingulum (cingula), 207
  presence, 209, 225
Circular ligament, 191f
Circumpulpal dentin, 162, 165f
Circumvallate lingual papilla (papillae), 15, 117–118
  clinical features, 117
  histologic features, 118
  presence, 118f
Class I malocclusion, 291–292
  neutroclusion, 291–292
  permanent dentition, 291f

Class II malocclusion (distoclusion), 292–298
  division I, permanent dentition, 292–293, 294f
  division II, permanent dentition, 293, 294f
  permanent dentition, 293f
Class III malocclusion (mesioclusion), 293–294
  permanent dentition, 295f
Cleavage, 20
Cleft lip
  deformities, types, 38f
  disfigurement/disability, 37–38
Cleft palate, 45
  degrees, 48f
Cleft uvula, 48f
Clenching, 296
Clinical crown, 199
  importance, 200
Clinical root, 199
Cloacal membrane, 27
Clot
  formation, 89f
  importance, 89
Col, 123
  faciolingual microscopic section, 124f
Collagen
  anchoring collagen fibers, 89
  bundle, composition, 91f
  fibers, 90–91
  types, 91t
Collagenous connective tissue, 90–91
Columnar cells, 88t
Compact bone, 94
  close-up view, 94f
  Haversian system, 95f
  histology, 95f
Concrescence, 66–67
Condylar cartilage, appearance, 180
Condyle, articulating surface, 272
Congenital malformations, 18
  teratogens, involvement, 19t
Connective tissue, 89–90
  adipose connective tissue, 93
  classification, 91–92
  dense connective tissue, 92
  elastic connective tissue, 93
  histology, 90–91
  loose connective tissue, 92
  papillae, 92, 92f
  proper, 92
  properties, 93–100, 89–93
  reticular connective tissue, 93
  turnover/repair, 92–93
Contact area, 201
  example, 209f
Contour
  gingival apex, 125
  height, 201, 201f
    identification, 209f
    permanent posterior tooth, 230f
  lines of Owen, 166–167, 166f
Copula, 47
Coronal fused epithelial tissue, 72f
Coronal pulp, 167
Coronoid notch, 2
Coronoid process, 2
Cortical bone, 180
CPP-ACP. See Casein phosphopeptide-amorphous calcium phosphate
Cribiform plate, 180

Crooked teeth (crowding), 292, 293f
Crossbites, 293f
  inclusion, 292
Crowding (crooked teeth), 292, 293f
  problems, 292
Crown, 10–12
  dentigerous cyst, radiograph, 76f
  lengthening, 200
  outlines
    occlusal views, 253f
    types, 253–254
  superior surface, masticatory surface, 200
  thirds, 203
  tooth forms, 203
  types, occlusal views, 252f
  wave patterns, 150f
Cuboidal cells, 88t
Curve of Spee, 285
Curve of Wilson, 285
Cuspids, 220
Cusp of Carabelli, 249–250
  groove, 249–250
Cusp ridges, 228
Cusp tip, 221
  distobuccal cusp, 250
Cytodifferentiation, 22
Cytoplasm, 79
Cytoskeleton (CSK), 81

D

D-A-Q-T System, 197
Deciduous dentition, 193
Dendrites, 102f
Dense connective tissue, 92
Dense layer, 92
Dens in dente, 60
Dental anatomy
  study, considerations, 205–206
  terminology, 197–203
Dental anomalies, syphilis (impact), 30f
Dental arches, 12–13
  eruption, sequence
    permanent dentition, 284f
    primary dentition, 284f
  landmarks, diagram, 11f
  midline, 197
Dental curvatures/angulations, 284–286
Dental development disturbances, 55b–57b
Dental fluorosis, 152, 152f
Dental hard tissue, 53t
Dental implant, placement, 184
Dental lamina, 54
  development, 54f
  initiation stage disturbances, clinical considerations, 54
  layer, production, 54
  proliferation, 58f
  successional dental lamina, 59
Dental mannikin, usage, 286
Dental papilla, 59
  central cells, 62
  differentiation, 60f–61f
  outer cells, close-up view, 62, 63f
Dental pulp stem cells (DPSCs), 168, 171
Dental sac, 59

Dental tissue, involvement, 199f
Dentigerous cyst, 73
  radiograph, 76f
Dentin, 10–12, 127f
  aging, 167
  apposition, 160
  appositional growth, 60f
    root area, 68f
  circumpulpal dentin, 162, 165f
  components, 160–161
  cross section, microscopic view, 189f
  dentinal tubules, curvature, 163f
  dysplasia, 66
  exposure, phase-contrast image, 175f
  formation, 66
    photomicrographs, 65f
  globular dentin, 160
    photomicrograph, 161f
  histology, 166–167
  interglobular dentin, 160
    photomicrograph, 161f
  intertubular dentin, 161–162
  invasion, 174f
  mantle dentin, 162, 165f
  maturation, photomicrograph, 160f
  pathology, clinical considerations,
    162–166
  peritubular dentin, 161–162
  physical properties, comparison, 148t
  predentin, appositional growth, 63f
  primary dentin, 165f
    formation, 162
  properties, 158–167
  reactive dentin, 163
  reparative dentin, 163
  sclerotic dentin, 163
  secondary dentin, 165f
    formation, 162
  structure, clinical considerations, 158–159
  tertiary dentin, 162, 165f
  Tomes granular layer, 167f
  types, 161–166, 163t
    enamel/pulp, relationship, 165f
    microscopic view, 165f
Dentinal caries, 162–163
  photomicrograph, 165f
Dentinal fluid, 160
Dentinal hypersensitivity
  cause, 163–164
  hydrodynamic theory, 165–166, 166f
  treatment, 166
Dentinal tubule, 64
  components, microscopic view, 162f
  cross sections, 164f
  curvature, 163f
  exposure, stimulation, 166f
  photomicrograph, 162f
  primary/secondary curvature, 163f
  secondary curvature, 160–161
Dentin matrix
  appositional growth, 63
  maturation, 160
Dentin matrix, formation, 63, 159–160
  apposition stage, 64f
    photomicrograph, 64f
  photomicrographs, 149f
Dentinocemental junction (DCJ), 66
  dentin, Tomes granular layer, 167f

Dentinoenamel junction (DEJ), 153–154
  ameloblast, relationship, 150
  formation, 63–66, 64f
  microscopic view, 154f
Dentinogenesis, 63
Dentinogenesis imperfecta, 66, 66f
Dentinogenesis, initiation, 63f
Dentin-pulp complex, 158
  vitality, 171
Dentition, 193–194
  mixed dentition period, 195
    primary/permanent teeth, identification, 197f
  overjet pressure, 282f
  periods, 194–197
    clinical considerations, 196–197, 196t
  permanent dentition, 51, 194f
    anterior/posterior teeth, identification, 198f
    maxillary/mandibular arch, identification, 198f
    period, 195–197
  primary dentition, 194f
    development, 51
    period, 194–195
  term, usage, 51
Dentogingival junction, 125
Dentogingival junctional tissue, 125
  development, 130
  epithelium, pathology (clinical considerations),
    130–132
  histology, 126–129
  photomicrograph, 125f
  properties, 125–132
  schematic diagram, 124f
  turnover time, 130–132
Dentogingival ligament, 191f
Dentoperiosteal ligament, 191f
Dermis, 92, 104
  layer, 92f
Desmosome, 83
Developmental groove, 208
Developmental pits, 208
Development depressions, 207
Diastema (open contact), 215
Differentiation, process, 22
Dilaceration, 68
Distal step, 289, 289f
Distal surface, 200
Distal tongue buds (lateral lingual swellings), 46
Distocclusion (Class II malocclusion), 292
Down syndrome (trisomy 21), 21–22, 21f
DPSCs. *See* Dental pulp stem cells
Dry mouth (xerostomia), 139, 139f
Ductal epithelium, 136f
Ductal system, 136–137
Ducts, 133
  excretory duct, 137
  intercalated duct, 136
  short ducts, 137
  striated duct, 136–137
  thyroglossal duct, 140

E

Early childhood caries, 265f
Ectoderm, 24, 25f
Ectodermal dysplasia, 27–29, 30f
Ectomesenchyme, 53
  deepening, 53f
  dental lamina, proliferation, 58f

Ectopic pregnancy, 22
Edentulous states, 183
  impact, 185f
Efferent nerves (motor nerves), 102, 187
Efferent vessels, 143
Elastic cartilage, 94
Elastic connective tissue, 93
Elastic fibers, 91
Embrasures, 201–202
  presence, 201f
Embryo, 22
  central nervous system, 26f
  developmental processes, 22t
  fourth week
    prenatal development, 39f–40f
    scanning electron micrograph, 33f
    schematic, 33f
  longitudinal section, photomicrograph, 23f
  surfaces, swellings/tissue, 27f
  trilaminar disc, folding, 29f
Embryoblast layer, 21, 21f
Embryology, 18
Embryonic cell layers (germ layers), 23
  development, 26t
  fourth embryonic cell layer, 26–27
Embryonic folding, 27, 29f
Embryonic orofacial development, 33t
Embryonic period, 19t, 22–31
  clinical considerations, 27–31
Enamel, 10–12
  abfraction, 148–149
  abrasion, 148
  appositional growth, 60f
    completion, 71f
  attrition, 148
  caries, 148
    process, 151f
  demarcation, 155f
  dental procedures, clinical considerations,
    156–157
  dysplasia, 152
    hereditary type, 65f
    result, 64
  erosion, 148
  formation
    clinical considerations, 150
    photomicrographs, 65f
  gnarled enamel, 153
  histology, 152–157
  intrinsic staining, 152f
  knot, 58–59
  lamella (lamellae), 156
    presence, 156f
  loss, 149f
  matrix, formation, 149–150
    crown, wave patterns, 150f
    photomicrographs, 149f
  matrix, maturation, 150–152
    ameloblasts, movement, 150
  matrix, production, 149f
  maturation, crown (wave patterns),
    150f
  pathology, clinical considerations,
    151–152
  pearl, production, 68
  physical properties, comparison, 148t
  properties, 147–149
  remineralization, 151

Enamel (Continued)
rods (prisms), 152, 154f
diagram, 153f
electron micrograph, 153f
photomicrograph, 156f
sealant, flow, 156f
shade, variation, 147–148
spindles, 155
microscopic views, 156f
structure
clinical considerations, 148–149
loss, 148t
surface, layers (compression), 71f
translucency, 158
transverse section, microscopic
view, 156f
tufts, 155
presence, 156f
Enamel epithelium, 67f
reduction, 71f, 130, 151
fusion, 72f
photomicrograph, 72f
Enamel matrix
appositional growth, 64
apposition stage, photomicrograph, 64f
formation, 63–66
apposition stage, 64f
secretion, 62f
Enamel organ, 58–59
close-up view, 62f
differentiation, 60f–61f
layers, 63f
Endochondral ossification, 97f
osteoid formation, 96
Endocrine gland, 133
Endocytosis, 77
Endoderm, 24, 25f
Endoplasmic reticulum, 80
Endosteum, 95
Endothelium, 86
End-to-end bites, 293f
presence, 292
Eosinophil, 99
Epiblast layer, 23f, 24
cells, migration, 25f
Epidermis, 87, 104
interdigitating rete ridges, 92f
layer, 92f
Epiglottic swelling, 47
Epithelial attachment (EA), 126
electron micrographs, 128f
Epithelial rests of Malassez (ERM), 66
Epithelium (epithelia), 86
cell types, 88t, 107t
classification, 86–87
histology, 86
presence, 125f
properties, 86–89
pseudostratified columnar epithelium,
88f
regeneration, 87–89
repair, 87–89
simple epithelium, 86
stratified epithelium, 86
stratified squamous epithelium, 86
turnover, 87–89
types, 107t
Erectile tissue, 144

Erosion, 148
Eruption cyst, 73, 76f
Eruption process, 75f
clinical considerations, 73
Ethmoidal paranasal sinuses, 145f
Excretory duct, 137
Exocrine gland, 133
Exocytosis, 77
Exostoses, 13
variation, 13f
External basal lamina, 128
External nose, 1–2
Extracellular materials, 81–83
Extracellular matrix (ECM) degradation, 186

F
Face, 1
adult face, facial processes
(embryonic derivatives), 34f
buccal region, 2
cervical development, 38–42
compact bone, removal, 74f
development, 32–38
fourth week, 33b
esthetics, clinical considerations, 2–6
features, 6f
frontal regions, 1–2
fusion, furrow (elimination), 34f
Golden Proportions, divisions, 6f
inferior third, vertical dimension
(loss), 185f
infraorbital regions, 2
landmarks, 4f
lower face, formation, 34–35
mental region, 2–6
mesognathic profile, 292, 292f
midface, formation, 36
nasal regions, 1–2
landmarks, 4f
oral region, 2
orbital regions, 1–2
profiles, 292f
prognathic profile, 292f, 294
regions, 1–6
schematic, 2f
retrognathic profile, 292f
structures, 9
upper face, formation, 35–36
vermilion zone, 2
vertical dimension, 2–6
considerations, 6f
divisions, 4f
zygomatic regions, 2
Faciolingual microscopic section, 124f
Fascicles, 102f
Fauces, 14
Fertilization, 20
Fetal alcohol syndrome (FAS), 30
presentation, 30f
Fetal period, 19t, 31
clinical considerations, 31
Fetus, 31
Fibroblasts, 90
diagram/photomicrograph, 91f
Fibrocartilage, 94
Fifth branchial arch, 38
Fight-or-flight responses, 103

Filiform lingual papilla (papillae), 15, 117
clinical appearance, 117
histologic features, 117
sensitivity, display, 118f
First branchial arch, 38
First mandibular molar, mesiobuccal
groove, 256
First molar, size, 245
Flexion, disturbance, 68
Floss, usage, 288f
Flush terminal plane, 289, 289f
Fluting, 256
Foliate lingual papillae, 15, 117
clinical appearance, 117
histologic features, 117
microscopic section, 117f
Follicles, 140
Foramen cecum, 15
Fordyce spots, 10
visibility, 11f
Foregut, 27
Fossa (fossae), 208, 228–229
Fourth branchial arch, 41
Fourth embryonic cell layer, 26–27
Free gingiva
crest, 14
groove, 14
Free gingival graft (FGG), 129
Freeway space, 288
Frontal paranasal sinuses, 145f
Frontonasal process, 35
enlargement, 35f
formation, 35–36
Fungiform lingual papilla (papillae), 15, 117
clinical appearance, 117
histologic features, 117
microscopic section, 117f
Furcations, 230
crotches, 230, 231t
Furrow, elimination, 34f
Fusion process, 26, 27f, 60

G
Ganglion (ganglia), 101–102
Gemination, 60
Generalized resorption, occurrence, 98
Geographic tongue, 118, 118f
Germinal center, 143
Gingiva, 13
attached gingiva, 13
free gingiva, 14
interdental gingiva, 14
marginal gingiva, 14
Gingival apex, 125
Gingival contour, 125
Gingival crevicular fluid (GCF), 125
increase, 130
Gingival fiber group, 190–192
fiber subgroups, 191f
Gingival hyperplasia, 128–129
cause, 129f
Gingival recession, 129
clinical view, 159f
parafunctional habits, impact, 296
Gingival sulcus, 14–15
location, 14f
probing measurements, 126

Gingival tissue, 13–14, 123–125
 anatomy, 123–124
 close-up, 14f
 esthetics, clinical considerations, 125
 histology, 124–125
 landmarks, 13f–14f
 pathology, clinical considerations, 128–129
 photomicrograph, 125f
 schematic diagram, 124f
Gingivitis, 130
Glands
 properties, 133–141
 structure, 133
Globular dentin, 160
 photomicrographs, 161f
Gnarled enamel, 153–154
Gnathic index, 292
Goblet cells, 144
Goiter, 141, 142f
Golden Proportions, 2–6
 divisions, 6f
 usage, 183–184
Golgi complex (Golgi apparatus), 80
Granular layer (stratum granulosum), 106f, 108
Granulation tissue, 92–93, 119–120
 formation, 89f
 postoperative excess, 122f
Grinding (bruxism), 288, 296
Groove caries, 151
Grooves, location, 245
Grooves of perikymata, 154
Group function, 287
Gubernacular canal, widening, 73
Guided tissue regeneration (GTR) membrane,
 usage, 186–187, 192
Gummy smile, 125, 295

H

Hard palate, 15, 112
 clinical appearance, 112
 histologic features, 112
 medial zone, submucosa (absence), 113f
 midline, 15f
 photomicrograph, 113f
 soft palate, junction (photomicrograph),
 112f
Haversian canal (central canal), 96
Haversian system, 95, 95f
 cortical bone location, 182f
Head
 development, coronal section
 (photomicrographs), 46f
 lymph nodes, 3f
 midsagittal section, 17f
 pharynx, divisions, 17f
 sagittal sections, 37f, 44f
 intermaxillary segment, display, 44f
 structures, 133
Hemidesmosome, 83
 impact, 84f
 schematic diagram, 90f
Hertwig epithelial root sheath (HERS),
 formation, 66, 67f
Hindgut, 27
Histodifferentiation, 22
Histology, 77
Horizontal group, 183f, 189

Howship lacunae, 97
 presence, 97f
Hunter-Schreger bands (HSB), 152, 154f
Hutchinson incisors, 30f
 occurrence, 212
Hyaline cartilage, 93–94
Hyoid arch, 38
Hyoid bone, 6
Hypercementosis, 178
 causes, 178f
Hyperdontia (supernumerary teeth), 54
Hyperkeratinization, 109
 palatal mucosa, 140f
Hypoblast layer, 23f, 24
 epiblast layer cells, migration, 25f
Hypodermis, 92
 presence, 92f
Hyposalivation, 103, 139

I

Imbrication lines, 154
 raised characteristic, 155f
 von Ebner, 166, 166f
Immunogens, 99
Immunoglobulins (antibodies), 99, 101t
Impacted maxillary canines, 225
Impacted permanent mandibular third molar,
 radiograph, 261f
Implantation, 21
Incisal angles, 209
Incisal edge, 210–212
Incisal ridge, 207
Incisal surface, 200
 attrition, 212f
 example, 208f
Incisive papilla, 15
Incisors, 12
 clinical considerations, 209–212
 features, 209–212
 permanent incisors, 209–219
 permanent mandibular incisors, 217–219
 permanent maxillary incisors, 212–217
 permanent maxillary lateral incisors,
 215–217
Inclined cuspal planes, 228
Inclusions, 81
Induction, process, 22
Initiation stage, 53–54, 53f
Inner enamel epithelium (IEE), 61, 67f
 close-up view, 62f
Inner junctional epithelium, photomicrograph,
 127f
Intercalated duct, 136
Intercellular junctions, 83, 83f
 hemidesmosome, impact, 84f
Intercellular substance, 83
Interdental gingiva, 14
Interdental ligament, 190
 insertion, 190f
 microscopic view, 190f
 transseptal ligament, 190
Interdental papilla, 14
Interdental septum/bone, 180–182
 microscopic view, 183f
Interglobular dentin, 160
 photomicrograph, 161f
Interlabial gap, 289

Intermaxillary segment, 36
 development, 37f
 display, 44f
 presence, 44f
Intermediate filaments, 81
Intermediate layer (stratum intermedium), 107–108
Internal basal lamina, 127
International Numbering System (INS), 194,
 195f–196f
International Standards Organization (ISO), oral
 cavity designation, 198, 198t
Interocclusal clearance, 288, 288f
Interphase process, 81, 82t
Interproximal space, 201
Interradicular group, 190
Interradicular septum/bone, 180–182
 microscopic view, 184f
Interrod enamel, 153
 demineralization, 156f
Interstitial fluid (tissue fluid), 81
Interstitial growth, occurrence, 22
Intertubular dentin, 161–162
Intramembranous ossification, 96, 96f

J

Jaw, 10–17
 alignment, 295
 anatomy, 180–187
 development, 179–180
 growth, 195
 histology, 180–187
 orientational terms, 10f
 permanent dentition, eruption, 74f
Joint disc, 274–275
 abnormalities, 277
 inferior section, 275f
 temporomandibular joint, 274f
Joints
 bones, 272–273
 capsule, 274
 example, 274f
 dislocation, lateral radiographic view, 280f
 movement, 275–278
 types, 279t
 pathology, clinical considerations, 275–278
 sounds, occurrence, 277
Junctional epithelium (JE), 72f
 cells, organelles (presence), 128
 electron micrographs, 128f
 epithelial attachment, 127f
 inner junctional epithelium, photomicrograph,
 127f
 ulceration, 131f
 impact, 130f

K

Karyotype, 20
 example, 20f
Keratin
 presence, 106
Keratinized attached gingiva, nonkeratinized
 alveolar mucosa (junction), 115f
Keratinized epithelium, electron micrograph,
 106f
Keratin layer (stratum corneum), 106f, 108
Keratohyaline granules, 108

L

Labial commissure, 2
Labial developmental depressions, 207
Labial frenum, 10
Labial mucosa, 9–10, 110
    clinical appearance, 110
    histologic features, 110
    variations, 11f
Labial ridge, 221
Labial structures, 9
Lacuna (lacunae), 93
    orientation, 175f
Lamella (lamellae), 95
Lamina dura, 180
Lamina propia, 107f, 108–109
    blood vessels, increase, 130f
    histologic features, 109f
    photomicrograph, 113f
    presence, 125f
    stratified squamous epithelium, relationship,
        105f
    vascular lamina propia, presence, 111f
Laryngopharynx, 17
Larynx (voice box), 6
Lateral deviation, 221
    occurrence, 288f
Lateral excursion, 288f
Lateral lingual swellings (distal tongue buds), 46
    impact, 49f
Lateral nasal processes, 36
    fusion, 36f
Lateral occlusion, 287–288
    evaluation, 287
Lateral pterygoid muscle, 276f–277f
Leeway space, 283
    holding, removable maxillary space maintainer
        (usage), 284f
    maxillary arch, 283f
Lens placodes, 35
Linea alba, 10
    visibility, 11f
Line angles
    designation, 202f
    formation, 202
Lines of Owen. *See* Contour
Lines of Retzius, 154
    incremental lines (striae), 154
    microscopic views, 154f
    neonatal line, microscopic view, 155f
Lingual erosion, 149f
Lingual frenum, 15
    attachment, 50f
Lingual papilla (papillae), 15
    comparison, 116t
    properties, 113–118
Lingual pit
    caries, presence, 212f
    permanent maxillary first molar, lingual pit, 247f
Lingual ridge, 221–222
Lingual structures, 9
Lingual surface
    example, 209f
    features, examples, 210f
    variations
        permanent maxillary right central incisor,
            214f
        permanent maxillary right lateral incisor,
            217f

Lingual triangular ridge, 236
Linguogingival groove, 216
Lining mucosa, 104–105
    histologic features, 106f
Lips
    bilateral cleft, 48f
    clinical considerations, 2
    incompetence, 297, 298f
    lower lips
        formation, 36–38
        vermilion zones/mucocutaneous junctions,
            5f
            disruption, 5f
    mucocutaneous junction, 2
    resting posture, 289
    solar damage, 5f
    unilateral cleft, 48f
    upper lips
        formation, 36–38
        vermilion zones/mucocutaneous junctions,
            5f
    vermilion zone, 2
Lobes, 134
    development, example, 208f
Lobule, microscopic section, 134f
Localized resorption, occurrence, 98
Loose connective tissue, 92
Lower face, formation, 34–35
Lower lips
    formation, 36–38
    mucocele, 140f
    photograph, 37f
    vermilion zones/mucocutaneous junctions, 5f
        disruption, 5f
Lumen, 134–135
Lymph, 142
Lymphadenopathy, 143
Lymphatic ducts, 142
Lymphatic nodule (LN), 143
    photomicrograph, 142f, 144f
Lymphatics, 141–142
    properties, 141–143
Lymphatic vessels, 142
Lymph nodes, 142–143
    development, 143
    head, 3f
    histology, 143
    location, 1
    neck, 7f
    structures, 142f
Lymphocytes, 99
Lymphoid tissue pathology, clinical considera-
    tions, 143
Lysosomes, 80
Lysosomes, impact, 97f

M

Macrodontia, 54
Macrophages, 99, 99f
Major salivary glands, 4f, 137
    comparison, 136t
    types, 137
Malocclusion, 290–298
    Angle classification, 290, 290t
    Angle system, assumptions, 291
    classification, 291–292
    Class I malocclusion, 291–292

Malocclusion (*Continued*)
    Class II malocclusion, 292–298
    Class III malocclusion, 293–294
    subdivisions, 294–298
Mamelons, 209
    absence, 221, 265
    presence, 211f
Mandible, 2, 272–273
    alveolar process, radiographic landmarks,
        182f
    angle, 2
    body, 10
    cross section, 181f
    depression, 275
    development, 179–180
    elevation, 275
    embryonic mandible, 180
    facial compact bone, removal, 74f
    hinge movement, establishment, 287f
    interocclusal clearance, 288, 288f
    landmarks, 5f
        facial features, 6f
    lateral deviation, 275, 288f
    movements, 278f, 279t
    physiological rest position, 288f
    protrusion, 275
    protrusive occlusion, 288
    range of motion (ROM), 282
    resting posture, 289
    rest position, 285f, 288–289
    retraction, 275
    single-tooth implant, placement, 185f
Mandibular anterior tooth, gingival recession,
    129f
Mandibular arch, 2, 12
    development, 34–35, 53f
    eruption, 258
    formation, 34–35
    identification, 198f
    lingual surface, bilateral mandibular tori (vari-
        ation), 13f
    teeth, removal, 181f
Mandibular canines
    clinical considerations, 227
    pulp cavity, 225
    single root, length, 225
Mandibular central incisors, clinical considera-
    tions, 219
Mandibular condyle, 2
    growth center, 273f
    inferior section, 275f
Mandibular first molars
    clinical considerations, 257–258
    crown, 256
    pulp cavity, 256
Mandibular first premolars, clinical considera-
    tions, 240–241
Mandibular incisors
    clinical considerations, 217–218
    lingual surfaces, concavities, 217
Mandibular lateral incisors, clinical considera-
    tions, 219
Mandibular molars
    clinical considerations, 256
    teeth, occlusal forces (impact), 178f
Mandibular premolars
    clinical considerations, 238
    permanent mandibular premolars, 238

Mandibular processes, 34
Mandibular right canine, distinction, 226–227
Mandibular right central incisor, distinction, 218–219
Mandibular right first molar, distinction, 257
Mandibular right first premolar, distinction, 240
Mandibular second molars
   mesial position, 289f
   pulp cavity, 259
Mandibular second premolars
   three-cusp types/two-cusp types, 243
Mandibular second premolars, clinical considerations, 244
Mandibular symphysis, 2
Mandibular teeth, 12
Mandibular third molars, clinical considerations, 261
Mandibular torus (tori), 13
Mantle dentin, 162, 165f
Marginal gingiva, 14
   edema, 129f
   lamina propia, 126f
Marginal groove, 229
Marginal ridge, 207
Masseter muscle, 2, 276f–277f
   overdevelopment, bilateral enlargement (accompaniment), 296f
Mastication, 10
   muscles, 275, 276f–277f
      origin/insertion, 279t
Masticatory mucosa, 105
   histologic features, 106f–107f
Masticatory surface
   attrition, 285f
   mechanical wear, 185f, 285f
Matrix metalloproteinase (MMP), 186
Matrix, secretion, 62
Maturation, process, 22
Maturation stage, 62–66
   disturbances, clinical considerations, 64–66
Mature dentin components, 160–161
Maxilla, 2
   alveolar process, 48f
   body, 10
   development, 179
   facial compact bone, removal, 74f
   growth, subdivision, 179
   landmarks, 5f
   teeth, removal, 181f
Maxillary anterior teeth, protrusion, 294f
Maxillary arch, 12
   facial surface, exostoses (variation), 13f
   gingival tissue, landmarks, 13f
   identification, 198f
   leeway space, 283f
Maxillary canines
   cingula, presence, 225
   clinical considerations, 225
   impaction, 225
   mandibular canine, comparison, 223
   micrograph, 155f
Maxillary central incisors
   clinical considerations, 215
   conical root, presence, 213
   proximal surfaces, 265–266

Maxillary first molar
   clinical considerations, 251
   furcations, 249
   loss, 251f
   mesial furcation, 249
   mesiobuccal cusp, 291f, 293f
   roots, 249
Maxillary first premolars
   bifurcation, 233
   crown
      angular shape, 233
      mesial/distal outlines, 235
Maxillary incisors
   clinical considerations, 212–213
   permanent maxillary incisors, 212–217
Maxillary lateral incisors
   clinical considerations, 215–217
   upper right quadrant, abfraction, 149f
Maxillary molars
   arch position, 248
   clinical considerations, 247–248
   roots
      branches, 247
      penetration, 248
Maxillary paranasal sinuses, 145f
Maxillary posterior teeth, roots (panoramic radiograph), 146f
Maxillary premolars, 203
   clinical considerations, 233
   cusps, size, 233
Maxillary process, 36
   formation, 36
Maxillary right canine, distinction, 223–224
Maxillary right central incisor, distinction, 214–215
Maxillary right first premolar, distinction, 235
Maxillary right second premolar, distinction, 237
Maxillary second molars
   furcations, layout, 251
   pulp cavity, 251
Maxillary second premolars, clinical considerations, 238
Maxillary sinus, 10
Maxillary space maintainer, removability, 284f
Maxillary third molars, clinical considerations, 254
Maxillary tuberosity, 12
Maximum mouth opening (MMO), 283
Meckel cartilage, formation, 34
Medial nasal processes, 36
   fusion, 36f–37f
Median lingual sulcus, 15
Median palatine raphe, 15
Medical pterygoid muscles, 276f–277f
Meiosis
   occurrence, 20
   process, 20f
Melanin pigmentation, 14–15
Melanocytes, 119
   electron micrograph, 120f
Melanosomes, 119
Mentalis muscle, hyperactivity, 298f
Mesenchyme, 26–27, 27f, 53
Mesial drift (physiological drift), 182–183
   occurrence, 293f
Mesial marginal groove, notches, 257
Mesial root concavity, presence, 234
Mesial step, 289, 289f
Mesial surface, 200

Mesiobuccal cusp, 250
   distal cusp ridge, 250
   maxillary first molar, 291f
Mesioclusion (Class III malocclusion), 293–294
Mesiolabial, term (usage), 202
Mesiolingual cusp, 250
Mesio-occlusal, term (usage), 202
Mesoderm, 24, 25f
   differentiation, 28f
   layer, formation, 25f
   middle layer, formation, 25f
Mesognathic facial profile, 292, 292f
Metaphase, 81, 82t
Microdontia, 54
Microfilaments, 81
Microplicae, 107
Microtubules, 81
Midface, formation, 36
Midgut, 27
Military Tooth Numbering System (Palmer Notation Method), 194
Mineralization, occurrence, 160
Minerals, deposition (remineralization), 151
Minor salivary glands, 137
   photomicrograph, 139f
   size, comparison, 137
Mitochondria, 80
Mitosis (cell division)
   anaphase, 81, 82t
   interphase, 81
   metaphase, 81, 82t
   process, 20–21
      phases, 82t
   prophase, 81, 82t
   telophase, 81, 82t
Mitotic cleavage, 21f
Mixed dentition
   mandibular sagittal section, photomicrograph, 75f
   period, 195
      primary/permanent teeth, identification, 197f
Molars, 12
   clinical considerations, 245–246
   etymology, 244
   features, 244–246
   permanent molars, 244–261
   primary molars, 268–270
   types, 244
Monocytes, 99, 99f
Morphodifferentiation, 22
Morphogenesis, 22
Morphology, 22
Morula, 20
Mouth
   edentulous case, 185f
   maximum mouth opening (MMO), 283
Mouth, floor, 15–17, 111–112
   clinical appearance, 111
   histologic features, 111–112
   landmarks, 17f
   ranula, 140f
Mucobuccal fold, 10
Mucocele, 139, 140f
Mucocutaneous junctions, 2, 5f
   disruption, 5f
Mucogingival junction, 13, 13f
   histologic features, 114f
   photomicrograph, 115f

Mucoperiosteum, 112
Mucous acinus (acini), 134f, 135
Mucous cells, 134
Mulberry molar, 30f
Mulberry molars, 246
Multirooted premolars/molars, origination, 230
Multirooted teeth, 12f
    development, 67–68
        apical view, 69f
        pulp stones, microscopic view/radiograph, 170f
        sagittal section, diagram, 188f
Muscles
    bundles, 102f
    classification, 100–101
    properties, 100–101
Myoepithelial cells, 135–136
Myofibers/myofibrils, 102f
Myofilaments, 102f

N

Naris (nares), 1–2
Nasal cavity, 145f
    development, 45
    histology, 144
    nose, inner space, 143
    pathology, clinical considerations, 146
    properties, 143
    respiratory mucosa lining, histology, 145f
Nasal conchae, 143, 145f
Nasal pits, 35
Nasal placodes, 35
Nasal septum, 1–2
    development, 45
        inferior view, 47f
    fusion, 47f
    highlights, 4f
    vertical nasal septum, fusion, 45
Nasmyth membrane, 73
    extrinsic staining, 76f
Nasopharynx, 17
Natural killer (NK) cells, 99
Neck, 1
    landmarks, 6f
    lymph nodes, 7f
    regions, 6
    structures, 133
Neonatal line, 155
    microscopic view, 155f
Nerves, types, 102
Nerve tissue
    histology, 101–102
    properties, 101–103
Nervous system, 103
    development, 28f
    divisions, 103t
Neural crest cells (NCCs), 26, 27f
    migration, failure, 30f
Neural folds, 26, 26f
    neural crest cells, 27f
Neural groove, 26
    deepening, 26f
Neural plate, 26
Neural tube, 26
Neuroectoderm, 26
    formation, 26f

Neurons, 101
    synaptic relationship, 102f
Neutroclusion (Class I malocclusion), 291–292
Neutrophils, 99f
    electron micrograph, 101f
Nicotinic stomatitis, 139
    palatal mucosa, 140f
Nonkeratinized alveolar mucosa, keratinized attached gingiva (junction), 115f
Nonkeratinized epithelium, 109f
    presence, 111f
Nonkeratinized stratified squamous epithelium, 107–108
    photomicrograph, 111f
Nonkeratinocytes, 106–107
Nonsuccedaneous permanent molars, 59
Nose
    ala (alae), 1–2
    apex, location, 1–2
    development, 36f
    external nose, 1–2
    formation, 35–36
    root, location, 1–2
Nuclear envelope, 79, 79f
Nuclear pores, 79, 79f
Nucleolus, 79, 79t
Nucleoplasm, 79, 79f
Nucleus (nuclei), 79
    cell data bank, 79
    components, 79f

O

Oblique group, 189
    location, 189f
Oblique ridge, 246–247
Occlusal drift (supereruption), 183
Occlusal pits, 228–229
Occlusal plane, 285
Occlusal surface, 200
    example, 229f
        pit and groove pattern, example, 232f
        supplemental grooves, 229f
Occlusal table, 228
    features, 229f
Occlusal trauma, 187, 289
    advanced occlusal trauma, 191
    early occlusal trauma, 191f
    effects, irreversibility, 289
Occlusion, 197
    centric occlusion (CO), 281–289
    clinical considerations, 289
    development, 281
    lateral occlusion, 287–288
    malocclusion, 290–298
    patterns, 297f
    primary occlusion, 289
    properties, 281
    protrusive occlusion, 287–288
Odontoblastic layer, 169
Odontoblastic process, 64, 162f
Odontoblasts
    differentiation, 63, 66
    formation, 63
    impact, 63f
    microscopic view, 159f
    presence, 160f

Odontoclasts, formation, 69
Odontogenesis
    apposition stage, 62–66
    initiation stage, 53–54, 53f
    maturation stage, 62–66
    process, 51
Odontogenesis, bell stage, 60–62
    outer to inner, 61t
    photomicrograph, 61f
    transition, 60f
Odontogenesis, bud stage, 54
    dental lamina, proliferation, 58f
    photomicrograph, 58f
Odontogenesis, cap stage, 54–60
    disturbances, clinical considerations, 60
    fusion, 60
    photomicrograph, 59f
    tooth germ, 59t
        formation, 58f
        transition, 60f
Olfactory mucosa, 144
Open bite, 293f
    anterior open bite, result, 296f
    impact, 297f
    mixed dentition, 297f
    presence, 292
Open contact (diastema), 215
Oral cavity
    aging process, changes, 121f
    areas, International Standards Organization designation, 198t
    divisions, 9–17
    formation, 33–34
    landmarks, 14f
    orientational terms, 10f
    permanent mandibular first premolar, metallic restorations, 241f
    pharyngeal divisions, 17
    proper, 14–17, 14f
    properties, 9
    vestibules, landmarks, 10f
Oral epithelium, 53
Oral mucosa, 9–10
    aging, 119–122
    clinical considerations, 10
    epithelium, 106–108
        types, 107t
    histologic features, 105f
    lamina propia, 108–109
        histologic features, 109f
    pathology, clinical considerations, 109, 121–122
    pigmentation, 118–119
        clinical considerations, 119
    properties, 104–109
    regional differences, 110–113, 110t
    repair, 119–122
    turnover time, 119–122
    types, 105t
Oral mucosa, repair process, 89f
Oral tissue, mean turnover time, 120t
Oral vestibules, 9–10
Organelles, 78f, 79–81
    metabolic activity, 79
Organ, formation, 77
Orientational tooth terms, 200–203

Orofacial development, 43
Orofacial myofunctional disorder (OMD)
  behaviors/patterns, involvement, 296
  identification/treatment, 298
  mentalis muscle, hyperactivity, 298f
  mixed dentition, open bite, 297f
  open bites, impact, 297f
Orofacial myofunctional therapy (OMT),
    297f
  usage, 296
Orofacial myology, 296
Oronasal membrane, 35
Oropharyngeal membrane, 27
  disintegration, 35f
Oropharynx, 17
Orthognathic surgical intervention, requirement,
    295
Orthokeratinized epithelium, photomicrograph,
    113f
Orthokeratinized stratified squamous epithelium,
    106f, 108
Ossification, 96
Osteoblasts, 95
  inclusion, 188f
  penetration, 97f
  presence, 95f
Osteoclasts, 97
  Howship lacunae, presence, 97f
Osteocytes, 95
  presence, 95f
Osteoid, 95
  endochondral ossification, 96
  formation, 96f–97f
Osteons, 95–96
Otic placodes, 35
Outer enamel epithelium (OEE), 61,
    67f
Overbites, 293f
  maxillary arch overlap, 282
  measurement, 282
Overjet, 282
  comparison, 282f
  measurement, 282
  pressure, 282f
Ovum, 20
  sperm fertilization, 20f

P

Palatal mucosa, nicotinic stomatitis/
    hyperkeratinization, 140f
Palatal torus, 15
  variation, 15f
Palate, 15
  adult palate, derivative developmental
      structures (diagram), 47f
  anterior part, appearance, 112
  clinical considerations, 15
  completion, 44–45
  development, 43–45, 44t
    clinical considerations, 45
    coronal section, 45f
    inferior view, 47f
  hard palate, 15
  landmarks, 15f
  posterior palate, bilateral cleft, 48f
  primary plate formation, 43–44
  secondary palate formation, 44

Palate (Continued)
  shelves, 44
    flipping, 45f
    fusion, failure, 45
    growth, 45f
  soft palate, 15
  structures, 9
Palatine rugae, 15
Palatine tonsils, 14–15
  histology, diagram, 144f
  lymphadenopathy, 145f
Palmer Notation Method (Military Tooth Num-
    bering System), 194, 195f–196f
Parafunctional habits, clinical considerations,
    296–298
Parakeratinized epithelium, presence, 114f
Parakeratinized stratified squamous epithelium,
    108
Paranasal sinuses, 145
  development, 146
  formation, 35–36
  histology, 145
  pathology, clinical considerations, 146
  properties, 145–146
Parasympathetic nervous system, 103
Parathyroid gland, 6
Parotid duct, opening (protection), 10
Parotid papilla, 10
Parotid salivary gland, 2, 138f
  photomicrograph, 135f
Passive eruption, 68–69
Pathological tooth migration, causes, 191f
Peg lateral, 216
Peg molar, 254
Peg third molar, 254f
Perichondrium, 93
Perikymata, grooves, 154
Periodontal debridement, performing, 200, 245
Periodontal inflammation, 130
Periodontal ligament (PDL), 10, 169f
  alveolar crest fibers, 183f
  cells, 187–188
  cementicle, attachment, 178f
  development, 69
  fiber groups, 188–192
  formation, 68
  horizontal group, 183f
  interdental ligament, microscopic view, 190f
  interradicular group, 184f
  microscopic view, 187f
    osteoblasts, inclusion, 188f
  pathology, clinical considerations, 190–192
  process, 68
  properties, 187–192
  repair, clinical considerations, 190–192
  sagittal section, diagram, 188f
  Sharpey fibers, insertion (microscopic view), 182f
  space, 187
    early occlusal trauma, 191f
  teeth, oblique group location
      (photomicrograph), 189f
  tension zone, development, 182
  vascular supply, 187
Periodontal pocket, 131
  endoscopic evaluation, 131–132
  probing, bleeding, 130f
  suprabody periodontal pockets, microscopic
      view, 192f

Periodontal tissue support, loss, 245
Periodontitis, 131
  photomicrographs, 131f
Periodontium
  arterial supply, 168t
  components, 173f
  involvement, 172
  nerve supply, 168t
  properties, 172
Periosteum, 94
  close-up view, 94f
Peripheral nervous system (PNS), 101–102
Peritubular dentin, 161–162
Permanent anterior teeth
  contact area, identification, 209f
  contour heights, example, 209f
  identification, 208f
  incisal surface, example, 208f
  lingual surface
    example, 209f
    features, examples, 210f
  lobe development, example, 208f
  properties, 207–208
Permanent canines, 220–227
  eruption, labial views, 222f
  features, 220–223
  lateral view, 223f
  lingual views, 222f
  types, 221t
Permanent dental arches, teeth (curves), 285f
Permanent dentition, 51, 193, 194f
  anterior/posterior teeth, identification,
      198f
  arches, 285f
  attached gingiva, association, 119f
  centric occlusion, 282f
  changes, occurrence, 251f, 258f
  Class I malocclusion, 291f
  Class II malocclusion, 293f
    division I, 292–293, 294f
    division II, 293, 294f
  Class III malocclusion, 295f
  dental arch, eruption sequence, 284f
  dentinogenesis imperfecta, 65f–66f
  eruption
    chronological order, 70f–71f
    sequence, 284
  maxillary/mandibular arch, identification,
      198f
  period, 195–197
  tooth types, identification, 194f
Permanent incisors, 209–219
  features, 211f
  incisal surface, 211f
  types, 210t
Permanent mandibular canines, 225–227
  features, 225
  incisal view features, 227
  labial view features, 225–227
  lingual view features, 227
  proximal view features, 227
Permanent mandibular central incisors,
    218–219
  features, 218
  incisal view features, 219
  labial view features, 218
  lingual view features, 218–219
  proximal view features, 219

Permanent mandibular first molars,
  256–258
  buccal view features, 256
  dilaceration, 246f
  eruption, 271f
  features, 256
  lingual view features, 256
  occlusal features, 257f
  occlusal view features, 257
  proximal view features, 257
  root surface, exposure, 245f
  skull, buccal pit, 257f
Permanent mandibular first premolars,
  238–241
  buccal view features, 239–240
  features, 238–239
  lingual view features, 240
  occlusal table components, 240
  occlusal view features, 240
  oral cavity, metallic restorations, 241f
  proximal view features, 240
Permanent mandibular incisors, 217–219
  features, 217–218
  incisal surface, attrition (occlusal view),
    217t
Permanent mandibular lateral incisors, 219
  features, 219
  incisal view features, 219
  lingual view features, 219
  proximal view features, 219
Permanent mandibular molars, 254–261
  features, 254–256
  types, 255t
Permanent mandibular premolars, 238–244
  features, 238
Permanent mandibular right canine, pulp cavity,
  227f
Permanent mandibular right central incisor,
  views, 218f
Permanent mandibular right first molar
  occlusal features, 257f
  pulp cavity, 256f
  views, 255f
Permanent mandibular right first premolar
  lingual features, 240f
  occlusal features, 240f
    fossae, presence, 241f
  pulp cavity, 239f
  views, 239f
Permanent mandibular right lateral incisor
  pulp cavity, 220f
  views, 220f
Permanent mandibular right second molars
  occlusal features, 259f
  pulp cavity, 259f
  views, 258f
Permanent mandibular right second premolars
  lingual views, 243f
  three-cusp type
    occlusal features, 243f
    occlusal view, 243f
    pulp cavity, 242f
    views, 242f
  two-cusp type, occlusal views, 244f
  types, occlusal views, 242f
Permanent mandibular right third molar
  pulp cavity, 260f
  views, 260f

Permanent mandibular second molars,
  258–259
  buccal view features, 259
  dilaceration, 246f
  features, 258–259
  lingual view features, 259
  occlusal table components, 259
  occlusal view features, 259
  proximal view features, 259
Permanent mandibular second premolars,
  241–244
  buccal view features, 241
  features, 241
  lingual view features, 241
  occlusal table components, 243–244
  occlusal view features, 243
  proximal view features, 241–243
  three-cusp type, views, 242f
Permanent mandibular third molars, 259–261
  crown, dentigerous cyst (radiograph), 76f
  features, 259–260
  impaction, radiograph, 261f
Permanent maxillary anterior teeth, lingual view
  (tetracycline stain), 31f
Permanent maxillary arch, peg third molar,
  251f
Permanent maxillary canines, 223–225
  features, 223
  incisal view features, 224–225
  labial view features, 223
  lingual view features, 223
  proximal view features, 223–224
Permanent maxillary central incisors, 213–215
  facial surface, restoration, 149f
  features, 213–214
  incisal view features, 214–215
  labial view features, 214
  proximal view features, 214
Permanent maxillary first molar, 248–251
  distobuccal surfaces, 251
  lingual pit, 247f
Permanent maxillary first premolars, 233–236
  buccal view features, 235
  lingual view features, 235
  occlusal view features, 235–236
  proximal view features, 235
Permanent maxillary incisors, 212–217
  features, 212–213
  lingual views, 212f
Permanent maxillary lateral incisors, 215–217
  features, 215
  incisal view features, 215
  labial view features, 215
  lingual view features, 215
  proximal view features, 215
Permanent maxillary/mandibular incisors, lateral
  view, 211f
Permanent maxillary/mandibular molar, buccal
  root features, 230f
Permanent maxillary molars, 69f, 246–254
  features, 246–254
  occlusal view, 247f
  types, 247t
Permanent maxillary premolars, 233–238
  features, 233
Permanent maxillary right canine
  lingual view, 225f
  views, 224f

Permanent maxillary right central incisor
  lingual surface variations, 214f
  pulp cavity, 214f
  views, 213f
Permanent maxillary right first molar
  occlusal features, 250f
    fossae, presence, 250f
  pulp cavity, 249f
  views, 248f
Permanent maxillary right first premolar
  buccal features, 235f
  mesial features, 235f
  occlusal features, 235f
    fossae, presence, 236f
  occlusal table components, 236
  occlusal view features, 235–236
  pulp cavity, 234f
  views, 234f
Permanent maxillary right lateral incisor
  lingual surface, variations, 217f
  pulp cavity, 216f
  views, 216f
Permanent maxillary right second molar
  crowns, occlusal views, 252f
  pulp cavity, 252f
  views, 252f
Permanent maxillary right second premolar
  pulp cavity, 237f
  views, 237f
Permanent maxillary right third molars
  crown outlines, occlusal views, 253f
  pulp cavity, 254f
  views, 253f
Permanent maxillary second molars, 251–253
  buccal view features, 251
  features, 251
  lingual view features, 251
  occlusal table components, 251–253
  occlusal view features, 251
  proximal view features, 251
Permanent maxillary second premolars,
  236–238
  buccal view features, 236–237
  features, 236
  lingual view features, 237
  occlusal table components, 238
  occlusal view features, 238
  proximal view features, 237–238
Permanent maxillary third molars, 253–254
  features, 253–254
Permanent molars, 244–261
  occlusal view, 245f
Permanent posterior teeth
  contour height, 230f
  furcations/furcation crotches, 231t
  identification, 229f
  occlusal surface
    example, 229f
    supplemental grooves, 229f
  occlusal table, features, 229f
  occlusal views, 229f
  pit and groove pattern, example, 232f
  properties, 228–230
Permanent premolars, 230–244
  buccal features, 233f
  identification, 233f
  types, 232t
Permanent succedaneous tooth, primordium, 58f

Permanent teeth (adult teeth), 12–13, 193
  color differences, 195
  crowns, differences, 263f–264f
  designation, 194
  eruption, 70–73
    clinical considerations, 73
  eruption/root completion ages, 197t
  landmarks, diagram, 11f
  primary teeth, differences, 264f
  pulp chambers/horns, differences, 264f
  roots, differences, 264f
  succedaneous permanent teeth, development, 73f
Phagocytosis, 77, 81f
Pharyngeal divisions, 17
Pharyngeal pouches, 41
  derivative structures, 41t
Pharyngeal tonsils, 143
Pharynx, 17
  primitive pharynx, formation, 38
Philtrum, 2
Physiological drift (mesial drift), 182–183
Physiological rest position, 288f
Pigmentation, 119f
  process, 120f
Pit and groove pattern, example, 232f
Pit caries, 151
Pits, location, 245
Placenta, 24
Placodes
  development, 35
  lens placodes, 35
  nasal placodes, 35
  otic placodes, 35
Plasma, 98
  cells, 99
    immunoglobulins, 101t
  membrane (cell membrane), 77–79
Platelets, 98
Plica fimbriata (plicae fimbriatae), 15
Plunging cusps, 283
Pocket epithelium (PE), 131
  magnification, 131f
Point angles, 202
  designation, 202f
Polymorphonuclear leukocyte (PMN), 99, 99f, 127
  electron micrograph, 101f
Porphyromonas gingivalis (Pg), 131
Posterior faucial pillar, 14–15
Posterior palate, bilateral cleft, 48f
Posterior teeth, 12–13
  anatomical crown/root, presence, 199f
  clinical considerations, 230
  contour height, 201f
  crown
    line angles, designation, 202f
    point angles, designation, 202f
    thirds, identification, 203f
  dental tissue, involvement, 199f
  identification, 198f
  mixed dentition, mandibular sagittal section
    (photomicrograph), 75f
  occlusal surface, 200
  root thirds, identification, 203f
Postglenoid process, 272
Preameloblasts
  differentiation, 62
  formation, 62–63
  induction, 64f

Predentin, 63, 159
  appositional growth, 63f
  formation, photomicrograph, 63f
  maturation, 160f
Preimplantation period, 19t, 20–22
  clinical considerations, 21–22
  occurrence, 20
Premature contacts, impact, 287
Premolars, 12–13
  clinical considerations, 232
  features, 230–232
  permanent maxillary first premolars, 233–236
  permanent maxillary premolars, 233–238
  permanent premolars, 230–244
Prenatal development, 18–19
  clinical considerations, 18–19
  embryo, fourth week, 39f–40f
    scanning electron micrograph, 33f
    schematic, 33f
  embryonic period, 19t, 22–31
    clinical considerations, 27–31
  facial development, fourth week, 33b
  fetal period, 19t, 31
    clinical considerations, 31
  fourth week, 27–31
  initiation, 18
  periods, 19t
  preimplantation period, 19t, 20–22
    clinical considerations, 21–22
    occurrence, 20
  second week, 23–24
  third week, 24–27
Primary bone, 96, 97f
Primary canines, 267–268
  features, 267
Primary cementum, 175
Primary dentin, 165f, 193
  formation, 162
Primary dentition, 194f
  clinical considerations, 263–265
  completion, 262
  crowns, impact, 76f
  dental arch, eruption sequence, 284f
  dental care, importance, 265
  development, 51
  eruption
    chronological order, 70f–71f
    sequence, 284
  evaluation, buccal view, 289f
  labial view, 263f
  period, 194–195
  tooth types, identification, 194f
Primary incisors, 265–267
  features, 265
Primary mandibular canines, 268
Primary mandibular central incisor, 266–267
  features, 266–267
  lingual surface, 267
Primary mandibular first molars, 270
  crown, appearance, 270
Primary mandibular lateral incisor, 267
Primary mandibular right canine, views, 268f
Primary mandibular right central incisor, views,
  266f
Primary mandibular right first molar, views, 270f
Primary mandibular right lateral incisor, views, 267f
Primary mandibular right second molar, views,
  271f

Primary mandibular second molars, 270
  distal step, 289f
  eruption, 271f
Primary maxillary anterior teeth, acute caries,
  265f
Primary maxillary canines, 267–268
  crown, 267
Primary maxillary central incisor, 265–266
  mamelons, absence, 265
Primary maxillary first molars, 268
  roots, number/position, 268
Primary maxillary first right molar, views, 269f
Primary maxillary lateral incisor, 266
Primary maxillary right canine, views, 267f
Primary maxillary right central incisor, views,
  266f
Primary maxillary right lateral incisor, views,
  266f
Primary maxillary right second molar, views,
  269f
Primary maxillary second molar, 268
  features, 268
Primary molars, 268–270
  clinical considerations, 270
  features, 268
  occlusal table, 268
Primary occlusion, 289
Primary palate
  bilateral cleft, 48f
  formation, 43–44
Primary second molars, loss, 284
Primary teeth (baby teeth), 12, 193
  bell stage, photomicrograph, 61f
  cervical loop, 67f
  cervical ridge, bulging, 265
  color differences, 195
  crowns, differences, 263f–264f
  eruption/shedding, 68–70
    ages, 263t
  microscopic images, 156
  mixed dentition, 74f
  odontogenesis, initiation stage, 53f
  permanent teeth, differences, 264f
  properties, 262–270
  pulp chambers/horns, differences, 264f
  resorption, 75f
  roots, 263
    differences, 264f
  succedaneous primary teeth, 59
  value, 265
Primate spaces, 262
  presence, 289
Primitive mouth, formation, 32
Primitive pharynx, formation, 38
Primitive streak, 24f
  formation, 24
Primordium, 18
Principal fibers, 188
Prognathic facial profile, 292f, 294
Proliferation, process, 22
Prophase, 81, 82t
Protrusive occlusion, 287–288
  evaluation, 288f
  mandible, 288
Proximal surface, 201
Pseudostratified columnar epithelium, 88f
  consideration, 86
Pterygomandibular fold, extension, 15

Pulp, 10–12
  aging, 170–171
  anatomy, 167–168, 168f
  chamber, 167
  coronal pulp, 167
  formation, 66–67
  histology, 168–169
  horns, 167
  inflammation, 191
  microscopic zones, 170t
  pathology, clinical considerations, 170–171
  properties, 167–171
  radicular pulp, 168
  repair, clinical considerations, 170–171
  stones, microscopic view/radiograph,
    170f
  zones, 169–170, 169f
Pulpal core, 169, 169f
Pulp cavity
  bifurcated cavity, 234
  mandibular canine, 225
  mandibular first molar, 256
  mandibular second molar, 259
  maxillary second molar, 251
  permanent mandibular right canine, 227f
  permanent mandibular right central incisor,
    219f
  permanent mandibular right first molar, 256f
  permanent mandibular right first premolar,
    239f
  permanent mandibular right lateral incisor,
    220f
  permanent mandibular right second molar,
    259f
  permanent mandibular right second premolar,
    three-cusp type, 242f
  permanent mandibular right third molar, 254f,
    260f
  permanent maxillary right central incisor,
    214f
  permanent maxillary right first molar, 249f
  permanent maxillary right first premolar, 234f
  permanent maxillary right lateral incisor, 216f
  permanent maxillary right second molar, 252f
  permanent maxillary right second premolar,
    237f
  tooth shape, mirroring, 214
Pulp chambers, differences, 264f
Pulp horns, differences, 264f
Pulpitis, 170–171, 191

Q
Quadrants, 197

R
Radicular pulp, 168
Ramus (rami), 2
Range of motion (ROM), mandible, 282
Ranula, 139
  submandibular salivary gland duct blockage,
    140f
Reactive dentin, 163
Red blood cells (RBCs), 98
Reduced enamel epithelium (REE), 130, 151
  formation, 69
Regeneration, 85

Reichert cartilage, 38
Removable maxillary space maintainer, usage,
  284f
Reparative dentin, 163
Repolarization, 62
Respiratory mucosa, 144
  lining, histology, 145f
Resting posture, 289
Rest position, 285f, 288–289
Retained sucking habit, 297, 297f
Rete ridges, 86, 92f
Reticular connective tissue, 93
Reticular fibers, 91
Reticular lamina, schematic diagram, 90f
Retrognathic facial profile, 292f
Retromolar pad, 12
Retzius, lines, 154
Reversal lines, 98, 179f
  cementum, 177f
Ribosomes, 80
Rods, 168
  long section, close-up view, 154f
Root, 10–12
  accessory canal, 169f
  accessory roots, 68
  alveolar bone proper (ABP), relationship, 183f
  angulations, 285f
  apices, hypercementosis (causes), 178f
  area
    cementum, appositional growth, 68f
    dentin, appositional growth, 68f
  concavities, 199–200
  dentin
    exposure, 159f
    formation, 66
  development, 66–68, 67f
  dilaceration, 246
  formation disturbances, clinical considera-
    tions, 68
  periodontal debridement, performing, 200
  presence, 199f
  primary tooth resorption, 75f
  sheath, microscopic view, 67f
  trunk, 230
    cervical cross section, 233
    dimensions, awareness, 246
Root axis line (RAL), 199, 285
Rough endoplasmic reticulum (RER), 80
Rubella, 29–30
Ruffled borders, 69

S
Saliva, production, 133
Salivary glands, 4f, 133
  aging, 139
  blockage, 139
  comparison, 136t
  development, 137–139
  ductal system, 136
  histology, 134
  major salivary glands, 4f, 137, 138f
  micrograph/diagram, 134f
  minor salivary glands, 137
    photomicrograph, 139f
  parotid salivary gland, 2, 138f
    photomicrograph, 135f
  pathology, clinical considerations, 139

Salivary glands (Continued)
  properties, 133–139
  serous demilunes, presence, 136f
  sublingual salivary gland, 6, 138f
    photomicrograph, 135f
  submandibular salivary gland, 6
    photomicrograph, 135f
  von Ebner salivary glands, 137
Sclerotic dentin, 163
Secondary bone, 96, 97f
Secondary cementum, 175
Secondary dentin, 165f
  formation, 162
Secondary dentition, 193
Secondary palate
  bilateral cleft, 48f
  formation, 44
Second branchial arch, 38
Second mandibular premolar, three-cusp type,
  243
Second premolars, impaction, 284
Secretory cells, 134–136
Septum (septa), 134
Septum development, 45
Serous acinus (acini), 134f, 135
Serous demilunes, 135
  presence, 136f
Sextants, 197–198
Sharpey fibers, 174
  impact, 173f
  insertion, microscopic view, 182f
Shedding, process, 69–70
Simple epithelium, 86
Single-tooth implant, placement, 185f
Sinusitis, 146
Sixth branchial arch, 41
Skeletal discrepancies, clinical considerations,
  295
Skeletal muscle, 101
  histology, 101
  striations, 102f
Skin
  aging, clinical considerations, 93–98
  epidermis/dermis layers, 92f
  microscopic sections, 87f
  repair process, 89f
Skull
  alveolar process, anatomy, 181f
  permanent mandibular first molar
    buccal pit, 257f
    root surface exposure, 245f
  permanent maxillary first molar, lingual pit,
    247f
  permanent posterior teeth, identification,
    229f
  permanent premolars, identification, 233f
Smooth endoplasmic reticulum (SER), 80
Smooth surface caries, 151f
Soft palate, 15, 112
  clinical appearance, 112
  hard palate, junction (photomicrograph),
    112f
  histologic appearance, 112
Somites, 27
  development/location, 28f
Specialized connective tissue, properties,
  93–100
Specialized mucosa, 105

Sperm, 20
    impact, 20f
Spina bifida, 31
Squames, 86
Squamous cells, 88t
Stellate reticulum, 61, 65f
Sternocleidomastoid muscle (SCM), 6
Stippling, 112
Stomodeum (stomatodeum), 33–34
    enlargement, 35f
Stratified epithelium, 86
Stratified squamous epithelium, 86
    lamina propia, relationship, 105f
Stratum basale (basal layer), 107–108
Stratum corneum (keratin layer), 106f, 108
Stratum granulosum (granular layer), 106f, 108
Stratum intermedium (intermediate layer), 61,
    65f, 107–108
Stratum superficiale (superficial layer), 108
Striated duct, 136–137
Subepithelial connective tissue graft (SECTG),
    129
Subgingival dental biofilm, scanning electron
    micrograph, 174f
Sublingual caruncle, 17
Sublingual duct, 17
Sublingual fold, 17
Sublingual salivary gland, 6, 138f
    appearance, 138
    photomicrograph, 135f
Subluxation, 278
    dislocation, lateral radiographic view, 280f
Submandibular duct, 17
Submandibular gland, cords, 138
Submandibular salivary gland, 6, 138f
    photomicrograph, 135f
Submucosa
    absence, 112, 113f
    presence, 109
Succedaneous dentition, 193
Succedaneous permanent teeth, development, 73f
Succedaneous primary teeth, 59
Successional dental lamina, 59
Sucking habit, retention (occlusion), 297f
Sulcular epithelium (SE), 125
    extension, 126
    inner SE, nonkeratinized epithelium (close-up
        view), 126f
    photomicrographs, 126f
Sulcus terminalis, 15, 113–115
    direction, 50
Supereruption (occlusal drift), 183
Superficial layer (stratum superficiale), 108
Supernumerary teeth (hyperdontia), 54
Supplemental groove, 208
Supporting alveolar bone (SAB), 180
Supporting cusps, 286
Suprabony periodontal pockets, microscopic
    view, 192f
Sympathetic nervous system, 103
Synapse, 101–102
Synovial cavities, 274f
    compartments, 274
Synovial fluid, 274
Synovial membrane, 274
Syphilis, cause, 29–30
System, 77
Systemic fluoride action, theory, 152

T
Talon cusp, 212
Taste buds, 115
    location, 117f
    microscopic sections, 116f
    taste sensation, events, 116f
Taste cells, 115
T-cell lymphocytes, travel, 99f
T cells, 99
Teeth, 10–17
    accessory canals, 168
    anatomy
        clinical considerations, 200
        terms, 198–200
    anterior teeth, 12–13
    arterial supply, 168t
    balancing interferences (confirmation), floss
        (usage), 288f
    bisection, 285
    cementum, 10–12
        relationship, 173f
    clenching, 296
    cross section, microscopic view, 189f
    crowding (crooked teeth), 292, 293f
    crown, 10–12
    curves, 285f
    dentin, 10–12
    designation, 193–194
        systems, 195f–196f
    development, 51–66
        stages, 52t
    developmental disturbances, 55b–57b
    developmental lobes, 249
    enamel, 10–12
    eruption, process, 72f
    forces, impact, 188
    form, 203–205, 204t–205t
        clinical considerations, 205
    function, 204t–205t
    germ, 59
        cap stage, 59t
        creation, 58f
        formation, 58f
    gross specimen, 12f
    height, reduction, 185f
    incisors, 12
    initiation stage, 53–54
    International Numbering System (INS), 194,
        195f–196f
    interproximal contact, interdental ligament
        (impact), 190f
    labial surface, scanning electron micrograph,
        155f
    loss, 251
    mandibular anterior tooth, gingival recession,
        129f
    mandibular teeth, 12
    masticatory surfaces
        attrition/mechanical wear, 285f
        flat planes, absence, 286
    matrix formation, photomicrographs, 149f
    maturation, waves, 150–151
    maxillary posterior teeth, roots (panoramic
        radiograph), 146f
    mesial contact, 253
    molars, 12
    movement (process), orthodontic therapy
        (impact), 184f

Teeth (Continued)
    multirooted teeth, 12f
    nerve supply, 168t
    oblique group location, photomicrograph,
        189f
    orientational tooth terms, 200–203
    Palmer Notation Method, 194, 195f–196f
    pathological tooth migration, causes,
        191f
    permanent teeth, 12–13
    posterior teeth, 12–13
    premolars, 12–13
    primary teeth, 12
    pulp, 10–12
    radiograph, 12f
    roots, 10–12
    surfaces
        clinical considerations, 203
        orientational relationship, 200f
        wearing, 217
    tissue types, distribution, 12f
    types, 193
        form/function, 204t–205t
        identification, 194f
    Universal Numbering System (UNS), 193–194,
        195f–196f
    vital whitening, 157
Telophase, 81, 82t
Temporal bones, 272
    articulating area, 273f
Temporalis muscle, 276f–277f
Temporomandibular disorder/dysfunction
        (TMD), 275
    abnormalities, 277
    treatment, controversies, 277
Temporomandibular joint (TMJ), 2
    block dissection, 273f
    bony components, 273f
    coronal MRI, 280f
    joint capsule, 274f
    joint disc, 274f
    mandible, movements, 278f
    microscopic appearance, 275f
    properties, 272
    ROM patterning, 287
    sagittal section, 273f
Tension zone, development, 182
Teratogens, 19
    involvement, 19t
Terminal plane, 289
    flush terminal plane, 289, 289f
Tertiary dentin, 162, 165f
Tetracycline, 31
    stain, usage, 31f
Third branchial arch, 41
Third median swelling, projection, 47
Thirds, 203
Three-rooted tooth, 69f
Thyroglossal duct, 140
Thyroid cartilage, 6
Thyroid gland, 6, 8f
    development, 140–141, 141f
    enlargement, 142f
    histology, 140–141
        photomicrograph/diagram, 141f
    pathology, clinical considerations, 141
    properties, 140
Thyroxine, 140

Tissue
  cells, blood cells (relationship), 100t
  classification, 86t
  connective tissue, properties, 89–93
  development, 27f
  fluid (interstitial fluid), 81
  formation, 77
  properties, 85
Toll-like receptors (TLRs), 130
Tomes granular layer, 167, 167f
Tomes process, 64, 64f, 149f
  impact, 150
Tongue, 15
  apex, lingual frenum (extension), 50f
  base, 15
  black hairy tongue, 118, 119f
  body, 15
    formation, 49f
  development, 45–50, 49t
    clinical considerations, 50
    diagram, 49f
  dorsal surface, 15
    landmarks, 16f
    microscopic section, 117f
    posterior part, histologic section, 118f
  formation
    base, 47
    body, 45–47
    completion, 49–50
  geographic tongue, 118, 118f
  lateral surface, 15
    landmarks, 16f
    microscopic section, 117f
  median downgrowth, 141f
  muscular core, photomicrographs, 115f
  pathology, clinical considerations, 118
  properties, 113–118
  resting posture, 289
  thrust, 296–297
  ventral surface, 15, 111–112
    clinical appearance, 111
    histologic features, 111–112
    landmarks, 17f
    lingual varicosities, 121f
    photomicrograph, 111f
Tonofilament, 81
  schematic diagram, 90f

Tonsillar tissue, 141–142
Tooth fairy, 69–70
Trabeculae, 143
  formation, 96
Trabecular bone, 180
Transseptal ligament (interdental ligament), 190
Transverse ridge, 228, 236
Treacher Collins syndrome (TCS), 29
  neural crest cells, migration (failure), 30f
Treponema pallidum
  impact, 29–30
  transmission, 246
Triangular fossa, 228–229
  shallowness, 243
Triangular groove, 229
Triangular ridges, 228
Trifurcated teeth, 230
Trilaminar disc, folding, 29f
Trilaminar embryonic disc, 24
  cephalic/caudal ends, 25–26, 25f
  components, 25f
Trismus, 278
Trisomy 21 (Down syndrome), 21–22, 21f
Trophoblast layer, 21, 21f
Tubercle, 2
Tuberculum impar, 45–46, 49f
Turnover time, 85
  elevation, 89

U
Underbite, 282–283
Unilateral cleft lip
  deformities, types, 38f
  location, 38f
Universal Numbering System (UNS), 193–194,
    195f–196f
Upper face, formation, 35–36
Upper lips
  development, clinical considerations, 37–38
  formation, 36–38
  photograph, 37f
  tubercle, 2
  vermilion zones/mucocutaneous
      junctions, 5f
Upper right quadrant, abfraction, 149f
Uvula, 15

V
Vacuoles, 79
Vascular lamina propia, presence, 111f
Ventral tongue surface. See Tongue
Vermilion zones, 2, 5f
  disruption, 2, 5f
Vertical nasal septum, fusion, 45
Vestibular fornix, 10
Vestibules, 9–10
  landmarks, 10f
  oral vestibules, 9–10
Vital whitening (bleaching), 159
Voice box (larynx), 6
Volkmann canal, 96
  communication, 95f
von Ebner, imbrication lines, 166, 166f
von Ebner salivary glands, 137
von Korff fibers, 162

W
Wear facets, 286, 296
White blood cells (WBCs), 98–99, 126
Working side, 287

X
Xerostomia (dry mouth), 139, 139f

Y
Yolk sac, 24

Z
Zygomatic arch, 2
Zygote, 20
  formation, 20f
  mitotic cleavage, 21f